Radiopharmaceuticals in Nuclear Medicine Practice

Titles in the Series

Current Practice in Nuclear Medicine

Series Editor: Sheldon Baum, M.D.

Published

Front: Radionuclide Brain Imaging
Kim and Haynie: Nuclear Imaging in Oncology
Kowalsky and Perry: Radiopharmaceuticals in Nuclear Medicine Practice
Loken: Pulmonary Nuclear Medicine
Rosenthall and Lisbona: Skeletal Imaging
Sty, Starshak, and Miller: Pediatric Nuclear Medicine
Tauxe and Dubovsky: Nuclear Medicine in Clinical Urology and Nephrology

Forthcoming

Lyons: Cardiovascular Nuclear Medicine

Radiopharmaceuticals in Nuclear Medicine Practice

Richard J. Kowalsky, Pharm. D.
Associate Professor of Pharmacy
School of Pharmacy
Associate Professor of Radiology
Director of Nuclear Pharmacy
North Carolina Memorial Hospital
University of North Carolina
Chapel Hill, North Carolina

J. Randolph Perry, M.D.
Associate Professor of Radiology
Director of Cardiovascular Nuclear Medicine
North Carolina Memorial Hospital
University of North Carolina
Chapel Hill, North Carolina

Appleton & Lange
Norwalk, Connecticut / Los Altos, California

0-8385-8263-X

Notice: Our knowledge in clinical sciences is constantly changing. As new information becomes available, changes in treatment and in the use of drugs become necessary. The author(s) and the publisher of this volume have taken care to make certain that the doses of drugs and schedules of treatment are correct and compatible with the standards generally accepted at the time of publication. The reader is advised to consult carefully the instruction and information material included in the package insert of each drug or therapeutic agent before administration. This advice is especially important when using new or infrequently used drugs.

Copyright © 1987 by Appleton & Lange
A Publishing Division of Prentice-Hall

All rights reserved. This book, or any parts thereof, may not be used or reproduced in any manner without written permission. For information, address Appleton & Lange, 25 Van Zant Street, East Norwalk, Connecticut 06855.

87 88 89 90 91 / 10 9 8 7 6 5 4 3 2 1

Prentice-Hall of Australia, Pty. Ltd., Sydney
Prentice-Hall Canada, Inc.
Prentice-Hall Hispanoamericana, S.A., Mexico
Prentice-Hall of India Private Limited, New Delhi
Prentice-Hall International (UK) Limited, London
Prentice-Hall of Japan, Inc., Tokyo
Prentice-Hall of Southeast Asia (Pte.) Ltd., Singapore
Whitehall Books Ltd., Wellington, New Zealand
Editora Prentice-Hall do Brasil Ltda., Rio de Janeiro

Library of Congress Cataloging-in-Publication Data
Kowalsky, Richard J.
  Radiopharmaceuticals in nuclear medicine practice.

  1. Radioisotope scanning. 2. Radiopharmaceuticals.
3. Radioisotopes in pharmacology. I. Perry, J. Randolph. II. Title. [DNLM: 1. Nuclear Medicine.
2. Radioisotopes—diagnostic use. WN 440 K88r]
RC78.7.R4K69 1987   616.07´575   87-1048
ISBN 0-8385-8263-X

PRINTED IN THE UNITED STATES OF AMERICA

To the residents and students who encouraged
us to put our lectures in writing,
to our wives, Louise and Carol,
whose patient encouragement
sustained us, and to our children,
Jennifer and Gregory, Christina and Brett,
who make everything worthwhile.

Contents

Preface and Acknowledgments ix

1. Radiopharmaceuticals in Nuclear Medicine: An Overview 1
2. Physics of Radiopharmaceuticals 13
3. Radionuclide Generators 59
4. Chemistry of Radiopharmaceuticals 75
5. The Nuclear Pharmacy 97
6. Quality Control of Radiopharmaceuticals 123
7. Brain and Cerebrospinal Fluid 147
8. Thyroid 181
9. Heart 211
10. Lung 235
11. Liver, Gallbladder, Spleen, and Bone Marrow 271
12. Kidney and Genitourinary System 315
13. Bone 351
14. Total Body Imaging: Gallium and Indium Radiopharmaceuticals .. 379
15. In Vivo Function Studies 411
16. In Vitro Radioassay Tests 435
17. Miscellaneous Radiopharmaceuticals and Applications 443
18. Licensing, Regulatory Control, and Radiation Safety 473

Index 501

Preface

This book is intended to be used as an informational text about radiopharmaceuticals used in nuclear medicine practice. The content is structured around courses on radiopharmaceutical science and nuclear medicine taught for several years to students in pharmacy and the radiological sciences. It is expected, therefore, that the greatest benefit will be derived by radiology residents and fellows, nuclear medicine technologists, and nuclear pharmacists. Students in these disciplines may find this text a useful adjunct to their regular classroom lectures.

The overriding theme in this book is the emphasis on application of basic principles to practice. The first four chapters, therefore, are dedicated to fundamental principles involving the physical and chemical aspects of radiopharmaceuticals. It is intended that these chapters provide basic information needed for greater comprehension of the clinical applications of radiopharmaceuticals presented in subsequent chapters. Since each of the latter is written as a separate entity, however, the more experienced reader may choose to skip the beginning chapters and refer directly to those chapters that deal with specific areas of interest.

The first chapter presents a perspective look at radiopharmaceuticals. Nuclear medicine and the radiopharmaceutical are defined. The essential properties of radiopharmaceuticals and their patterns of biodistribution are discussed. The types of procedures performed in nuclear medicine and how radioactive tracers are applied in these procedures are described. The intent is to present an overall "picture" before delving into more specific topics.

Chapter 2 presents a discussion of atomic physics applied to radiopharmaceuticals. The content covers atomic properties, radioactive decay, radioactivity, radiation interactions, detection and measurement, and radionuclide production.

Chapter 3 deals with radionuclide generators with particular emphasis on the Tc-99m generator. The chapter begins with a discussion of the practical aspects of generator construction, operation and quality control, and concludes with a detailed theoretical discussion of generator physics for the reader desiring a greater depth of understanding.

Chapter 4 describes the ideal properties of radiopharmaceuticals, focusing on technetium and iodine chemistry, radiopharmaceutical design, radiolabeling methods, and stability.

Chapter 5 presents information about the nuclear pharmacy and the operational functions important to the safe handling of radioactive material and the accurate measurement of radiopharmaceutical dosages. The main points covered are pharmacy design and equipment, instrumentation, "hot lab" techniques, receipt, disposition and disposal of radioactive material, preparation and quality control of radiopharmaceutical kits, radioactive waste management, and record keeping.

Throughout these first chapters are several example problems and situations to illustrate the practical application of nuclear science principles.

The next eight chapters consider radiopharmaceutical use in evaluating the major systems in the body. The systems are brain and cerebrospinal fluid, thyroid, heart, lung, liver, gallbladder, spleen, and bone marrow, kidney and genitourinary system, bone, and total body imaging. These chapters are organized in a similar format beginning with a short introduction. This is followed by a review of physiologic anatomy to provide pertinent information for the rational selection and use of radiopharmaceuticals and for understanding their mechanisms of localization. A brief historical chronology of the development of radiopharmaceuticals used to study the organ system follows. The subsequent discussion focuses on the current agents of choice with a consideration of their methods of production, stability, quality control, physical, chemical and biologic properties, potential toxicity, and radiation dose. Each chapter ends with a discussion of the clinical application of radiopharmaceuticals used in studying the particular organ system and considers rationale for use, typical procedures, pharmaceutical choices, and interpretation of results. Images, tables, and graphs are used to illustrate normal and abnormal studies.

Chapter 15 discusses the nonimaging use of radiopharmaceuticals for in vivo function studies. Those studies performed routinely in nuclear medicine are covered with a focus on the underlying principle involved and the radiopharmaceuticals used.

Chapter 16 discusses in vitro studies performed with radioassay tests, primarily radioimmunoassays (RIA). This chapter covers the basic principles involved with RIA and illustrates a few of the common tests used.

Chapter 17 is a collection of miscellaneous radiopharmaceutical agents or applications not included in other chapters, but which nonetheless find a useful place in nuclear medicine practice.

The final chapter is an attempt to excerpt from experience and the literature those licensing, regulatory, and radiation safety aspects which apply to nuclear medicine practice involving the use of radioactive material in human studies.

The overall content of this text is one of an introductory to intermediate–advanced nature depending on one's background. References are given at the end of each chapter to provide the reader with a more detailed treatment of particular areas of interest.

ACKNOWLEDGMENTS

A great debt of gratitude is owed to many individuals for their time, patience, and personal efforts in helping bring this book to fruition.

A special appreciation is extended to Eva M. Henderson, Joyce McEachern, and Nancy Jenkins of the School of Pharmacy, University of North Carolina, Chapel Hill, North Carolina, who worked diligently and tirelessly typing the manuscript throughout several revisions.

An equal appreciation is extended to two very capable photographic specialists, Mr. Robert Strain and Miss Karen Curran of the Department of Radiology, North Carolina Memorial Hospital, Chapel Hill, North Carolina, for their steadfast efforts and technical expertise in preparing the illustrations.

A special thank you is due to Mrs. Marilyn Parrish, Educational Coordinator, Nuclear Medicine Technology Program, North Carolina Memorial Hospital, Chapel

Hill, North Carolina, for her generosity of time and collaborative effort in obtaining the excellent nuclear medicine images used as clinical illustrations.

Finally, a deep appreciation is expressed to all those residents, technologists, and students who have contributed greatly to our knowledge and understanding as practitioner–educators through their inciteful questions into the "whys" and "hows" of nuclear pharmacy and nuclear medicine practice.

Richard J. Kowalsky
J. Randolph Perry

CHAPTER 1

Radiopharmaceuticals in Nuclear Medicine: An Overview

The beginning of nuclear medicine and its definition depend upon one's perspective of time in the application of radiation to human disease. If one focuses on the use of either natural or artificial radioactive material, then nuclear medicine implicitly started in 1901[1] when the French physician Henri Danlos used radium (a natural element) to treat a tuberculous skin lesion. If the definition requires artificial radioisotopes, then nuclear medicine started after 1934 when the French radiochemists Frederic Joliot and his wife Irene Curie Joliot produced the first artificial radioisotope, phosphorus-30. In this case the choice of nuclear medicine's beginning is either with George Hevesy's successful use of radiophosphorus in healthy animals in 1935 or with Joseph Hamilton's attempts at treating leukemic patients with sodium-24 in 1936. The introduction of the cyclotron at this time created an investigative ferment that produced numerous radionuclides that were applied to diagnosis and therapy. It was thus natural that the official definition of nuclear medicine be adopted in 1967 as "the specialty of the practice of medicine dealing with the diagnostic, therapeutic (exclusive of sealed radiation sources) and investigative use of radionuclides." Since that time, however, the field of nuclear medicine has grown rapidly and has undergone many changes.

The recent application of nuclear magnetic resonance (NMR) imaging methods to diagnosis in nuclear medicine without the use of radioactive material has inspired a new definition to reflect the use of nuclear properties from stable nuclides as well. In February 1983 the Board of Trustees of the Society of Nuclear Medicine adopted the new definition of nuclear medicine as "the medical specialty which utilizes the nuclear properties of radioactive and stable nuclides for diagnostic evaluation of the anatomic and/or physiologic conditions of the body and provides therapy with unsealed radioactive sources." With the exception of NMR the practice of nuclear medicine is accomplished primarily through the application of radiopharmaceutical agents and in vitro tests in diagnosis and therapy and will be the focal point of this book on radiopharmaceuticals in nuclear medicine practice.

THE RADIOPHARMACEUTICAL

A radiopharmaceutical may be defined simply as a chemical substance that contains radioactive atoms within its structure and is suitable for administration to humans for diagnosis or treatment of disease. There are more sophisticated and all-inclusive definitions, but this one should suffice at this point. Radiopharmaceuticals are formulated in various chemical and physical forms to deliver their radioactivity to particular parts of the body. Furthermore, the gamma radiation emitted from these drug molecules readily penetrates the tissues and escapes from the body, thus allowing external detection and measurement. In this way the nuclear physician can evaluate the functional and morphologic characteristics of various organs in the body.

NUCLEAR MEDICINE PROCEDURES

It will be helpful in understanding how radiopharmaceuticals are used if we examine the types of procedures routinely performed in nuclear medicine. These procedures can be classified into four groups as (1) imaging procedures, (2) in vivo function studies, (3) in vitro tests, and (4) therapeutic procedures. The first three procedures are purely diagnostic in nature and make up most studies performed in nuclear medicine.

Imaging Procedures

Imaging procedures provide diagnostic information about organs or body systems based upon the distribution pattern of radioactivity in the body. Imaging procedures are either dynamic or static. Dynamic studies provide functional information through measurement of the rate of accumulation and removal of the radiopharmaceutical by the organ. Static studies provide morphologic information regarding organ size, shape, position, or the presence of space occupying lesions, and in some cases relative function.

Detection and measurement of organ radioactivity is usually made with a gamma camera. This is a stationary electronic device with a radiation detector large enough (8 to 20 inches in diameter) to visualize, in most cases, the entire organ of interest (Fig. 1-1). Before the use of gamma cameras, images were made with rectilinear scanners. The rectilinear scanner detector was small, usually 3 to 5 inches in diameter, and required multiple passes or scans over the area of interest in a rectangular and linear fashion to obtain an image of the entire organ. Because of this technique one still hears imaging procedures referred to as scans.

Dynamic imaging studies require that the camera detector be positioned over the organ of interest before injection of the radiopharmaceutical. In this way the camera will be able to record the radioactivity as it enters and leaves the organ. Information collected may be stored in a computer for further analysis or permanently recorded on photographic film. An example of a dynamic study is the renogram, which is performed to assess kidney function. This is accomplished by the intravenous injection of radioiodinated Hippuran and measuring the time course of its concentration and excretion by the renal tubular cells. With normal kidney function the time to peak renal concentration is 3 to 5 minutes after injection, and the half-time of renal clearance of activity is 12 to 15 minutes. The presence of kidney disease will be reflected by a change in these times.

Static imaging studies are performed after a radiopharmaceutical is allowed to accumulate in the organ of interest. Individual images or "pictures" of the organ are made, typically in the anterior, posterior, and right and left lateral and oblique views to visualize the organ and lesions from several angles. Each view requires several minutes to produce a satisfactory image. Gamma camera images are somewhat analogous to making a conventional photograph under low-light conditions where a prolonged shutter speed is required to collect enough light for a good picture. Motion artifacts are therefore of concern with nuclear medicine images.

The pattern of radiopharmaceutical distribution in an organ varies with and depends on the particular organ studied and the presence or absence of disease. In some studies, the normal organ readily concentrates the radiopharmaceutical and appears uniformly radioactive or "hot." In these organs, diseased tissue excludes the radiopharmaceutical, and lesions will appear as "cold" areas within a "hot" organ. An example is the liver colloid scan obtained after injection of radioactive colloidal particles that localize in the phagocytic cells of the liver. If a tumor or other lesion is present that destroys the colloid localizing ability, it will be visualized as an area of decreased or absent radioactivity. In other organ studies, the normal organ excludes the radiopharmaceutical, but diseased tissue concentrates it so that lesions appear as "hot" spots within a "cold" organ. An example is the brain scan whereby the blood-brain barrier normally prevents blood radioactivity from entering the brain. In disease states in which the blood–brain barrier is disrupted, radioactivity concentrates in the lesion. In still other instances a normal organ may accumulate the radiopharmaceutical, but diseased tissue may concentrate it either to a higher degree because of increased function or to a lesser degree because of decreased function. An example is thyroid imaging with radioactive iodine. The normal gland readily accumulates iodine, but a diseased gland with either hyper- or hypofunctioning thyroid tissue demonstrates increased or decreased concentration, respectively. Examples of these aforementioned static studies are illustrated in Figure 1–2. They were obtained using a conventional planar imaging camera that produces two-dimensional images. A disadvantage of planar imaging is that lesion detection may be impaired, especially when target-to-background ratios are low or there are overlying structures that obscure the view. The new emission computed tomographic (ECT) cameras, however, are able to construct slice images through an organ in transverse, sagittal, and coronal planes and allows one to

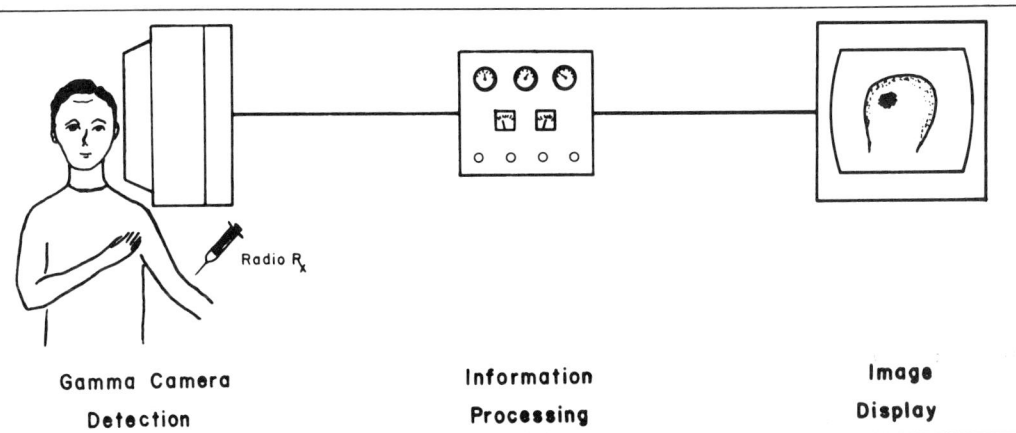

Figure 1-1. Schematic illustration of a scintillation gamma camera system demonstrating radiopharmaceutical injection, detection of radioactivity, electronic processing of information, and image display of the information obtained.

visualize an organ in three dimensions (Fig. 1–3). ECT, therefore, provides greater depth resolution and delineation of the structural and functional information present.

In Vivo Function Studies

In vivo function studies measure the function of a particular organ or body system based upon the absorption, dilution, concentration, or excretion of radioactivity after administration of radiopharmaceuticals. These studies do not require imaging, but analysis and interpretation is based on counting radioactivity either directly from organs within the body or from blood or urine samples. Some examples of in vivo function studies include the following: (1) the radioactive iodine uptake (RAIU) study to assess thyroid gland function by determining the percentage of a dose of radioiodine taken up by the gland within a given time period, (2) the determination of whole blood volume by measuring the dilution of a known amount of intravenously injected chromium-51-labeled red blood cells to determine the red cell volume and the dilution of radioiodinated serum albumin (RISA) labeled with iodine-125 to measure plasma volume, (3) assessing cyanocobalamin (vitamin B_{12}) absorption from the gastrointestinal (GI) tract indirectly by measuring the fraction of orally administered radioactive cobalt-57- or

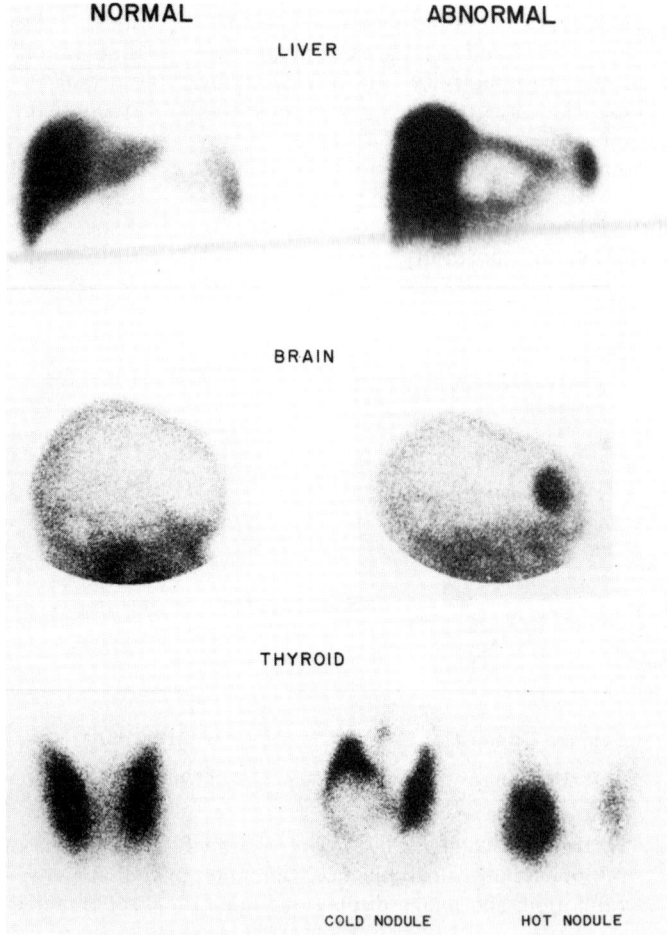

Figure 1-2. Illustration of typical normal and abnormal static images of various organs obtained with a conventional planar imaging gamma camera: anterior view of the liver, lateral view of the brain, and anterior view of the thyroid.

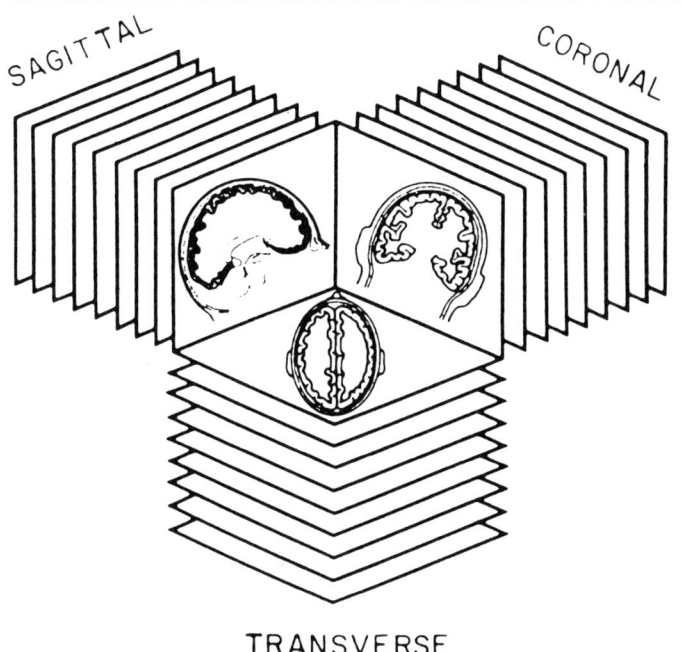

Figure 1-3. Diagram illustrating the three-dimensional imaging technique of an ECT gamma camera that is able to construct slice images through an organ in transverse, sagittal, and coronal planes. *(Copyright, Siemens Medical Systems, Inc., with permission.)*

cobalt-58-labeled vitamin that is excreted in the urine over a defined period of time (the Schilling test). Other studies of this type may also be performed. With all in vivo function studies, however, the radiopharmaceutical must be a true physiologic tracer, i.e., it must function in the system being studied as would its nonradioactive counterpart. Radioiodide thus physiologically mimics stable dietary iodide in thyroid function, radiolabeled red cells and albumin are prevented from being denatured so that they will act similarly to native cells and protein during the time of blood volume measurement, and radiocyanocobalamin is absorbed and excreted identically to natural cyanocobalamin. In all of these instances the radiolabeling does not significantly alter the chemical and biologic properties of the agents used to make functional measurements.

In Vitro Studies

In vitro studies differ from all other nuclear medicine procedures because they do not involve the administration of radioactive material to the patient. These studies require only a small sample of blood that contains the drug or chemical substance to be measured. The blood is then subjected to specific tests using radioactive reagents to measure the unknown amount of substance present. The majority of in vitro tests are based on the radioimmunoassay (RIA) principle because the amount of substance to be measured is usually present in a low concentration in the blood. The radioactivity makes RIA tests highly sensitive, and the antigen–antibody immune reaction gives the test specificity. The different RIA tests may vary in the manipulative technique for obtaining a final result, but the principle is based upon an antigen–antibody reaction. These tests are frequently used to measure plasma levels of thyroid hormones, cortisol, digoxin, and numerous other substances.

Therapeutic Procedures

Therapeutic procedures in nuclear medicine are limited, in most instances, to the treatment of thyroid disease with iodine-131 and occasionally to the treatment of polycythemia with phosphorus-32 as sodium phosphate. The intent in these procedures is to use the beta radiation to selectively destroy diseased tissue. Beta particle radiation is completely absorbed by the tissue in which it resides and will produce a high radiation dose and localized destruction of diseased tissue when present in sufficient amounts. Because I-131 is a beta and gamma emitter, it can be used both diagnostically and therapeutically in thyroid disease; however, the therapeutic dose of radioactivity administered is 1000 to 10,000 times larger than the diagnostic radioactivity used in measuring thyroid function. It is the emission of beta radiation by I-131 that places a limit on the amount of activity that can be administered for diagnostic studies because it contributes about 90 percent of the absorbed radiation dose to the gland compared with about 10 percent from the gamma radiation.

PERSPECTIVE ON RADIOPHARMACEUTICAL USE

One objective in nuclear medicine is to keep the radiation absorbed dose as low as reasonably achievable (ALARA) while obtaining the desired diagnostic information. This is accomplished primarily by limiting the amount of radioactivity administered and decreasing exposure time by using short-lived radionuclides. Radionuclide is a name that refers to any radioactive nuclide or atom. Radionuclides with short half-lives are preferred because larger amounts of radioactivity can be administered. This improves the information obtained because more photons are available for the "nuclear photograph." The radiation dose may also be reduced because the radioactivity decays quickly with short half-life radionuclides.

The common radionuclide used in many nuclear medicine studies is technetium-99m. It has a half-life of 6 hours. It would be difficult for a commercial drug manufacturer to prepare Tc-99m radiopharmaceuticals and adequately test them before use because greater than 90 percent of the radioactivity is lost by decay after 1 day. Tc-99m and other short-lived radiopharmaceuticals therefore require local or in-hospital preparation. Each Tc-99m agent is prepared daily and involves incorporation of Tc-99m atoms into the desired chemical form. Additionally, adequate quality control testing must be done to assure a pure product. This requires measuring the labeling yield as well as maintaining strict aseptic conditions during preparation because these agents are administered by intravenous injection. The personnel who perform these functions may be radiochemists, radiopharmacists, or nuclear medicine technologists. Radiochemists and radiopharmacists are usually employed at large medical center hospitals and are instrumental in developing new agents and procedures. Radiopharmacists also practice in centralized nuclear pharmacies located in large cities and supply radiopharmaceuticals to nuclear medicine departments at several local hospitals. Nuclear medicine technologists usually have the responsibility of preparing and controlling radiopharmaceuticals in smaller community hospitals.

Radiopharmaceuticals with a longer half-life are also used in nuclear medicine because their chemical and physiologic properties outweigh any undesirable physical properties. An example is I-131, which as an 8-day half-life. This is long enough to permit commercial manufacture and testing of I-131 radiopharmaceuticals before use and allows storage in the nuclear medicine laboratory for use when needed. Although I-131 has somewhat undesirable physical properties from a radiation dose viewpoint, such as long half-life, high-energy gamma rays, and beta radiation, iodine's physiologic importance in thyroid work and its chemical reactivity allow it to be labeled to different chemical molecules, making it a valuable radionuclide in nuclear medicine.

Table 1–1 lists the general classification of chemical and physical forms of radio-

TABLE 1-1. CHEMICAL AND PHYSICAL FORMS OF RADIOPHARMACEUTICALS

Elemental	^{133}Xe	^{127}Xe	^{81m}Kr
Simple ions	$^{131}I^-$	$^{99m}TcO_4^-$	$^{111}In^{3+}$
Labeled small molecules	O-iodohippuric acid-I-131 (covalently bonded)		^{111}In-diethylene triamine penta acetic acid (In-111-DTPA) (complexation)
Labeled macromolecules	Proteins (I-125-human serum albumin)		
Labeled particles	Colloids (Tc-99m-sulfur colloid) Albumin aggregates and microspheres (Tc-99m)		
Labeled cells	Erythrocytes (Cr-51, Tc-99m) Leukocytes (In-111) Platelets (In-111)		

pharmaceuticals used in nuclear medicine and illustrates the diverse nature of these agents. These include elemental radionuclides such as the inert gases, simple inorganic ions, radiolabeled molecules, and specialized forms such as labeled particles and blood cells.

Table 1-2 lists the usual routes of administration of radiopharmaceuticals. Noteworthy is the fact that, contrary to the usual requirement that intravenous injections be true solutions without particle contamination, some radiopharmaceuticals are deliberately particulate to achieve site-specific localization of radioactivity. In this way the reticuloendothelial system, comprising mainly the liver, spleen, and bone marrow, can be imaged after administration of radiolabeled colloidal particles. The cardiac blood pool can be imaged following injection of radiolabeled red blood cells. A list of commonly used radiopharmaceuticals and their approved uses is given in Table 1-3.

There are other unique properties of radiopharmaceuticals when compared with conventional therapeutic drugs. Intrinsically, they are radioactive and have the potential for radiation-induced biologic damage. Therefore, before they are used in humans, tissue distribution studies are performed in animal species to estimate the radiation dose and to identify the critical organs. Critical organs are those that receive the highest radiation absorbed dose from a particular radiopharmaceutical. The magnitude of this estimate will set limits on the amount of radioactivity that can be safely administered to humans in diagnostic studies.

Radiopharmaceuticals are administered in extremely small amounts so that chemical toxicity is not the same degree of concern as it is with traditional pharmaceuticals. In fact, the amount of radiopharmaceuticals given is not enough to produce a pharmacologic response. Therefore, the testing required for traditional drugs to identify acute and chronic toxic effects is usually not as extensive for radiopharmaceuticals. One can readily appreciate this fact by considering that a typical 10-μCi diagnostic dose of sodium iodide I-131 con-

TABLE 1-2. TYPICAL ROUTES AND FORMS OF RADIOPHARMACEUTICAL ADMINISTRATION

Route	Form
Oral	Capsules and solutions
Injection	Intrathecal
	Intravenous
	True solutions
	Colloidal dispersions
	Suspensions
Inhalation	Gases and aerosols
Miscellaneous	Subcutaneous
	Intraperitoneal
	Instillation (eye drops)
	Urethral

TABLE 1-3. COMMONLY USED RADIOPHARMACEUTICALS, APPROVED USES, AND RADIATION DOSE ESTIMATES

Radionuclide	Chemical Form	Use	Adm Activity (Adult)	Route	Critical Organ	Radiation Dose mrad/μCi Adm	Reference
1. Chromium-51	Sodium chromate injection	Labeling red blood cells for measuring RBC volume, survival and splenic sequestration	150 μCi	IV	Spleen	4.0	2
2. Chromium-51	Albumin injection	Detection and quantitation of GI protein loss	30 μCi	IV	Spleen	23.0	2
3. Cobalt-57, Co-58	Cyanocobalamin capsules and solution	Diagnosis of pernicious anemia and defects of intestinal absorption	0.5–0.8 μCi	PO	Liver	110.0	2
4. Gallium-67	Gallium citrate injection	Tumor imaging; localization of inflammatory lesions	3 mCi	IV	Spleen	0.60	2
5. Indium-111	Indium pentetate (DTPA) injection	Radionuclide cisternography	500 μCi	IT	Brain surface	14.0	2
6. Iodine-123	Sodium iodide capsules and solution	Diagnosis of thyroid function Thyroid imaging	100–400 μCi	PO	Thyroid	13 (25% uptake) 7.5 (15%) 2.4 (5%)	2
7. Iodine-125	Albumin injection	Blood and plasma volume determination metabolism and turnover studies	5–10 μCi	IV	Ovaries Total body	0.78 0.60	2
8. Iodine-125	Iothalamate injection	Evaluation of glomerular filtration rate	30 μCi	IV	Ovaries Kidneys	0.14 0.11	3
9. Iodine-125	Fibrinogen injection	Diagnosis of deep venous thrombosis of the legs	100 μCi	IV	Thyroid (unblocked) (blocked)	13.0 0.2	2
10. Iodine-131	Sodium iodide capsules and solution	Diagnosis of thyroic function Thyroid imaging (neck)	5–10 μCi 50–100 μCi	PO PO	Thyroid	1300 (25% uptake) 800 (15%)	2

#	Radionuclide	Compound	Use	Dose	Route	Organ	Value	Note
			Thyroid imaging (substernal) Localization of thyroid metastasis	100–200 µCi	PO		260 (5%)	
			Treatment of hyperthyroidism	1–2 mCi	PO			
			Treatment of thyroid carcinoma	5–30 mCi	PO			
11.	Iodine-131	Rose bengal injection	Diagnosis of liver function	150–200 mCi	PO			
				250 µCi	IV	Lower large intestine	35	2
12.	Iodine-131	Orthoiodohippurate injection	Diagnostic aid for determining renal function, renal blood flow, and urinary tract obstruction	75 µCi (1 kidney) 200 µCi (2 kidney)	IV	Bladder wall (no iodide) Thyroid (3% maximum iodide)	3.3 40.5	4
13.	Iron-59	Ferrous citrate injection	Ferrokinetic studies of iron metabolism	10 µCi	IV	Spleen	130	2
14.	Krypton-81m	Gas	Pulmonary ventilation studies	1–10 mCi	Inhalation	Lungs	2.5 (mrad/mCi·min)	5
15.	Phosphorus-32	Chromic phosphate suspension	Treatment of peritoneal or pleural effusions caused by metastatic disease	10–20 mCi	IP	Pleura (surface) Peritoneum (surface)	1150 900	6
16.	Phosphorus-32	Sodium phosphate injection	Treatment of polycythemia vera	1–8 mCi	IV	Skeleton	63	7
17.	Selenium-75	Selenomethionine injection	Pancreas imaging	250 µCi	IV	Liver	25	2
18.	Technetium-99m	Sodium pertechnetate injection	Brain imaging	20 mCi	IV	Resting pop	(stomach wall) 0.25	8
			Thyroid imaging	10 mCi	IV	Active pop	(thyroid) 0.13	
			Salivary gland imaging	5 mCi	IV			
			Blood pool imaging	20 mCi	IV	Bladder wall	0.03 (30 min void)	9
			Vesico-ureteral reflux	1 mCi	Urethral	Eye lens	0.14 (normal)	
			Lacrimal gland imaging	0.1 mCi	Eye drops		4 (tot obs)	10
			Placenta localization	3 mCi	IV			

(continued)

TABLE 1-3. (Continued)

Radionuclide	Chemical Form	Use	Adm Activity (Adult)	Route	Critical Organ	Radiation Dose mrad/μCi Adm	Reference
19. Technetium-99m	Albumin (HSA) injection	Heart blood pool imaging	20 mCi	IV	Blood	0.05	2
20. Technetium-99m	Albumin aggregated (MAA) Albumin microspheres (HAM) Injections	Lung perfusion imaging for pulmonary embolus; radionuclide venography for deep-vein thrombosis	3 mCi	IV	Lungs	0.25	11
21. Technetium-99m	Albumin colloid injection	Diagnostic imaging of liver, spleen, and bone marrow	5 mCi	IV	Liver	0.33	2
22. Technetium-99m	Disofenin (DISIDA) injection	Hepatobiliary imaging	5 mCi	IV	Upper large intestine	3.9	12
23. Technetium-99m	Etidronate (EHDP) injection	Bone imaging	15 mCi	IV	Bladder wall Bladder wall	0.13 (2 hr void) 0.31 (4.8 hr void)	2
24. Technetium-99m	Gluceptate (GH) injection	Brain imaging Kidney imaging	20 mCi 15 mCi	IV IV	Bladder wall Bladder wall Renal cortex	0.12 (2 hr void) 0.28 (4.8 hr void) 0.24	13
25. Technetium-99m	Medronate (MDP) injection	Bone imaging	15 mCi	IV	Bladder wall Bladder wall	0.13 (2 hr void) 0.31 (4.8 hr void)	2
26. Technetium-99m	Oxidronate (HMDP) injection	Bone imaging	15 mCi	IV	Bladder wall Bladder wall	0.13 (2 hr void) 0.31 (4.8 hr void)	2
27. Technetium-99m	Pentetate (DTPA) injection	Brain imaging, renal perfusion Kidney imaging renograms Estimation of GFR Lung inhalation imaging	10–20 mCi 3–5 mCi 3–5 mCi 1–2 mCi	IV IV IV Aerosol inhalation	Bladder wall	0.45	2
28. Technetium-99m	Pyrophosphate (PPi) injection	Bone imaging Infarction avid imaging	15 mCi 15 mCi	IV IV	Bladder wall Bladder wall	0.10 (2 h void) 0.23 (4.8 h void)	14

#	Radionuclide	Form	Use	Dose	Route	Organ	Value	Ref
			Heart blood pool (Tc-RBC)	20 mCi	IV	Bladder wall	0.12	2
29.	Technetium-99m	Sulfur colloid (SC) injection	Liver-spleen imaging Bone marrow imaging Gastroesophageal transit and reflux, pulmonary aspiration	5 mCi 10 mCi 0.3–0.5 mCi	IV IV PO	Liver	0.34	2
30.	Technetium-99m	Succimer (DMSA) injection	Kidney imaging	5 mCi	IV	Renal cortices Bladder wall	0.85 0.07	15
31.	Thallium-201	Thallous chloride injection	Myocardial perfusion imaging for diagnosis and localization of myocardial infarction	2 mCi	IV	Kidneys	1.25	16
32.	Xenon-127	Gas	Pulmonary inhalation imaging	5–10 mCi	Inhalation	Airway mucosa Lung	0.015 (1 mc/L conc) 0.0044 (1 mc/L conc)	17 18
33.	Xenon-133	Gas	Pulmonary inhalation imaging, cerebral blood flow studies	10–20 mCi	Inhalation	Airway mucosa Lung	0.116 (1 mc/L conc) 0.0065 (1 mc/L conc)	17 18
34.	Xenon-133	Saline injection	Cardiac abnormalities Cerebral blood flow studies Pulmonary function studies Muscle and skin blood flow studies	1–30 mCi 1.0 mCi 2–30 mCi 0.1–0.2 mCi	IV IV IV IM, ID	Brain Brain Lung Whole body	0.013 0.020 0.008 0.002	19 19 19 19
35.	Ytterbium-169	Pentetate (DTPA) injection	Radionuclide cisternography	0.5–1.0 mCi	IT	Brain Spinal cord (NL) Spinal cord (NPH)	3.2 15.0 25.0	2

tains only 8×10^{-11} g of iodine. By comparison this is one eighty-millionth of the normal total-body iodine stores and about one two-millionth of the daily dietary intake of iodine. One can readily see that this amount of radioiodine poses no threat to patients, even to those who are allergic to iodine.

The radioactive nature of radiopharmaceuticals gives them a very special significance regarding their safe and efficacious use. This translates into the need for protecting patients from unnecessary radiation exposure, personnel from the radioactive material that they handle, and the general public from unnecessary exposure to radioactive environmental waste. The use of radioactive material is therefore strictly controlled by state and federal agencies. Because radiopharmaceuticals are radioactive drugs, they are regulated by the Food and Drug Administration regarding their safety and efficacy from a drug viewpoint and by the Nuclear Regulatory Commission or appropriate state licensing agency, which regulates the safe use of radioactive material. The use of radioactive material in human subjects requires that physicians and other technical and paramedical personnel be properly trained and experienced to handle such materials and be recognized in this regard by specific licensure.

All of the topics discussed in this introductory chapter will be covered in greater detail in subsequent chapters of this book. Fundamental principles will be discussed, but always with application to the practical use of radiopharmaceuticals in nuclear medicine.

REFERENCES

1. Grigg ERN: The beginnings of nuclear medicine. In Gottschalk A, Potchen, EJ (eds): Diagnostic Nuclear Medicine. Baltimore, Williams & Wilkins, 1976, p 1
2. Kereiakes JG, Rosenstein M: Handbook of Radiation Doses in Nuclear Medicine and Diagnostic X-ray. Boca Raton, Fla, CRC Press, 1980
3. Package insert: Glofil-125. Iso-tex Diagnostics, Inc, Friendswood, Tex., 1979
4. Eliott AT, Britton KE, Brown NJG, et al: Dosimetry of current radiopharmaceuticals used in renal investigations. In Clutier RJ, Coffey JL, Snyder WS, Watson EE (eds): Radiopharmaceutical Dosimetry Symposium. Washington, DC, DHEW Publication (FDA) 76-8044, 1976, pp 293–304
5. Package insert: MPI Krypton-81m Gas Generator. Mediphysics, Inc, Emeryville, Calif, 1980
6. Package insert: Phosphocol P-32. Mallinckrodt Diagnostics, Inc, St Louis, 1980
7. Package insert: Sodium Phosphate P-32. Millinckrodt Diagnostics, Inc, St Louis, 1981
8. Package insert: Technetium-99m Generator. Mallinckrodt Diagnostics, Inc, St Louis, 1984
9. Conway JJ, Belman AB, King LR: Direct and indirect radionuclide cystography. Semin Nucl Med 4:197, 1974
10. Robertson JS, Brown ML, Colvard DM: Radiation absorbed dose to the lens in dacryoscintigraphy with pertechnetate. Radiology 113:747, 1979
11. Package insert: TechneScan MAA. Mallinckrodt Diagnostics, Inc, St Louis, 1080
12. Package insert: Hepatolite. Dupont NEN Medical Products, N Billerica, Mass, 1984
13. Package insert: TechneScan Gluceptate. Mallinckrodt Diagnostics, Inc, St Louis, 1983
14. Package insert: TechneScan PYP. Mallinckrodt Diagnotics, Inc, St Louis, 1984
15. Package insert: MPI DMSA Kidney Reagent. Medi-Physics, Inc, Emeryville, Calif, 1984
16. Package insert: Thallous Chloride Tl-201. Mallinckrodt Diagnostics, Inc, St Louis, 1980
17. Goddard BA, Ackery DM: Xenon-133, Xe-127 and Xe-125 for lung function investigations. A dosimetric comparison. J Nucl Med 16:780, 1975
18. Atkins, HL, Robertson JS, Croft BY, et al: Estimates of radiation absorbed doses from radioxenons in lung imaging. J Nucl Med 21:459, 1980
19. Package insert: Xeneisol. Mallinckrodt Diagnostics, Inc, St Louis, 1980

CHAPTER 2

Physics of Radiopharmaceuticals

The physical and chemical properties of a radiopharmaceutical are important to its use in nuclear medicine. The chemical properties are largely responsible for localization within the body, whereas the physical properties associated with the radionuclide provide a means of detection and measurement. This chapter will consider the radionuclide properties in some detail.

NUCLIDES

An atom is the smallest particle of an element possessing the properties of the element. We know from elementary chemistry that atoms are made up of protons and neutrons within the nucleus, which is surrounded by electrons in orbitals or shells. These shells are designated with the letters K, L, M, etc., with the K shell closest to the nucleus. Electrons fill these shells in this order with a specified number per shell. A neutral atom has the same number of electrons as protons in the nucleus (Fig. 2–1). Removal of one or more electrons will produce an ionized atom. Ionization can occur by several processes. One of these is through the interaction of radiation with matter, which will be discussed later in this chapter.

A nuclide is an atom characterized by the number of protons and neutrons in its nucleus. Nuclides are designated by a symbol notation as follows:

$$^{A}_{Z}X_{N}$$

where X is the elemental symbol, Z is the number of protons and N is the number of neutrons. The mass number A is equal to the sum of protons and neutrons.

Nuclides are classified according to their A, Z, and N values as follows:

- Isotopes = nuclides with the same Z, but different A and N

$$^{1}_{1}H_{0} \qquad ^{2}_{1}H_{1} \qquad ^{3}_{1}H_{2}$$

- Isobars = nuclides with the same A, but different Z and N

$$^{64}_{28}Ni_{36} \qquad ^{64}_{30}Zn_{24}$$

- Isotones = nuclides with the same N, but different Z and A

$$\begin{array}{cc} {}^{41}K & {}^{42}Ca \\ {}_{19}{}_{22} & {}_{20}{}_{22} \end{array}$$

- Isomers = nuclides with the same A, Z, and N, but different nuclear energy states

$$\begin{array}{cc} {}^{99}Tc & {}^{99m}Tc \\ {}_{43}{}_{56} & {}_{43}{}_{56} \end{array}$$

The lowercase *m* in the mass number denotes the metastable state, one sustaining an excited condition for a measurable period of time.

The periodic table lists 103 elements. If one considers the isotopes of each element, the total number of nuclides is in excess of 1900 species. Of this number only 266 are stable. The unstable species are called radionuclides. A radioisotope is a radionuclide of a particular element. Figure 2–2 illustrates a portion of the chart of the nuclides in the region of the light elements.

ORBITAL ENERGY LEVELS

Electrons are bound in their shells by an electron binding energy. The binding energy is the work that must be applied to remove an electron from the atom. The K-shell electrons have the highest binding energy because they are closest to the positive attractive force of the nucleus. Inner shells fill with electrons first, and if one of these electrons is removed, an outer-shell electron will fall into its place to fill the vacancy. After such an event the release of energy from the atom is equal to the difference between the binding energies of the two shells. Consider, for example, the tungsten (W) atom shown in Figure 2–3. If a K-shell electron is removed and subsequently filled in by an L-shell electron, a characteristic x-ray is produced equal to 59,000 electron volts (eV) (Fig. 2–3A). An electron volt is a unit of energy equal to the energy acquired by an electron falling through a potential difference of 1 volt (V). In lieu of the characteristic x-ray, an Auger electron may be emitted (Fig. 2–3B). In this case, the atom transfers its energy to an outer-shell electron that is ejected from the atom. The Auger electron has an energy equal to that of the x-ray minus the electron's binding energy. A 59,000-eV x-ray will thus produce a 56,000-eV Auger electron from the tungsten M-shell. In some radionuclides such as iodine-125, characteristic x-ray production is significant and is the principal radiation that is detected.

Optical radiation may also be produced but is only of academic interest in nuclear medicine (Fig. 2–3C). This occurs when outer-shell valence electrons are excited to higher-energy suborbits. When the electrons return to their ground state, visible light is emitted. An example is the excitation of minerals with ultraviolet light causing fluorescence.

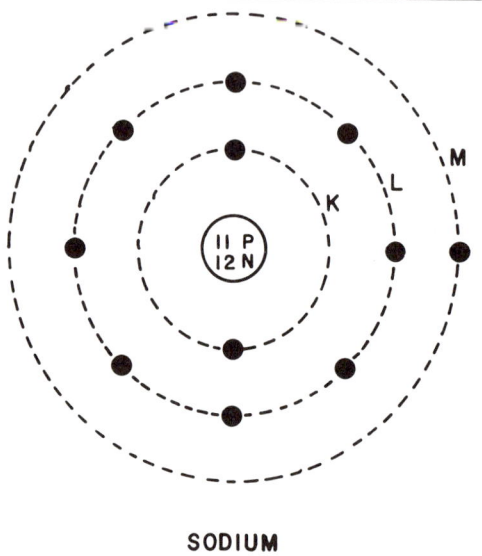

Figure 2-1. Bohr model of the sodium atom.

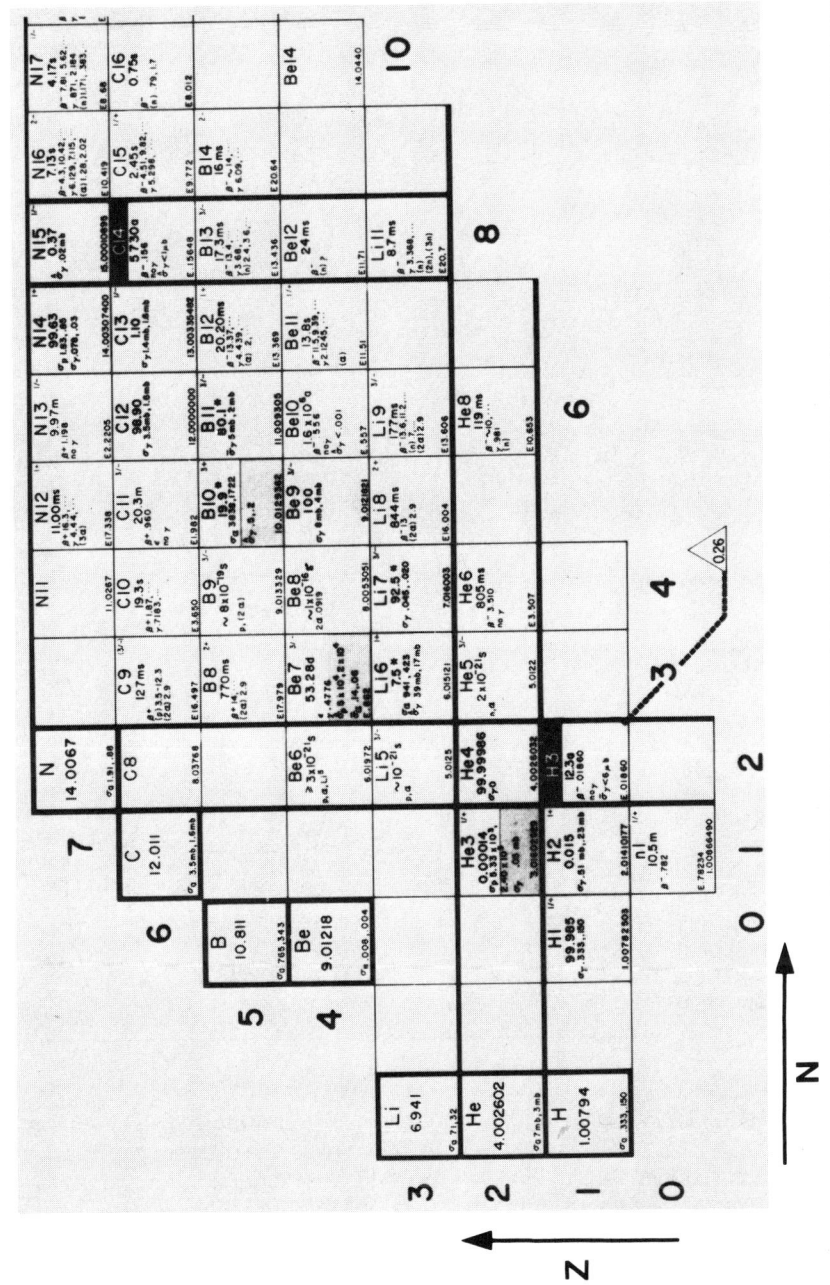

Figure 2-2. Chart of the nuclides in the region of the light elements. *(From the General Electric Co, San Jose, Calif, with permission.)*

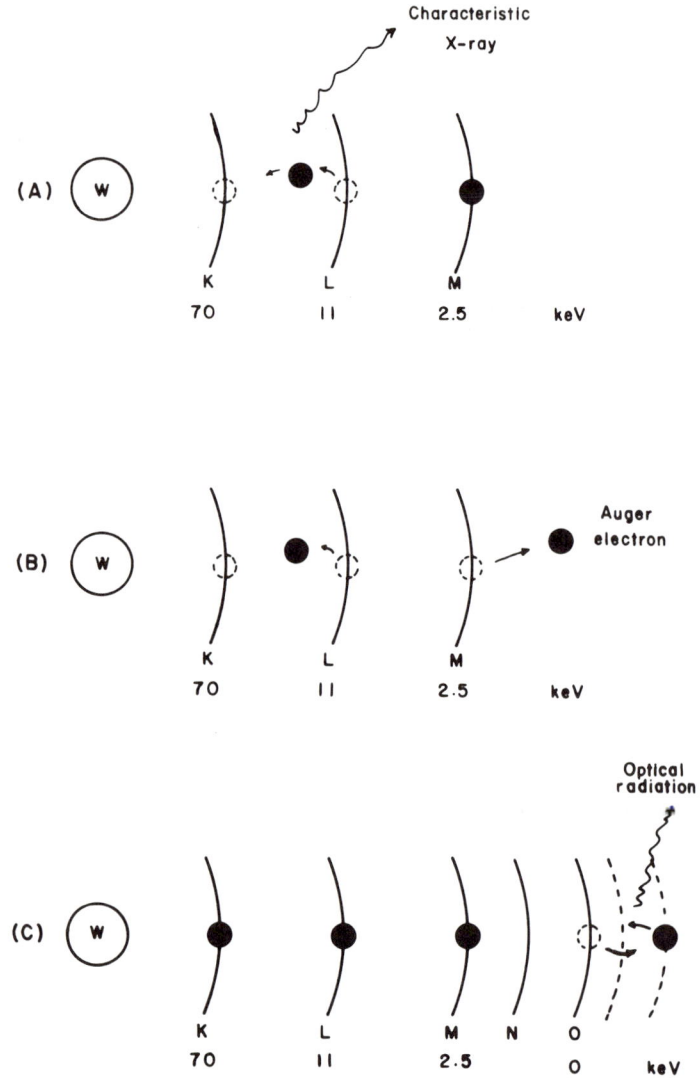

Figure 2-3. Perturbations of the tungsten electron shells: (A) characteristic x-ray production after ejection of a K-shell electron, (B) Auger electron production following ejection of a K-shell electron, (C) optical radiation production after excitation of the valence shell electron.

NUCLEAR ENERGY LEVELS

Neutrons and protons (collectively called nucleons) exist in the nucleus of an atom in discrete energy levels. In a stable atom nucleons are in their ground state. They may, however, be excited to higher-energy states, for example, by interaction with a high-speed particle or after radioactive decay. When these excited nucleons return to their ground state, energy is emitted from the nucleus as a gamma ray. The energy may be released as one discrete gamma ray or in cascade as several smaller gamma rays of different energies (Fig. 2-4). The nuclear deexcitation process is analogous to the electron shell changes discussed previously, but certain differences exist. First, the electron shell deexcitation process immediately follows atomic excitation whereas nuclear deexcitation may be immediate or delayed. When nuclear deexcitation is delayed, the

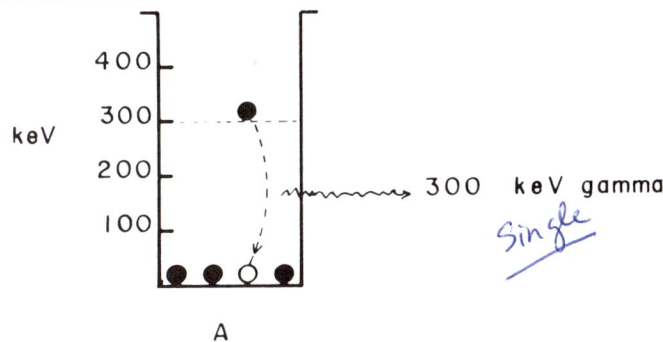

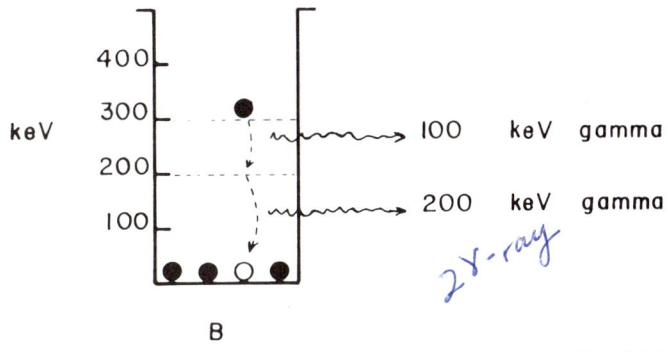

Figure 2-4. Nuclear deexcitation by emission of gamma rays after the return of excited nucleons to their ground state. Energy is emitted as a single gamma ray or as a cascade of two gamma rays.

excited nucleus is said to be metastable. It should be noted also that although characteristic x-rays and gamma rays are high-energy electromagnetic radiation, they differ in that gamma rays typically have much higher energy and originate from nuclear energy changes, whereas characteristic x-rays are lower in energy and arise from electron shell energy changes.

NUCLEAR MASS AND ENERGY

In 1905 Albert Einstein proposed his famous equation that equates mass and energy, $E = mc^2$, where E is energy in erg units, m is mass in gram units, and c is the velocity of light (2.998×10^{10} cm/sec). The standard atomic mass unit (AMU) is defined as one twelfth the mass of a carbon-12 atom. The weight in grams of 1 AMU may thus be calculated as follows:

$$\frac{12 \text{ g}}{6.023 \times 10^{23} \text{ atoms}} \times \frac{1 \text{ atom}}{12 \text{ AMU}}$$
$$= 1.66 \times 10^{-24} \text{ g/AMU}$$

The energy equivalent of this small mass can be calculated from Einstein's equation as follows:

$$E = (1.66 \times 10^{-24} \text{ g/AMU})(2.998 \times 10^{10} \text{ cm/sec})^2$$

$$E = 1.49232 \times 10^{-3} \text{ ergs/AMU}$$

In the radiation sciences the basic energy unit used is the electron volt (eV), previously defined, and its multiples, the kiloelectron volt (keV) and the million electron volt (MeV). The energy equivalent of 1 AMU is as follows:

$$\frac{1.4923 \times 10^{-3} \text{ ergs/AMU}}{1.602 \times 10^{-6} \text{ ergs/MeV}}$$
$$= 931.5 \text{ MeV/AMU} \quad (2\text{-}1)$$

TABLE 2-1. MASS-ENERGY RELATIONSHIP OF ATOMIC PARTICLES

Particle	Mass (AMU)	Energy (MeV)
Electron	5.48597×10^{-4}	0.511
Proton	1.0072766	938.278
Neutron	1.0086654	939.572
Hydrogen atom	1.0078252	938.789

This simple relationship between mass and energy allows one to easily calculate the energy released in a nuclear reaction or in a radioactive decay process. Some useful atomic mass–energy relationships are listed in Table 2-1.

NUCLEAR FORCES

Opposite poles of a magnet attract each other, and like poles repel. The attractive and repulsive forces become greater as the poles come close together. A similar phenomenon occurs with protons and electrons. Protons, however, may exist in close proximity within the nucleus of an atom without repulsion. This can only be possible if an attractive force is present that is much greater than the electrostatic repulsive force. This attractive force is called the nuclear force and is about 100 times greater than the electrostatic force. It is responsible for holding the neutrons and protons in the nucleus.

The nuclear force is greatest between unlike and uncharged particles, i.e., the attraction between n,p > n,n > p,p. The nuclear attractive force is appreciable only over a finite range and is strongest when nucleons are 1×10^{-13} cm apart. The force becomes repulsive at distances less than 0.4×10^{-13} cm and becomes negligible at 2.4×10^{-13} cm.

NUCLEAR BINDING ENERGY

Suppose you are able to create atoms from their component parts of neutrons, protons, and electrons. If you created a C-12 atom, you would find that the sum of its individual parts, i.e., six neutrons, six protons, and six electrons, is as follows:

Mass:
n	= 6 (1.0086654 AMU) =	6.0519924 AMU
p	= 6 (1.0072766 AMU) =	6.0436596 AMU
e^-	= 6 (0.0005486 AMU) =	0.0032916 AMU
Sum of individual components		= 12.0989436 AMU

If you reweigh the finished atom of C-12, you will find that its nuclidic mass is only 12.0000000 AMU, which is 0.0989436 AMU less than the sum of its individual components. This mass that is apparently lost is called the mass defect and occurs each time atoms are created from individual atomic particles. Because most of the atom's mass is in the nucleus, this mass defect is associated with the nucleus and in actuality is not lost but converted into an equivalent amount of energy called the nuclear binding energy. The amount of this energy for C-12 can be calculated as follows:

$$0.0989436 \text{ AMU} \times 931.5 \text{ MeV/AMU} = 92.166 \text{ MeV}$$

The nuclear binding energy is thus the energy released when a nucleus is produced from its component nucleons. It may also be defined as the energy required to break a nucleus apart into its individual components. The average binding energy (BE_{avg}) per nucleon for C-12 is as follows:

$$BE_{avg} = \frac{92.166 \text{ MeV}}{12 \text{ nucleons}} = 7.68 \text{ MeV/nucleon}$$

The average binding energy per nucleon has been determined for all stable nuclides and is plotted as a function of mass number in Figure 2-5. For an A greater than 11 it ranges between 7.4 and 8.8 MeV throughout the table of elements, with the maximum values near 8.8 MeV occurring in the vicinity of A = 60 for iron and nickel nuclei. The higher the average binding energy, the more stable is the nucleus because it takes more energy to break it apart. This is significant in that the trend in nature

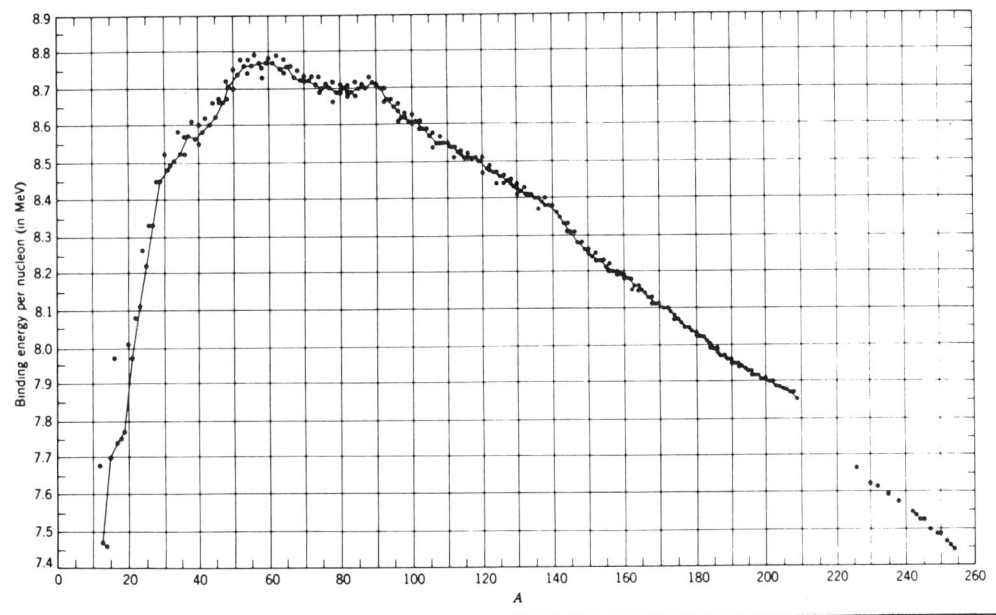

Figure 2-5. The average binding energy per nucleon as a function of mass number, A. The line drawn connects the odd A points. *(From Friedlander G, et al, 1966, with permission.²)*

is to achieve the greatest nuclear stability and is evident by the fisson of heavy nuclei to form lighter, more stable ones having higher average binding energies and by the fusion of light nuclei (occurring in the stars) to form heavier ones with more nuclear stability.

RADIATION AND RADIOACTIVE DECAY

Radiation can be defined as the emission and propagation of energy through space. Radiation may be particulate or electromagnetic. The principal forms of radiation emitted from radionuclides are alpha particles, beta particles, gamma rays, and x-rays. An alpha particle is a helium nucleus, $^4He^{2+}$, i.e., a helium atom stripped of its two orbital electrons. Alpha particles are emitted primarily from heavier nuclei such as uranium, thorium, plutonium, and radium, but a few lighter nuclides are alpha emitters. Beta particles are electrons generated in and emitted from the nuclei of unstable atoms. Negatively charged beta particles are called negatrons; positively charged beta particles are called positrons. Beta particles have the same mass as orbital electrons and a rest-mass energy equivalent to 0.511 MeV. Gamma rays are high-energy electromagnetic radiation. They have no mass or charge and are emitted from unstable nuclei secondary to particle decay.

The ratio of neutrons to protons in the nucleus determines whether a nuclide will be stable or radioactive. For the light nuclei, stability is achieved when the N/P ratio is 1. Above atomic number 20, however, the N/P ratio must be greater than 1 for stability because the repulsive force of additional protons becomes more prominent and extra neutrons are required to "buffer" this proton interaction (Fig. 2–6). Stable nuclides fall on the line of beta

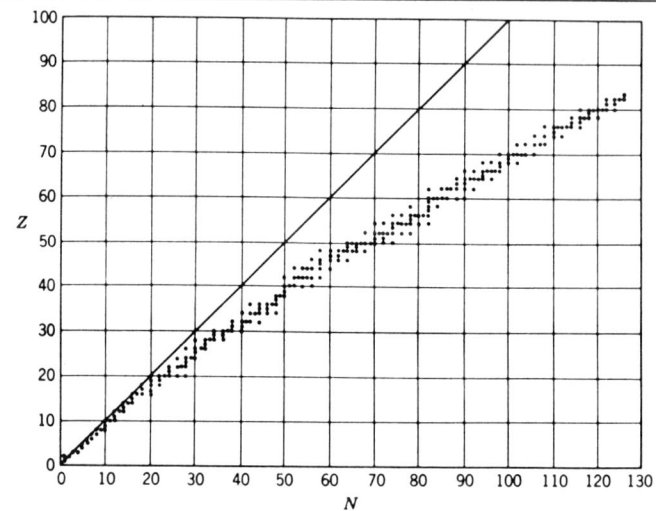

Figure 2-6. Plot of Z versus N of the stable nuclei. The solid line represents a neutron-to-proton ratio of unity. Note the increase in this ratio for nuclides of Z greater than 20. (From Friedlander G, et al, 1966, with permission.[2])

stability. Nuclides that fall in regions above or below this line are radioactive and undergo radioactive decay until a stable N/P ratio is achieved. Nuclides further away from the line of beta stability, in general, have shorter half-lives, indicating their tendency toward greater instability than those closer to it. This is illustrated in Table 2-2, which lists the isotopes of carbon and indicates that proton-rich nuclides with N/P ratios less than 1 undergo positron decay, whereas neutron-rich nuclides undergo negatron decay. In positron decay excess nuclear positive charge is reduced by ejecting a positive electron from the nucleus, and in negatron decay the positive charge is increased in the nucleus by ejecting a negative electron.

Negatron Decay

Neutron-rich nuclides undergo negatron or beta-minus decay. Negatron decay begins when a neutron is converted into a proton, an electron, and a neutrino according to the following transformation:

$$n \longrightarrow p^+ + e^- + \bar{\nu}$$

Because the electron is not part of the nucleus, it is ejected as beta radiation. The neutrino will be discussed later. Consider,

TABLE 2-2. CARBON ISOTOPES

Isotope	N:P Ratio	Radiation	Half-life	Isotopic Abundance (%)
C-9	0.50	β^+	0.13 sec	—
C-10	0.67	β^+	19 sec	—
C-11	0.83	β^+	20.5 min	—
C-12	1.00	—	Stable	98.89
C-13	1.17	—	Stable	1.11
C-14	1.33	β^-	5730 yr	—
C-15	1.50	β^-	2.25 sec	—
C-16	1.67	β^-	0.74 sec	—

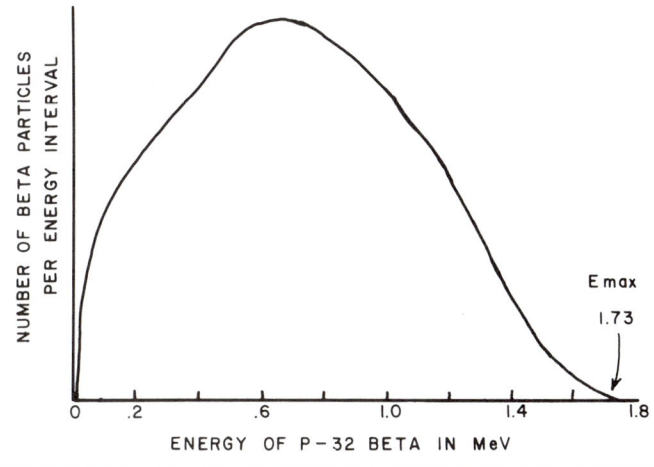

Figure 2-7. Beta energy spectrum for P-32 decay. The vertical coordinate gives the relative number of beta particles that are emitted at each energy on the horizontal coordinate up to the maximum of 1.73 MeV. For example, there are about twice as many particles emitted with an energy of 0.6 MeV compared with 1.2 MeV.

for example, the decay of phosphorus-32 shown in the following decay equation.

$$^{32}_{15}P_{17} \xrightarrow{14.3\ d} {}^{32}_{16}S_{16} + E\ (\beta, \bar{\nu})$$

31.973908 AMU   31.972047 AMU

P-32 is the parent nuclide and sulfur-32 is the daughter nuclide. We will examine this decay and account for all particles, mass, and energy. Consider for a moment that you could visually observe a P-32 atom and are able to count the numbers of protons and neutrons in its nucleus and the number of orbital electrons. You would observe 15 protons, 17 neutrons, and 15 orbital electrons. The instant after it decays it no longer is phosphorus but sulfur. You now observe 16 protons (atomic number of sulfur), 16 neutrons, and 16 orbital electrons. Additionally, you would have observed the beta particle escaping from the P-32 nucleus just before it changed into S-32. If the P-32 atom rested on an atomic balance, it would have registered 31.973908 AMU before decay to S-32 and 31.972047 AMU afterwards. The difference is a mass defect of 0.001861 AMU and is equivalent to 1.73 MeV of energy. This is known as the transition energy (E_{max}). The transition energy is the total energy released when a parent radionuclide decays to its daughter nuclide. This energy comes from the small amount of mass lost by the parent. Parent nuclides are always "heavier" than their daughters.

In negatron decay the transition energy is dissipated as kinetic energy of the beta particle and the neutrino. The maximum energy a P-32 beta particle can have is 1.73 MeV. Measurements made by scientists, however, have demonstrated that on the average only about one third of the transition energy is associated with the beta particle when P-32 decays. Because this is in contradiction to the law of conservation of matter and energy, scientists postulated that another particle must dissipate the remaining two thirds of the energy. This particle was subsequently found to be the neutrino.* The neutrino is essentially a massless, chargeless particle emitted from the nucleus in all beta decay processes and carries away the energy not used by the beta particle.[3] If one were to measure the energy of each particle from thousands of P-32 atoms and plot their frequency of occurrence versus

---

* It appears to be a general rule that a matter–antimatter pair is formed whenever energy is converted to mass. Since the negatron is a member of the matter system, we write $\bar{\nu}$ for the antineutrino. The neutrino, ν, is associated with the emission of the positron, which is antimatter, so that again a matter–antimatter pair is created. Typically, both are referred to simply as neutrinos.

energy, a beta energy spectrum would result similar to the one in Figure 2–7. If a decaying P-32 atom emits a 0.73-MeV beta particle, the neutrino will thus carry away 1.00 MeV.

In negatron decay one need not account for the electron mass lost from the nucleus of the P-32 atom because an equivalent electron mass is acquired in the electron shell of S-32 to offset it.

Decay schemes are often used to provide a ready reference to a variety of data such as mode of decay, transition energy, radiation energies and abundances, and parent and daughter nuclides. Transitions are indicated by diagonal arrows drawn from the parent to the daughter nuclide to either the right or left. Isomeric transitions with emission of gamma radiation are indicated by vertically drawn arrows. As a rule, the diagonal arrow depicting transitions from parent to daughter is drawn to the right when the daughter nuclide has a higher atomic number than the parent (negatron decay). When the daughter nuclide is of lower atomic number as in alpha particle decay, positron decay, or electron capture decay, the arrow is drawn to the left.

The decay scheme for P-32 is shown in Figure 2–8. P-32 is called a pure beta emitter because all of the transition energy is distributed between the beta particle and the neutrino. The nucleus does not receive any of this energy and is therefore not raised to an excited state that would lead to gamma emission. For this reason, P-32 is not a useful diagnostic radionuclide but is used

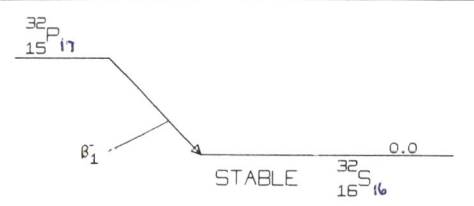

Figure 2-8. Decay scheme for P-32. *(From Dillman LT, et al, 1975, with permission.*[4]*)*

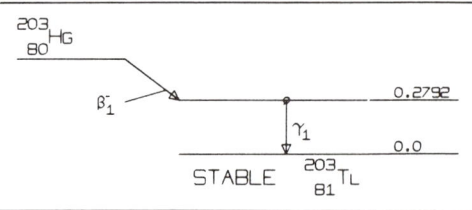

Figure 2-9. Decay scheme for Hg-203. *(From Dillman LT, et al, 1975, with permission.*[4]*)*

for various types of interstitial therapies where all of its energy is absorbed by the tissues. Other examples of pure beta emitters are C-14, H-3, and S-35.

Some radionuclides are beta–gamma emitters. Examples of those used in nuclear medicine are I-131, Mo-99, Xe-133, Au-198, and Hg-203. The last two are no longer routinely used, but the decay of Hg-203 will be illustrated because it is simple. The decay equation for Hg-203 is as follows:

$$^{203}_{80}\text{Hg}_{123} \xrightarrow{46.5 \text{ d}} {}^{203}_{81}\text{Tl}_{122} + E\,(\beta, \bar{\nu}, \gamma)$$
$$202.972857 \text{ AMU} \qquad 202.972330 \text{ AMU}$$

The mass defect for this decay is 0.000527 AMU, which is equivalent to a transition energy of 0.471 MeV. The decay scheme is shown in Figure 2–9. Hg-203 does not decay directly to the ground state of thallium-203 but to its excited state of 0.279 MeV. That is, in each decay of Hg-203, 0.192 MeV of the transition energy is distributed between the beta particle and neutrino, and 0.279 MeV is released as a gamma ray when the excited Tl-203 nucleus deexcites to its ground state. The gamma ray is emitted instantaneously after beta particle emission.

Positron Decay

Positron decay occurs when the N/P ratio is too low for stability. These proton-rich nuclides decay by converting a proton into a neutron and a positron–neutrino pair, which are ejected from the nucleus. The transformation is as follows:

$$p^+ \longrightarrow n + e^+ + \nu$$

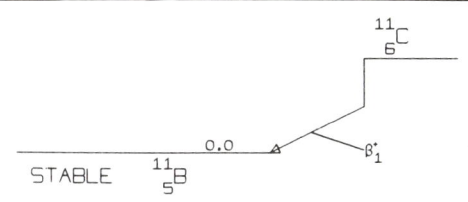

Figure 2-10. Decay scheme for C-11. (From Dillman, LT, et al, 1975, with permission.[4])

Because positron emission decreases the atomic number by one unit, the electron orbitals must lose one electron as soon as the nucleus ejects the positron. The atomic mass of the daughter nuclide will thus be at least two electron masses less than the parent. The loss of two electron masses in positron decay requires that at least 1.022 MeV (2 × 0.511 MeV/electron) of transition energy be available for the process to occur.

Carbon-11 is a positron emitter whose decay equation is shown below:

$$^{11}_{6}C_5 \xrightarrow{20.3 \text{ min}} {}^{11}_{5}B_6 + E\ (\beta^+, \nu)$$

11.011433 AMU   11.009305 AMU

The mass defect for this decay is 0.002128 AMU, which is equivalent to a transition energy of 1.982 MeV. Because 1.022 MeV of this energy must be used for the positron–electron masses, 0.960 MeV is dissipated between the positron kinetic energy and the neutrino in roughly a one-third–two-thirds distribution. The decay scheme is shown in Figure 2–10. The vertical line leading directly down from the C-11 energy level represents the 1.022 MeV of energy emitted as two 0.511-MeV gamma rays. This occurs from the annihilation reaction of the positron with an electron. Positrons are antimatter and exist for very short periods of time. After ejection from the nucleus, the positron's energy moves it through as distance of a few millimeters in about 1 microsecond. After this time it has lost most of its energy and will combine with a negative electron. The two electron masses are converted into two 0.511-MeV photons called annihilation radiation emit-

ted in opposite directions (Fig. 2–11). Positron emitters will always produce 0.511 MeV photons. There are a few positron emitters used in nuclear medicine, but they are mostly for investigative purposes because they require specialized equipment for detection. Some examples include C-11, F-18, N-13, and O-15. It should be noted also that some positron emitters decay to excited states of the daughter nuclide, and therefore nuclear gamma rays will also accompany the decay process.

Electron Capture Decay

Electron capture is the second way that proton-rich nuclides can decay to decrease the excess positive nuclear charge. The change occurring in the nucleus is the same as in positron decay, only the mechanism is different. Therefore, electron capture and positron decay are competing processes. In fact, in some radionuclides that have transition energies greater than 1.022 MeV, both processes of decay can occur. If a proton-rich nuclide does not have at least 1.022 MeV of transition energy, however, a posi-

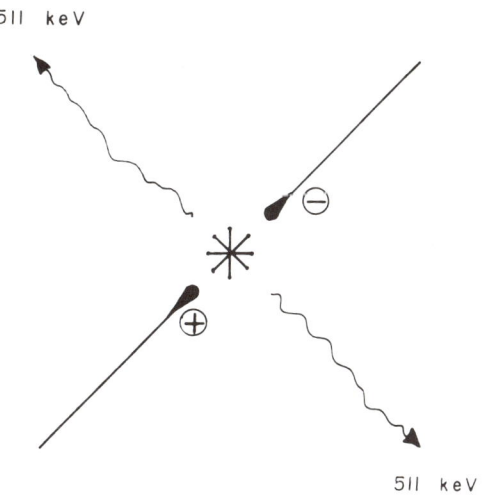

Figure 2-11. Positron annihilation reaction. Two electron masses, one positron and one negatron, are converted into their equivalent electromagnetic energy of two 0.5-MeV photons.

tron cannot be created, and electron capture decay will occur.

In electron capture decay an orbital electron, usually the K-shell electron, is captured by the nucleus whereby it combines with a proton to produce a neutron and a neutrino. The positive nuclear charge is thus reduced by one unit. The nuclear transformation that occurs is as follows:

$$p^+ + e^- \longrightarrow n + \nu$$

For most cases of electron capture the process involves a K-shell electron unless the transition energy is less than the K-shell binding energy, in which case L-shell capture occurs.

The neutrino carries off all of the transition energy released in the electron capture decay process unless an excited daughter is produced, in which case the energy is shared between the neutrino and the gamma ray.

Several radionuclides used in nuclear medicine decay by electron capture: gallium-67, thallium-201, iodine-123, cobalt-57, indium-111, xenon-127, iodine-125, and chromium-51. Electron capture is a desirable decay mode because no particulate radiation is produced and this potentially lowers the radiaton absorbed dose. The decay equation for Cr-51 is as follows:

$$^{51}_{24}Cr_{27} \xrightarrow{27.7 \text{ d}} {}^{51}_{23}V_{28} + E(\nu, \gamma)$$

50.944786 AMU   50.943978 AMU

The mass defect for this transition is 0.000808 AMU and is equivalent to a transition energy of 0.753 MeV. The decay scheme is shown in Figure 2–12. It demonstrates that 91 percent of Cr-51 atoms decay directly to the ground state of vanadium-51 by emitting a 0.753-MeV neutrino. In 9 percent of decays, however, the neutrino carries only 0.433 MeV, and a gamma ray of 0.320 MeV is emitted from the excited V-51 daughter. One must also keep in mind that secondary radiations of characteristic x-rays and Auger electrons will also be produced.

Each of the decay processes previously discussed is called an isobaric transition because in every case of negatron, positron, or electron capture decay the parent and daughter nuclides have the same mass number and only the number of protons and neutrons change.

Isomeric Transitions and Metastable States

An isomeric transition occurs when an excited nucleus loses its excess energy by emission of only a gamma ray with no change in the atomic or neutron number. Reference was made to this process earlier in the chapter during the discussion of nuclear energy levels. A nucleus can become excited in several ways, but the most common one is through a radioactive decay process whereby some of the transition energy remains in the nucleus. This excess nuclear energy can be emitted either promptly or in a delayed manner. Prompt deexcitaton occurs when gamma rays are emitted immediately after the decay process, usually within 10^{-13} seconds. Delayed deexcitation occurs when the excited nucleus persists for a measurable time period with a half-life on the order of 10^{-9} seconds to several months. These nuclei are called metastable states and are designated by writing a lowercase *m* after the mass number. Most of the radionuclides used in nuclear medicine are prompt gamma emitters such as I-131 and Cr-51. Some metastable species have a long enough half-life that they can be separated and isolated from the parent radionuclide. These isolated species are sometimes called pure gamma emitters. A good example is technetium-99m produced by the decay of Mo-99. A simplified decay scheme is shown in Figure 2–13. When

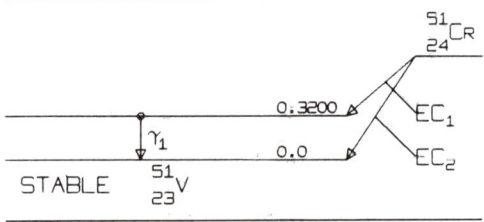

Figure 2-12. Decay scheme for Cr-51. *(From Dillman LT, et al, 1975, with permission.[4])*

PHYSICS OF RADIOPHARMACEUTICALS

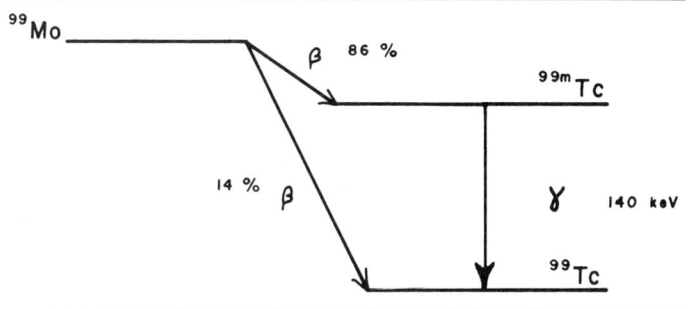

Figure 2-13. Simplified decay scheme for Mo-99.

Mo-99 decays, 13.95 percent of the decays occur to the Tc-99 ground state, but 86.05 percent of decays yield the metastable Tc-99m, which has a half-life of 6 hours. It will deexcite by emitting a monoenergetic 0.140-MeV gamma ray to its isomer Tc-99.

Internal Conversion

In some isomeric transitions the energy released may be transferred to an inner-shell electron instead of emitting a gamma ray. According to quantum mechanics, some of the orbital electrons, particularly the K-

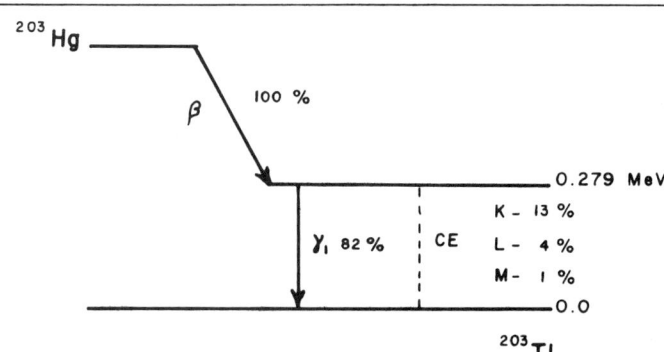

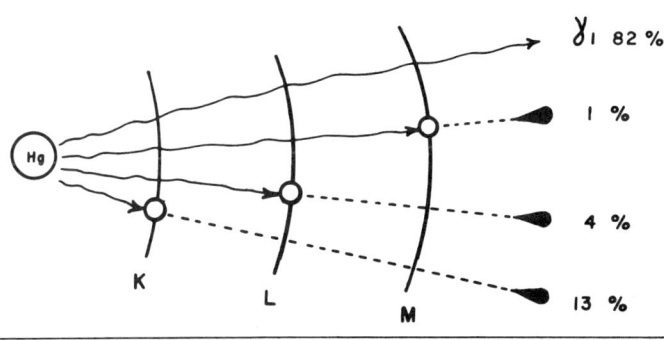

Figure 2-14. Decay scheme for Hg-203 illustrating the percentage of internal conversion in the K, L, and M shells.

shell electrons, spend an appreciable amount of time near or actually within the nucleus. If an electron absorbs the nuclear energy, it is ejected from the atom with a kinetic energy equal to the difference between the energy available in the nucleus and the binding energy of the electron. Such an electron is called a conversion electron and the process, internal conversion. Nuclides in the isomeric state may therefore emit either gamma rays or conversion electrons during their deexcitation. This can be illustrated by reexamining the decay scheme for Hg-203 (Fig. 2–14). It illustrates the internal conversion process as an internal photoelectric effect whereby the 0.279-MeV gamma ray undergoes K-, L-, and M-shell conversion. Because 100 percent of Hg-203 atoms decay by beta emission to the excited state of Tl-203, theoretically, one should be able to detect 100 gamma rays of 0.279 MeV for every 100 atoms decayed. Only 82 gamma rays, however, are detectable (so-called 82 percent photon abundance) because 18 percent undergo internal conversion in the K, L, and M shells.

Alpha Particle Decay

Although alpha radiation holds no current clinical usefulness, some alpha-emitting radionuclides have been used in medicine. Radium-226 and its radioactive daughter radon-222 have been used in medicine since the time of radium's discovery by Marie and Pierre Curie in 1898. The greatest use has been in radiation therapy in the form of sealed sources in glass or platinum seeds that can be implanted within cancerous tissue for radiation treatment and removed at the end of treatment. Presently, other radionuclides are used for such purposes.

Alpha emitters are not used in radiopharmaceuticals because alpha particles produce dense ionization within tissue accompanied by severe radiation damage. For completeness and because of historical interest, the decay of Ra-226 will be discussed. The decay equation is as follows:

$$^{226}_{88}Ra_{138} \xrightarrow{1600 \text{ y}} {}^{222}_{86}Rn_{136} + {}^{4}_{2}He_{2}$$

226.0254 AMU   222.0175 AMU

4.0026 AMU

Alpha decay usually occurs in heavy nuclei where four nucleons (two protons plus two neutrons) can achieve an energy greater than the nuclear binding energy to escape from the nucleus. In the previous equation the alpha particle is shown as a neutral helium atom with its orbital electrons, but alpha particles do not assume this state until they are almost exhausted of their kinetic energy. The sum of the Rn-222 and He-4 masses is 0.0053 AMU less than the mass of Ra-226. This mass defect is equivalent to a transition energy of 4.94 MeV.

A simplified decay scheme depicting the principal decay routes for Ra-226 is shown in Figure 2–15. A branching decay occurs, with 98.8 percent of the decays directly to Rn-222 and 1.2 percent to the excited state of Rn-222, which subsequently deexcites by emission of a 0.187-MeV gamma ray. The difference between the alpha-1

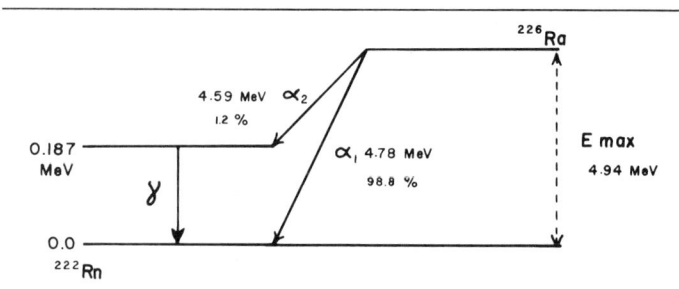

Figure 2-15. Simplified decay scheme for radium-226.

energy of 4.78 MeV and the transition energy of 4.94 MeV is 0.16 MeV. This is known as the recoil energy, which is given to the nucleus as the massive alpha particle is ejected. This occurs with all alpha emitters and is required for the conservation of energy and momentum. Recoil energy is usually on the order of 0.1 MeV.

Table 2–3 lists several radionuclides used in nuclear medicine along with some

TABLE 2-3. RADIONUCLIDES USED IN NUCLEAR MEDICINE

Radionuclide	Decay Mode	Half-life		Photon Energy (keV)		Abundance (%)
C - 11	β^+	20.3	min	511		200
F - 18	β^+	109.0	min	511		194
P - 32	β^-	14.3	d	None		—
Cr - 51	EC	27.7	d	320		10
Co - 57	EC	270.0	d	122		86
				136		10
Co - 58	EC, β^+	71.3	d	811		99
				511		31
Fe - 59	β^-	45.0	d	1099		55
				1292		44
Ga - 57	EC	78.1	hr	93		38
				185		24
				300		16
Se - 75	EC	120.0	d	121		16
				136		54
				265		57
				280		24
				401		12
Kr - 81m	IT	13.0	sec	191		66
Mo - 99	β^-	66.7	hr	740		14
				778		4
Tc - 99m	IT	6.0	hr	140		88
In - 111	EC	2.8	d	172		90
				247		94
In - 113m	IT	99.4	min	392		62
I - 123	EC	13.0	hr	159		84
				27	(x-rays)	71
I - 125	EC	60.0	d	35		7
				27	(x-rays)	115
Xe - 127	EC	36.4	d	172		25
				203		68
				375		18
I - 131	β^-	8.1	d	364		82
				637		7
Xe - 133	β^-	5.3	d	81		36
Hg - 197	EC	65.0	hr	77		25
Hg - 203	β^-	46.5	d	279		82
Tl - 201	EC	73.0	hr	69	(x-rays)	27
				71	(x-rays)	47
				80	(x-rays)	20

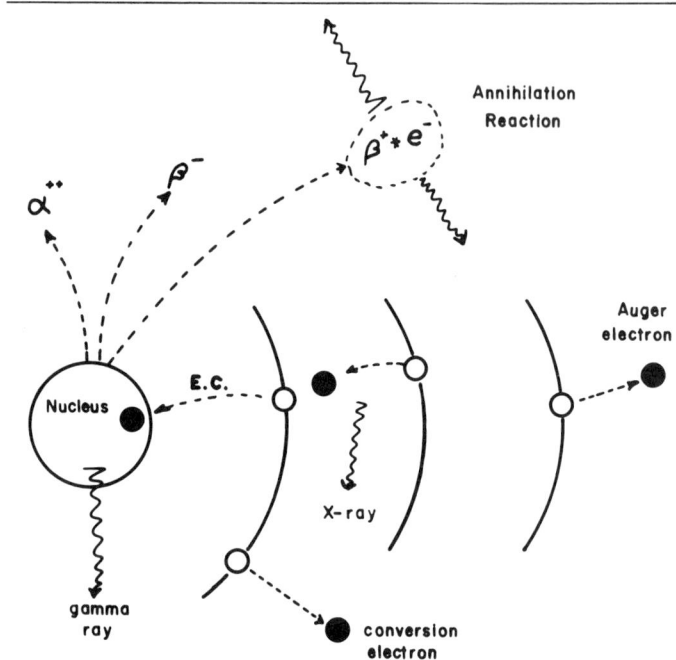

Figure 2-16. Composite radionuclide illustrating the principal modes of decay and the variety of possible electron shell interactions.

properties of interest. Figure 2-16 illustrates a composite radionuclide that summarizes the principal modes of radioactive decay and the various electron shell interactions that may occur.

RADIOACTIVITY

Up to this point we have discussed some basic properties of all atoms and those unique to unstable ones by considering the ways in which they transform into stable nuclei. Soon after the discovery of radioactivity by Henri Becquerel in 1896 it was observed that some elements lost their radioactive properties in a consistent fashion that varied from one element to another. The terms *decay* or *disintegrate* used to describe this process were coined by Rutherford in early 1900 before atomic structure was known. It is now known that radioactivity is a nuclear process and the more exacting description is nuclear transformation. However, use of the older terms still prevails.

Radioactivity is defined as the process whereby unstable nuclei undergo spontaneous transformation by releasing excess energy in the form of radiation. The key words in this definition are *spontaneous transformation*. If one were able to observe a single radioactive atom, one could not predict at what point in time it would transform or decay because radioactive decay is a spontaneous or random process. If, however, one were to observe the decay of a large number of radioactive atoms of a particular radionuclide, one would find that some of them decay immediately, some at intermediate times, and some very late. In this way, however, it is possible to observe that a certain fraction of the total number of atoms will decay within a certain time. If this observation is made for any radionuclide in pure form, it will be found that the number that decay per unit of time, dN/dt, is proportional to the number originally present, N, and a proportionality constant, λ. This relationship describes the *radioactive decay law* and is expressed as follows:

$$-\frac{dN}{dt} = \lambda N \quad (2\text{-}2)$$

The negative sign indicates a decreasing number with time. This first-order differential equation provides the rate of decay for only infinitely small periods of time, and to obtain the rate of decay for any period of time the equation must be integrated into the following form:

$$N = N_0 e^{-\lambda t} \quad (2\text{-}3)$$

where:

N_0 = original number of atoms at t = 0

N = number of atoms remaining after decay time t = t

$N_0 - N$ = number of atoms that decayed in time t = t

λ = decay constant in reciprocal time (t^{-1})

t = time of decay

The rate of decay of a radionuclide is described by its activity A, which is the number of nuclear transformations or disintegrations per second of time; therefore, A equals $-dN/dt$, and we may write

$$A = \lambda N \quad (2\text{-}4)$$

where:

A = number of disintegrations per unit time

N = number of radioactive atoms

λ = decay constant

The *decay constant* is roughly defined as the fraction of atoms or activity that decays per unit time. For example, a decay constant of 0.01 sec^{-1} means approximately 1 percent of the atoms decay per second. This is not an absolutely accurate statement, however, because radioactive decay is a logarithmic rather than linear function. A linear function interpretation gives a falsely high decay rate, but it helps to make the decay constant a more tangible concept. The decay constant is peculiar to the radionuclide in question. No two radionuclides are identical. As we shall see in a subsequent section, the decay constant is related to the radionuclide half-life.

Activity, then, is directly proportional to the number of radioactive atoms present and the decay constant. This expression allows one to relate activity, which is simply a rate, to a definite weight of radioactive substance.

In working with radioactive substances it is more convenient to know how much activity is present in the sample at various periods of time. Because activity is directly proportional to the number of atoms, we may substitute the expression A/λ for N in Equation 2–3 and arrive at the exponential expression for radioactive decay in terms of activity as follows:

$$A = A_0 e^{-\lambda t} \quad (2\text{-}5)$$

where the terms are defined as before.

Units of Activity

There are three ways to express radioactivity: (1) as nuclear transformations per second, frequently referred to as decays or disintegrations per second (dps); (2) as curies, millicuries, microcuries, or nanocuries; and (3) as becquerels. Originally the curie was defined as the number of disintegrations per second occurring in 1 g of Ra-226. This standard, however, was affected by the purity of radium used, and the curie was subject to slight change. Experiments determined that 1 g of "pure" radium had a disintegration rate close to 3.7×10^{10} dps, and this value was officially adopted in 1950. More recently the International System of Units (SI) has adopted the becquerel (Bq) as the official unit of radioactivity. One Bq is defined as one nuclear transformation per second. Therefore, the following expressions are considered to be equivalent:

1 becquerel (Bq) = 1 dps

1 curie (Ci) = 3.7×10^{10} dps (Bq) or 37 gigabecquerels (GBq)

1 millicurie (mCi) = 3.7×10^7 dps (Bq) or 37 megabecquerels (MBq)

1 microcurie (μCi) = 3.7×10^4 dps (Bq) or 37 kilobecquerels (KBq)

1 nanocurie (nCi) = 37 dps (Bq) or 37 Bq

By definition we also have the following equivalent expression:

$$1 \text{ Bq} = 2.7 \times 10^{-11} \text{ Ci}$$

Although the Bq is the official new unit of radioactivity, we will use the traditional curie units, which are more familiar to most readers. Conversions can be made readily from the previous expressions.

Half-life

In 1902 Ernest Rutherford noted in his measurements of thorium-234 that half of any quantity was gone in 24 days. He coined the term half-life, which is the time it takes for any quantity of radionuclide to decrease to half the original quantity. Mathematically it is expressed as follows:

$$T_{1/2} = \frac{0.693}{\lambda} \qquad (2\text{-}6)$$

It is evident that half-life and the decay constant are inversely proportional. The derivation of this expression is given in Table 2-4.

The half-life of a radionuclide can be determined experimentally by measuring the activity of a sample over time, assuming the half-life is reasonably short. Radionuclides with very short or very long half-lives require special techniques. Figure 2-17 illustrates graphic plots of activity versus time on linear–linear and log–linear coordinates. Because radioactive decay is a first-order rate process, the log–linear plot is a straight line from which the half-life is easily determined.

TABLE 2-4. MATHEMATICAL DETERMINATION OF HALF-LIFE

Accept the time of decay t in the following expression to be that of the half-life so that $A = A_o/2$:

$$A = A_o\, e^{-\lambda t}$$

or

$$A_o/2 = A_o\, e^{-\lambda t_{1/2}}$$

$$1/2 = e^{-\lambda t_{1/2}}$$

$$2 = e^{+\lambda t_{1/2}}$$

$$\ln 2 = \lambda t_{1/2}$$

$$t_{1/2} = \frac{\ln 2}{\lambda} = \frac{0.693}{\lambda}$$

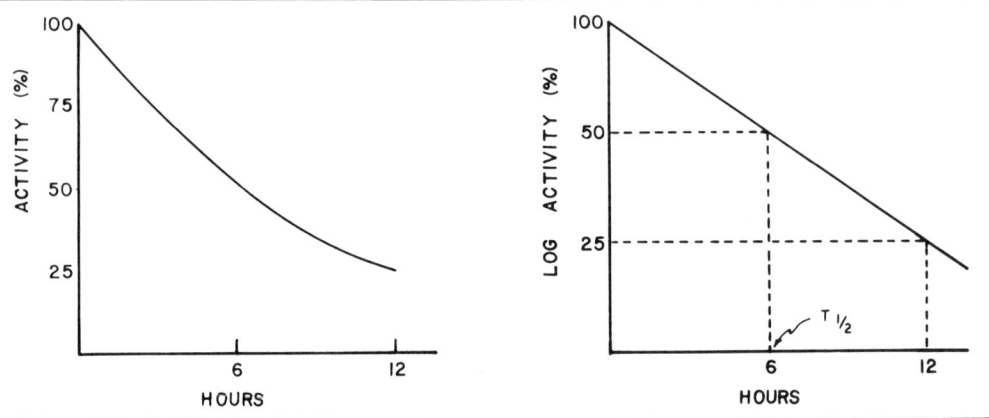

Figure 2-17. Half-life determination illustrated by a plot of the decay of Tc-99m over time on linear coordinates (left) and log–linear coordinates (right) that yields a straight line characteristic of a first-order rate process.

Examples of radioactivity calculations:
1. To illustrate the random nature of radioactive decay
   A. Estimate the probability of the decay of one atom in 1 second for a radionuclide with a half-life of 69.3 seconds.

   $$\lambda = \frac{0.693}{T_{1/2}} = \frac{0.693}{69.3 \text{ sec}} = 0.01 \text{ sec}^{-1}$$

   This means that one atom out of 100 has a chance of decaying in 1 second.
   B. Would a longer half-life increase or decrease the probability of decay? Consider what it would be for I-131 whose half-life is 8.05 days.

   $$T_{1/2} = 8.05 \text{ d} \times \frac{24 \text{ hr}}{\text{d}}$$
   $$\times \frac{3600 \text{ sec}}{\text{hr}} = 6.95 \times 10^5 \text{ sec}$$

   $$\lambda = \frac{0.693}{6.95 \times 10^5 \text{ sec}}$$
   $$= 1 \times 10^{-6} \text{ sec}^{-1}$$

   This means that one atom out of 1 million has a chance of decaying in 1 second; therefore, longer half-lives decrease the probability of decay.

2. What is the weight in grams of iodine in a 10-μCi dose of sodium iodide I-131? The formula $A = \lambda N$ relates activity to atoms.
   Thus

   $$N = A/\lambda = \frac{A \times T_{1/2}}{0.693}$$
   $$= (A)(T_{1/2})(1.443)$$
   $$N = (10 \text{ μCi})(3.7 \times 10^4 \text{ dps/μCi})$$
   $$(6.95 \times 10^5 \text{ sec})(1.443)$$
   $$N = 3.71 \times 10^{11} \text{ disintegrations (atoms)}$$

   Recall that by definition

   1 gram atomic weight (GAW) I-131
   (131 g) = 6.023×10^{23} atoms I-131

   Therefore

   $$\frac{3.71 \times 10^{11} \text{ atoms} \times 131 \text{ g/GAW}}{6.023 \times 10^{23} \text{ atoms/GAW}}$$
   $$= 8.07 \times 10^{-11} \text{ g}$$

The total amount of iodine in the body is approximately 6.5 mg. A 10-μCi I-131 dose is thus only about one eighty-millionth of the body's iodine stores and demonstrates the extremely small amounts of radionuclide tracer required for a diagnostic study.

Note the following: The expression (A) $(T_{1/2})$ (1.443) will always give the total number of atoms equivalent to a given activity. The term $(T_{1/2}\ 1.443)$ is equivalent to $1/\lambda$ and is called the *mean life* of the radionuclide. Consider a sample decaying at a rate of 1 mCi. During the first second 3.7×10^7 atoms decay, but during the next second less than this number decay and during the third second even less, etc., so that the decay rate decreases with time. Consider an alternative hypothetical situation where we assume the sample decay rate does not decrease with time but continues at its initial rate until all the atoms have decayed. The time for this to occur is the mean life. The mean life is a useful term in calculating the radiation dose to the body because one must know the total number of atoms and therefore the total energy that will eventually be deposited after complete decay. Note in Example 2 that 10 μCi I-131 is equal to 3.7×10^{11} atoms. This means that after complete radioactive decay this many atoms of I-131 will have transformed into Xenon-131. If each I-131 atom emits one beta particle and one gamma ray, then 3.7×10^{11} beta particles and gamma rays would have been emitted.

3. A vial contains 100 mCi of I-131 sodium iodide in a 10-ml volume on Monday at 12 noon. Calculate the volume of solution required for a 12-mCi dose on Friday noon.
   This problem requires use of the exponential decay Equation 2–5. First calculate the radioactive concentration on Monday noon.

   100 mCi/10 ml = 10 mCi/ml

Next, calculate the new concentration on Friday noon (4 days later).

$$A = A_o e^{-\lambda t}$$

$$A = (10 \text{ mCi/ml}) e^{-\frac{0.693}{8.05 \text{ d}} (4 \text{ d})}$$

$$A = (10 \text{ mCi/ml}) (0.7087)$$

$$A = 7.09 \text{ mCi/ml}$$

A 12-mCi dose requires

$$\frac{12 \text{ mCi}}{7.09 \text{ mCi/ml}} = 1.7 \text{ ml}$$

4. A vial contains 50-μCi I-131 sodium iodide capsules. How many days are required for the capsules to decay to an acceptable thyroid uptake dose of 5 μCi?

As an approximation one may use the half-life rule to estimate the time required.

Number of days	0	8	16	24	32
Number of half-lives	0	1	2	3	4
Capsule activity (μCi)	50	25	12.5	6.25	3.125

Thus, between 24 and 32 days is required. To arrive at the exact answer, use Equation 2-5 in logarithmic form.

$$A = A_o e^{-\lambda t}$$

$$\ln A = \ln A_o - \lambda t$$

$$\ln (5 \ \mu\text{Ci}) = \ln (50 \ \mu\text{Ci}) - \frac{0.693}{8.05 \text{ d}} (t)$$

$$1.61 = 3.91 - 0.0861 \ t$$

$$t = \frac{2.3}{0.0861 \text{ d}^{-1}} = 26.7 \text{ d}$$

Decay Tables

When making decay calculations on a routine basis in the radiopharmacy lab, it is more convenient to use decay tables rather than the exponential equation. A decay table is a tabulation of specified times and the respective fraction of activity remaining at those times. It is prepared using the exponential decay equation. Rearrangement of Equation 2-5 yields the following expression.

$$A/A_o = e^{-\lambda t} \quad (2\text{-}7)$$

If A is the activity remaining after a period of decay (t), then A/A_o is the fraction of the original amount remaining. For example, prepare a decay table for I-131 for days 1 through 8. Substituting the values 1, 2, 3,...8 days for t in the equation yields the following table:

t (days)	$e^{-\lambda t}$
0	1.0000
1	0.9175
2	0.8418
3	0.7724
4	0.7087
5	0.6502
6	0.5966
7	0.5474
8	0.5022

Example calculations:

1. Calculate the activity in a 10-μCi capsule of I-131.
   a. After 5 days decay?

   Answer: 10 μCi (0.6502) = 6.5 μCi

   b. After 9 days decay?

   Answer: 10 μCi (0.5022) (0.9175) = 4.6 μCi

Radiopharmaceuticals are labeled listing the total amount of activity at a specified date and time called the calibration date and time. Only at this time will the vial contain the labeled activity. At times after the calibration date it will contain less activity because of radioactive decay, and at times before the calibration date it will contain proportionately more activity. Radiopharmaceuticals are frequently received into the nuclear medicine lab before the calibration date.

2. Calculate the activity in a capsule of I-131 at 12 noon on January 1 if the label states "10 μCi per capsule as of 12 noon January 6."

Since the capsule must obviously contain more than 10 μCi on January 1 we must divide by the decay factor for 5 days:

Answer: $\dfrac{10 \ \mu Ci}{0.6502} = 15.38 \ \mu Ci$

The same answer can be obtained using the reciprocal of the postcalibration decay factor, i.e., 1/0.6502, to yield a precalibration decay factor of 1.538, which is found in some decay tables. The answer to the previous question would thus be calculated as follows:

10 μCi (1.538) = 15.38 μCi

Precalibration factors can be readily calculated for any times before the calibration date using the following rearrangement of Equation 2–5.

$$A_o/A = e^{+\lambda t} \quad (2\text{--}8)$$

A precalibration decay table for I-131 would be as follows:

t (days)	$e^{+\lambda t}$
8	1.9912
7	1.8268
6	1.6762
5	1.5380
4	1.4110
3	1.2947
2	1.1879
1	1.0899
0	1.0000

Radioactive Concentration

The concentration of radioactivity is expressed in several ways. *Specific concentration* is the radioactivity per unit weight or volume of diluent, which is usually water or normal saline, but it may be a solid diluent such as an ointment. It is expressed, for example, as millicuries or microcuries per milliliter of solution or milligrams of solid. *Specific activity* is the radioactivity per unit weight of radionuclide or labeled compound. It will be expressed in units appropriate to the sample in question, for example, millicuries per milligram or micromole of element or compound. Theoretically, the highest specific activity of an elemental substance is achieved if every atom in the sample is that of the radionuclide of interest, or for a labeled compound, every potential labeling site in the molecule contains only the radionuclide of interest. The theoretic specific activity can be calculated using Equation 2–4, which is modified to yield Equation 2–9.

Example: Calculate the specific activity of isotopically pure C-14 in mCi/mg.

$$A \ mCi/mg = \dfrac{\lambda N}{3.7 \times 10^7 \ dps/mCi} \quad (2\text{--}9)$$

$$A = [0.693/(5730 \ y) \ (3.15 \times 10^7 \ sec/y)] \\ \times \ [(6.023 \times 10^{23} \ disintegrations/mole)/(14 \ g/mole) \\ (10^3 \ mg/g)] \div 3.7 \times 10^7 \ dps/mCi$$

$$A = 4.46 \ mCi/mg \ C\text{-}14$$

A natural source of carbon contains mostly stable C-12 and C-13 atoms so that its specific activity with respect to the trace amount of C-14 present is extremely low because almost all of the sample weight is stable carbon.

The extremely small amounts of material present in radioisotopically pure radioactive substances sometimes create a problem with recovery in chemical methods. A technique was thus developed by radiochemists to mitigate this problem by adding a sufficient amount of the stable isotope of the radionuclide being analyzed to "carry" it through the reactions. The stable isotope used was called a "carrier." The term *carrier-free* was then defined to mean "radioactive preparations to which no isotopic carrier had been intentionally added and containing no isotopic material detectable by chemical or spectrographic means."[5] Subsequently the term *carrier-free* has been misunderstood and misused in relation to its original definition. In more recent years scientists and manufacturers have applied the term to mean radionuclide samples that contain only the radionuclide of interest and no stable isotope present, i.e., one of absolute theoretic specific activity. Whether this could actually be measured is questionable because of the limitations of analytic methods. As a result, some new terminology has been proposed to clear up the ambiguous terms. According to Wolf,[5] "*carrier-free* (CF) should mean that the radionuclide or stable nuclide is not contaminated with any other stable or radioactive nuclide of the same element; *no carrier added* (NCA) should apply to an element or compound to which no carrier of the same element has been intentionally or otherwise added during its preparation; *carrier added* (CA) should apply to any element or compound to which a known amount of carrier has been added."

INTERACTIONS OF RADIATION WITH MATTER

Radiation interacts with matter, causing excitation and ionization of atoms. During excitation orbital electrons may be raised to higher-energy suborbits emitting visible and UV light when they return to the ground state. If an electron is removed from the atom, ionization has occurred, thus producing an ion pair: the negatively charged orbital electron and the remaining positively charged atom. Radiation produces thousands of excitations and ionizations before total loss of energy. It requires an average energy (W) of 34 eV to produce an ion pair in air. Actually, only about 20 percent of this energy is needed for the ionization; the remainder is dissipated as excitation energy. A 340-keV beta particle will thus produce about 10,000 ion pairs before it comes to rest.

The number of ion pairs produced per millimeter of path traveled by radiation is termed *specific ionization* (SI). The energy dissipated per millimeter of path is termed the *linear energy transfer* (LET). The SI and LET are directly related as follows:

$$LET = SI \times W \quad (2\text{--}10)$$

Specific ionization is inversely proportional to particle velocity so that most of the radiation energy is released near the end of a particle's path.

The interaction of radiation with matter is important because it is the initiating event leading to biologic damage and is the basis for detection and measurement of radiation.

Alpha Particles

Alpha particles are fast-moving monoenergetic helium nuclei. Relative to other radiation, they are quite massive. They are not easily deflected by interaction with electrons and travel in straight-line paths with a definite range into an absorber. An alpha particle produces ionization by electrostatic attraction of electrons. It eventually acquires two electrons to become a neutral helium atom. Alpha particles have high SI and LET. This is illustrated in Figures 2–18 and 2–19. In tissue this dense concentration of energy results in a high probability for biologic damage and essentially excludes alpha emitters for diagnostic applications.

Positrons

Positrons produce ionization by electrostatic attraction of electrons similar to alpha particles; however, because of their small mass

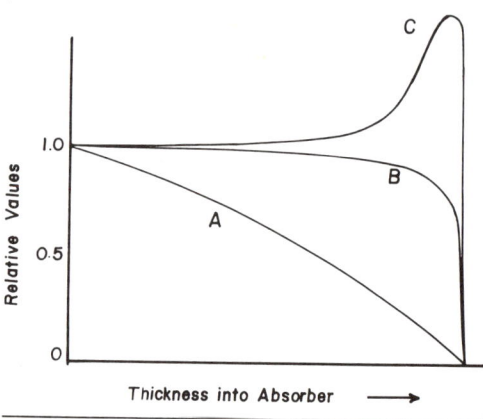

Figure 2-18. Composite diagram of alpha particle interactions in matter: A, particle velocity; B, particle range; C, particle SI and LET.

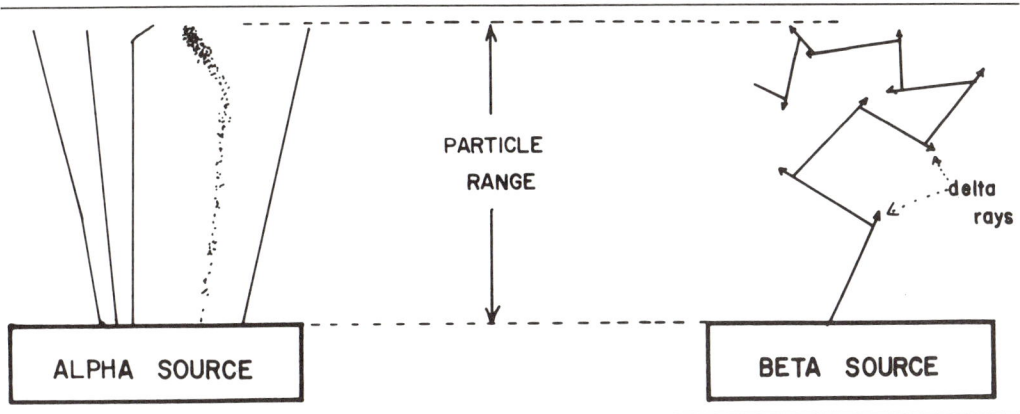

Figure 2-19. Pathways of alpha and beta particle interactions with matter.

positrons are easily deflected during interaction. Their paths through matter are tortuous and meandering similar to that of negatrons (Fig. 2-19). When the positron comes to rest, it is annihilated along with a negative electron, thus producing 0.511-MeV photons.

Negatrons

Negatrons cause ionization by electrostatic repulsion of orbital electrons. Their path of interaction is tortuous similar to positrons. Additionally, a high-speed electron may decelerate near the nuclear force field of an atom, thus releasing electromagnetic radiation called bremsstrahlung. Bremsstrahlung production increases directly as the electron energy and atomic number of the absorber increases. For this reason, it is helpful to shield high-energy beta emitters such as P-32 in low Z plastic or glass containers with an outer shield of lead to absorb the bremsstrahlung.

Gamma and X-Rays

Although electromagnetic radiation exhibits wave-like properties, the nature of interaction with matter depends upon energy, which is described as follows:

$$E \text{ (keV)} = \frac{12.4}{\lambda \text{ (Å)}} \quad (2-11)$$

Long-wavelength, low-energy sound waves and visible light are readily stopped by simple objects. Short-wavelength, high-energy radiation such as gamma and x-rays do not behave as waves but more as discrete packets of energy, which are called quanta or photons. Photons interact with matter as if they were small particles. The three processes of photon interaction with matter are the photoelectric effect, Compton scatter, and pair production. Each process produces ionization of matter.

Photoelectric Effect. Photoelectric absorption is illustrated in Figure 2-20. This process involves a relatively low energy photon interacting with and ejecting an inner-shell electron, usually the K shell. The photon disappears, with all of its energy used to overcome the electron's binding energy and to impart the remainder as kinetic energy to the ejected electron. If the photon had an initial energy of 50 keV and the K-shell binding energy of the interacting atom was 40 keV, the photoelectron would thus be ejected with 10 keV of energy. Photoelectric absorption produces an ion pair, and characteristic x-radiation and Auger electrons will be emitted when the electron shell vacancy is filled. The total energy emitted from the atom by all processes is equal to the incident photon energy.

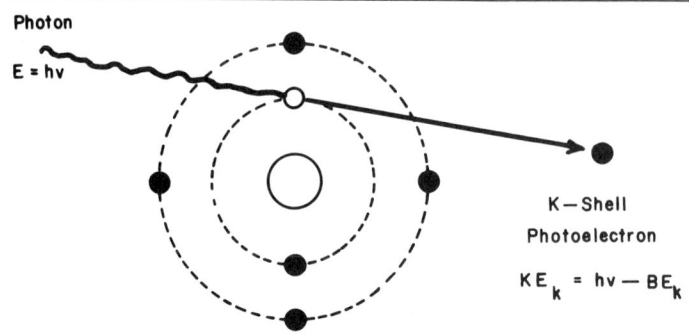

Figure 2-20. Photoelectric absorption. The entire photon energy is transferred to the ejected electron. The kinetic energy of the ejected electron, KE (k), is equal to the initial photon energy, hv, minus the electron's binding energy, BE (k).

In soft tissue, photoelectric absorption is the predominant interactive process for photon energies up to 50 keV. The probability for the interaction increases as the photon energy decreases below 50 keV and as the atomic number and density of the absorber increase. Bone with an average Z value of 13.8 and a density of 1.85 will absorb about six times more energy than soft tissue with an average Z of 7.4 and density of 1. Radionuclides with photon energies below 50 keV such as I-125 (30 keV) are poor diagnostic tracers because of high tissue absorption by the photoelectric effect.

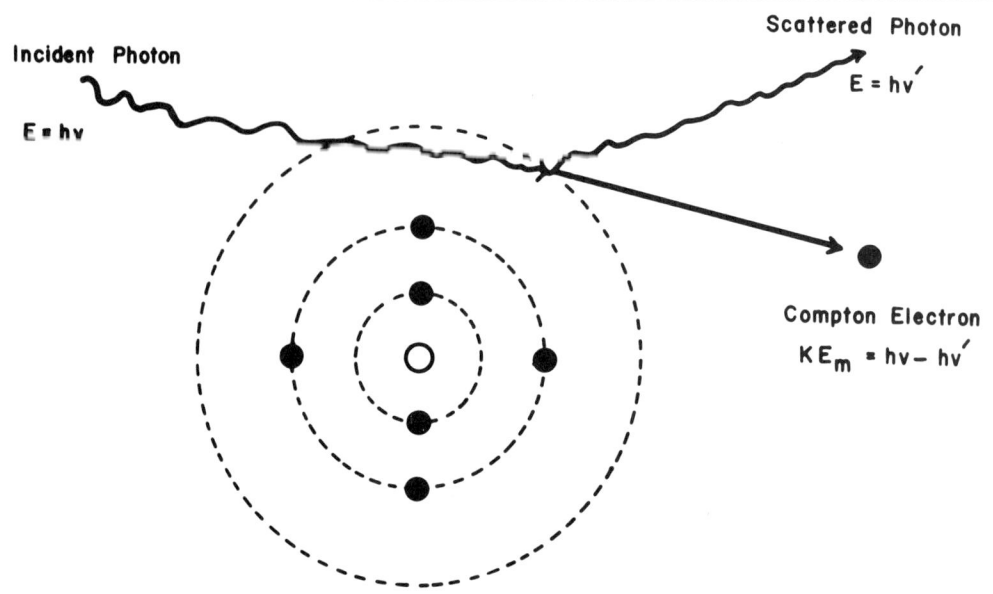

Figure 2-21. Compton effect. An incident photon transfers part of its energy to a loosely bound free electron that is ejected from the atom. The remaining energy is associated with the scattered photon. The kinetic energy of the ejected electron, KE (m), is equal to the difference between the incident and scattered photon energies because the orbital binding energy is insignificant.

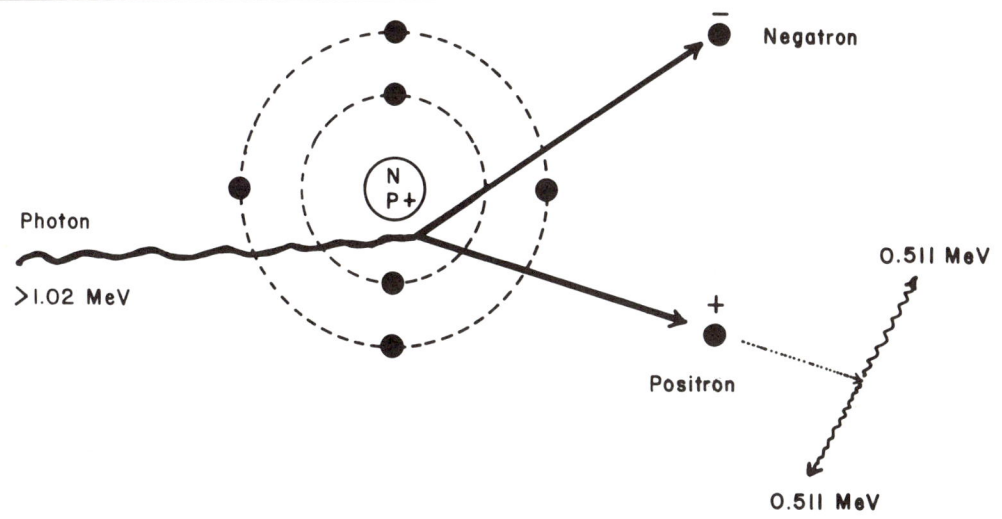

Figure 2-22. Pair production. An incident photon of at least 1.022 MeV disappears in the vicinity of the nuclear force field, and two electrons are produced, one negative and one positive. The positron eventually is annihilated outside the atom, and two 0.511-MeV photons are produced.

Compton Scatter. Compton scatter involves a medium-energy photon that interacts with a loosely bound outer-shell electron that is ejected, and an ion pair is produced. As shown in Figure 2–21, only a portion of the incident photon energy is transferred to the electron. The kinetic energy given to the ejected electron depends on the angle at which the photon hits the electron. A direct hit transfers the largest amount of energy. The incident photon is scattered in a different direction at a reduced energy equivalent to its initial energy minus the energy used to overcome the electron binding energy (very small) and the kinetic energy imparted to the ejected electron. The secondary or Compton-scattered photon continues on to undergo additional Compton interactions that are eventually totally absorbed by the photoelectric effect.

Between 60 and 90 keV the probability for photon interaction by the photoelectric effect and Compton scatter is about equal, and from 100 keV to 2 MeV the Compton process predominates. Most diagnostic radionuclides used in nuclear medicine initially interact with tissue by Compton scatter because their photon energies are greater than 100 keV. The probability of Compton interaction depends upon electron density. High-density material provides more stopping power because more atoms (and electrons) are present per unit volume of absorber compared with low-density material. For this reason, lead (density, 11.1) is a good absorber of gamma radiation.

Pair Production. This process involves the interaction of a very high energy photon with the nuclear force field whereby the photon is converted into electronic mass: one positron and one negatron (Fig. 2–22). Because two electron masses are produced, the minimum energy required is 1.02 MeV. Photon energy in excess of 1.02 MeV is distributed to the electrons as kinetic energy. The probability for pair production increases with increasing atomic number of the absorber because of the increased nuclear force field present with high-Z material. Pair production begins to be significant in soft tissue with photon energies of 5 to 10 MeV, and therefore it is not an important mode of photon absorption with diagnostic radionuclides.

RADIATION DETECTION INSTRUMENTATION

Detection and measurement of radiation is an important part of nuclear pharmacy and medicine operation from both the radiation protection viewpoint and that of accurate assessment of radiopharmaceutical activity. Proper use of radiation detection equipment requires an understanding of basic construction and operation. This section will cover the two basic methods to detect and measure radiation, namely, ion collection and scintillation.

Ion Collection Methods

The ion collection method is based on the ability of radiation to ionize the atoms of a gas. The gases used are usually air, helium, or argon. The gas is contained in an ionization chamber, which is a sealed vessel containing a positive and negative electrode (Fig. 2-23). A power supply creates the potential across the electrodes. An ammeter measures the current produced by the collection of ionized gas atoms. The amount of current is directly proportional to the number of ion pairs produced by the radiation source.[6]

The electrode potential must be adjusted to a proper operating voltage that depends on how the instrument will be used. Ionization chambers used to measure high-intensity sources have operating voltages in the range of 50 to 500 V. Instruments that operate in this range include the hand-held "Cutie-Pie" ionization chamber, which is useful for measuring output from x-ray tubes and Curie sources of radionuclides, and dose calibrators, which are used to measure the activity of radiopharmaceuticals. Geiger–Müller detectors used to measure low-intensity radiation, such as for radiation safety surveys, have operating voltages near 1000 V.

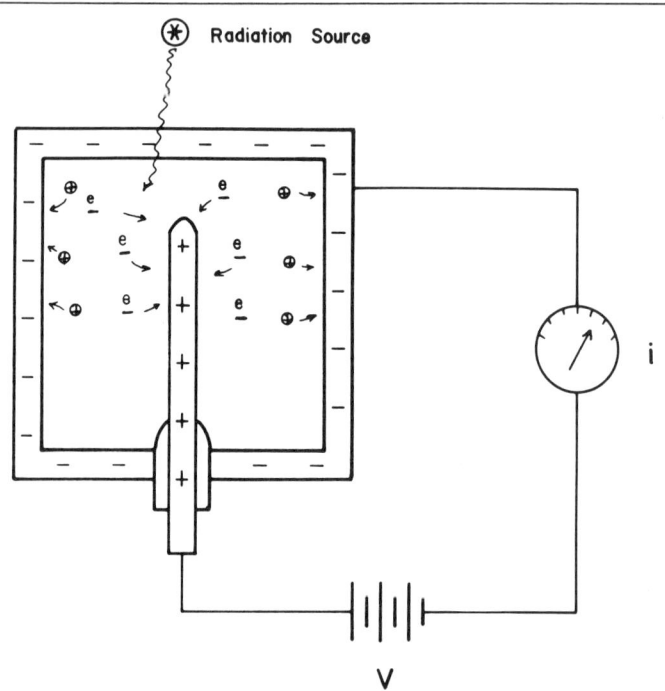

Figure 2-23. A simple ionization chamber.

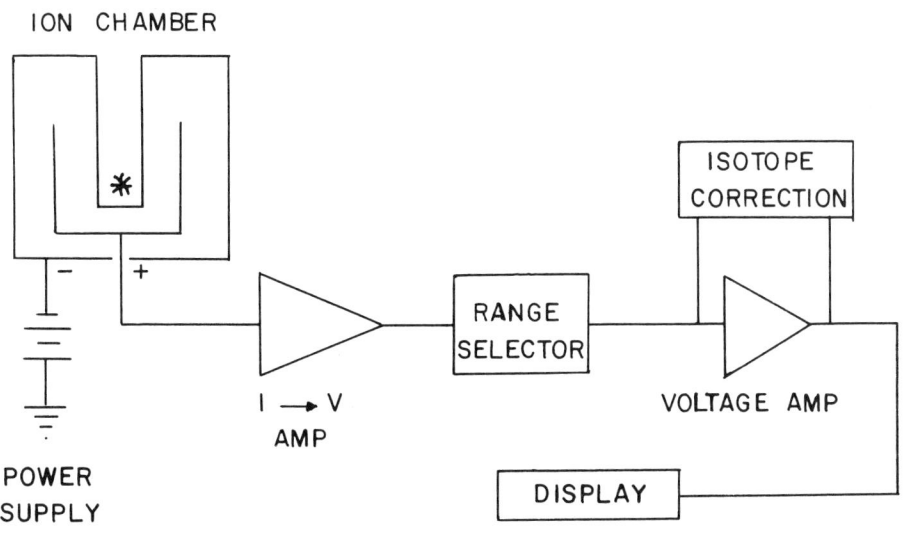

Figure 2-24. Block diagram of a dose calibrator. *(From Kowalsky RJ, et al, 1977, with permission.[7])*

Radionuclide Dose Calibrator. The dose calibrator is an instrument used routinely in nuclear medicine to measure the activity of radiopharmaceuticals. Figure 2–24 illustrates a block diagram of a dose calibrator.[7] The electrodes operate at about 150 V in a sealed chamber of argon gas. It is constructed with a central well for accepting vials and syringes containing radioactivity. The current-to-voltage amplifier converts the small current to a usable voltage. The range selector is a variable resistor circuit that adjusts the activity range (μCi, mCi, Ci) being measured. The isotope correction amplifier is a resistance feedback circuit that compensates for detector sensitivity to the various photon energies and intensities of different radionuclides. In this way activities of all radionuclides will display a true value on the readout. Thus, 1 mCi of Tc-99m, I-131, or any other radionuclide will display a reading of 1 mCi when the correct radionuclide calibration factor is selected.

When a dose calibrator is manufactured, its operating voltage is established and its ion chamber response and sensitivity are determined for a wide range of radionuclides.[8] From this information radionuclide calibration factors are determined.

To measure the activity of a source the proper calibration factor is selected and the instrument "zeroed" to remove background activity. The source is then placed into the chamber well whereupon the activity is read out on the meter. Daily quality control requires assay of a long-lived reference source such as cesium-137 to assure precision. Other quality control tests will be discussed in detail in Chapter 6.

Geiger-Müller Detectors. A Geiger-Müller detector is a device used for detection and measurement of low-level beta and gamma radiation. Some units can also detect alpha radiation. Its high operating voltage (1000 V) makes it a very sensitive detector, useful for radiation safety surveys.

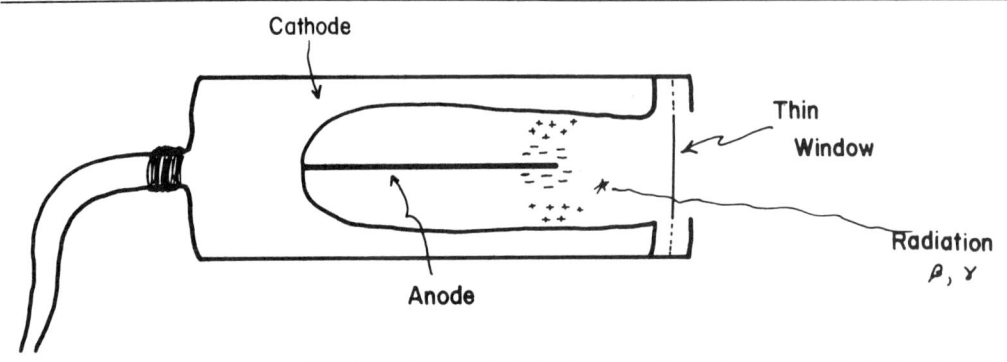

Figure 2-25. Cutaway diagram of an end-window Geiger-Müller detector.

Geiger–Müller tubes are supplied in several configurations. A typical end-window tube is shown in Figure 2–25. The thin mica window allows passage of beta particles and weak gamma rays that normally would be stopped by the metal casing of the tube. Radiation entering the tube produces an initial ionization that proceeds to ionize the entire gas because of the high potential. A quenching agent absorbs energy to momentarily stop discharge between ionizing events. This alternating ionization–quenching sequence produces current pulses that are recorded on a meter and can be audibly heard through a ticking device. Geiger–Müller detectors have no energy-discriminating ability but are useful for determining exposure rate in roentgens per hour from gamma ray sources if they are calibrated against a reference source such as Ra-226.

SCINTILLATION METHODS

There are two types of scintillation detection methods: solid-crystal scintillation and liquid scintillation. In solid crystal detection a sodium iodide crystal is hermetically sealed in a metal casing. Although gamma radiation of sufficient energy can readily penetrate this casing to interact with the crystal, particulate radiation cannot do so. Consequently, the counting of pure beta emitters such as H-3 and C-14 is best accomplished by liquid scintillation. The sample to be counted is dissolved or suspended in a scintillation "cocktail" that consists of a solvent (usually toluene) and scintillator compounds. The intimate admixture of sample and scintillator molecules provides for the most efficient detection of beta radiation. Except for the difference in initial scintillation detection, the operating principles of liquid and solid crystal scintillation detectors are basically the same. Because almost all nuclear medicine counting is done with gamma emitters, further discussion will focus on solid-crystal detectors.

A scintillation spectrometer consists of a detector and an electronic processing unit (Fig. 2–26). The detector is the sodium iodide crystal where photon energy is converted into visible light after the absorption of gamma rays by Compton scatter and the photoelectric effect. A photomultiplier (PM) tube converts the visible light photons into electrical pulses. The processing unit consists of an amplifier that magnifies linearly the small electrical pulses, a pulse height analyzer that selects or rejects pulses for counting, and a variety of display devices such as rate meters, scalers, oscilloscopes, photographic film, and computer memory to record and store information.

Figure 2–27 illustrates the sodium iodide (NaI) detector and PM tube. The

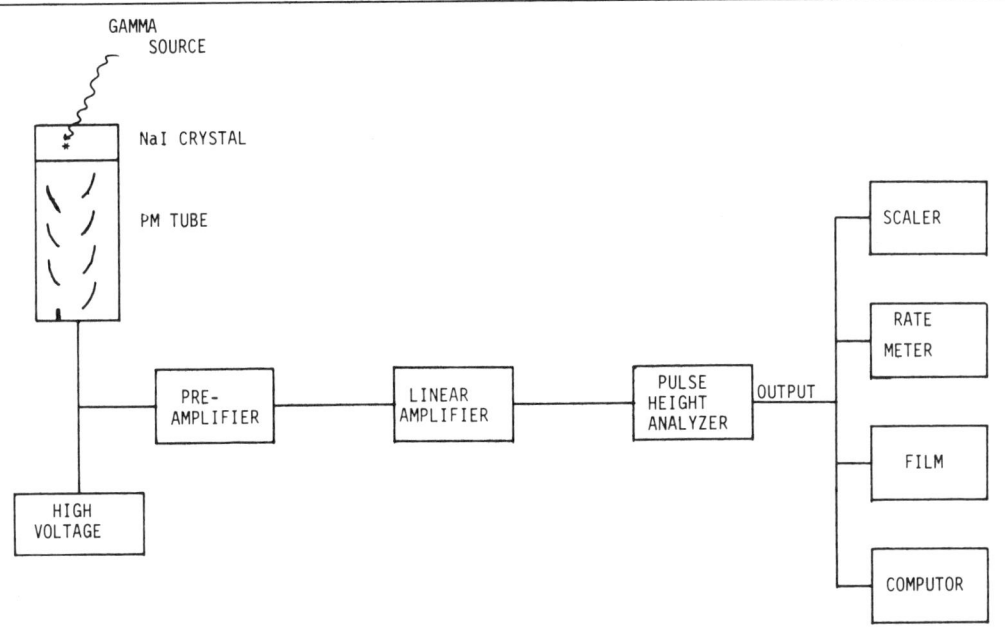

Figure 2-26. Block diagram of a scintillation spectrometer.

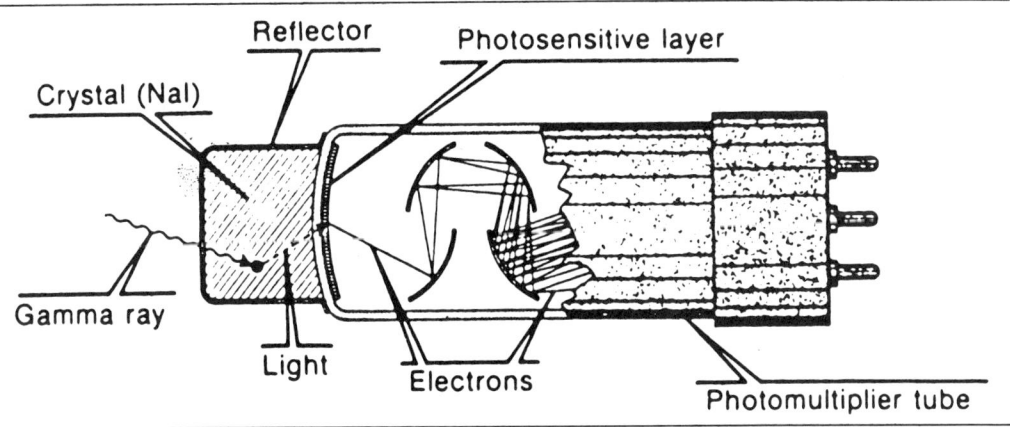

Figure 2-27. Sodium iodide crystal-PM tube scintillation detector. Total light to tube nearly proportional to gamma ray energy. If 1 electron ejects 5 from a dynode, 11 dynodes result in 5^{11} or about 50 million electrons output. *(From Early PJ, Razzak MA, Sodee DB: Textbook of Nuclear Medicine Technology, 3rd ed. St Louis, C.V. Mosby, 1979, with permission, and courtesy of the US Nuclear Regulatory Commission.)*

crystal is doped with 0.1 percent thallium because pure crystals do not scintillate well. The number of scintillations and thus the amount of visible light photons is proportional to the amount of gamma energy deposited in the crystal. The light photons cause electrons to be ejected from a photosensitive cathode. The electrons are attracted to a series of dynodes that are about 100 V positive with respect to each other. An average of four electrons are ejected for each incident electron on a dynode so that electron multiplication occurs. A series of ten dynodes will result in 4^{10} or about 1 million electrons, which produce a small electrical pulse at the collecting anode.

In summary, the magnitude of the output pulse of the PM tube is proportional to the intensity of light photons and the gamma ray energy deposited in the crystal. A 200-keV gamma ray would thus produce a pulse with twice the height of a 100-keV gamma ray.

Processing of the output pulse from the PM tube involves amplification and discrimination. A preamplifier serves to match impedence between the PM tube and the amplifier, which amplifies each pulse so it can be measured. The pulse height analyzer (PHA) consists of an electronic circuit containing an upper-level energy discriminator (ULD) and a lower-level energy discriminator (LLD) in an anticoincidence circuit. The only pulses counted are those that fall within the "window" between the LLD and ULD settings. The PHA operates to allow certain pulse heights to be counted and others to be rejected. Different radionuclides with different photon energies may thus be counted independently by adjusting the window (Fig. 2-28).

Various display units record events. A scaler is a digital counter that totals the number of counts detected by the crystal and PHA. A rate meter displays counts per unit time whereas a strip chart recorder produces a hard copy of count rate versus time. An oscilloscope is a cathode ray tube visual display of radioactivity distribution in an organ and is usually a part of a gamma camera that is used to position patients. A film recording device activates a light that exposes a photographic film and provides a permanent record of organ distribution of radioactivity. Last, detector output can be stored in computer memory.

Gamma Energy Spectrum

When a radionuclide is counted with a scintillation spectrometer and the count rate plotted versus energy, a gamma energy spectrum is produced (Fig. 2-29). This "gamma fingerprint" may be used as an analytic tool to identify radionuclides in an unknown source. Alternatively, if the spectrum is already known, it can be used to establish the best instrument settings for counting or imaging with scintillation

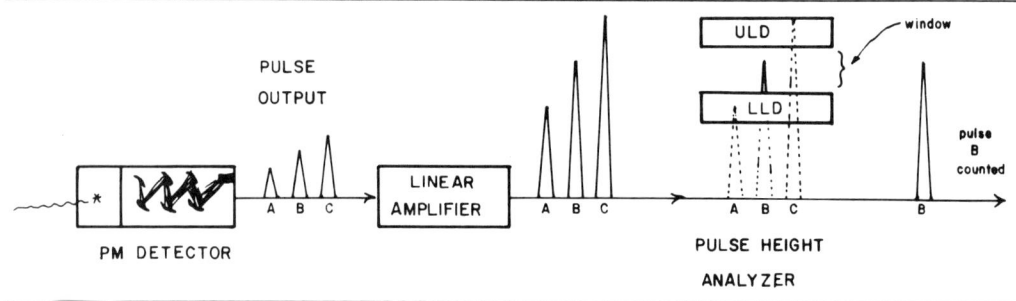

Figure 2-28. Schematic of pulse height processing in a scintillation spectrometer. Pulses A, B, and C are amplified linearly before processing by the pulse height analyzer. Only pulse B falls within the window and is counted; pulse A is discriminated out by the LLD and pulse C by the ULD.

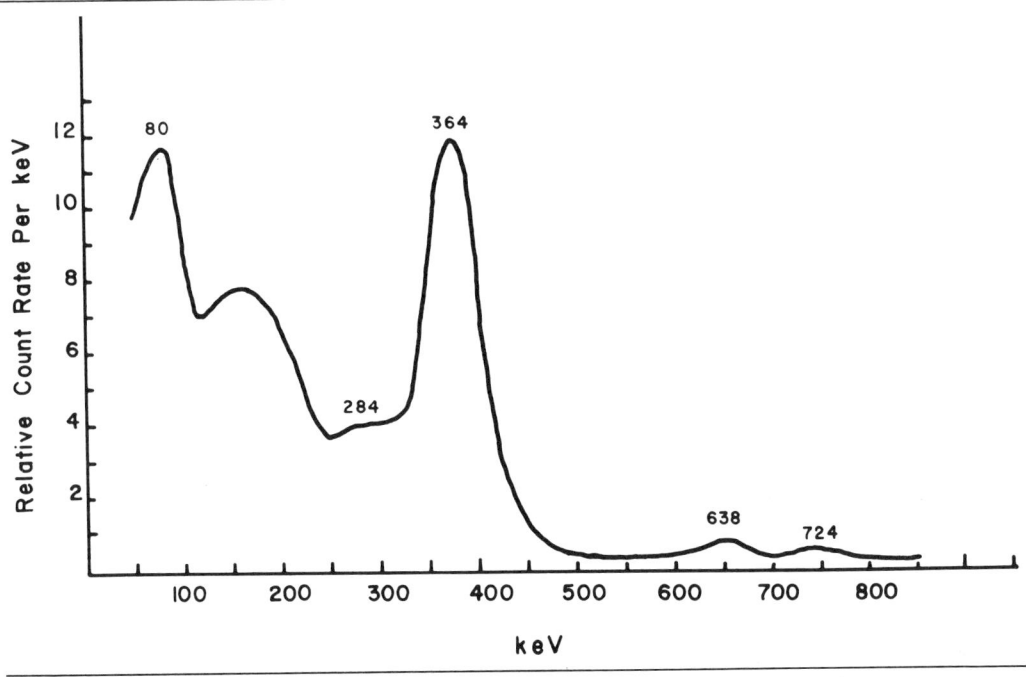

Figure 2-29. Gamma energy spectrum for I-131 in a 2 × 2-inch sodium iodide crystal.

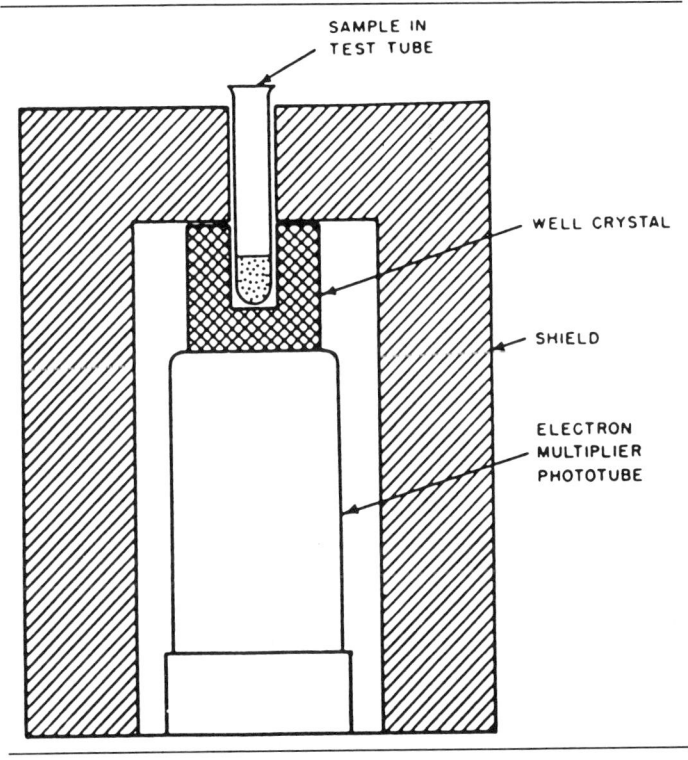

Figure 2-30. Scintillation well counter. *(From US Department of Commerce, National Bureau of Standards, Handbook 80, A Manual of Radioactivity Procedures, 1963.)*

instruments. The instruments most frequently used in nuclear medicine are the scintillation well counter, probe, and gamma camera.

Well Counter

A well counter is a scintillation spectrometer system for counting test tube samples. It is an extremely sensitive device, and generally samples containing not more than 1 µCi are counted. The sodium iodide crystal varies in size, generally being 1.5 to 3 inches in diameter and 2 to 3 inches deep. It has a cylindrical well drilled into it for accepting test tubes. Figure 2-30 illustrates the configuration of a well counter detector. The major advantage of this arrangement is the increased counting efficiency that results from surrounding the sample by the detector. It is heavily shielded with lead to reduce background radiation.

Scintillation Probe

A probe is similar to the well counter except that it has no well. The crystal may be of various sizes depending on the intended use. Thicker crystals are more efficient detectors and are necessary for high-energy gamma rays. Probes with crystals 1.5 to 2 inches in diameter and 1 inch thick are routinely used for thyroid uptake measurements. Smaller hand-held portable probes are used to monitor radioactivity over various body parts, for example, in the detection of deep venous thrombi in the leg veins after the administration of fibrinogen labeled with I-125. Examples of probe detectors are shown in Figures 2-31 and 2-32.

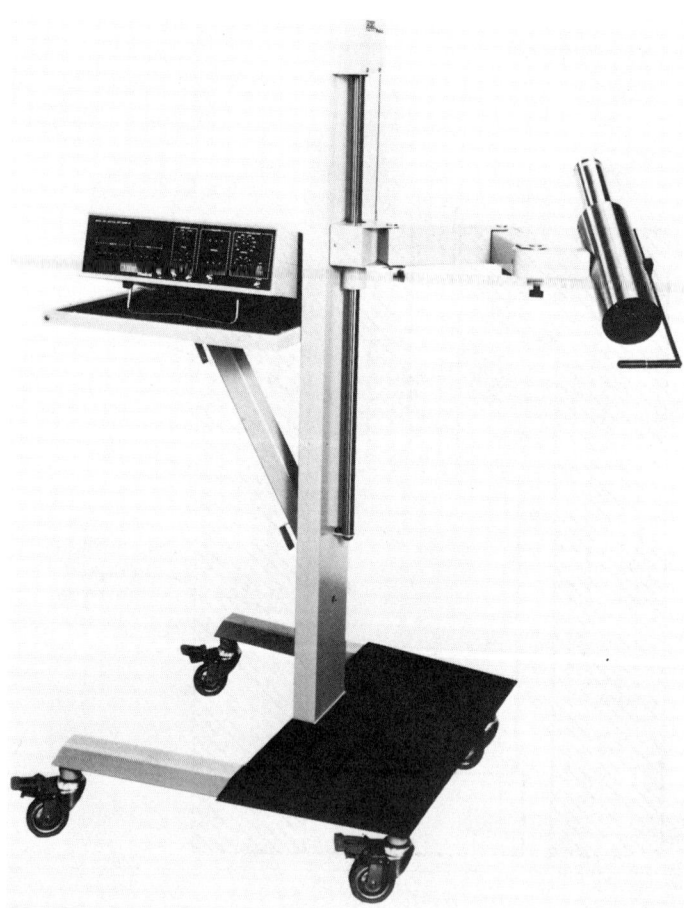

Figure 2-31. Stationary scintillation thyroid uptake probe and counter. *(From ADC Medical, Farmingdale, NY, with permission.)*

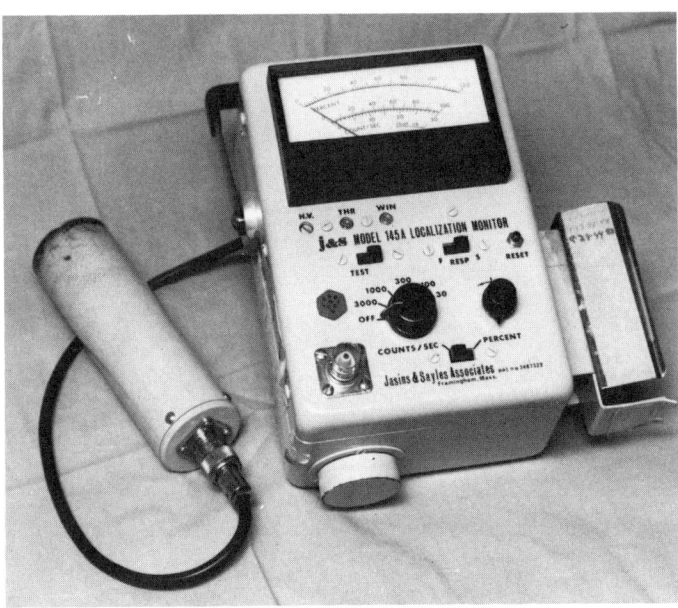

Figure 2-32. Hand-held portable scintillation probe and counter. (From Jasins and Sayles Associates, Natick, Mass, with permission.)

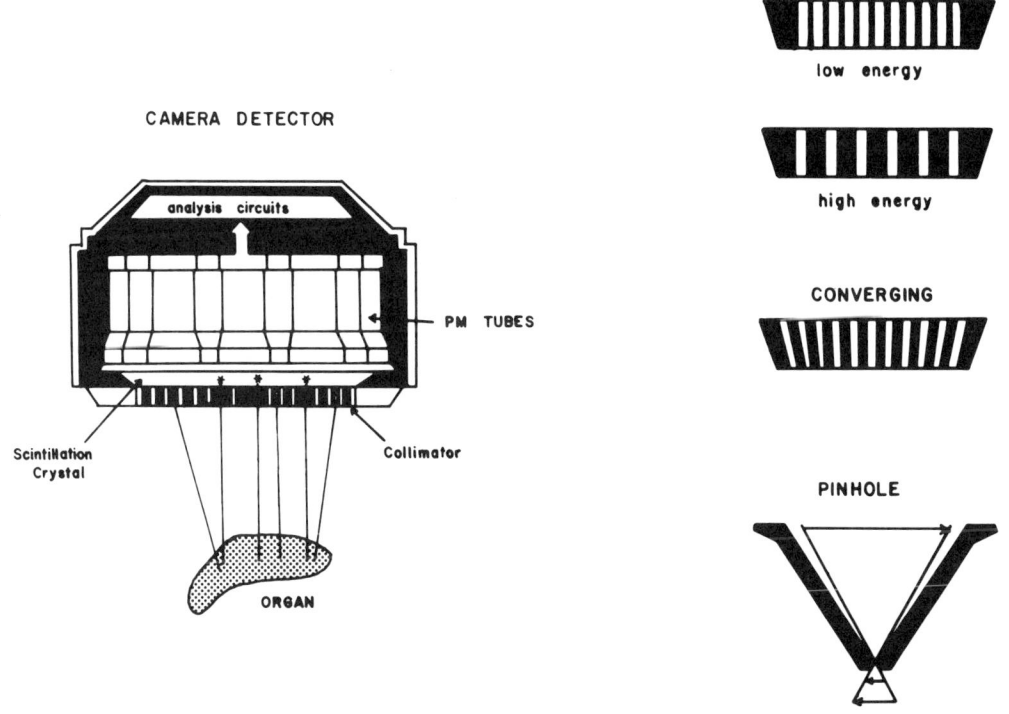

Figure 2-33. Diagram of a gamma camera detector with several types of collimators.

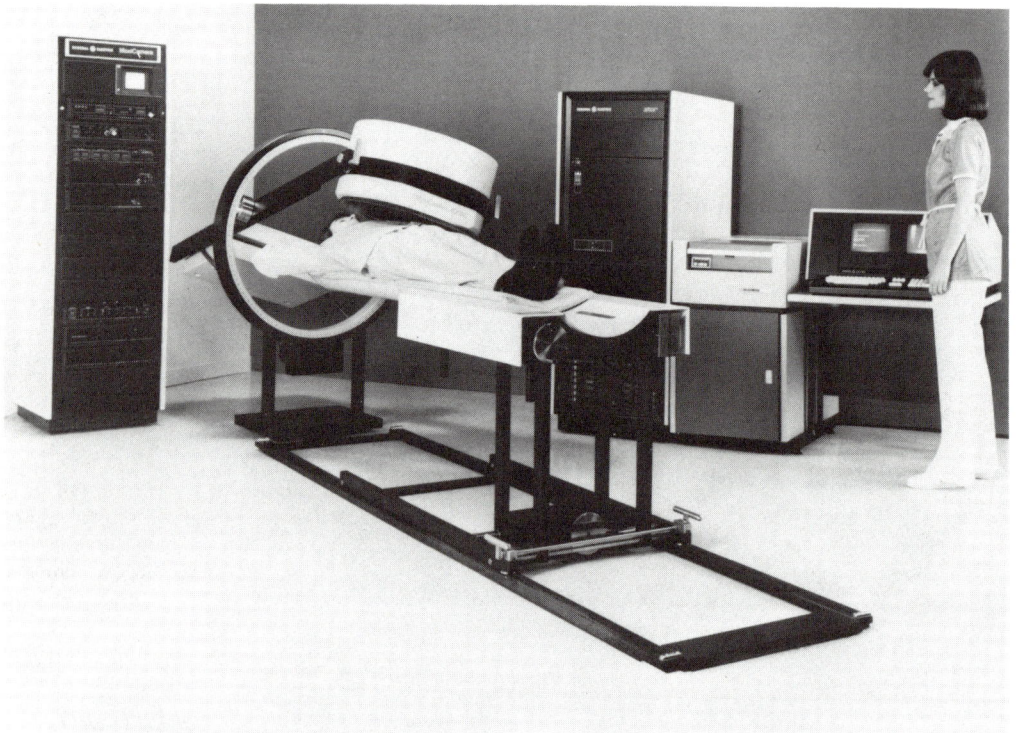

Figure 2-34. A gamma camera system. *(Maxicamera-Star system, from General Electric Medical Systems, with permission.)*

Gamma Cameras

A gamma camera is a stationary imaging device. The detection head contains a sodium iodide crystal optically coupled to an array of several photomultiplier tubes. Gamma camera detectors are available in several sizes. A typical camera uses a sodium iodide crystal that is 0.5 inches thick and 15 inches in diameter coupled to 37 PM tubes. Attached to the face of the crystal is a collimator that is made of lead. Collimators are made in different configurations to provide some latitude with regard to resolution and size of the image. The basic configurations are the pinhole, parallel-hole, and diverging collimators. Figure 2-33 demonstrates a camera detector with a parallel-hole collimator in place.

The detector is connected to a module that contains camera controls and the display devices. Figure 2-34 shows a complete gamma camera system.

RADIATION MEASUREMENT AND PROTECTION

Soon after the discovery of radioactivity the biologic effects of radiation were demonstrated. In the first instance Becquerel suffered an erythema from a radioactive preparation kept in his side coat pocket. In another, Pierre Curie exposed radium radiation to his hand, which developed an ulcer that was slow to heal. Many other instances like these occurred in the early years of radiation use, often because of ignorance of its biologic interactions. From these experiences a respect for radiation developed, and ways of measuring radiation dose became important.

There are two parameters used to define the various terms of radiation measurement: the ionization of matter by radiation and the energy absorbed by matter from radiation. There are several terms used in the measurement of radiation: the curie (Ci), the roentgen (r), the radiation absorbed dose (rad), and the roentgen equivalent man (rem).

The Curie
This term was previously discussed under radioactivity and is defined as the amount of radioactive material that produces 3.7×10^{10} disintegrating atoms per second. It is used when measuring the quantity of radioactive material present in a source and is related to a definite number of radioactive atoms.

The Roentgen
The roentgen is that quantity of x- or gamma radiation such that the associated corpuscular emission per 1 cc (0.001293 g) of air produces, in air, ions carrying 1 electrostatic unit of charge of either sign. The roentgen is measured at standard temperature and pressure (STP). The corpuscular emissions are the photoelectrons and Compton electrons that are produced by photon interactions with the atoms of air. The passage of one roentgen of radiation will result in the production of 2.082×10^9 ion pairs (IP) per cubic centimeter of air under STP. The roentgen relates only to x- and gamma rays and does not include particulate radiation. Additionally, it relates only to an exposure quantity with no qualification of the time of exposure.

The Radiation Absorbed Dose
The radiation absorbed dose (rad) is that quantity of any ionizing radiation required to produce 100 ergs of energy absorbed per 1 g of absorber. This term is more practical because it relates to the radiation dose absorbed, not just exposure, and to any ionizing radiation, not just x- or gamma rays. One can, however, convert the roentgen to rads as in Equation 2–12.

$$1\ R = \frac{2.082 \times 10^9\ \text{IP}}{0.001293\ \text{g air}} \times \frac{33.7\ \text{eV}}{1\ \text{IP}}$$

$$\times\ 1.602 \times 10^{-12}\ \frac{\text{erg}}{\text{eV}} \times \frac{1\ \text{rad}}{100\ \text{ergs/g}}$$

$$= 0.869\ \text{rad} \qquad (2\text{–}12)$$

Because tissue is denser than air, the absorbed dose in tissue is greater by a factor 1.108. One roentgen is therefore equal to (1.108) (0.869 rad) or 0.96 rad in tissue.

The Relative Biologic Effectiveness
The biologic effect of radiation not only relates to how much energy is absorbed but how it is distributed within the absorber (tissue). Certainly, if 100 ergs of energy is concentrated within a few cells in 1 g of tissue, the damage will be greater than if it was spread uniformly throughout the gram. The relative biologic effectiveness (RBE) is a term used to describe the degree of biologic effect produced by different types of radiation at the same absorbed dose. It is defined as follows:

$$\text{RBE} = \frac{\text{Dose in rads of x- or gamma radiation required to produce a given biologic effect}}{\text{Dose in rads of any ionizing radiation required to produce the same biologic effect}}$$

Gamma rays of cobalt-60 (1.25 MeV average E) and 200 to 300-keV x-rays have been used as the reference radiation in determining RBE. The RBE depends on the LET of a given radiation. Generally, the larger the LET, the greater will be the biologic effect of a given absorbed dose. There is no one RBE for a given type of radiation; the value depends on the tissue, the cell, the biologic effect being studied, the total dose, and the dose rate. It is a term restricted to experimental biology. In radiation protection where it is convenient to add up the dose contributions from different radiation types, a modifier known as quality factor (QF) is used. The QF is of the nature of a somewhat arbitrarily chosen conservative round-off of the range of RBEs depending on the LET. A practical guide to quality factors is shown in Table 2–5.

The Roentgen Equivalent Man
The roentgen equivalent man (rem) is a unit of biologic dose used in personnel radiation monitoring. It is equal to the absorbed dose in rads times the QF for the particular

TABLE 2-5. PRACTICAL QUALITY FACTORS

Radiation Type	Rounded QF
X-rays, gamma rays, electrons, or positrons	1
Neutrons <10 keV	3
Neutrons >10 keV	10
Protons	1-10
Alpha particles	1-20
Fission fragments, recoil nuclei	20

(From NCRP Report No. 39, 1971.[9])

radiation. We thus have the expression:

$$\text{Dose (rems)} = \text{Dose (rads)} \times QF \quad (2\text{–}13)$$

This equation indicates that an absorbed dose of 1 rad from an alpha particle emitter in tissue may produce up to 20 times the biologic effect as 1 rad of gamma or beta radiation. The significant difference is due to the high LET of alpha particles.

In summary, r may be considered a unit of exposure dose, rad a unit of absorbed dose, and rem a unit of biologic dose. As a general rule for gamma ray sources used in nuclear medicine, 1 r ≅ 1 rad ≅ 1 rem.

Limits of Radiation Exposure

Each person receives a certain amount of radiation dose per year as a result of exposure to natural, background sources of radiation. This amounts to a dose of about 0.15 rem per year from exposure to radioactive air pollution, cosmic rays, radiation from building materials, and traces of body radionuclides such as potassium-40 and C-14.

Persons who work with radiation are permitted to receive amounts not to exceed 5 rem per year total body dose. This is called the maximum permissible dose (MPD) and is determined for persons over 18 years of age by the following formula:

$$\text{MPD} = 5 (N - 18) \quad (2\text{–}14)$$

where N is the age in years. This implies that one cannot work with radiation before age 18.

The *Radiation Protection Guides* is a tabulation of radiation doses in rems that must not be exceeded for various body parts during a specified time and is listed in Table 2–6. The MPD formula is applicable to radiation exposure to the whole body, head and trunk, lens of the eye, active blood-forming organs, and gonads. The formula indicates that the cumulative maximum permissible dose to these organs shall not exceed 5 rem multiplied by the number of years beyond age 18. It also states in the protection guide that the dose in any 1 quarter year (13 consecutive weeks) could be as large as 3 rem, i.e., 12 rem per year, but only if the total occupational exposure during the workers' lifetime does not exceed the MPD value. For example, a radiation worker aged 22 has a lifetime exposure limit of 5 (22 – 18) = 20 rem. If the worker received 11 rem in the 3 years before age 22,

TABLE 2-6. RADIATION PROTECTION GUIDES

Organ	Permissible Dose	
Whole body (includes gonads, lens of the eye, and red bone marrow)	5 rem/yr	(3/quarter)
Skin	15 rem/yr	
Hands	75 rem/yr	(25/quarter)
Forearms	30 rem/yr	(10/quarter)
Other organs, tissues, and organ systems	15 rem/yr	(5/quarter)
Fertile women (with respect to fetus)	0.5 rem/gestation period	
General public	0.5 rem/yr	

(Data from Glasstone S, 1967.[10])

9 rem could be received during the 22nd year. Up to 3 rem per quarter could be received, and if this were the case, the 9 rem would be received during the first 3 quarters. The worker would, however, be required to abstain from any exposure during the last quarter because any exposure would then exceed the MPD of 20 rem for 4 years of occupational exposure.

Protection from Radiation

There is little hazard to the body from external exposure to particulate radiation except for neutrons, which penetrate tissue deeply, but neutron sources are not used in nuclear medicine. Electrons and alpha particles are easily stopped by air, by the container they are in, or by a few millimeters of skin in cases of personal contact. These particles are a major concern from internally deposited radiation sources however. The major concern from external exposure arises from gamma and x-radiations because of their ability to penetrate tissue and ionize atoms. Table 2–7 compares the penetrating ability for various radiations in tissue.

Potential sources of radiation exposure are from inadvertent internally deposited sources of external exposure. Internal deposition can be caused by ingestion of contaminated food and water but most likely will be due to inhalation of airborne radionuclides. The most common example of this is radioiodine vapor. Other examples include radioaerosols and radiogases used in lung imaging studies. For the most part, however, radiation dose is mainly due to exposure from gamma radiation from radiation sources in the laboratory and from patients who have received radiopharmaceuticals. Protection from all these sources requires vigilance and the use of a combination of techniques. Airborne contamination can be controlled by use of exhaust hoods during dose preparation and negative pressure rooms for the administration and imaging procedures. Additionally, traps and filters can be used to effectively limit air contamination. The three most important considerations for protection from external exposure to gamma radiation are time, distance, and shielding.

Time of Exposure. Obviously the shorter the time of exposure, the lower will be the radiation dose. This requires that the work be well planned out and performed as quickly as possible when unshielded sources are handled. The Nuclear Regulatory Commission (NRC) states in its regulations that "no licensee shall possess, use or transfer licensed (radioactive) material in such a manner as to create in an unrestricted area radiation levels which if an individual were continuously present in the area, could result in his receiving a dose in excess of 2 mrems/hr or a dose of 100 mrems in 7 consecutive days." It should be remembered, however, that these limits are intended only for short-term exposures over periods of not more than 50 hours per week. In this way both limits of the regulation are

TABLE 2-7. RADIATION RANGE IN TISSUE

	Radiation (MeV)		Range in Tissue (cm)
Alpha Particles		1	0.0006
		5	0.0037
		7.5	Will penetrate skin
Beta Particles		1	0.42
		5	2.20
	^{3}H	0.018	0.0006
	^{14}C	0.155	0.30
	^{32}P	1.7	0.80
Gamma Rays		0.15	2.8% absorbed per cm
		0.50	3.3% absorbed per cm

met, i.e., 100 mrem ÷ 50 hours = 2 mrem/hr. For nonoccupational personnel such as nurses, visitors, and adjacent patients the maximum yearly dose is not more than 500 mrem, which places a top limit on exposure. If nonoccupational personnel will be exposed to an extended chronic-type exposure such as that from patients treated with a radioactive source, the hourly limit must be reduced. In these circumstances the dose rate is based upon a 168-hour week whereby the limit is 100 mrem ÷ 168 hours = 0.6 mrem/hr. Again, the maximum limit of whole-body exposure is 500 mrem in 1 year. Another example of where chronic radiation exposure may threaten hospital personnel is in such instances where their work place is adjacent to a radiation therapy department that uses a linear accelerator for patient treatment. Adequate shielding of floors, walls, and ceiling around the accelerator must be provided so that nonoccupational exposure does not exceed 500 mrem per year.

Distance. Maintaining as much distance as practicable from a radioactive source is an effective method for reducing radiation exposure because of the *inverse square law*. This law states that the amount of radiation from a point source is inversely proportional to the square of the distance from the source. Simply stated, if you double the distance from a source, the exposure is reduced to one fourth the original. Of course, this law applies only to electromagnetic radiation.

To apply the inverse square law for exposure from a radionuclide source, its specific gamma ray dose constant Γ must be known. This relates the exposure rate from an amount of activity at a defined distance from the source as follows: Γ = R/hr/mCi at 1 cm. Table 2–8 lists Γ for several radionuclides of interest. For any given number of millicuries N, the dose rate at any distance d from the source is given by the following equation:

$$\frac{N\Gamma}{d^2} \text{ R/hr} \qquad (2\text{--}15)$$

Example:

1. Calculate the dose rate from a 10-mCi I-131 source at 1 cm and at 2 cm.

$$\text{R/hr at 1 cm} = \frac{N\Gamma}{d^2}$$

$$= \frac{(10 \text{ mCi})(2.2 \text{ R/hr/mCi/cm})}{(1 \text{ cm})^2}$$

$$= 22 \text{ R/hr}$$

$$\text{R/hr at 2 cm} = \frac{22 \text{ R/hr}}{(2 \text{ cm})^2} = 5.5 \text{ R/hr}$$

2. What distance would lower the dose rate to 2 mR/hr?

$$\frac{N\Gamma}{d^2} = 2 \text{ mR/hr}$$

$$\frac{22,000 \text{ mR/hr}}{2 \text{ mR/hr}} = d^2$$

$$d = 105 \text{ cm or about 1 m}$$

Although maintaining distance from a source provides significant reduction in exposure, it does not provide adequate safety when handling highly active sources, and shielding of the source must be provided.

Shielding. The effectiveness of shielding material depends upon its atomic number, its density, and its thickness. Material of high density and high Z has many atoms (and electrons) packed into a small volume, which produces high stopping power. As energy of gamma radiation increases, thicker shields are required.

If one interposes an absorber between a radiation source and a Geiger–Müller detector, the fraction of the original intensity transmitted through the shield will be a function of the absorber thickness x and the linear attenuation coefficient u. This coefficient depends on the Z of the absorber and the photon energy (E), but for given values of Z and E, u has a constant value. The relationship between original intensity and transmitted intensity after shielding is given by the formula:

$$I = I_o e^{-ux} \qquad (2\text{--}16)$$

PHYSICS OF RADIOPHARMACEUTICALS

TABLE 2-8. GAMMA RAY DOSE CONSTANTS AND HALF-VALUE LAYERS IN LEAD FOR SEVERAL RADIONUCLIDES

Radionuclide	HVL mm Pb	R/hr/mCi at 1 cm
Iodine-131	3.0	2.2
Chromium-51	2.00	0.15
Iodine-125	0.04	1.23
Iron-59	11.00	6.40
Cobalt-57	0.20	1.00
Xenon-133	0.04	0.56
Technetium-99m	0.30	0.80
Gallium-67	0.04	1.60
Thallium-201	0.0006	4.70
Selenium-75	3.00	2.00
Xenon-127	0.23	2.20
Indium-111	0.21	3.30
Krypton-81m	0.019	1.60
Iodine-123	0.50	1.50

where

- I is the transmitted intensity after shielding
- I_o is the original intensity before shielding
- u is the linear attenuation coefficient (mm^{-1})
- x is the absorber thickness (mm)

If one measures and then plots I for various absorber thicknesses, a linear relationship is obtained on semilog paper as shown in Figure 2–35. The thickness of absorber required to reduce the original intensity to half the value is called the *half-value layer* (HVL). Mathematically HVL is inversely related to the linear attenuation coefficient as follows:

$$u = \frac{0.693}{HVL} \quad (2\text{-}17)$$

Example:

How much lead is required to reduce the radiation intensity from a 100-mCi point source of Tc-99m to 2 mR/hr?

HVL Tc-99m in Pb = 0.2 mm

$$\Gamma = 0.8 \text{ R/hr/mCi at 1 cm}$$

Original Intensity, I_o = (0.8 R/hr/mCi) (100 mCi) (1000 mR/R) = 80,000 mR/hr
Using the natural log form of $I = I_o\, e^{-ux}$ we have

$$\ln I = \ln I_o - ux$$

$$\ln 2 \text{ mR/hr} = \ln 80{,}000 \text{ mR/hr} - \frac{0.693}{0.2 \text{ mm}}(x)$$

$$0.693 = 11.29 - 3.465\, x$$

$$x = 3.06 \text{ mm of Pb}$$

Monitoring of Personnel Radiation Exposure

The greatest concern regarding radiation exposure to nuclear medicine personnel arises from external gamma ray sources, namely, radiopharmaceuticals and patients who have received radioactive material for diagnostic studies and radiation treatment. There are several ways to monitor personnel radiation exposure. One must keep in mind, however, that accuracy depends on the methods used and on stringent quality control procedures. Measurements will give a reasonably accurate determination of radiation exposure only to the area of the body where the monitor is worn. In general, monitors will document that a signifi-

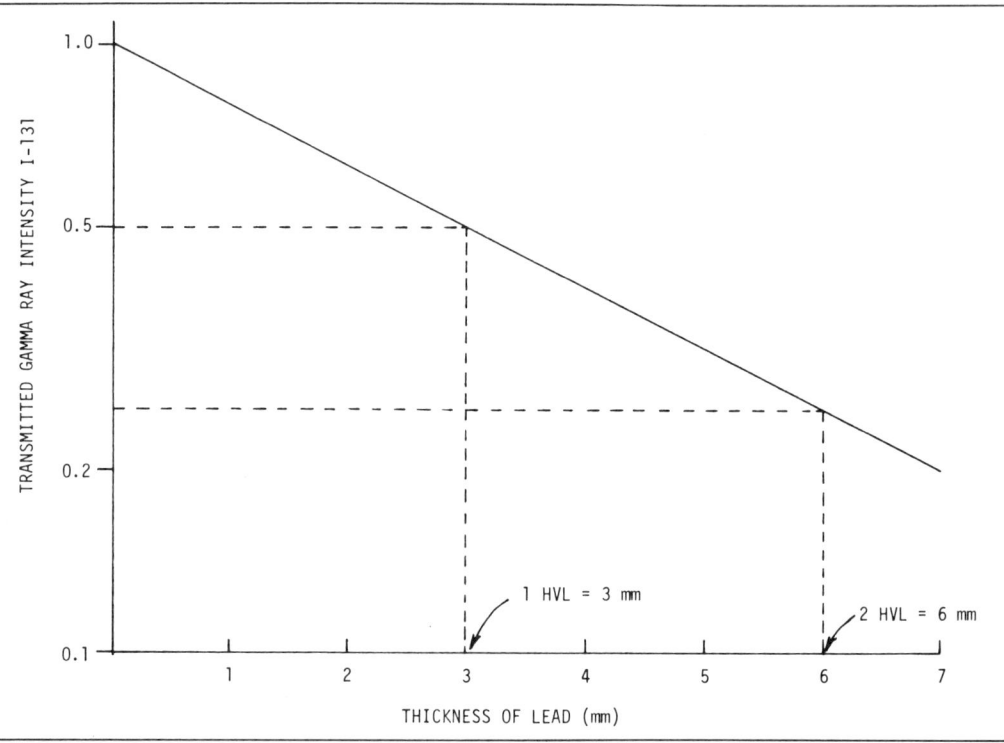

Figure 2-35. Plot of log transmitted gamma ray intensity (ordinate) versus absorber thickness (abscissa) for I-131 in lead.

cant radiation dose has not been acquired by the worker. Such measurements are important for use in detecting unusual radiation exposure conditions so that corrective measures can be instituted to prevent significant radiation exposure to the individual in excess of the radiation protection guides.

There are a variety of personnel dosimeters used for monitoring radiation exposure. Such devices are worn on some position of the body to record the radiation exposure to that portion. In general, collar badges are worn to measure exposure to the eyes and thyroid gland, waste badges for gonadal exposure, and ring badges for the hands and fingers. Badges contain either a photographic film or a fluorescent chemical to quantitate radiation exposure. Photographic film badges consist of a plastic holder containing radiation sensitive film and an arrangement of filters that allows identification of a specified type of radiation. The film is processed and read with special optical density sensing instruments to determine the radiation exposure. Thermoluminescent dosimeter (TLD) badges contain a fluorescent chemical, usually lithium fluoride, arranged in a plastic holder. For example, a badge may contain a LiF chip, LiF powder, or both. Radiation is quantitated by heating the exposed LiF, which then emits light in proportion to the radiation absorbed by it. Ring badges usually are of the TLD type.

Another device that is used occasionally is a direct-reading pocket dosimeter. This dosimeter contains an ionization chamber as the radiation detector. The unit must be charged initially using a power

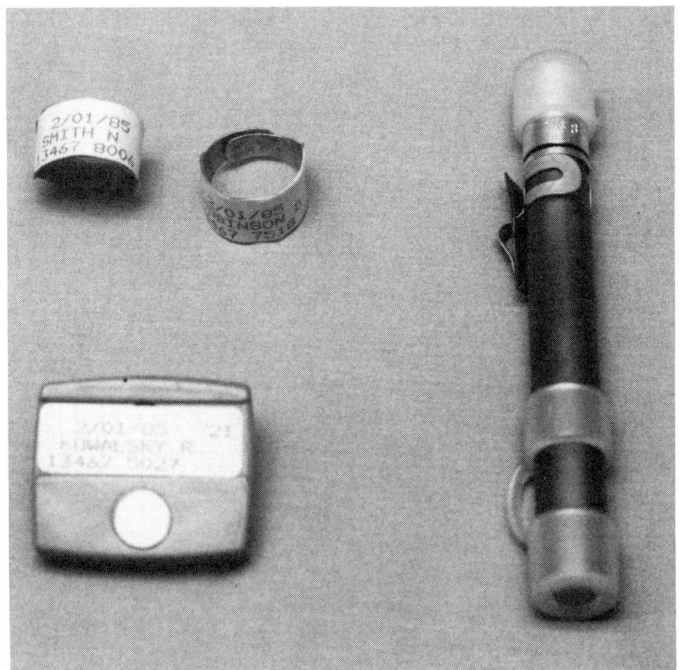

Figure 2-36. Radiation monitoring devices: ring badges, film badge, and quartz fiber pocket dosimeter.

source. Radiation exposure discharges the unit, thus causing a quartz fiber to move along a calibrated scale that can be read at will by looking through the viewing lens at the end of the dosimeter barrel. Examples of radiation monitoring devices are shown in Figure 2–36.

PRODUCTION OF RADIONUCLIDES

The majority of radionuclides used in nuclear medicine are artificially produced. This is accomplished by bombarding a stable target nucleus with a particle, which changes the target into a different nuclide. This process is called transmutation. A nuclear reaction occurs in two stages. In the first stage, the bombarding particle penetrates into and is captured by the target nucleus, which adds to the nucleus its kinetic energy and its binding energy. The newly formed intermediate nucleus contains an extra allotment of energy that is transferred among the nucleons. In the second stage, by chance one or more nucleons acquire enough energy to overcome the nuclear binding energy, and they escape. The escaping particle may carry off all the extra energy or only enough to escape. Any energy remaining will be released as gamma radiation from the new nucleus. Note that this is not radioactivity but simply the second stage of the nuclear reaction. Bombarding and escaping particles vary and usually include protons $^1H^+$, deuterons $^2H^+$, neutrons, and alpha particles $^4He^{2+}$.

In 1934 Frederick Joliot and Irene Curie Joliot performed a nuclear reaction by bombarding a piece of aluminum foil with alpha particles. This produced the first artificially made radionuclide, P-30, according to the following reaction:

$$^{27}_{13}Al + ^4_2He \longrightarrow ^1_0n + ^{30}_{15}P$$

The shorthand notation for this reaction is $^{27}Al(\alpha,n)^{30}P$.

Medical radionuclides are produced either in a nuclear reactor or a particle accelerator.

The (n,γ) Reaction

This is the most common type of reaction with neutrons, and it has the following characteristics: (1) the reaction requires low-energy thermal neutrons with an energy of 0.025 eV. This energy is equivalent to that of an atom of air in equilibrium with its surroundings, and (2) The product nuclide is an isotope of the target. Chemical separation is therefore not possible, and a low specific activity product is obtained.

Examples of reactions include the following:

$^{98}Mo(n,\gamma)^{99}Mo$ $^{196}Hg(n,\gamma)^{197}Hg$
$^{50}Cr(n,\gamma)^{51}Cr$ $^{74}Se(n,\gamma)^{75}Se$
$^{58}Fe(n,\gamma)^{59}Fe$

A(n,γ)A* ⟶ B Reaction

In some instances product separation is possible with (n,γ) reactions because the primary radionuclide product A* has a short half-life and decays to a longer-lived radionuclide B that can be isolated. The following are some examples:

$^{124}Xe(n,\gamma)^{125}Xe \xrightarrow[18\ hr]{\beta^-} {}^{125}I\ (60\ d)$

$^{130}Te(n,\gamma)^{131}Te \xrightarrow[25\ min]{\beta^-} {}^{131}I\ (8\ d)$

A(n,p) B Reaction

In (n,p) reactions the neutron energy is increased. This provides extra energy in the intermediate nucleus so that a proton is able to overcome the nuclear binding energy to escape. The radionuclide product therefore is not an isotope of the target but an isobar; chemical separation of product from the target atoms is possible, and high specific activities are obtained. The following is an example:

$^{32}S(n,p)^{32}P$

^{235}U(n,f) By-products Reaction

When uranium-235 captures a thermal neutron, the intermediate nucleus is very active and fissions into radioactive fragment nuclides as follows:

$^{235}U + {}^1n$
↓
$^{236}U + 2\ {}^1n$

^{131}Sn ← → ^{103}Mo
↓ ↓
^{131}Sb ^{103}Tc
↓ ↓
^{131}Te ^{103}Ru
↓ ↓
^{131}I ^{103}Rh
↓
^{131}Xe

Because the fragments are not isotopes, they may be separated chemically. Many radionuclides are made this way. Some typical examples are Xe-133, I-131, and Mo-99.

Particle Accelerator Methods

Accelerator radionuclides are produced either in a cyclotron or linear accelerator. The method used depends upon the type of nuclear reaction and the yield desired. Generally, cyclotrons can accelerate positively charged ions up to about 30 MeV before relativistic problems become a concern. Higher-energy particles require the use of linear accelerators that can readily compensate for the increase in mass of very high energy particles. Linear accelerators can produce particles in the 100- to 200-MeV range. The high energy of positively charged bombarding particles is required to overcome the repulsive coulomb barrier of the target nucleus. The product nuclei formed with charged particle nuclear reactions are not isotopes of the target nuclei so that high specific activity is achieved after chemical separation. Some typical accelerator-produced radionuclides used in nuclear medicine are as follows:

$^{58}Ni(p,pn)^{57}Ni \xrightarrow[37\ hr]{EC} {}^{57}Co\ (270\ d)$

$^{127}I(p,5n)^{123}Xe \xrightarrow[2\ hr]{EC} {}^{123}I\ (13\ hr)$

$^{111}Cd(p,n)^{111}In$

$^{133}Cs(p,2p5n)^{127}Xe$ (linear accelerator)

Nuclear Reactors

In the reactor, nuclear fuel of enriched U-235 is positioned in the reactor core. The fuel rods are surrounded by a moderator that slows fast neutrons to thermal energy. The thermal neutrons are captured by other uranium atoms that fission, producing more neutrons that can sustain a chain reaction. The moderators used to slow fast neutrons are usually heavy water or graphite. The rate of thermal neutron capture by fissionable nuclei determines the fission rate in the reactor and is controlled by the use of boron or cadmium control rods, which serve as inert absorbers of neutrons. For a fast reaction the rods are pulled out further, and to shut the reaction down the rods are pushed completely into the reactor core. Heat generated in the reactor is carried off by water or other coolants through heat exchangers. For isotope production, ports are provided where target material may be inserted into the reactor.

Cyclotrons and Linear Accelerators

The cyclotron consists of two hollow semicircular chambers called Dees. They resemble an empty tuna fish can cut in half. The Dees are coupled to a very high frequency electrical system so that they are oppositely charged and the charge on each Dee is alternately positive and negative, changing sign about 10^7 times per second. The whole chamber, in a shield that can be evacuated to a low pressure, is placed between the pole pieces of a large electromagnet. At the center of the space between the Dees some arrangement is made for releasing protons or deuterons. When a proton is generated, it is attracted into the negative Dee and repelled by the positive Dee. It therefore accelerates into the negative Dee, but its path is circular because of the magnetic field. When the proton again reaches the gap between the Dees and the Dee charges are reversed, it will be accelerated faster into the opposite Dee, and the radius of its circular path will be larger. But because it is moving faster, the proton will again arrive at the gap precisely when the Dee polarity is reversed, thus causing further acceleration of the proton. Eventually the proton gains great energy and reaches the periphery of the Dees where it exits and is deflected onto a target where the nuclear reaction takes place.

As the proton attains speeds approaching the speed of light, its mass becomes relativistic and increases with increasing energy. As a result of the increased mass the proton spends more time in the Dee and arrives at the gap after the polarity has changed. Because of this problem an alternative method of producing very high energy particles was conceived. One of these methods was the linear accelerator (linac). The linac is a series of cylindrical drift tubes through which electromagnetic waves pass, along with their associated oscillating electric and magnetic fields. A charged particle (e.g., a proton) injected into the drift tube will be carried forward by the traveling wave. The length of the drift tubes changes in accordance with the increase in particle speed and relativistic mass. In this way the particle arrives at the gap between drift tubes always in phase, and very high energy particles can be achieved.

Figure 2-37 illustrates diagrams of a cyclotron and linear accelerator.

Other Methods of Radionuclide Production

Most radionuclides produced in nuclear reactors, cyclotrons, and linear accelerators have half-lives long enough that allow them to be produced and processed into a chemical form ready for use in nuclear medicine. There are, however, some very useful radionuclides that have half-lives too short to allow this fabrication into useful radiopharmaceuticals by commercial manufacturers. Fortunately for some of these radionuclides, generator systems have been developed to allow short-lived radionuclide production in the hospital. Because of their importance radionuclide generator systems will be discussed in the next chapter.

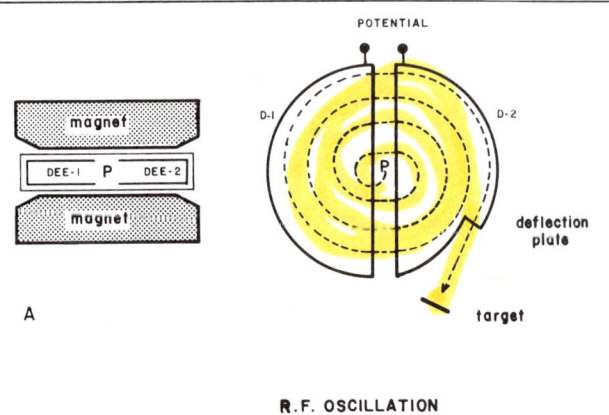

Figure 2-37. Schematic diagram of a cyclotron (**A**) and a linear accelerator (**B**).

RADIATION DOSIMETRY

The radiation dose to an organ from an internally administered radionuclide is given by the expression

$$\overline{D}\,(r_k \leftarrow r_h) = \tilde{A}_h \cdot S\,(r_k \leftarrow r_h) \quad (2\text{-}18)$$

where $\overline{D}$ is the mean absorbed dose in rad to a target organ r_k from a radionuclide distributed uniformly in a source organ r_h. Intuitively one would expect the absorbed dose to an organ to depend on several factors: the amount of radioactivity in the organ, the type and energy of the radiation, the amount of energy absorbed by the organ, the residence time of radiation in the organ, the distribution of radiation in the organ, and the organ mass.

In Equation 2-18 the $\tilde{A}_h$ term is the cumulated activity (μCi-hr) in the source region r_h. It is a biologic data term that represents the time course of activity within the organ. More specifically $\tilde{A}_h$ is governed by the following factors: the amount of administered activity A_o, the site and rate of radiopharmaceutical uptake and removal, and the physical decay of the radionuclide. It is given by the expression

$$\tilde{A}_h(\mu\text{Ci-hr}) = \frac{A_o(\mu\text{Ci})}{\lambda_e}$$
$$= A_o(\mu\text{Ci}) \cdot 1.443 \cdot T_e\,(\text{hr}) \quad (2\text{-}19)$$

The value of $\tilde{A}_h$ depends on the fraction of the administered dose take up by the organ and the pathologic state of the organ.

The S term in Equation 2-18 relates to physical data regarding the radionuclide and the organ mass since the dose will be expressed in rad. It is given by the expression

$$S\,(r_k \leftarrow r_h) = \frac{\Sigma \Delta_i \Phi_i(r_k \leftarrow r_h)}{m_k} \quad (2\text{-}20)$$

where

$$\Delta_i = 2.13 \cdot n_i \cdot E_i \quad (2\text{-}21)$$

In Equation 2-21, 2.13 is a unit conversion constant, n_i is the mean number of particles or photons per nuclear transformation and E_i is the mean energy of the radiation in MeV. The units of Δ_i are g-rad/μCi-hr. The term m_k is the mass in grams of the target organ which makes the S term units rad/μCi-hr. The unit Φ_i is the absorbed fraction of radiation in the target organ. For nonpenetrating radiations such as beta particles, the fraction absorbed is 1. For photons the fraction absorbed is usually less than 1 and depends on photon energy.

The Medical Internal Radiation Dose (MIRD) Committee of the Society of Nuclear Medicine has tabulated values of S for several radionuclides, greatly facilitating radiation dose calculations using Equation 2-18.

Examples:

1. An investigational Tc-99m radiopharmaceutical for spleen imaging has the following distribution after intravenous administration: 80% to spleen, 15% to liver and 5% to total body. Estimate the radiation dose to the spleen from a 1 mCi dose.

Assume: Very slow biological elimination, i.e., $T_e = T_p$ or 6 hr

A spl = (1000 μCi) (0.80) (1.443) (6 hr)
= 6926 μCi-hr

A liv = (1000 μCi) (0.15) (1.443) (6 hr)
= 1299 μCi-hr

A tb = (1000 μCi) (0.05) (1.443) (6 hr)
= 433 μCi-hr

Using the S values from MIRD pamphlet 11 the total dose to the spleen is:

D spl = A spl · S(spl ← spl) + A liv · S(spl ← liv) + A tb · S(spl ← tb)
= (6926 μCi-hr) (3.3 × 10^{-4} rad/μCi-hr) +
(1299 μCi-hr) (9.2 × 10^{-7} rad/μCi-hr) +
(433 μCi-hr) (2.2 × 10^{-6} rad/μCi-hr)
= 2.286 rad + 0.001 rad + 0.001 rad

D spl = 2.288 rad

2. Estimate the radiation dose to the lungs from Tc-99m DTPA aerosol used for lung ventilation studies.

Assume: Instantaneous uptake in lungs of 1 mCi with 1.5%/min biologic removal from lungs into blood.

λ_b = 0.015 min^{-1} · 60 min/hr = 0.9000 hr^{-1}

λ_p = $\dfrac{0.693}{6.02 \text{ hr}}$ = 0.1151 hr^{-1}

λ_e = 0.9000 + 0.1151 = 1.015 hr^{-1}

$\tilde{A}_{lu}$ = $\dfrac{1000 \ \mu Ci}{1.015 \text{ hr}^{-1}}$ = 985 μCi-hr

$\overline{D}_{lu}$ = $\tilde{A}_{lu}$ · S (lu ← lu)
= 985 μCi-hr · 5.2 × 10^{-5} rad/μCi-hr
= 0.051 rad

REFERENCES

1. Chart of the Nuclides, 12th ed. Knolls Atomic Power Laboratory, Naval Reactors, US Department of Energy, 1977
2. Friedlander G, Kennedy JW, Miller JM: Nuclear and Radiochemistry, 2nd ed. New York, Wiley, 1966
3. Johns HE, Cunningham JR: The Physics of Radiology, 3rd ed. Springfield, Ill, Chas. C Thomas, 1969
4. Dillman LT, Von der Lage FC: MIRD Pamphlet No. 10: Radionuclide Decay Schemes. New York, Society of Nuclear Medicine, 1975
5. Wolf AP: Terminology concerning specific activity of radiopharmaceuticals: Reply. J Nucl Med 22:392, 1981
6. Chase CD, Rabinowitz JL: Principles of Radioisotope Methodology, 3rd ed. Minneapolis, Burgess, 1967
7. Kowalsky RJ, Johnston RE, Chan FH: Dose calibrator performance and quality control. J Nucl Med Tech 5:35, 1977
8. Suzuki A, Suzuki MN, Weis AM: Analysis of a radioisotope calibrator. J Nucl Med Tech 4:193, 1976
9. NCRP Report No. 39: Basic Radiation Protection Criteria, National Council on Radiation Protection and Measurements. Washington, DC, 1971
10. Glasstone S: Sourcebook on Atomic Energy, 3rd ed. New York, Van Nostrand Reinhold, 1967

CHAPTER 3

Radionuclide Generators

The introduction of radionuclide generators into nuclear medicine practice arose from the need to administer large amounts of radioactivity to achieve better-quality diagnostic images. Of necessity this requires the use of short-lived radionuclides so that the radiation dose to the patient is not prohibitive. For hospitals not located close to a radionuclide production facility, the only practical way to obtain short-lived radionuclides is by use of a generator. A generator is a system that contains a long-lived parent radionuclide that decays to a short-lived daughter that is used in preparing the desired radiopharmaceuticals. Because parent and daughter nuclides are not isotopes, chemical separation and isolation of the daughter from the parent is possible. After separation new daughter atoms are generated from the parent atoms remaining in the generator. A generator thus provides a fresh supply of short-lived daughter nuclides when needed until the parent activity is depleted. The useful life of a radionuclide generator therefore depends upon the parent half-life. Table 3–1 lists several parent–daughter generator systems.

The generator most prominent in nuclear medicine is the molybdenum-99–technetium-99m generator. It was developed in 1957 at the Brookhaven National Laboratory[1] and first used clinically in 1961 at the University of Chicago.[2] The 2.8-day Mo-99 parent provides a useful life of about 2 weeks. Typically, however, a new generator is received each week on a Monday morning, but midweek and end-of-the-week delivery schedules are also available to meet the diverse needs of a hospital.

PRODUCTION OF THE MO-99/TC-99M GENERATOR

Figure 3–1 outlines the general steps involved in the production of the Mo-99/Tc-99m generator. The Mo-99 in contemporary generators is obtained as a product from the fission of uranium in a nuclear reactor. Various chemical techniques are used to separate Mo-99 from the other radionuclides in the reactor product. The purified Mo-99 is then used to prepare the generator. In one reported method[3] the Mo-99 is adjusted to an acidic pH to form various anionic species such as molybdate

TABLE 3-1. RADIONUCLIDE GENERATOR SYSTEMS

Parent	Daughter
^{99}Mo 67 hr ⟶	^{99m}Tc 6 hr
^{113}Sn 115 d ⟶	^{113m}In 1.7 hr
^{132}Te 3.2 d ⟶	^{132}I 2.3 hr
^{68}Ge 270 d ⟶	^{68}Ga 68 min
^{87}Y 3.3 d ⟶	^{87m}Sr 2.8 hr
^{81}Rb 4.5 hr ⟶	^{81m}Kr 13 sec

(MoO_4^{2-}) and paramolybdate ($Mo_7O_{24}^{6-}$). The anionic molybdate solution is then loaded onto a generator column containing alumina (Al_2O_3). The alumina had been previously washed in pH 5 saline. At this pH, alumina has a positive charge so that the molybdate ions firmly adsorb to the alumina. The completed generators are then autoclaved to render them sterile. They are then assembled under aseptic conditions into their final form in the lead-shielded container. Each generator is then eluted with normal saline (0.9 percent NaCl). The eluate is subjected to several tests before the generator is released for use. Typical tests are generator elution efficiency, eluate volume, radionuclidic purity to detect the presence of Mo-99 and other radionuclide contaminants, radiochemical purity to assure Tc-99m in the proper chemical form as pertechnetate, aluminum

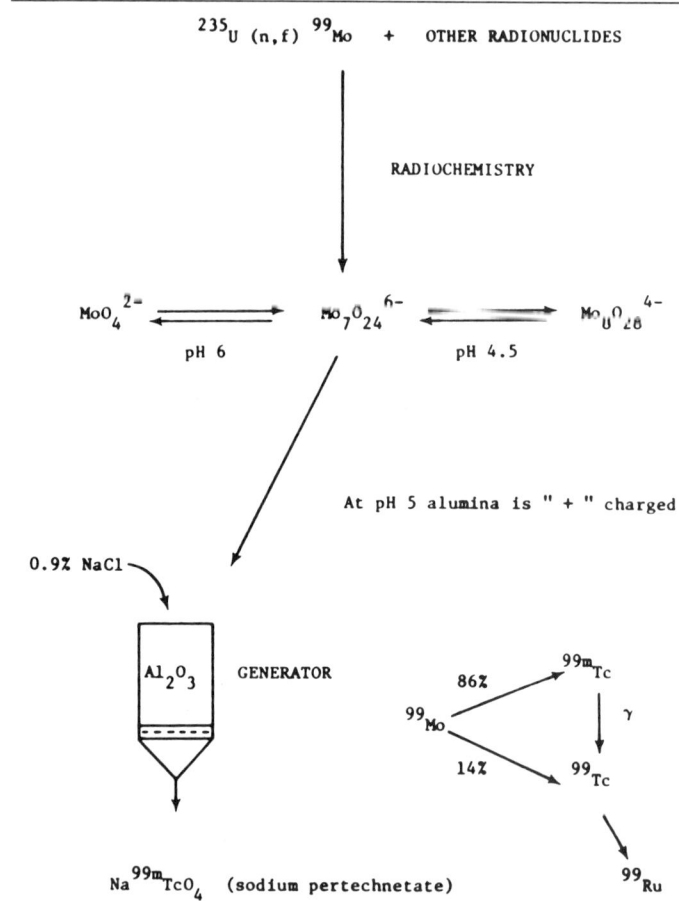

Figure 3-1. Schematic diagram of the steps involved in the production of a Mo-99/Tc-99m generator.

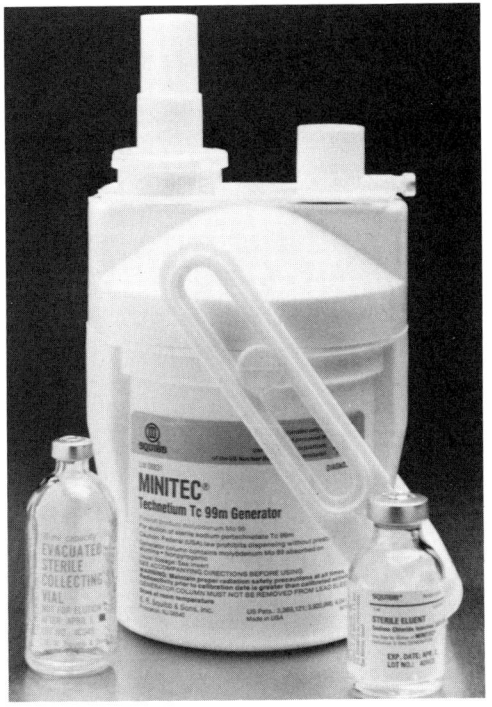 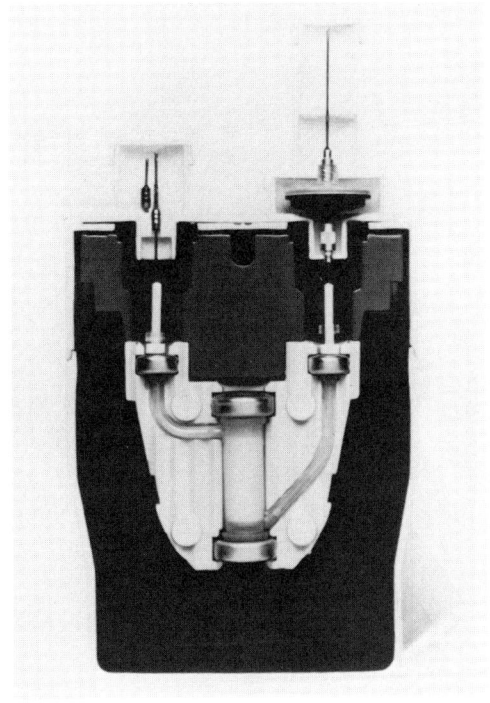

Figure 3-2. A commercial Mo-99/Tc-99m generator system (**A**) and cutaway view (**B**). *(From E.R. Squibb and Sons, Inc., New Brunswick, NJ, with permission.)*

ion contamination in the eluate, pH of the eluate, and finally pyrogen and sterility tests. Figure 3–2 illustrates a generator system.

GENERATOR OPERATION

Figure 3–1 illustrates the simplified decay scheme for the decay of Mo-99 to Tc-99m and Tc-99 within the generator. The relative amounts of Mo-99 and Tc-99m activity in the generator over time are shown in Figure 3–3. This figure illustrates the gradual decay of Mo-99 activity and the subsequent buildup of Tc-99m activity, which reaches a maximum in about 23 hours. About 50 percent of the maximum value is reached in 4.5 hours and 75 percent by 8.5 hours following generator elution.[4]

The accumulated activity is eluted by washing normal saline solution through the column. The Mo-99 activity remains firmly bound to the alumina, but the Tc-99m activity as the pertechnetate ion (TcO_4^-) is easily displaced by the chloride anion (Cl^-) in the saline solution. Typically 70 to 90 percent of the available Tc-99m activity is removed in one 5-ml elution. The remaining Mo-99 activity then continues to decay, generating more Tc-99m activity, but the maximum amount will be less on each subsequent day. Eventually the amount of Tc-99m activity obtained is less than that required to perform all the clinical studies, and the generator is replaced, usually on a weekly basis. Because the Tc-99m activity builds up rapidly immediately after generator elution, the generator may be eluted several times during the same day to

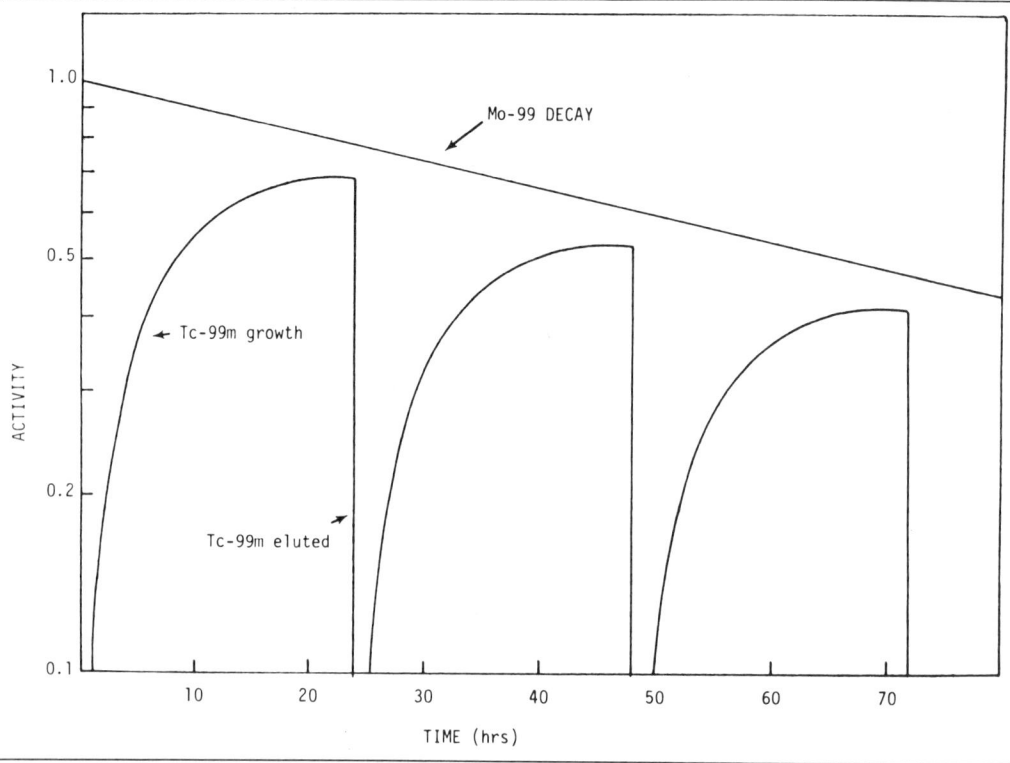

Figure 3-3. Decay of Mo-99 and growth of Tc-99m activities over time in a Mo-99/Tc-99m generator.

obtain more activity if needed. This would most likely occur during the last days of the week when the early morning elution is not sufficient for the daily need.

GENERATOR SYSTEMS

There are two basic types of generator systems: the *wet system* and the *dry system*. An illustration of each system is shown in Figure 3–4. In the *wet system* a large reservoir of saline is connected to the generator, which remains bathed in saline continuously. Technetium activity is eluted by simply connecting a sterile evacuated vial to the elution port. The vacuum draws the saline–pertechnetate solution into the vial. In the *dry system* a 5-ml saline charge is attached before attaching the evacuated vial.

The 30-ml evacuated vial then draws the 5 ml of saline through the generator to remove the Tc-99m activity followed by 25 ml of air to "dry" the column. In both systems the elution vial will end up containing Tc-99m and Tc-99 as sodium pertechnetate in normal saline.

GENERATOR YIELD

Early commercial generator systems were of the wet type. The rapid growth of nuclear medicine studies required larger amounts of Tc-99m activity, which in turn required larger generators with increased Mo-99 activity. This was not without problems, however. Occasionally the entire Tc-99m activity could not be removed dur-

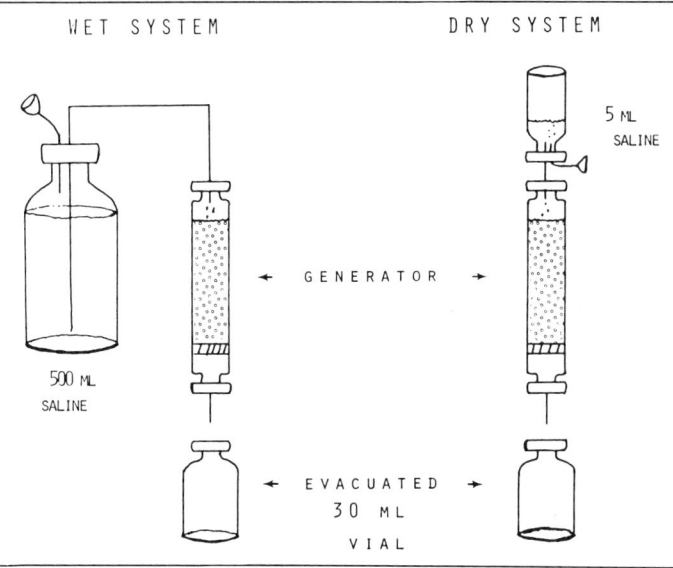

Figure 3-4. Diagram illustrating the two basic types of Mo-99/Tc-99m generator systems.

ing the first elution of a new generator. One reason for this problem was attributed to the change in the technetium oxidation state, causing it to bind more firmly to the alumina. This change in oxidation state (probably to Tc IV) was believed to be mediated through the production of peroxides and free radicals in the aqueous environment of the generator column by the high radiation intensity.[5] This effect is shown in Figure 3-5, which illustrates generator elution efficiency as a function of absorbed dose from a Cobalt-60 source equivalent to 100 mCi of Mo-99 for 1 hour. In Figure 3-5A a series of small generators was prepared, and after washing out the Tc-99m they were irradiated for various times and eluted. In Figure 3-5B small

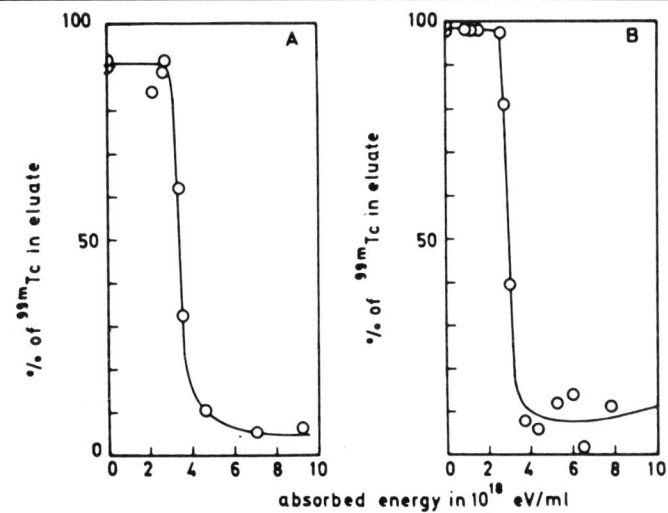

Figure 3-5. Percentage of Tc-99m in generator eluate as a function of absorbed energy of ionizing radiation. **A.** Irradiated alumina columns with absorbed Mo-99. **B.** Irradiated alumina columns soaked in pertechnetate without Mo-99. Columns eluted with 0.9 percent NaCl. *(From Vesely P, et al, 1971, p 71, with permission.[5])*

alumina columns were soaked in aliquots of sodium pertechnetate eluate from a commercial generator, and these columns were irradiated before elution. These experiments demonstrate that pertechnetate is altered to a state that binds to the column. In the past some generator manufacturers used oxidizing agents such as sodium hypochlorite in the saline eluant to keep technetium oxidized in the pertechnetate form to facilitate elution. This is no longer done, however, because of the interference by oxidizing agents in the radiolabeling reactions with Tc-99m radiopharmaceuticals. Other systems (e.g., Mallinckrodt) increase the titer of dissolved oxygen in the saline for the same purpose. This technique improves early elution yields and apparently does not adversely affect radiolabeling. Dry generator systems were developed to alleviate the poor elution problem of wet generators by removing most of the saline after elution to cut down on radiolysis products formed. The dry systems introduce air into the column to promote oxidation to the pertechnetate state.

The problem of incomplete elution rarely occurs with modern generator systems, wet or dry. When the problem does occur, it usually happens with new generators when the highest activity is present and the system has not been eluted for 2 to 3 days. Upon the first elution perhaps only 10 percent of the total activity is removed. The residual activity in the column can usually be eluted 1 hour later, however, because the first elution removes most of the radiolytic contaminants present and the fresh saline and oxygen introduced revert the reduced technetium back to the pertechnetate state.

QUALITY CONTROL OF GENERATOR ELUATE

There are three tests that should be performed daily on the generator eluate of sodium pertechnetate. These tests are illustrated in Figures 3–6A, 3–6B, and 3–6C. The first test is a *radioactivity calibration* with the dose calibrator to determine the activity eluted and the radioactive concentration. This may be accomplished in two ways: (1) assaying the whole vial to obtain the total activity, and from the total volume

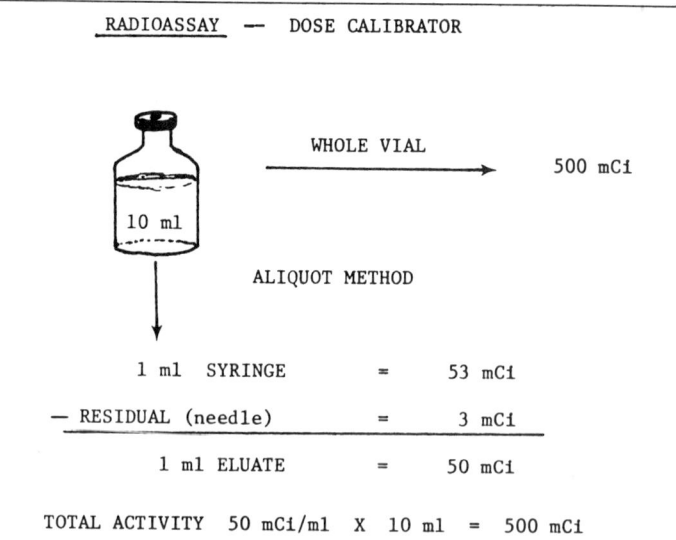

Figure 3-6. A. Generator eluate radioassay in dose calibrator by whole-vial method or aliquot method of assay.

COONH₄ / COONH₄ / OH / HO / C / O / COONH₄

ALUMINON

Forms a pink colored lake with Al^{3+}

Figure 3-6. B. Generator eluate test for aluminum ion chemical impurity by the colorimetric spot test. USP limits: NMT 10 μg Al/ml eluate.

eluted determining the concentration; (2) drawing a 1-ml aliquot into a syringe and assaying its contents. This measures the activity in the 1-ml volume plus that in the needle. Next, the 1 ml is expelled back into the eluate vial and the syringe reassayed to determine the needle activity. The difference between the two measurements provides the activity per milliliter. The total activity in the vial can be obtained from the activity per milliliter and the total volume in the vial. The aliquot method is preferred because the operator is exposed to only a small fraction of the total activity. Also, the concentration measurement using a syringe is more accurate than the whole-vial technique.

The second test of a generator eluate is a *chemical purity test* for the concentration of aluminum ion present. This can be done by several methods, but the most convenient method is a colorimetric spot test. With this test a small drop of sodium pertechnetate eluate is placed on a strip of filter paper impregnated with an indicator. The indicator is the ammonium salt of aurintricarboxylic acid, commonly called aluminon. A spot of a standard aluminum ion solution of known concentration, usually 10 μg Al^{3+}/ml, is placed next to the

MOLYBDENUM 99 " BREAKTHROUGH "

1. GAMMA SPECTROMETRY COUNTING: MCA or SCA with "moly equivalent" Cs-137 STD.

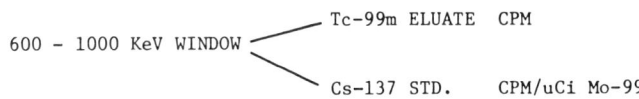

600 - 1000 KeV WINDOW — Tc-99m ELUATE CPM / Cs-137 STD. CPM/uCi Mo-99

2. LEAD SHIELD TECHNIQUE IN DOSE CALIBRATOR

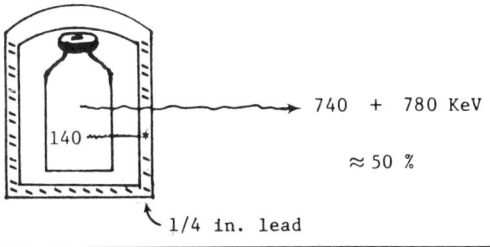

140 → 740 + 780 KeV
≈ 50 %
1/4 in. lead

Figure 3-6. C. Generator eluate test for molybdenum breakthrough by gamma spectrometry or the lead shield method.

pertechnetate spot. The aluminum ion present reacts with the indicator to produce a pink color the intensity of which is proportional to the amount of Al^{3+} ion present. If the color of the pertechnetate spot is less intense than the aluminum standard spot, the eluate passes the test. In the early days of nuclear medicine when neutron-activated Mo-99 generators were used, the upper limit was not more than 20 µg Al^{3+}/ml. Currently the limit is 10 µg Al^{3+}/ml for fission product Mo-99 generators because the generator column is much smaller and is not expected to yield as much aluminum contamination.

The third test of a generator eluate is the *radionuclide purity test* for the presence of Mo-99 contamination. This is the so-called moly-99 breakthrough test. This test can be accomplished by use of a scintillation spectrometer or the more routine lead shield technique.

With a scintillation spectrometer of the single-channel analyzer (SCA) type the whole vial of eluate in a specified shielded configuration is counted with a sodium iodide detector using a wide window encompassing the range of Mo-99 photon energy of 740 to 780 keV. After this a vial of "moly equivalent" cesium-137 is counted in the same configuration. Because the Cs-137 source is calibrated in cpm/µCi of Mo-99, the microcuries of Mo-99 in the eluate can be calculated from its count rate. Alternately, a multichannel analyzer (MCA) calibrated for Mo-99 can be used to perform this test.

The most common method used in hospitals is the lead shield dose calibrator technique.[6] With this method the whole vial of generator eluate is placed into a tightly sealed lead shield that is then placed into the dose calibrator adjusted to read Mo-99 activity. The shield is designed so that all of the 140-keV Tc-99m photons are absorbed by the lead, but approximately 50 percent of the more energetic 740- and 780-keV Mo-99 photons penetrate the shield. The photons that penetrate are counted in the ionization chamber to provide a direct reading in microcuries. The only deficiency in this method is that any radionuclide contaminant with gamma energies capable of penetrating the lead shield will also be counted, thus producing an erroneous reading. This is also true if the wide-window SCA method is used, but not so with the MCA method. In the past this has been a problem with generators contaminated with tellurium-132 that produced iodine-132 in the eluate. Activity levels of I-132 high enough to masquerade as Mo-99 breakthrough have been observed.[7] I-132 has gamma energies ranging from 668 keV to 1398 keV. Fortunately, I-132 has a short half-life, and the contamination quickly diminishes with time. A method to identify I-132 contamination by all three methods has been suggested.[7]

The limits for Mo-99 contamination in Tc-99m eluates have been set by the Nuclear Regulatory Commission (NRC) and the US Pharmacopeia (USP) as follows: Not more than 0.15 µCi Mo-99 per 1 mCi Tc-99m per administered dose at the time of administration.

Accordingly, a 20-mCi dose of Tc-99m could conceivably contain not more than 3 µCi of Mo-99. A convenient method for determining the expiration time for Tc-99m eluates has been devised based on these limits.[8] Table 3–2 lists the expiration time in hours for the Tc-99m based upon the initial ratio of Mo-99/Tc-99m activities at generator elution time. For example, if the initial ratio of Mo-99 microcuries to Tc-99m millicuries is 0.025, the Tc-99m eluate could not be used 17 hours after the time of elution.

The moly breakthrough test is usually negative, indicating no significant Mo-99 contamination. In the past 10 years we have noted only one positive test, but it was very significant and produced 7 mCi of Mo-99 in the generator eluate.[9] In this instance the moly breakthrough was caused by an improperly assembled generator. Without a

TABLE 3-2. EXPIRATION TIMES FOR Tc-99m FOLLOWING GENERATOR ELUTION

Initial µCi Mo-99/mCi Tc-99m	Expires (hr)	Initial µCi Mo-99/mCi Tc-99m	Expires (hr)
0.135	1	0.0108	25
0.122	2	0.0097	26
0.109	3	0.0088	27
0.098	4	0.0079	28
0.089	5	0.0071	29
0.080	6	0.0064	30
0.072	7	0.0058	31
0.065	8	0.0052	32
0.058	9	0.0047	33
0.052	10	0.0042	34
0.047	11	0.0038	35
0.042	12	0.0034	36
0.038	13	0.0031	37
0.034	14	0.0028	38
0.031	15	0.0025	39
0.028	16	0.0022	40
0.025	17	0.0020	41
0.023	18	0.0018	42
0.020	19	0.0016	43
0.018	20	0.0015	44
0.016	21	0.0013	45
0.015	22	0.0012	46
0.013	23	0.0011	47
0.012	24	< 0.0010	48

(Data from Ponto JA, 1981, p. 40.[8])

routine quality control procedure the Mo-99 contamination could easily have gone unnoticed.

TECHNETIUM CONTENT IN GENERATOR ELUATES

Because of the long half-life of Tc-99 the decay of Mo-99 and Tc-99m produces increasing amounts of Tc-99 over time in the generator. In a practical sense this means that eluates from all Mo-99/Tc-99m generators contain both Tc-99m and Tc-99 atoms. The mole fraction of the Tc-99m isomer in the eluate is given by the following relationship[10] where N_1 and N_2 are the number of atoms of Tc-99m and Tc-99 respectively:

$$\frac{N_1}{N \text{ (total)}} = \frac{N_1}{N_1 + N_2} \quad (3\text{-}1)$$

The mole fractions can be calculated from various periods of time from the following equation[8] and are listed in Table 3-3.

$$\frac{N_1}{N \text{ (total)}} = \frac{\lambda_1 (e^{-\lambda_1 t} - e^{-\lambda_2 t})}{\lambda_2 - \lambda_1 (1 - e^{-\lambda_1 t})} \quad (3\text{-}2)$$

TABLE 3-3. Tc-99m MOLE FRACTIONS IN Tc-99m GENERATOR ELUATES[a]

Days Since Prior Elution	Hours Since Prior Elution							
	0	3	6	9	12	15	18	21
0		0.7270	0.6191	0.5315	0.4599	0.4009	0.3520	0.3112
1	0.2769	0.2479	0.2232	0.2020	0.1838	0.1679	0.1540	0.1418
2	0.1311	0.1215	0.1129	0.1053	0.0984	0.0921	0.0865	0.1813
3	0.0766	0.0722	0.0682	0.0646	0.0612	0.0580	0.0551	0.0523
4	0.0498	0.0474	0.0452	0.0431	0.0411	0.0393	0.0375	0.0359

[a]Fraction of technetium in metastable form.

where λ_1 and λ_2 are the decay constants for Tc-99m and Tc-99 respectively. With increasing time of decay, the mole fraction of Tc-99m continuously decreases because of the buildup of Tc-99 atoms. For example, after a 1-day decay the mole fraction of Tc-99m in the generator is 0.2769. In other words, about 28 percent of the total number of technetium atoms in the generator eluate will be Tc-99m; the remainder will be Tc-99. The Tc-99m in generator eluates is not therefore "carrier free," and its specific activity continuously decreases as the period of time between generator elutions increases. This sometimes creates problems with the labeling efficiency in radiopharmaceutical kits that contain small amounts of reducing agent. This becomes most critical when a generator manufactured on a Friday is not eluted until the following Monday morning or over holiday weekends when it may not be eluted until Tuesday. The effect of carrier technetium on the preparation of Tc-99m–human serum albumin is a noteworthy example.[11] This is illustrated in Figure 3–7.

Because the labeling yield of some Tc-99m radiopharmaceuticals depends on the total number of atoms present in the reaction mixture, it is desirable to be able to determine quickly the total number of technetium atoms present in the eluate. This can be accomplished by knowing the Tc-99m activity and its mole fraction present according to the following formula[10]:

$$N \text{ (total)} = \frac{A \text{ (Tc-99m)} (T_{1/2}) (1.443)}{\text{Tc-99m mole fraction}} \quad (3\text{-}3)$$

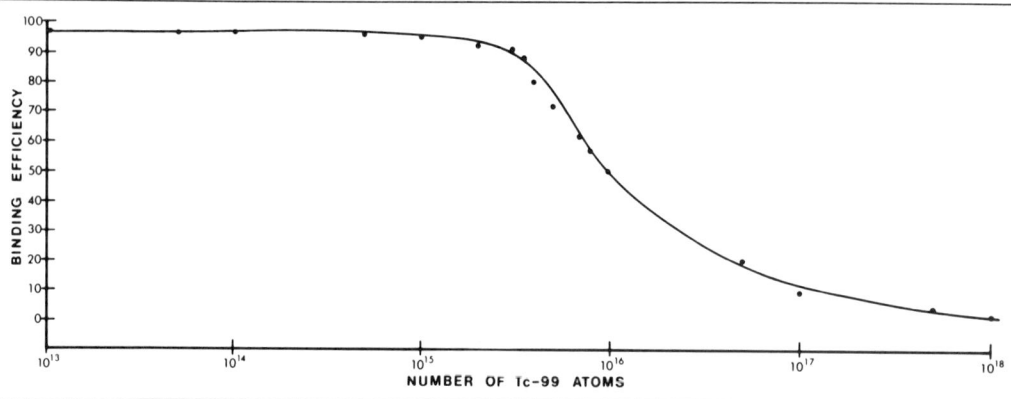

Figure 3–7. Effect of carrier technetium on the labeling efficiency of Tc-99m–albumin. (From Porter WC, et al, 1976, p 704, with permission of the Society of Nuclear Medicine.[11])

Thus, the total number of Tc atoms N (total) per mCi of Tc-99m is given by the following formulas:

N (total) = [1 mCi × (3.7 × 10^7 dps/mCi) × (6.02 hr × 3600 sec/hr) × 1.443] ÷ Tc-99m mole fraction

or

$$N \text{ (total)} = \frac{1.157 \times 10^{12}}{\text{Tc-99m mole fraction}} \text{ atoms/mCi} \quad (3\text{-}4)$$

Table 3–4 lists the total number of Tc atoms per mCi of Tc-99m eluted from a generator for various periods of time calculated from the mole fraction values listed in Table 3–3 and Equation 3–4. Table 3–4 can be used to determine how much Tc-99m eluate should be used for radiolabeling in cases where the Tc-atoms should be limited, such as with the Brookhaven Red Blood Cell Kit.[12] One should note also that Table 3–3 indicates the highest Tc-99m mole fraction is achieved when the generator elution interval is short; thus when preparing kits requiring small amounts of Tc, a practical method, particularly with new generators, is to reelute the generator within a few hours of the first elution and use the second eluate for kit preparation.

Example:

For efficient labeling the Brookhaven kit cannot exceed 1.48 × 10^{14} technetium atoms because of the small amount of stannous ion reducing agent. What is the maximum volume of generator eluate that can be used to label the kit if the generator was eluted 24 hours after the previous elution and the eluate contained 800 mCi Tc-99m in a 20-ml volume?

From Table 3–4 the total amount of Tc eluted per 800 mCi Tc-99m in 24 hours is

(4.18 × 10^{12} atoms/mCi) × 800 mCi
= 3.34 × 10^{15} atoms

The amount of eluate that can be used is

$$\frac{1.48 \times 10^{14}}{3.34 \times 10^{15}} \times 20 \text{ ml} = 0.9 \text{ ml}$$

GENERATOR PHYSICS

In Chapter 2 we considered the radioactive decay process where the daughter products were most often stable nuclides. With generators we must consider the situation when the daughter atoms are radioactive, represented by the following decay sequence:

$$N_1 \xrightarrow{\lambda_1} N_2 \xrightarrow{\lambda_2} N_3$$

where N_1 and N_2 are parent and daughter radionuclides respectively and N_3 is stable or very long-lived. Because we are interested in the daughter radionuclide, its decay rate, dN_2/dt, is described by the following expression:

$$\frac{dN_2}{dt} = \lambda_1 N_1 - \lambda_2 N_2 \quad (3\text{-}5)$$

TABLE 3-4. TOTAL TECHNETIUM ATOMS (Tc-99 + Tc-99m) × 10^{12} PER MILLICURIE Tc-99m ELUTED FROM A Mo-99/Tc-99m GENERATOR

Days Since Prior Elution	Hours Since Prior Elution							
	0	3	6	9	12	15	18	21
0	—	1.59	1.87	2.18	2.52	2.89	3.29	3.72
1	4.18	4.67	5.18	5.73	6.30	6.89	7.51	8.16
2	8.83	9.52	10.25	10.99	11.76	12.56	13.38	14.23
3	15.11	16.03	16.97	17.91	18.91	19.95	21.00	22.12
4	23.23	24.41	25.60	26.85	28.15	29.44	30.86	32.23

The net rate at which the daughter atoms build up is thus just the difference between the rate of their formation by the parent, $\lambda_1 N_1$, and the rate of their own decay, $\lambda_2 N_2$. For the Mo-99/Tc-99m generator, N_1 is the number of Mo-99 atoms and λ_1 its decay constant; N_2 is the number of Tc-99m atoms and λ_2 its decay constant. Even though the third product Tc-99 (N_3) is radioactive, its half-life is so long (2.1×10^5 years) that it is essentially stable and need not be considered in the decay calculations.

After appropriate rearrangement of Equation 3-5, solution of the first-order differential equation yields the following equation[13]:

$$N_2 = \frac{\lambda_1}{\lambda_2 - \lambda_1} N_1^0 (e^{-\lambda_1 t} - e^{-\lambda_2 t}) + N_2^0 e^{-\lambda_2 t} \quad (3-6)$$

$$\underbrace{}_{A} \quad \underbrace{}_{B}$$

where the expressions in bracket A describe the rate of production and decay of daughter Tc-99m atoms and the expression in B describes the contribution to N_2 from any daughter Tc-99m atoms present initially or remaining after generator elution. The last term is significant only if generator elution efficiency is low or if the generator is re-eluted within a few hours since the previous elution. Recalling the expression $N = A/\lambda$, one can substitute the appropriate activity expression into Equation 3-6 and derive the following activity equation:

$$A_2 = \frac{\lambda_2}{\lambda_2 - \lambda_1} A_1^0 (e^{-\lambda_1 t} - e^{-\lambda_2 t}) + A_2^0 e^{-\lambda_2 t} \quad (3-7)$$

Equation 3-7 presumes that 100 percent of parent decays to the daughter. For the Mo-99/Tc-99m generator, the decay to Tc-99m is only 86 percent; therefore, Equation 3-7 is modified as follows:

$$A_2 = \frac{0.86 \, \lambda_2}{\lambda_2 - \lambda_1} A_1^0 (e^{-\lambda_1 t} - e^{-\lambda_2 t}) + A_2^0 e^{-\lambda_2 t} \quad (3-8)$$

Equation 3-8 allows one to calculate the theoretic Tc-99m activity (A_2) present in the generator at any time, t, after the previous elution if one knows the Mo-99 activity (A_1^0) present at the time of the previous elution.

Transient Equilibrium Generators

If the half-life of the parent radionuclide is longer than the daughter half-life, say 10 to 100 times, and a sufficient period of time is allowed to elapse before the generator is eluted, a condition of transient equilibrium is established between the parent and daughter. This is illustrated in Figure 3-8 where line A_2 represents daughter ingrowth and line A_1, parent decay. Immediately after generator elution the rate of daughter production is greater than its rate of decay, and daughter activity increases rapidly with time. As daughter atoms accumulate, they begin to decay such that their rate of decay is equal to the rate of production, and a maximum activity is reached, i.e., $dN_2/dt = 0$ and $A_1 = A_2$ (point X). It should be noted that $A_1 = A_2$ only if 100 percent of the parent decays to the daughter. The broken line A_2 represents the situation with the Tc-99m generator where 86 percent of the Mo-99 decays to Tc-99m. The time required to reach the maximum daughter activity in a generator is derived from Equation 3-6 and is given by the following:

$$t_{max} = \frac{1}{\lambda_2 - \lambda_1} \ln \frac{\lambda_2}{\lambda_1} \quad (3-9)$$

In the Mo-99/Tc-99m generator the time to the maximum Tc-99m activity is 23 hours.[4] Beyond this point the daughter activity exceeds that of the parent but eventually reaches the point of *transient equilibrium* where the ratio of the daughter and parent activities is a constant (point Y) and the daughter from then on appears to decay with the parent half-life (66.7 hours). This is the case, however, only for a parent–daughter mixture in equilibrium. If the daughter is separated from the parent and its activity alone plotted with time, line B is obtained whose slope gives the true half-

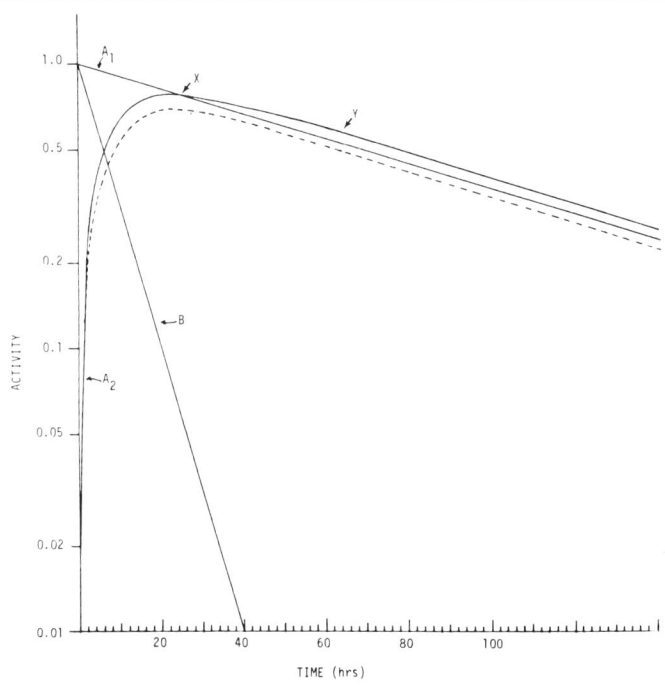

Figure 3-8. Transient equilibrium in the Mo-99/Tc-99m generator.

life of the daughter (6.03 hours for Tc-99m). The time required to achieve transient equilibrium in the Mo-99/Tc-99m generator is on the order of 48 to 72 hours. At this point, the time of decay since the previous elution has become so large that the value of the exponential term $e^{-\lambda_2 t}$ in equations 3-7 and 3-8 becomes very small compared with $e^{-\lambda_1 t}$ because λ_2 is much greater than λ_1. Equation 3-8 therefore simplifies to the following expression at transient equilibrium:

$$A_2 = \frac{0.86 \, \lambda_2}{\lambda_2 - \lambda_1} A_1^0 \, e^{-\lambda_1 t} \quad (3\text{-}10)$$

The ratio $\lambda_2/(\lambda_2 - \lambda_1)$ is numerically equal to 1.1, making the constant term in equation 3-10 equal to 0.946, i.e., (0.86 × 1.1). Furthermore, the term $A_1^0 e^{-\lambda_1 t}$ is equal to the activity of Mo-99 present in the generator after transient equilibrium is established. The actual Tc-99m activity present in the generator at transient equilibrium is therefore given as 0.946 times the Mo-99 activity present. Tc-99m activity can also be determined from broken line A_2 in Figure 3-8. It should be kept in mind that Equation 3-10 is valid for the calculation of Tc-99m activity only after extended decay time (48 to 72 hours) since the previous generator elution. For times less than 48 hours, Equation 3-8 should be used although Tc-99m activities calculated with Equation 3-10 at 24 hours will be about 92 percent of those calculated with Equation 3-8. Table 3-5 lists various relationships between Tc-99m and Mo-99 activities in the generator at various times after elution.

Examples:

1. A Mo-99/Tc-99m generator is manufactured on a Friday calibrated for 2.5 Ci of Mo-99 at 8:00 PM. Calculate the theoretic Tc-99m activity in the generator on the following Monday at 8:00 AM if

TABLE 3-5. RELATIONSHIP BETWEEN Tc-99m AND Mo-99 IN THE GENERATOR AT VARIOUS TIMES AFTER ELUTION

Time (hr)	Curies Mo-99	×	Ratio Tc-99m/Mo-99	=	Curies Tc-99m[a]
0	1.000		—		0
1	0.990		0.094		0.093
2	0.979		0.179		0.175
3	0.969		0.255		0.247
4	0.959		0.324		0.311
5	0.949		0.386		0.366
6	0.940		0.441		0.414
12	0.883		0.677		0.598
18	0.829		0.803		0.666
24	0.779		0.870		0.678
36	0.688		0.924		0.636
48	0.607		0.940		0.571
60	0.536		0.944		0.506
72	0.473		0.946		0.448
78	0.445		0.946		0.421

[a]Actual Tc-99m present based upon 86.05 percent Mo-99 decay to Tc-99m.

no previous elutions have been made. The decay constants are as follows:

$$\lambda_1 \text{ (Mo-99)} = \frac{0.693}{66.7 \text{ hr}} = 0.01039 \text{ hr}^{-1}$$

$$\lambda_2 \text{ (Tc-99m)} = \frac{0.693}{6.03 \text{ hr}} = 0.1149 \text{ hr}^{-1}$$

The time of decay is 60 hours, so Equation 3-10 can be used. Thus,

$$A \text{ (Tc-99m)} = (0.86) \frac{0.1149}{0.1149 - 0.01039}$$

$$2.5 \text{ Ci } e^{-0.01039 \text{ hr}^{-1} (60 \text{ hr})}$$

A (Tc-99m) = (0.86) (1.1) (2.5) (0.536)

A (Tc-99m) = 1.27 Ci

Alternatively, one may use the data in Table 3-5 to solve this problem. Mo-99 activity after a 60-hour decay is:

2.5 Ci (0.536) = 1.34 Ci

Multiply this value by the Tc-99m/Mo-99 ratio at 60 hours

1.34 Ci (0.944) = 1.27 Ci Tc-99m

2. If the activity actually eluted from the generator in Example 1 was 1.08 Ci, what is the elution efficiency?

$$\text{Percent elution efficiency} = \frac{\text{Measured activity}}{\text{Theoretic Activity}} \times 100$$

$$\frac{1.08 \text{ Ci}}{1.27 \text{ Ci}} \times 100 = 85 \text{ percent}$$

3. A Mo-99/Tc-99m generator is eluted at 11:00 AM. If a previous elution of 0.400 Ci was made at 6:00 AM the same day and the Mo-99 activity present at that time was 0.5 Ci, calculate the Tc-99m activity expected in the 11:00 AM elution if the generator elution efficiency is 85 percent.

Because transient equilibrium is not established since the previous elution, Equation 3-8 must be used. The residual Tc-99m activity remaining on the column after the 6:00 AM elution is estimated as follows:

$$\frac{0.400 \text{ Ci}}{0.85} = 0.470 \text{ Ci Tc-99m present on the column at 6:00 AM}$$

Therefore (0.470 Ci) − (0.400 Ci eluted) = (0.070 Ci retained. From Equation 3–8 the Tc-99m present on the column at 11:00 AM is as follows:

$$A(\text{Tc-99m}) = (0.86)(1.1)(0.5 \text{ Ci}) \\ (e^{-0.01039(5)} \\ - e^{-0.1149(5)}) \\ + 0.70 \text{Ci } e^{-0.1149(5)}$$

$$A(\text{Tc-99m}) = 0.183 \text{ Ci} + 0.039 \text{ Ci} \\ = 0.222 \text{ Ci}$$

Alternatively, one may use Table 3–5 to solve the problem.
Tc-99m activity from 5 hours of Mo-99 decay is:

(0.5 Ci) (0.949) (0.386) = 0.183 Ci

Tc-99m activity from 5 hours of residual Tc-99m decay is:

(0.070 Ci) (0.563) = 0.039 Ci

Total Tc-99m present = 0.183 Ci + 0.039 Ci = 0.222 Ci

Because the elution efficiency is 85 percent, the expected Tc-99m activity in the generator eluate is as follows:

(0.222 Ci) (0.85) = 0.189 Ci

Secular Equilibrium Generators

If the half-life of the parent is much longer than the daughter's, say 1000 times or more, the parent will not decay appreciably during several daughter half-lives, and a condition of secular equilibrium is established. As in the case with transient equilibrium generators, the rate of daughter production initially is greater than its rate of decay, and daughter activity increases rapidly over time (line A_2 in Figure 3–9). When the rate of production equals the rate of decay, secular equilibrium is established (intersection of lines A_1 and A_2). In this condition the daughter appears to decay with the parent half-life. Because of the large difference in decay constants ($\lambda_2 >>> \lambda_1$) the value of λ_1 is insignificant compared with λ_2, and the

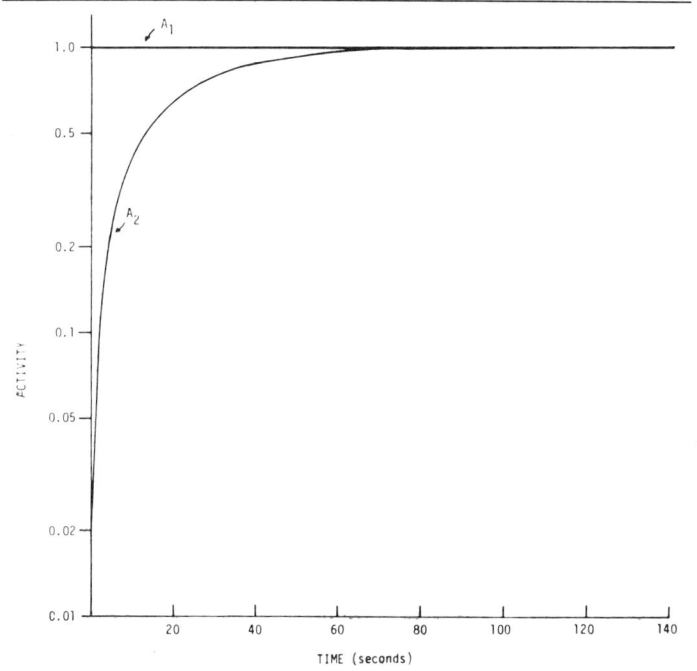

Figure 3-9. Secular equilibrium in the rubidium-81/krypton-81m generator.

constant term $\lambda_2/(\lambda_2 - \lambda_1)$ in Equation 3–7 approaches unity.

Additionally, at secular equilibrium the $e^{-\lambda_2 t}$ terms approach zero, and therefore Equation 3–7 is simplified to the following:

$$A_2 = A_1^0 e^{-\lambda_1 t} \qquad (3-11)$$

That is to say, at secular equilibrium the daughter activity is equal to the parent activity present in the generator.

Some examples of secular equilibrium generators are as follows:

$^{226}\text{Ra} \xrightarrow{1600 \text{ yr}} {}^{222m}\text{Rn} \xrightarrow{3.8 \text{ d}} {}^{218}\text{Po}$

$^{113}\text{Sn} \xrightarrow{115 \text{ d}} {}^{113m}\text{In} \xrightarrow{99.4 \text{ min}} {}^{113}\text{In}$

$^{81}\text{Rb} \xrightarrow{4.7 \text{ hr}} {}^{81m}\text{Kr} \xrightarrow{13 \text{ sec}} {}^{81}\text{Kr}$

Secular equilibrium for the Rb-81/Kr-81m generator is illustrated in Figure 3–9.

DISPOSAL OF GENERATORS

Generator manufacturers provide a return program for used Tc-99m generators. Usually when the new generator is received, the old one is placed into the empty shipping carton, sealed, surveyed, and shipped back to the manufacturer for credit. A certain amount of paperwork is involved for the proper shipment of used generators to comply with Department of Transportation regulations.

Some hospitals choose to decay the old generators to background levels of radioactivity, dismantle them, and discard the generator columns in regular trash. Because fission–moly generators may contain long-lived radiocontaminants such as ruthenium-103 (39.5 day half-life), it has been determined that old generators should be held for 14 weeks before discarding. After this time the generator columns may be removed, surveyed with a Geiger-Müller meter, and disposed of in regular trash if the surface exposure rate is 0.2 mR/hr or less.

REFERENCES

1. Stang LG Jr, Tucker WD, Doering RF, et al: Development of methods for the production of certain short-lived radioisotopes. Proceedings of the first UNESCO Conference, Vol 1, Paris, 1957, p 50
2. Harper PV, Andros G, Lathrop K: Preliminary observations on the use of six-hour Tc-99m as a tracer in biology and medicine. USAEC Report ACRH-18, 1962, p 788
3. Arino H, Kramer HH: Fission product Tc-99m generator. Int J Appl Radiat Isot 26:301, 1975
4. Lamson M III, Hotte CE, Ice RD: Practical generator kinetics. J Nucl Med Tech 4:21, 1976
5. Vesely P, Cifka J: Some chemical and analytical problems connected with technetium-99m generators. In Radiopharmaceuticals from Generator-Produced Radionuclides. Vienna, IAEA, 1971, p 71
6. Richards P, O'Brien MJ: Rapid determination of Mo-99 in separated Tc-99m. J Nucl Med 10:517, 1969
7. Briner WH, Harris CC: Radionuclidic contamination of eluates from fission product molybdenum–technetium generators. (Letter to Editor.) J Nucl Med 15:466, 1974
8. Ponto JA: Expiration times for Tc-99m. J Nucl Med Tech 9:40, 1981
9. Kowalsky RJ, Preslar J: Report of a positive Mo-99 breakthrough test. J Nucl Med Tech 2:108, 1979
10. Lamson ML III, Kirschner AS, Hotte CE, et al: Generator-produced 99m TcO_4^-: Carrier free? J Nucl Med 16:639, 1975
11. Porter WC, Dworkin HJ, Gutkowski RF: The effect of carrier technetium in the preparation of Tc-99m–human serum albumin. J Nucl Med 17:704, 1976
12. Smith TD, Richards P: A simple kit for the preparation of Tc-99m–labeled red blood cells. J Nucl Med 17:126, 1976
13. Friedlander G, Kennedy JW, Miller JM: Nuclear and Radiochemistry, 2nd ed. New York, Wiley, 1966

CHAPTER 4

Chemistry of Radiopharmaceuticals

A radiopharmaceutical is a chemical substance containing radioactive atoms within its structure that is administered to humans for diagnostic or therapeutic purposes. Furthermore, because radiopharmaceuticals undergo distribution, metabolism, and excretion within the body, sealed radionuclide sources are not considered to be radiopharmaceuticals. Additionally, radiopharmaceuticals differ from radiochemicals in that radiopharmaceuticals have met specific requirements of the Food and Drug Administration, permitting them to be used in humans in a safe and effective manner.

There are a few characteristics of radiopharmaceuticals that make them unique. Because of the trace amounts of substance administered, radiopharmaceuticals are considered to be subpharmacologic and therefore do not elicit a physiologic response. Although their chemical toxicity is nil, a radiation risk must be considered with their use. Radiopharmaceuticals are used almost exclusively for diagnostic purposes although a few therapeutic applications exist.

IDEAL PROPERTIES OF DIAGNOSTIC RADIOPHARMACEUTICALS

One may divide the diagnostic agents into two categories of use: in vivo function and imaging.

In vivo function agents trace or mimic certain bodily processes without altering the process in any way so that a true measure of function can be obtained. Noteworthy examples are the use of I-131 sodium iodide to measure thyroid function, cobalt-57 cyanocobalamin to assess vitamin B_{12} metabolism, and chromium-51-labeled red blood cells to determine blood volume. With such studies, the radioactive agent is administered to humans, and the specific bodily function is determined by counting radioactivity emanating directly from the body or from urine or blood samples. A most important aspect of these studies is that the chemical integrity of the radiotracer not be altered by the radiolabeling procedure.

Imaging agents are selected for use by virtue of their ability to localize within specific organs. Images may then be obtained with the gamma camera regarding organ morphology (size, shape, position, or presence of space-occupying lesions) and organ function. From a theoretic standpoint the ideal imaging agent should rapidly and avidly localize within the organ of interest, remain there for the duration of study, and be quickly excreted from the body thereafter. Clearly no such agent exists, and judicious selection of radionuclide and chemical form must be combined to achieve the best compromise. Table 4–1 lists several properties of the ideal radionuclide for diagnostic imaging.

Decay Mode and Energy

Electromagnetic radiation (gamma and x-rays) are the only suitable forms for external detection. Particulate radiation, being completely absorbed by tissue, renders a high radiation burden. The most desirable decay modes for diagnostic imaging therefore are electron capture and isomeric transition from metastable nuclides because there are no primary particle radiations associated with these processes. Additionally, to assure a high yield of detectable photons the extent of internal conversion should be minimal.

The energy of gamma rays should be high enough to readily penetrate and escape

TABLE 4-1. IDEAL PROPERTIES OF RADIONUCLIDES FOR DIAGNOSTIC IMAGING

1. **Decay Mode:** Electron capture or isomeric transition from metastable states; no particulate radiation; gamma or x-rays only.
2. **Photon Energy:** Ideally 100–200 keV; below 100 keV there is tissue absorption and scatter; above 200 keV there is low detection efficiency.
3. **Half-life:** Effective half-life equal to 1 to 1.5 times the imaging time.
4. **Chemical Reactivity:** Ability to be compounded into several chemical forms.

TABLE 4-2. PHOTON DETECTION EFFICIENCY IN A HALF-INCH SODIUM IODIDE CRYSTAL

Radionuclide	Photon Energy (keV)	Detector Efficiency %
Xenon-133	81	92
Technetium-99m	140	86
Indium-111	172	73
	247	45
Iodine-131	364	23
Positron emitters	511	13

(Adapted from Anger HO, 1967.[1])

from the body, yet low enough to be efficiently stopped by the gamma camera detector. Table 4–2 lists the detection efficiencies of different radionuclide photon energies in a sodium iodide crystal detector.

Half-life

The rate of loss of radioactivity from an organ or the body is directly proportional to the rates of physical decay of the radionuclide and of biologic excretion. Both processes are usually operational, and one typically refers to the effective rate of removal. Because the removal rate is inversely proportional to half-life, one may obtain an expression that relates effective half-life (Te) to physical half-life (Tp) and biologic half-life (Tb) as follows:

$$\text{Te} = \frac{\text{Tp} \times \text{Tb}}{\text{Tp} + \text{Tb}} \qquad (4\text{--}1)$$

The effective half-life is therefore the time required to remove half of the radioactivity from an organ by a combination of physical decay and biologic elimination. Te is always less than either Tp or Tb but will be nearly equal to the smaller function when the other is very large. This is illustrated by the following example: calculate the effective half-life for a radiopharmaceutical if (1) Tp is 1 hour and Tb is 10 hours, (2) Tp and Tb are equal, say 10 hours, and (3) Tp is 10 hours and Tb is 1 hour.

1. $Te = \dfrac{1 \times 10}{1 + 10} = \dfrac{10}{11} = 0.91$ hours

2. $Te = \dfrac{10 \times 10}{10 + 10} = \dfrac{100}{20} = 5.0$ hours

3. $Te = \dfrac{10 \times 1}{10 + 1} = \dfrac{10}{11} = 0.91$ hours

It is evident that if a radiopharmaceutical has a very long biologic elimination rate Te will be approximately equal to Tp. From an imaging standpoint the optimum Te should be about 1 to 1.5 times the period of observation or study time.[2] This time provides enough radioactivity for a good count rate and a removal rate that diminishes the radiation dose. In practice, however, it is very difficult to achieve an optimum balance between imaging time and Te.

One must be aware of Te in clinical studies. For instance, a radiopharmaceutical having a long Te will remain in the body for a prolonged time period and may interfere with subsequent diagnostic imaging or in vivo function studies.

In some instances, rapid biologic elimination of the tracer dominates so that the convenience of a long Tp (and shelf life) may be gained. An example is the use of xenon-127 (Tp = 36.4 days) in lieu of Xe-133 (Tp = 5.3 days) for lung ventilation studies. A trade-off, however, is that radioactive contamination may become a problem with long-half-lived nuclides.

The type of study sometimes dictates the half-life of the radionuclide selected for use. For example, cisternography studies may require 2 to 3 days for completion in which case 2.8-day In-111 DTPA is the agent of choice. Six-hour Tc-99m agents are generally unsatisfactory for studies beyond 1 day although Tc-99m DTPA may be a satisfactory choice for cerebrospinal fluid (CSF) leak studies, which require only a few hours to complete.

Desirable Chemistry

A radionuclide ideally should have chemical properties that allow it to be reacted into different chemical forms useful as biologic tracers. For example, radioiodine has the advantage of a diversified chemistry whereby it may be used as the simple iodide anion for thyroid studies or it may be incorporated as a radiolabel into other iodine-containing compounds such as radioiodinated Hippuran for kidney studies or into protein substances, antibodies, and antigens for a variety of biologic studies.

RADIOPHARMACEUTICAL DEVELOPMENT

Figure 4–1 illustrates the small number of elements available that have radioisotopes that possess the necessary properties for nuclear medicine studies. Because this number is limited, the development of radiopharmaceuticals has oftentimes followed the empiric approach. That is, select a radionuclide with favorable nuclear properties, manipulate its chemical and physical form, and perform biodistribution studies with the purpose of finding a useful tracer. Examples include the labeling of proteins, the complexation of radionuclide metals with chelating agents, or simply the adjustment of pH to form insoluble colloidal particles. This approach has been moderately successful with some of the earlier Tc-99m and In-113m nuclides.

A more rational approach is to combine knowledge of both the physiology and biochemistry of various organ systems and the properties of certain compounds to produce a suitable radiotracer. The replacement of a stable atom in a compound with its radioisotope is called *isotopic labeling*. It results in a radiotracer that is physiologically identical to the nonradioactive parent molecule. Although this approach is ideal, it is limited by the choice of radionuclides available. Biologic molecules and drugs are mostly composed of the elements carbon, hydrogen, oxygen, nitrogen, phosphorus, and sulfur; however, the physical properties of these elements are generally unsatisfactory for diagnostic

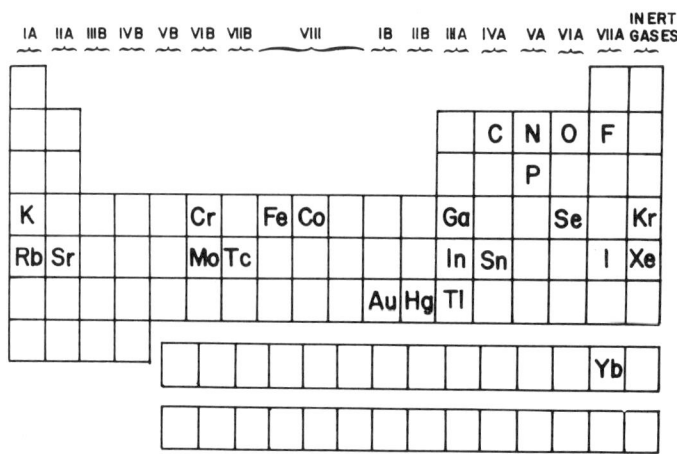

Figure 4-1. Elements that have radioisotopes useful for diagnostic application in nuclear medicine.

studies. The primary limitations are half-life, decay mode, photon energy, and availability. The limited properties of these nuclides are listed in Table 4-3.

A few of the isotopically labeled tracers that currently are or have been used in nuclear medicine are iodide I-131 for thyroid studies, cyanocobalamin Co-57 for vitamin B_{12} metabolism studies, ferrous citrate iron-59 for ferrokinetic studies, sodium phosphate P-32 for treatment of polycythemia vera, and chlormerodrin mercury-203 or mercury-197 for kidney scans. Compounds labeled with carbon-11, nitrogen-13, or oxygen-15 are not satisfactory for routine studies because they require a cyclotron for production, their half-lives are very short, and a positron camera is needed for detection. Studies with these agents are limited to major research centers.

Because of the aforementioned limitations, it is often necessary to introduce into a molecule a radionuclide not previously present—a process called *nonisotopic labeling* or "foreign labeling." Although this is not the ideal method of labeling, many useful radiopharmaceuticals have been developed using this technique.

Some examples of various types of radiopharmaceuticals developed for nuclear medicine studies based upon empiric and rational approaches to design are given as follows:

1. Many metallic radionuclides, if not chelated, will readily hydrolyze in neutral

TABLE 4-3. PROPERTIES OF ISOTOPIC LABELS FOR BIOLOGIC MOLECULES

Nuclide	Decay Mode	Half-life	Photon Energy
S-35	β^-	87 d	No photons
P-32	β^-	14.3 d	No photons
H-3	β^-	12.3 y	No photons
C-14	β^-	5730 y	No photons
C-11	β^+	20 min	511 keV
N-13	β^+	10 min	511 keV
O-15	β^+	2 min	511 keV

aqueous solution to form insoluble hydrated oxides or hydroxides. Because of the small mass present they do not precipitate from solution but disperse into fine colloidal particles. Examples include colloidal gold-198, indium-113m phosphate and hydroxide colloids, and tin-reduced Tc-99m colloid. The fact that foreign particles are removed from the blood by the phagocytic action of the reticuloendothelial system provides a means to evaluate the liver, spleen, and bone marrow with these radiocolloids.

2. The ability of sodium chromate Cr-51 to label red blood cells without significant elution provides a method to measure red cell mass by isotope dilution analysis.

3. Radioiodinated human serum albumin provided one of the first agents to image the blood pool and measure plasma volume by isotope dilution analysis.

4. The normal function of splenic sequestration of effete red blood cells provides a mechanism to image the spleen after the administration of radiolabeled, heat-denatured red blood cells.

5. Heat denaturation of radiolabeled human serum albumin produces aggregate particles large enough to be mechanically lodged in the lung arteriolar-capillary bed. These radiolabeled particles produce a lung scan and a method for evaluating regional pulmonary blood flow for the detection of pulmonary emboli.

6. Ion exchange and transport mechanisms in the body provide a means to evaluate various organs with radionuclides.
    a. Heart muscle perfusion can be studied with potassium-43 and potassium analogues such as thallium-201. These ions mimic the distribution of potassium ion in the myocardium, thus providing a means to evaluate ischemia and infarction.
    b. In bone imaging, fluoride-18 exchanges for hydroxyl ions in hydroxyapatite crystals in bone whereas Tc-99m phosphate and phosphonate complexes chemisorb to calcium ions on the bone surface.
    c. Imaging the thyroid gland is possible with pertechnetate ion, which is actively trapped in the gland because its ionic charge and molecular volume are similar to iodide.[3]
    d. Agents for evaluating liver and kidney function were developed based upon the ability of these organs to excrete certain ionic substances. When no suitable label for para-aminohippurate could be prepared to measure kidney function, a compound with similar properties, orthoiodohippurate, was used because it could be labeled with radioiodine. Similarly, the anionic radioiodinated fluorescein dye rose bengal is excreted into the bile by active transport through the hepatocytes and was the first radiopharmaceutical used in nuclear medicine to evaluate hepatobiliary function.

7. Radiotracer design based upon biochemical processes in the body led to several useful compounds.
    a. The classic example is the use of radioiodide to study thyroid function.
    b. Development of the radioactive methionine bioisostere selenomethionine Se-75 used to image the pancreas was based upon the high turnover of amino acids in this organ in the production of digestive enzymes.
    c. The ability to image the adrenal cortex was made possible with 19-iodocholesterol labeled with I-131. Its development was based on the incorporation of cholesterol precursors into steroid hormones by the adrenal gland.
    d. One can also include in this category the use of radiolabeled glucose and its analogues 2-deoxy-D-glucose labeled with C-11 and F-18 to map oxidative metabolism in the brain.

8. Many radiopharmaceuticals are chelates of radionuclide metals. Some of the chelates of DTPA (Tc-99m and In-111) were developed for kidney studies because of the well-known excretion of

chelates by glomerular filtration in the treatment of heavy-metal poisoning. The biodistribution of these monofunctional chelates is determined primarily by the properties of the chelating agent. An extension of this approach is the development of bifunctional chelates. These agents contain a chelating moiety to bind the radionuclide and a drug moiety that can be modified with various chemical substituents to alter the molecule's biodistribution. Noteworthy examples of this class of agents are the N-substituted iminodiacetic acid analogues labeled with Tc-99m used in hepatobiliary imaging. A most interesting finding with these agents is that the technetium atom present in the compound, although considered to be a foreign label, is essential for the radiopharmaceutical's excretion by the hepatocyte.

The desire for site-specific localization of radiotracers has placed more emphasis on the development of agents based upon the receptor-specific approach. This approach is based upon the well-known structure–activity relationship concept whereby a drug molecule reacts with a specific biologic receptor molecule because of their complimentary chemical structures, and the interaction produces a response. The development of receptor-binding radiotracers for the autonomic nervous system and radiolabeled monoclonal antibodies for tumor-associated antigens are examples. A useful classification of radiopharmaceuticals has been suggested based on their mechanism of localization that catagorizes them into two groups: substrate nonspecific and substrate specific.[4] Accordingly, substrate-nonspecific agents do not participate in a specific chemical reaction. Radiopharmaceuticals that localize by diffusion, compartmental confinement, capillary blockade, cell sequestration, and phagocytosis are examples. Substrate-specific agents must participate in a definite chemical reaction or take part in a specific ligand-substrate interaction. Examples are radiotracers that localize by entering into biochemical or metabolic processes involving enzyme systems, protein receptors, or antigen-antibody reactions. These approaches to radiopharmaceutical design present only some of the well-known examples and are not an exhaustive description of all methods used. A more complete discussion of this topic can be found in other reference works.[3,5]

CHEMICAL BONDING

The three basic types of chemical bonds, namely, the ionic or electrovalent bond, the covalent or electron-sharing bond, and the coordinate covalent bond, characterize the bonding of radionuclides in radiopharmaceutical agents.

Ionic bonds, characterized by the association of a negatively charged species with a positively charged species, are relatively weak bonds and are easily dissociated when a substance is dissolved in aqueous solution. Examples are I-131 sodium iodide and Tc-99m sodium pertechnetate, which yield iodide ($^{131}I^-$) and pertechnetate ($^{99m}TcO_4^-$) anions, respectively in aqueous solution.

Covalent bonds, whereby each of two species donates one electron to the bond, are much stronger and usually do not dissociate in solution unless the molecule is acted upon by some metabolic or chemical process. An example is I-131 O-iodohippurate in which the radioiodide is covalently bound at the *ortho* position of the aromatic ring. In the coordinate covalent bond one species donates a pair of electrons to the other species to form the bond.

A complex may be defined as a species formed by the association of two or more simpler species, each capable of independent existence. When one of the simpler species is a metal ion, the resulting entity is known as a metal complex. Many radiopharmaceuticals are characterized by complex formation between a metallic radionuclide and a complexing agent (ligand). A ligand is a molecule containing functional groups capable of bonding with a metal ion

Figure 4-2. Chemical structure of the disodium calcium EDTA chelate.

to form a complex. A complex may contain ionic, covalent, and coordinate covalent bonds. If several sites within the ligand bind to the metal ion, simultaneously forming a ring structure, the resultant species is called a *chelate*, and the ligand is called a chelating agent. An example is the chelation of calcium ion with ethylenediamine tetraacetic acid sodium salt (Na_2EDTA) (Fig. 4-2). Many natural substances are chelates including chlorophyll, hemoglobin, vitamin B_{12}, and insulin.

The formation of a metal complex or a chelate may result in precipitation of the metal or, usually, formation of a soluble compound. Chelation suppresses certain reactions of a metal without removal of the metal from the system. One example in nuclear medicine is the chelation of aluminum ion by EDTA in Tc-99m sulfur colloid injection, which prevents the aluminum ion from reacting with phosphate buffers to form insoluble aluminum phosphate. Another example is the chelation of tin and reduced species of technetium in radiopharmaceutical kits, which suppresses unwanted hydrolysis of these metal ions in neutral aqueous solutions. Chelation, however, does not suppress the desired redox reactions between tin and technetium and may even enhance them.

RADIOLABELING CHEMISTRY

This section will discuss the radiolabeling reactions involved with the most widely used radionuclides, technetium and iodine, because their radiopharmaceuticals represent greater than 90 percent of all agents used in nuclear medicine. The chemistry and preparation techniques of other radiopharmaceuticals will be covered in later chapters that deal specifically with them.

TECHNETIUM

Element 43, technetium, was discovered in 1937 by Perrier and Segrè[6] in a sample of molybdenum that was irradiated by deuterons. The new element was named after the Greek word *technetos*, meaning artificial, because technetium was the first element previously unknown on earth to be made artificially. Since then 21 isotopes of technetium have been discovered, ranging from Tc-90 through Tc-110. Tc-110 has the shortest half-life (0.86 sec) and Tc-97 the longest (2.6×10^6 years). All isotopes of technetium are radioactive.

In 1939 Seaborg and Segrè[7] observed that molybdenum-98 irradiated with slow neutrons gave rise to Tc-99 through decay of the metastable isomer, Tc-99m.

In the 1950s purification work on the tellurium-132/iodine-132 generator at Brookhaven National Laboratory (BNL) turned up a contaminant that proved to be technetium. Its presence was due to Mo-99, which also was present, because it had followed tellurium in the chemical separation process.[8] This discovery eventually led to the production of the Mo-99/Tc-99m generator in 1957 at BNL. Final improvements were made by Powell Richards.[8] The simplified decay scheme for Tc-99m production is shown in the following illustration. Mo-99 can be produced either by neutron activation or as a fission by-product. The latter method is now used in Tc-99m generator production.

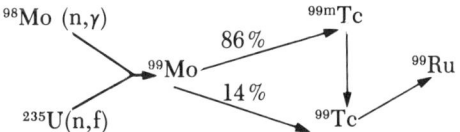

Technetium was introduced into clinical use at the University of Chicago by

Harper et al.[9] The generator yielded technetium as pertechnetate ion TcO_4^-. After injection into mice the activity was found to localize in the thyroid, salivary glands, stomach, and urinary bladder, similar to iodide ion. These early studies identified the advantages of Tc-99m:

1. Short but reasonable half-life of 6 hours
2. High photon yield (88 percent) of 140 keV gave good tissue penetration but was easily collimated and stopped by the detector
3. No beta radiation resulting in a low radiation dose
4. Availability in a generator for in-hospital use
5. Chemically reactive, yielding other chemical forms

Although the 6-hour half-life was advantageous from an imaging standpoint, it created the necessity for radiopharmaceutical preparation, purification, and testing within the hospital. This resulted in the employment of radiochemists and radiopharmacists in nuclear medicine who subsequently developed new technetium radiopharmaceuticals, kits, and techniques.

Technetium Chemistry

Technetium is positioned in the periodic table along with manganese and rhenium, but its chemistry is more similar to rhenium. As a transition metal in group VIIB, technetium has seven electrons beyond the noble gas configuration and readily loses these electrons to yield the 7 + oxidation state of pertechnetate, TcO_4^-. Although this is the most stable state in aqueous solution, oxidation states from 1 − to 7 + have been reported. For this reason technetium exhibits a diverse chemistry that allows it to be incorporated into a variety of chemical forms to be used as radiopharmaceuticals.

As pertechnetate, technetium will not bind to other chemical species. Being an oxidizing agent, however, it can be reduced to positively charged species that will complex to a variety of ligands. The only exception to this is Tc-99m sulfur colloid in which technetium is considered to maintain the 7 + oxidation state by virtue of its stability as insoluble technetium hepta-sulfide, Tc_2S_7.[10]

Reduced states of technetium can be achieved by suitable reducing agents, most notably stannous ion. Other systems have been used including ferrous ion, ferric ion with ascorbic acid, sodium borohydride, concentrated HCl, and electrolysis. The primary disadvantage of these latter methods is incomplete labeling yields necessitating a purification step to remove unbound pertechnetate. Stannous ion, however, is a powerful reducing agent capable of producing quantitative yields of technetium-labeled compounds. Its use ultimately led to the introduction of "instant" kits for the preparation of Tc-99m radiopharmaceuticals.[11]

Tc-99m Kits

A radiopharmaceutical kit is simply a sterile reaction vial containing the nonradioactive chemicals required to produce a specific radiopharmaceutical after reaction with Tc-99m pertechnetate. The primary chemical substances present in the kit are a complexing agent (ligand) and a reducing agent, usually stannous chloride. Other substances such as stabilizers and dispersing agents may be present.

The radiopharmaceutical kit is usually prepared by adding an acidified stannous chloride solution to a solution of the complexing agent at a defined pH. Aliquots of the final mixture are dispensed into presterilized serum vials and frozen. The frozen product is then lyophilized under vacuum to remove all water, and the vials are backfilled with nitrogen gas before sealing. See Figure 4–3 for stepwise kit production.

The complexing agent is present usually in a 10- to 20-molar excess over the amount of tin to assure that all of the tin, as stannous ion and any stannic ion, will be complexed. Uncomplexed tin at neutral pH will readily hydrolyze to form the insoluble hydroxide. In other words, the complexing agent sequesters the tin from the hydrolysis reaction. As we shall see, however, it does

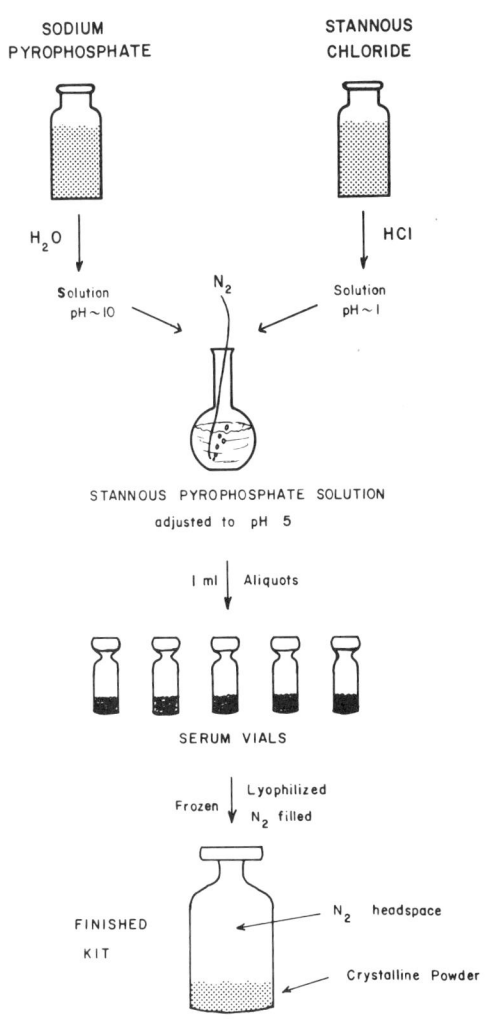

Figure 4-3. Stepwise procedure for production of the stannous pyrophosphate kit.

not prevent tin from entering into oxidation–reduction reactions.

Stannous ion is a strong reducing agent and is easily oxidized by atmospheric and dissolved oxygen. All solutions are therefore purged with nitrogen, and kits are prepared under a nitrogen atmosphere to exclude oxygen. To illustrate some of the problems encountered in the preparation of kits containing stannous tin, consider, as an example, the production of stannous pyrophosphate kits. During kit production a solution of stannous ion is prepared. This can be accomplished either by dissolving stannous chloride or high-purity elemental tin wire in concentrated HCl followed by dilution with water. The latter method produces higher initial titers of stannous ion. Some initial heating of the HCl solution is usually required to facilitate dissolution of the wire or any stannous oxychloride present in the stannous chloride crystals. A problem with either method, however, is that the stannous ion in solution will readily oxidize, and therefore the water used and the final tin solution must be kept under a nitrogen-purged condition. Other inert gases such as argon can be used in lieu of nitrogen. Bubbling nitrogen gas through water will readily dispel dissolved oxygen within a short time as shown in Figure 4-4. In the absence of a nitrogen blanket tin solutions readily degrade. This process is illustrated in Figure 4-5, which demonstrates the stability of stannous pyrophosphate solution prepared and stored under various conditions.

Once a stable solution of the stannous complex is formed, kits are prepared by dispensing small aliquots, usually 1 ml, into serum vials. This process is performed under aseptic conditions in a sterile air environment, usually in a laminar airflow hood. To preserve the kit for long-term storage the product is then frozen and freeze-dried. This process removes the water from the product, leaving a dried crystalline powder. Before the freeze-drying operation, however, while the kits are being prepared in the laminar air flow hood, significant oxidation of stannous ion can take place in the vials because of the moving air environment. One effective method of retarding oxidation in this situation is to precool the vials by some method. Placing vials on a bed of dry ice works very well because the solution freezes immediately after it is placed into the vials. Figure 4-6 illustrates the stability of stannous pyrophosphate vials filled in a laminar airflow hood under liquid and frozen conditions.

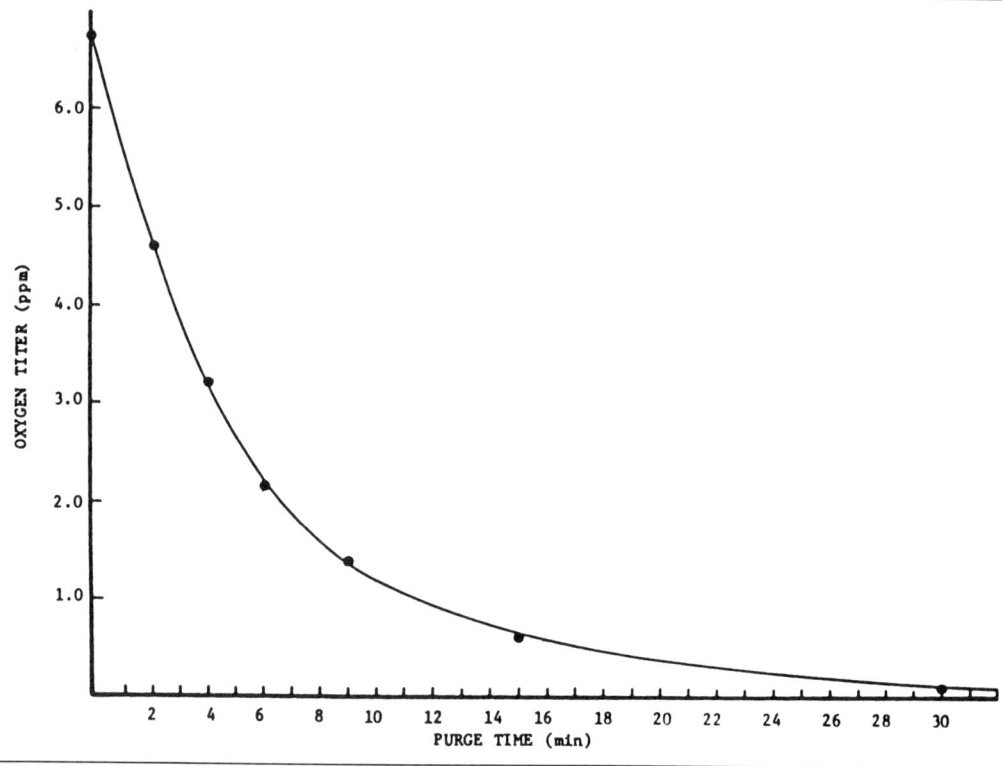

Figure 4-4. Reduction of dissolved oxygen concentration in distilled water as a function of nitrogen gas purge time.

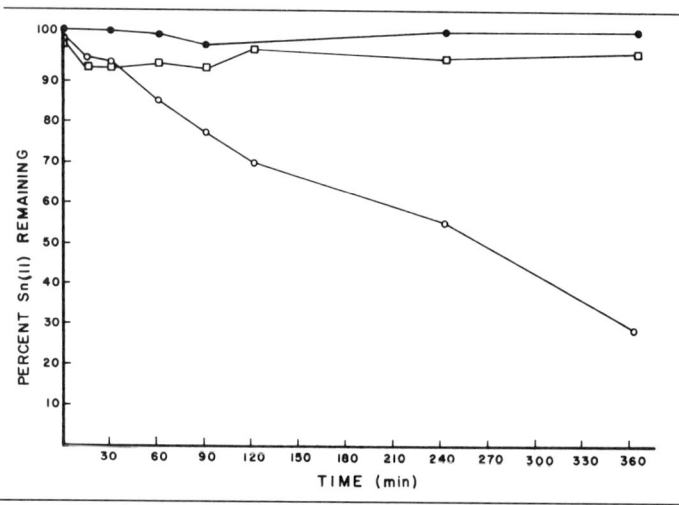

Figure 4-5. Influence of preparation and storage conditions on stability of stannous pyrophosphate solutions. □, oxygenated water, nitrogen atmosphere; ●, nitrogen-purged water, nitrogen atmosphere; ○, nitrogen-purged water, room air. *(From Kowalsky RJ, Dalton DR: Technical problems associated with the production of technetium Tc-99m tin (II) pyrophosphate kits. Am J Hosp Pharm 38:1722-1726, 1981, with permission.)*

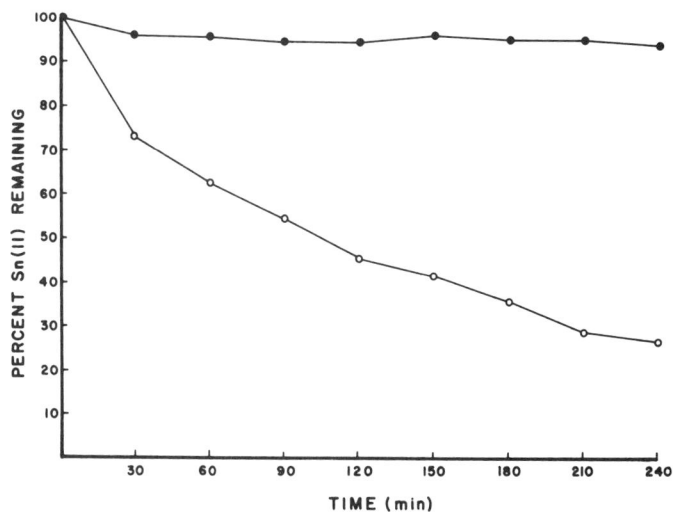

Figure 4-6. Effect of physical state on stability of stannous pyrophosphate. ●, frozen samples; ○, liquid samples. *(From Kowalsky RJ, Dalton DR: Technical problems associated with the production of technetium Tc-99m tin (II) pyrophosphate kits. Am J Hosp Pharm 38:1722–1726, 1981, with permission.)*

Freeze-dried kits will remain stable to oxidation for several months; however, when reconstituted with saline or Tc-99m pertechnetate, the oxidation problem will reoccur if air is not excluded from the vials. For this reason kits are filled with nitrogen gas before they are sealed.

Quantitative Assay of Tin (II). The ease with which Sn(II) is oxidized makes it quite difficult to prepare solutions accurately unless they are of high concentration. In practice, Sn(II) concentrations in radiopharmaceuticals are quite dilute, magnifying the problem of stability despite efforts to provide inert conditions during preparation. Because the usefulness of a Sn(II) radiopharmaceutical kit depends upon its titer of divalent tin, a representative sample of kits from a production run must be assayed to determine their reducing power. The most common method for the quantitative measurement of Sn(II) is by volumetric titration. This method is based on the oxidation of Sn(II) to the quadrivalent state by means of a standard oxidant solution such as ceric, dichromate, or iodate. Although all three oxidants are useful for analyzing stannous chloride solutions, iodate appears to offer the most versatility for solutions of Sn(II) in the presence of organic complexing agents.[12] Ceric and dichromate, because of their powerful oxidizing ability, may produce erroneous results when organic complexes are present. Iodate titrations of stannous complexes can be carried out effectively for kits containing Sn(II) in the range of 15 µg to 4 mg or more in a 10-ml volume. An alternative method based on spectrophotometrically measuring a blue complex produced upon reduction of phosphomolybdate by Sn(II) allows the determination of Sn(II) in the range of 2 to 10 µg/ml. The latter method was developed by Brookhaven National Labs to assay the small amounts of Sn(II) in its RBC kits. Details of these methods of Sn(II) analysis are reported in the literature.[12–14] Another useful method is analysis of the usable amounts of Sn(II) in kits by direct titration of kits with Tc-99m pertechnetate containing known amounts of carrier-added Tc-99 pertechnetate.[15]

Toxicity of Tin. Occasionally the question arises concerning the potential for toxicity from the administration of tin in radiopharmaceutical kits. Because information on the in vivo distribution and toxicity of tin in humans is scarce and not well documented, one must rely primarily on animal studies for determining acute toxicity. Additionally, one can consider the amounts of tin expected to be administered to humans and compare those numbers with the normal concentrations of tin in the body resulting from dietary sources to gain some perspective regarding safety.

Acute toxicity studies in rats demonstrate that when stannous chloride dihydrate is injected intravenously, the 24-hour lethal dose for 50 percent survival of the group (LD_{50}) is a 15.4 mg Sn/kg.[16] Some of the symptoms of toxicity are tremors, ataxia, muscle weakness, weight loss, and depression. At the tissue level, the most important toxic effect is found to be renal function impairment because of pathologic changes in the kidney.

The primary route of excretion of tin is urinary, and the principal organ that concentrates tin is bone.[17] From a single intravenous dose of 2 mg Sn(II) or Sn(IV)/kg, 30 percent is excreted in the urine and 11 percent of the Sn(II) but none of the Sn(IV) in the bile. Sn(IV), however, appears to show more of a preference for bone than Sn(II). Two days after an intravenous dose of tin citrate labeled with Sn-113, the total skeletal Sn-113 activity was 35 percent of the administered Sn(II) and 46 percent of Sn(IV). The biologic half-life in bone was calculated to be 20 to 40 days. In blood, 2 days after oral or intravenous dosing, the blood Sn-113 activity was very low and was limited entirely to the red cells.

Tissue studies in humans have demonstrated the normal presence of metals in the body, including tin.[18] The majority of tin is localized in bone.

Tissue distribution of tin from radiopharmaceuticals will depend upon the chemical form administered. Weak chelates that undergo in vivo hydrolysis are expected to deposit tin in the reticuloendothelial system (RES), whereas stable chelates will distribute tin more widely in the tissues or it will be excreted in the urine.[19]

If one considers the usual concentrations of tin administered in radiopharmaceutical doses, it becomes evident that the amounts appear to be quite safe. In general the largest single dose of tin expected to be administered intravenously in nuclear medicine is 2 mg, which is equivalent to about 0.03 mg/kg for a 70-kg adult. This is a dose 1/500 of the LD_{50} reported in rats. Typically, however, the dose of tin administered is one half to one tenth this amount, thus making the safety factor on the order of 1000 to 5000.

Preparation of Tc-99m Radiopharmaceuticals Using Kits

The complexing agent in the kit dictates the final chemical form of technetium and ultimately its biologic fate following intravenous injection. The functions of the complexing agent (ligand) are summarized in Table 4-4. Typical examples of complexing agents are illustrated in Figure 4-7.

The Tc-99m radiopharmaceutical is prepared by simply adding Tc-99m pertechnetate to the kit. This effects dissolution of the lyophilized powder. Subsequently the complexed stannous ion reduces the pertechnetate to a lower oxidation state, typically Tc(IV), whereby the reduced technetium binds to the complexing agent to produce the desired radiopharmaceutical. The reaction is complete within a few minutes. The reduction–oxidation reactions are shown in the following section for reduction of pertechnetate to the Tc(IV) state. Other oxidation states of technetium such as Tc(III) and Tc(V) may be produced depending upon the complexing agent and reaction conditions.

$$3\ Sn^{2+} \rightleftharpoons 3\ Sn^{4+} + 6\ e^{-} \quad (4\text{-}2)$$

TABLE 4-4. FUNCTION OF COMPLEXING AGENTS IN Tc-99m KITS

1. Complexes Sn^{2+} and Sn^{4+} ions
2. Complexes reduced Tc-99m and Tc-99
3. Determines technetium's biologic localization

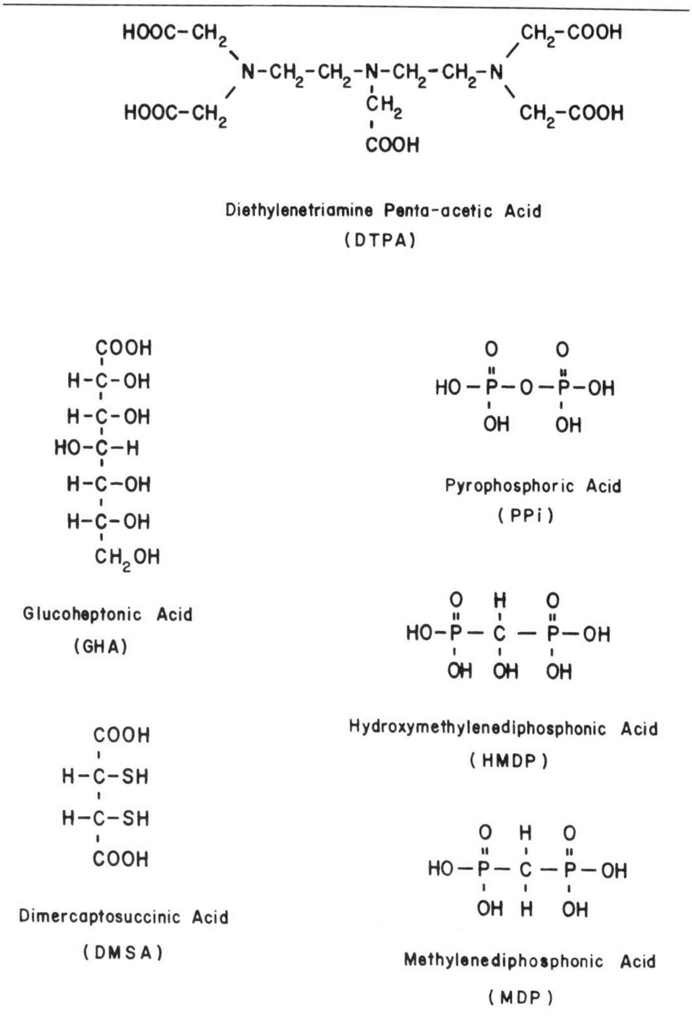

Figure 4-7. Chemical structures of several complexing agents (ligands) used in preparing Tc-99m kits.

$$2\ TcO_4^- + 12\ H^+ + 6\ e^- \rightleftharpoons$$
$$2\ TcO^{2+} + 6\ H_2O \quad (4\text{-}3)$$

The sum of Reactions 4-2 and 4-3 is as follows:

$$2\ TcO_4^- + 3\ Sn^{2+} + 12\ H^+ \rightleftharpoons$$
$$2\ TcO^{2+} + 3\ Sn^{4+} + 6\ H_2O \quad (4\text{-}4)$$

The generalized scheme for the binding of reduced technetium in kits containing stannous ion is shown in Figure 4-8 using DTPA as the exemplary ligand. As shown in this figure, technetium can be present in three chemical forms: technetium bound to ligand; unreduced pertechnetate; and reduced, hydrolyzed technetium. The latter two species are undesirable impurities.

Pertechnetate Impurity. There are at least two primary factors that may promote the development of pertechnetate impurity: oxygen and free radicals induced by radiolysis. Each of these substances can cause oxidation of stannous ion according to the

Figure 4-8. General scheme followed in Tc-99m kit labeling using DTPA as an exemplary ligand that illustrates the Tc-99m DTPA complex as the desired product and the potential undesirable impurities that can be expected.

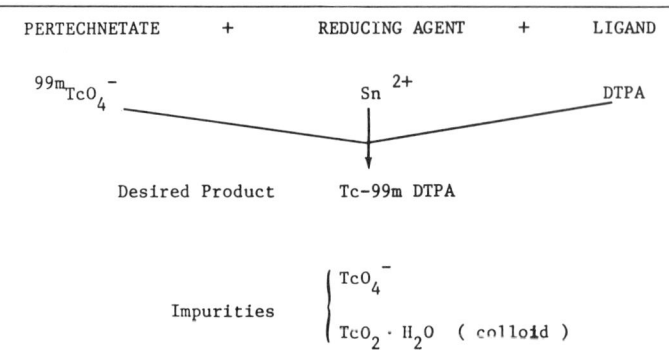

following reactions. An insufficient stannous ion concentration decreases the reducing power in the kit.

$$Sn^{2+} + O_2 + 4 H^+ \rightleftharpoons Sn^{4+} + 2 H_2O \quad (4\text{-}5)$$

$$Sn^{2+} + 2 OH^\bullet \rightleftharpoons Sn^{4+} + 2 OH^- \quad (4\text{-}6)$$

Additionally, radiolytic decomposition of reduced–complexed technetium may also occur by interaction of free radical species, $RO^\bullet$, with the complex by an undefined mechanism.

$$Tc\text{-Ligand} \xrightarrow{RO^\bullet_2} Ligand + TcO_4^- \quad (4\text{-}7)$$

Reaction 4–5 is important during the kit production process because it causes a loss of stannous ion before kit use, but it is also important after kit reconstitution, particularly if air is introduced into the kit. Reactions 4–6 and 4–7 are only significant after kit reconstitution with pertechnetate and become more pronounced if increased amounts of radioactivity are added to the kit and if the kit contains low amounts of stannous ion initially. It has been demonstrated that radiation-induced decomposition is catalyzed by the presence of dissolved oxygen and that the presence of excess stannous ion acts as an inhibitor of this reaction.[20] It is therefore of utmost importance that a sufficient level of stannous ion be maintained throughout the useful life of the Tc-labeled kit. The oxygen-catalyzed reaction probably occurs through the generation of two free radical oxidation intermediates.[21] The first intermediates are alkoxy or hydroxy radicals produced by the scission of the oxygen–oxygen bond of peroxides according to Reaction 4–8. The other intermediate is the peroxy radical formed from oxygen and radiolysis by-products according to Reaction 4–9.

$$RO\text{-}OH \longrightarrow RO^\bullet + {}^\bullet OH \quad (4\text{-}8)$$

$$R^\bullet + O_2 \longrightarrow RO^\bullet_2 \quad (4\text{-}9)$$

These free radical species then degrade the Tc complex with the generation of free pertechnetate (Reaction 4–7).

Some technetium-labeled chelates are more stable than others. The bone imaging agents are fairly weak chelates, and those kits containing low levels of stannous ion can be stabilized against oxidation by adding antioxidants to the kits. Ascorbic acid and gentisic acid have been used as effective antioxidants in bone kits. As shown in Reactions 4–10 and 4–11, they function by donating reactive hydrogen atoms to the free radical intermediates to yield a resonance-stabilized and nonreactive molecule, RO_2H.[21] The free radical is thus neutralized to a chemical state that cannot attack the Tc complex.

Ascorbic acid (4-10)

$$\underset{\text{Gentisic acid}}{\ce{HO-\chemfig{6(-(-CH(-OH)=[::60]O)=-(-OH)=-=)}}} \xrightarrow[\ce{RO^\bullet}]{\ce{RO_2^\bullet}} \underset{}{\ce{HO-\chemfig{6(-(-CH(-OH)=[::60]O)=-(-O^\bullet)=-=)}}} + \ce{RO_2H} \quad (4\text{-}11)$$

Hydrolyzed-Reduced Technetium Impurity. The hydrolyzed-reduced technetium (HR-Tc) impurity is characterized by the formation of an insoluble colloidal species according to Reaction 4-12.

$$\ce{TcO^{2+} + 2 OH- -> TcO2 . H2O (s)} \quad (4\text{-}12)$$

This reaction is favored at pH values close to neutrality and at low concentrations of chelating agent.[15] Increased concentration of hydroxyl ion present will compete with the chelating agent for reduced technetium, thus forming the colloid. Additionally, any uncomplexed stannous ion can also hydrolyze to form insoluble colloidal tin hydroxide as shown in Reaction 4-13.

$$\ce{Sn^{2+} + 2 OH- -> Sn(OH)2 (s)} \quad (4\text{-}13)$$

This presents a problem because this tin colloid will also bind reduced technetium and compete with the chelating agent during the labeling reaction.

These hydrolysis problems can be mitigated by ensuring that a sufficient excess of chelating agent is present and maintaining favorable pH conditions.

Methods of analyzing Tc-99m radiopharmaceuticals for pertechnetate and HR-Tc impurities will be discussed in Chapter 6.

Technetium-Ligand Complexation. The character of the complexation between reduced technetium and the ligand depends upon the type of ligand and the reduction conditions, although the process involves ionic, covalent, and coordinate covalent bonding. Many chelating ligands in Tc-99m radiopharmaceuticals contain ionized oxygen atoms that can provide ionic bonding and nitrogen and sulfur atoms that can provide covalent-type bonding with technetium. Technetium exhibits various coordination numbers that can be satisfied through a combination of binding sites on the ligand and through hydroxyl species in solution. Many technetium complexes are dimeric and others polymeric in character, with a technetium atom bridging two ligand molecules. This provides stability to the complex. Figure 4-9 illustrates the binding of two N-substituted iminodiacetate ligands to hexa-coordinate technetium as a representative example. The chemical structures of specific Tc-99m radiopharmaceuticals and other properties of these agents will be covered individually in subsequent chapters.

Summary of Technetium Chemistry. Technetium can exist in a number of valence (oxidation) states, but Tc(VII) is the most stable. It is obtained in this form from the Tc-99m generator. Technetium must be reduced to a lower valence state, typically Tc(IV), before it will bind with complexing agents to form useful radiopharmaceu-

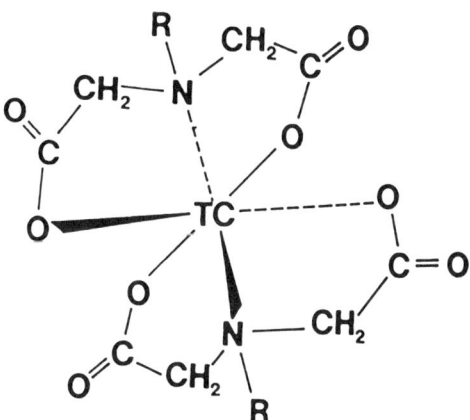

Figure 4-9. The dimeric structure typical of several technetium-ligand complexes characterized by a technetium atom bridging two ligand molecules. *(From Loberg MD, Porter DW, Ryan JW: In Radiopharmaceuticals II. New York, Society of Nuclear Medicine, 1979, p 530, with permission.)*

ticals. Chemical reduction is usually accomplished with stannous tin as the reducing agent. Radiopharmaceutical preparation is usually accomplished by adding Tc-99m pertechnetate to a vial (kit) containing the complexing agent and stannous tin. The chemical species of technetium that can form during kit radiolabeling are Tc complex (desired species) and various undesirable impurities that include technetium dioxide colloid, technetium tin hydroxide colloid, and pertechnetate. The colloidal impurities can be minimized by the use of sufficient excess complexing agent and proper pH adjustment. Pertechnetate impurity can be minimized by maintaining sufficient stannous ion concentration, excluding oxygen and the use of antioxidants. The various technetium species present in Tc-99m radiopharmaceuticals can be readily determined by simple radiochromatography procedures.

IODINE

The most useful radioisotopes of iodine for nuclear medicine studies are I-123, I-125, and I-131 because of their favorable physical properties. The choice of which isotope to use is determined by the ultimate application. I-131 has been widely used for clinical diagnosis for several reasons. Its 8-day half-life provides a reasonable shelf life of commercially prepared radiopharmaceuticals ready for use, it is inexpensive, and its 364-keV gamma radiation provides good tissue penetration for organ imaging. Undesirable properties of I-131 are the high radiation dose from the beta emission and the requirement for heavy collimation and shielding of high-energy gammas. I-125 has been used clinically to evaluate superficial organs such as the thyroid gland, but its weak photons severely limit its usefulness for deep-seated organs because of photon absorption by tissue. Its lack of beta radiation, however, makes it a good choice for labeling organic compounds to avoid the problem of radiolytic decomposition encountered with I-131. Its 60-day half-life is desirable for long-term studies of the metabolism of its compounds and also provides a long shelf life for such compounds, thus obviating the need for frequent preparation. I-123 is an ideal isotope for clinical studies because of the 159-keV gamma radiation, 13.3-hour half-life, and lack of beta radiation. Its main disadvantages are availability and cost because it must be produced in a cyclotron. Additional properties of iodine isotopes are discussed in Chapter 8.

An important advantage of iodine in nuclear medicine is its ability to react with a number of compounds to produce many useful radiopharmaceuticals.

Solution Chemistry of Radioiodide

Radioiodine is usually obtained as sodium iodide. Under favorable conditions, iodide will enter into oxidation reactions in aqueous solution, producing volatile forms that are a potential safety hazard. The most significant oxidative reactions are with oxygen or radiolysis products, namely, peroxides and free radicals as shown in the following:

$$4\ I^- + O_2 + 4\ H^+ \rightleftharpoons 2\ I_2 + 2\ H_2O \tag{4-14}$$

$$2\ HI + H_2O_2 \rightleftharpoons I_2 + 2\ H_2O \tag{4-15}$$

$$2\ I^- + 2\ OH^\bullet \rightleftharpoons I_2 + 2\ OH^- \tag{4-16}$$

Reaction 4–14 can be effectively retarded by buffering the radioiodide solution to an alkaline pH and by use of reducing agents such as sodium thiosulfate that reverse the reaction. Reactions 4–15 and 4–16 are radiation-induced reactions and are difficult to prevent entirely but can be minimized by lowering the radioactive concentration. Some practical considerations for handling radioiodine are discussed in Chapter 8.

Iodine Labeling

Like technetium, the chemical and biologic behavior of iodine depends upon whether it is in the oxidized state (iodine) or the reduced state (iodide). In contrast to technetium, however, is the fact that iodine's reduced state does not label molecules but the oxidized state does. Labeling with radioiodine is usually accomplished by introducing the electrophilic species I^+ into an aromatic ring in the molecule of interest. This occurs either by a substitution reaction where iodine replaces hydrogen or by isotope exchange where the radioiodine atom is exchanged with a stable iodine atom already present in the molecule. These reactions are as follows:

Substitution:
$$R\text{-}H + I_2^* \rightleftharpoons R\text{-}I^* + HI \qquad (4\text{-}17)$$

Isotope exchange:
$$R\text{-}I + I_2^* \rightleftharpoons R\text{-}I^* + I_2 \qquad (4\text{-}18)$$

In free molecular iodine, I_2, the structure $I^-\text{-}I^+$ is presumed. The I^+ ion does not exist alone, however, but usually forms a complex with a nucleophilic species in aqueous solution. The following reactions in water are possible:

$$I_2 + H_2O \rightleftharpoons H_2OI^+ + I^- \qquad (4\text{-}19)$$

$$I_2 + OH^- \rightleftharpoons HOI + I^- \qquad (4\text{-}20)$$

It is believed that the iodinating species in iodine labeling reactions is either the hydrated complex H_2OI^{+22} or hypoiodous acid, HOI.[23]

Protein iodination is one of the most important radiolabeling techniques in nuclear medicine. Typical iodination sites in protein molecules include the aromatic ring of tyrosine as the primary site of iodination or the imidazole ring of histidine as a secondary site. Because the anionic form of the molecule to be labeled seems to be the reactive species with I^+, close attention must be paid to the pKa value and the pH of the reaction mixture. At low pH tyrosine is protonated, and labeling yields are low. Basic pH, however, promotes dissociation of tyrosine hydrogens to form the desired tyrosinate anion[24] and also promotes the hydrolysis of I_2 according to Reaction 4-20. This greatly facilitates the rate of iodination into the tyrosine ring. Solutions of pH 7 to 9 are usually used in protein iodination. One must avoid higher pH values (>10) because of the irreversible disproportionation of HOI to iodate as is shown in the following reaction:

$$3\ HOI + 3\ OH^- \longrightarrow 2\ I^- + IO_3^- + 3\ H_2O \qquad (4\text{-}21)$$

Even at pH 7 to 9 iodate formation can occur.

The order of mixing reagents is important in achieving high iodination yield. This depends, of course, on the method used for radioiodination, but in general, the molecule to be labeled is added first, followed by buffer, radioiodide, and iodinating agent. To retard protein damage mild iodinating conditions must be used. More concern must be given when using iodinating agents that are fairly strong oxidizing agents because they may attack the protein. In general it is recommended that not more than one atom of iodine per molecule of protein on the average be introduced to preserve protein integrity; however, this too depends upon the protein, the iodinating method, and the ultimate use or application of the iodinated protein.[25] For example, iodinated albumin prepared by the iodine monochloride method should contain not more than one atom of iodine per molecule, but ten atoms per molecule are permitted if the electrolytic method is used. When iodinating insulin with the iodine monochloride method, not more than one atom of iodine per molecule of insulin is permitted to retain hormonal activity, but seven atoms per molecule are permitted if only immunologic activity is required.

RADIOIODINATION METHODS

One of several methods can be used to generate the I^+ species. These include (1) iodine, (2) iodine monochloride, (3) chloramine-T, (4) lactoperoxidase, (5) electrolysis, (6) prelabeled ligands, and (7) miscellaneous methods.

Iodine

In this method the radioiodide is mixed with the compound to be labeled and an iodine–potassium iodide solution. The KI serves to solubilize the I_2 as the triiodide complex. After hydrolysis of I_2 to HOI the radioiodide I* undergoes isotope exchange with HOI to produce HOI*, which iodinates the compound. Theoretically, only half of the radioiodide is converted to the I^+ form so that labeling yields are usually only 10 to 20 percent. Reaction conditions are mild, however, and protein denaturation is low. Both stable iodinated and radioiodinated compounds are formed. This method is no longer widely used.

Iodine Monochloride

In iodine monochloride (ICl) the iodine is in the I^+ form because of chlorine's greater electronegativity. Iodine monochloride is formed by the oxidation of iodide with iodate in strong acid according to Reaction 4–22.

$$2\ NaI + NaIO_3 + 6\ HCl \rightleftharpoons 3\ ICl + H_2O + 3\ NaCl \quad (4\text{-}22)$$

When mixed with ICl, radioiodide undergoes isotope exchange. Because the ICl is in excess and all of its iodine is in the I^+ form, essentially all of the radioiodide is converted to I^+ accordingly:

$$ICl + NaI^* \rightleftharpoons I^*Cl + NaI \quad (4\text{-}23)$$

Subsequently, the I*Cl hydrolyzes to HOI*, which iodinates the compound.[24] Higher radiolabeling yields are possible (about 75 percent), but the specific activity of the product is low because stable iodine is also incorporated into the compound because of the excess stable ICl present. In this labeling technique radioiodide is added to the buffered compound, and ICl is jetted into the mixture. If ICl is added before the radioiodide, labeling yields are lowered considerably because the isotope exchange reaction is impaired because of the reaction of ICl directly with the compound. Rapid addition of ICl (jetting) is done to dispense the mixture quickly to reduce the degree of multiple labeling within the same molecule created by localized concentrations of reactive iodine. An advantage of using ICl, however, is that the amount of iodine incorporated into the compound is controlled by the amount of ICl used. This is an advantage if excessive substitution must be avoided.

Chloramine-T

This method uses N-chloro-4-methyl benzene sulfonamide sodium salt (chloramine-T) as the iodinating agent.[25,26] Chloramine-T undergoes hydrolysis at pH 7 to 8, liberating sodium hypochlorite, which then oxidizes the radioiodide to hypoiodous acid according to the following reactions:

$$CH_3\text{-}C_6H_4SO_2NaNCl + H_2O \rightleftharpoons$$
$$CH_3\text{-}C_6H_4SO_2NH_2 + NaOCl \quad (4\text{-}24)$$

$$NaOCl + HI^* \rightleftharpoons HOI^* + NaCl \quad (4\text{-}25)$$

The general technique is to mix the compound to be labeled with buffer and radioiodide and then to rapidly add the fresh chloramine-T solution. Because chloramine-T is a powerful oxidizing agent, it may damage proteins; however, if labeling conditions are carefully controlled, high radioiodination yields can be obtained.[27] The advantage of chloramine-T is that no carrier iodide is needed, and therefore high specific activities can be obtained. Additionally, virtually complete utilization of the isotope can be achieved.

Lactoperoxidase

In this method lactoperoxidase enzyme and hydrogen peroxide react to form a species that in turn oxidizes radioiodide to iodine.[28] Usually the protein is mixed with the radioiodide and lactoperoxidase. Small quantities of hydrogen peroxide are then added to effect the labeling reaction. The reaction is terminated by the addition of cysteine or by dilution. This method is claimed to be less destructive to proteins. The enzyme itself can be labeled with iodine, which may reduce the labeling yield, but this is not significant when a sufficient concentration of protein is present.

Electrolysis

Iodide can be oxidized by electrons generated at an inert electrode in solution.[29] This would seem to be ideal in that no chemical iodinating species need be present that might adversely affect the protein molecules. This method is thus relatively mild. A slow and controlled rate of electrolysis results in a steady release of iodine that can result in a uniform labeling of the compound. This method is more complex than other methods and is not widely used.

Prelabeled Ligands

To circumvent the problem of protein damage by direct iodination procedures and to be able to label proteins that lack the tyrosine moiety, indirect radioiodination can be accomplished using the Bolton–Hunter reagent.[30] This method uses a reactive conjugate prelabeled with radioiodine that is then reacted with the protein, thus eliminating contact with oxidizing and reducing agents. The reagent used is an I-125–labeled acylating agent, iodinated 3-(4-hydroxyphenyl) propionic acid N-hydroxysuccinimide ester, which reacts with free amino groups of lysine in the protein through amide bonds.[30] This method is mild, producing proteins that retain immunoreactivity, and is therefore useful for radioimmunoassay development. The reactions presented below illustrate this method.

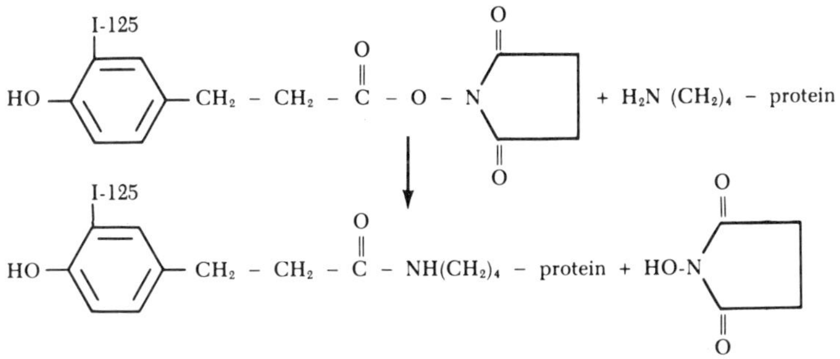

Miscellaneous Methods

Molecules that cannot be labeled with iodine directly or indirectly can sometimes be labeled after the introduction of a tyrosine-containing reactive group into the molecule. Radioiodinated digoxin used in the digoxin radioimmunoassay can be prepared by replacing the digitoxose sugars of digoxin with a succinyltyrosine moiety. The result is 3-0-succinyl digoxigenin tyrosine, which can be radioiodinated in the tyrosine ring as shown in the following reaction:

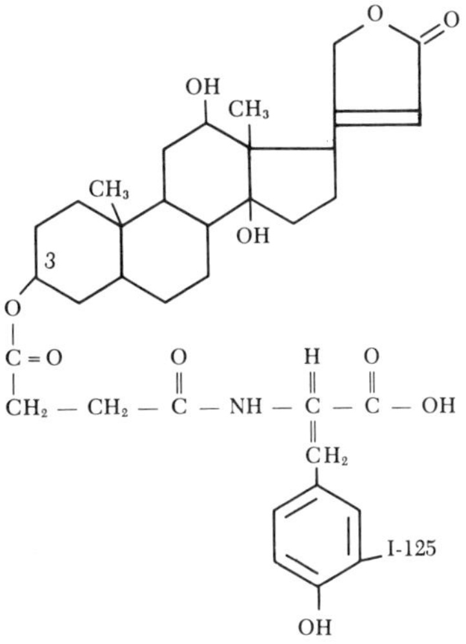

3-0-Succinyl digoxigenin tyrosine iodine-125

RADIOIODINATED PHARMACEUTICALS

Several radioiodinated compounds have been or are currently being used in nuclear medicine. Those labeled by direct iodination include radioiodinated human serum albumin I-125 for plasma volume measurements and radioiodinated fibrinogen I-125 for detection of venous thromboses. These proteins are usually labeled with a modified chloramine-T procedure.

A large number of agents have been labeled by isotope exchange. In the past many of these were iodinated contrast agents including iodopyracet (Diodrast) and diatrizoate (Hypaque), which were used for renal function studies and rose bengal for hepatobiliary studies. Two agents in current use prepared by isotope exchange are O-iodohippurate I-131 (Hippuran) for the assessment of renal tubular function and iothalamate I-125 (Glofil) used for glomerular filtration rate (GFR) studies. The structures of these compounds can be found in Chapter 12.

OTHER LABELING METHODS FOR PREPARING RADIOPHARMACEUTICALS

There are of course numerous radiolabeling methods used to produce compounds with isotopic labels containing C-14, H-3, P-32, and S-35.[25] Although such compounds are of no value as diagnostic imaging agents, they are very useful for studying the metabolic and pharmacokinetic pathways of drugs. Most of these compounds are produced by chemical synthesis. Some radiolabeled compounds are produced by biosynthesis, and two of those used in nuclear medicine are cyanocobalamin labeled with Co-57, Co-58, Co-60, and selenomethionine Se-75.

REFERENCES

1. Anger HO: Radioisotope cameras. In Hine GJ (ed): Instrumentation in Nuclear Medicine. New York, Academic Press, 1967
2. Maynard CD: Clinical Nuclear Medicine. Philadelphia, Lea & Febiger, 1969, p. 9
3. McAfee JG, Subramanian G: Radioactive agents for imaging. In Freeman LM, Johnson PM (eds): Clinical Scintillation Imaging, 2nd ed. New York, Grun & Stratton, 1975, p 56
4. Eckelman WC, Reba RC: The classification of radiotracers. J Nucl Med 19:1179, 1978
5. Counsell RE, Ice RD: The design of organ imaging radiopharmaceuticals. In Ariens EJ (ed): Drug Design, 6th ed. New York, Academic Press, 1975, Vol 2, p 172
6. Perrier AC, Segrè E: Some chemical properties of element 43. J Chem Physiol 5: 712, 1937
7. Seaborg GR, Segrè E: Nuclear isomerism of element 43. Physiol Rev 55: 808, 1939
8. Richards P: Nuclide generators. In Andrews GA, Knisely RM, Wagner HN Jr (eds): Radioactive Pharmaceuticals. Oak Ridge, Tenn, US Atomic Energy Commission, 1965, p 155
9. Harper PV, Lathrop KA, Gottschalk A: Pharmacodynamics of some technetium-99m preparations. In Andrews GA, Knisely RM, Wagner HN Jr (eds): Oak Ridge, Tenn, Radioactive Pharmaceuticals. US Atomic Energy Commission, 1965, p 335
10. Richards P, Steigman J: Chemistry of technetium as applied to radiopharmaceuticals. In Subramanian G, Rhodes BA, Cooper JF, Sodd VJ (eds): Radiopharmaceuticals. New York, Society of Nuclear Medicine, 1975, p 23
11. Eckelman W, Richards P: Instant Tc-99m DTPA. J Nucl Med 11:761, 1970
12. Srivastava SC, Richards P: Technetium-labeled compounds. In Rayudu GVS (ed): Radiotracers for Medical Applications. Boca Raton, Fla, CRC Press, 1981
13. Meinken GE, Srivastava SC, Richards P: Determination of microgram amounts of stannous tin in technetium labeling kits. J Nucl Med 21:78, 1980
14. Chervu LR, Vallabhajosyula B, Mani J, et al: Stannous ion quantitation in Tc-99m radiopharmaceutical kits. Eur J Nucl Med 7:291, 1982
15. Srivastava SC, Meinken G, Smith TD, et al: Problems associated with stannous Tc-99m radiopharmaceuticals. Int J Appl Radiat Isot 28:83, 1977
16. Conine DL, Yum M, Martz RC, et al: Toxicity of sodium pentafluorostannite, a new anticariogenic agent. Comparison of the acute toxicity of sodium pentafluorostannite, sodium fluoride, and stannous chlo-

ride in mice and/or rats. Toxicol Appl Pharmacol 33:21, 1975
17. Hiles RA: Absorption, distribution, and excretion of inorganic tin in rats. Toxicol Appl Pharmacol. 27:366, 1974
18. Kehoe RA, Cholak J, Story RV: A spectrochemical study of the normal ranges of concentration of certain trace metals in biological materials. J Nutr 19:579, 1940
19. Zalutsky MR, Rayudu GVS, Friedman AM: The biological behavior of tin following administration of nine Tc99m-Sn-complexes. Int J Nucl Med Biol 4:224, 1977
20. Billinghurst MW, Rempel S, Westendorf BA: Radiation decomposition of technetium-99m radiopharmaceuticals. J Nucl Med 20:138, 1979
21. Tofe AJ, Francis MD: In vitro stabilization of a low-tin bone imaging agent (Tc-99m-Sn-HEDP) by ascorbic acid. J Nucl Med 17:820, 1976
22. Hughes WL: The chemistry of iodination. Ann NY Acad Sci 70:3, 1957
23. McFarlane AS: Efficient trace-labeling of proteins with iodine. Nature 182:53, 1958
24. Helmkemp RW, Contreras MA, Bale WF: I-131 labeling of proteins by the iodine monochloride method. Int J Appl Radiat Isot 18:737, 1967
25. Bayly RJ, Anthony E, Evans JS, et al: Synthesis of labeled compounds. In Tubis M, Wolf W (eds): Radiopharmacy. New York, Wiley, 1976
26. Hunter WM, Greenwood FC: Preparation of iodine-131 labeled human growth hormones of high specific activity. Nature 194:495, 1962
27. McConahey PJ, Dixon EJ: A method of trace iodination of proteins for immunological studies. Int Arch Allergy 29:185, 1966
28. Marchalonis JJ: An enzymatic method for the trace iodination of immunoglobulins and other proteins. Biochem J 113:299, 1969
29. Katz J, Bonorris G: Electrolytic iodination of proteins with I-125 and I-131. J Lab Clin Med 72:966, 1968
30. Bolton AE, Hunter WM: The labeling of proteins to high specific radioactivities by conjugation to a I-125 containing acylating agent. Biochem J 133:529, 1973

CHAPTER 5

The Nuclear Pharmacy

The nuclear pharmacy is the area in a nuclear medicine department where radioactive material is handled. The design of a nuclear pharmacy depends on the type and extent of the procedures to be performed. The nuclear medicine department that provides only routine services will not require the more extensive design needed for a department that also is involved with research applications using radiopharmaceuticals. As an alternative to having its own nuclear pharmacy, the nuclear medicine department may elect to obtain its radiopharmaceuticals from a commercial nuclear pharmacy. In this case the local space needs within the nuclear medicine department may be quite modest. This chapter will describe a routine service-type facility that performs primarily imaging procedures, in vivo function studies, and radionuclide therapy and represents what is found in many nuclear medicine departments. It should be pointed out that in vitro studies do not involve the administration of radioactive material to human subjects and these procedures are oftentimes performed by another department of the hospital such as endocrinology or pathology or by hospital laboratories. If these studies are performed in nuclear medicine, the nuclear pharmacy lab may need to be expanded beyond the space allocation described in this chapter. More complete information on nuclear pharmacy planning and design can be found elsewhere.[1,2]

SPACE AND EQUIPMENT NEEDS IN THE NUCLEAR PHARMACY

Floor Plan

The primary functions listed previously require a defined space allocation within the nuclear medicine department. Ideally the nuclear pharmacy space should be designed at the inception of a new nuclear medicine department to provide a safe and efficient work area. Unfortunately, this is not always possible, and the pharmacy oftentimes is relegated to an existing space within the department. Despite any constraints on space the nuclear pharmacy should be divided into at least four areas: a "hot" storage area, the dispensing and work area, the counting and quality control area, and an office. There are several ways these areas can be arranged, but in concept they should be designed so that the areas of higher

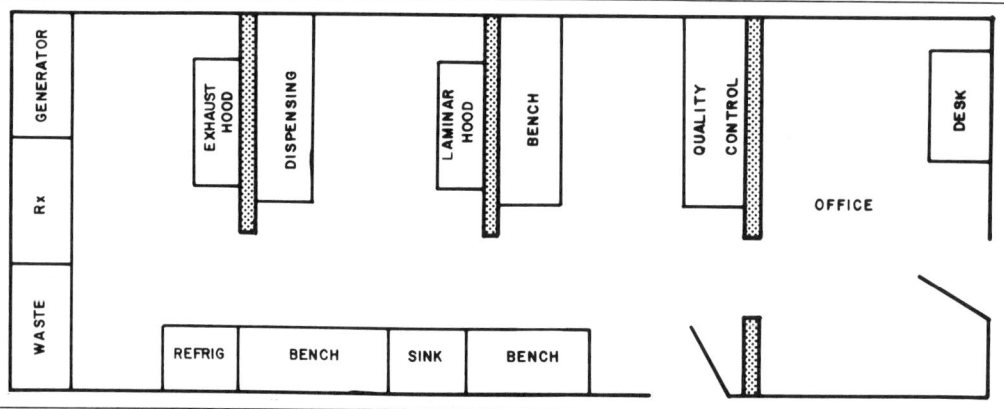

Figure 5-1. Nuclear pharmacy floor plan.

radiation intensity are farthest away from the areas used for low-level radioactive counting procedures and the office. Figure 5-1 is a floor plan that exemplifies this flow pattern. The "hot" storage area should be placed in the most remote area to limit traffic flow and personnel radiation exposure.

Storage and Shielding Equipment for Radioactive Material

The nature of radioactive material dictates that it must be contained and stored in a manner that minimizes radiation exposure to the workers. Basic equipment needs in this area are listed in Table 5-1. Storage cabinets are available in a variety of sizes and design to accommodate particular needs. A functional set of cabinets includes a drawer module for the storage of individual radiopharmaceuticals; a shelf module for radioactive sources such as flood sources used to calibrate cameras, organ phantoms, and reference standards; and a waste module containing a fiber drum into which used vials, syringes, needles, etc., can be stored before final waste disposal. Typical units are shown in Figure 5-2.

Lead bricks of various sizes, usually $2 \times 4 \times 8$ inches, are useful for providing extra shielding on countertops or other areas where extemporaneous shielding is required such as around Tc-99m generators. Lead bricks provide the versatility of a movable shielded area that can be built up and taken down as the need arises. Lead bricks are available from commercial suppliers.

Lead vial shields, sometimes referred to as lead "pigs", can be purchased but more frequently are obtained by saving the shields supplied with radiopharmaceuticals. They are available in various sizes and are easily adaptable for most needs in the nuclear pharmacy. One should match the thickness of lead with the gamma energy of the source to provide adequate shielding. For example, the radiation intensity from technetium-99m (half-value layer [HVL] = 0.3 mm Pb) will be reduced by a factor of nearly 1000 by one-eighth inch (3.2 mm)

TABLE 5-1. BASIC STORAGE AND SHIELDING EQUIPMENT FOR RADIOACTIVE MATERIAL

1. Lead-lined storage cabinets
   A. Radiopharmaceuticals
   B. Radioactive sources
   C. Radioactive waste
2. Lead L-block shields
3. Leaded glass bricks and view screens
4. Lead bricks
5. Lead vial shields and syringe shields
6. Lead foil or sheeting of various thickness

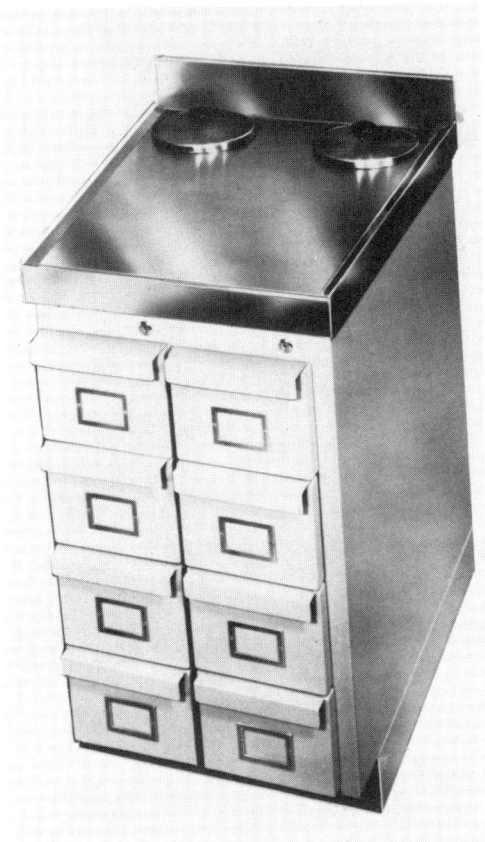

Figure 5-2. A. Lead-lined storage drawers for radiopharmaceuticals. *(Figures 5-2 A-D are from ADC Medical, Farmingdale, NY, with permission.)*

Shields are rather expensive and somewhat cumbersome to use at first, but a little practice will overcome the initial inconvenience. Several studies have demonstrated the extent of radiation dose to the hands and fingertips from sources in syringes, which points out the importance of using syringe shields.[3-6] Figure 5-3 illustrates various types of syringe shields.

A lead L-block is an L-shaped piece of lead affixed with a piece of leaded glass. It is used at dispensing stations in particular to shield the worker's body and head while preparing radioactive material. Figure 5-4 illustrates such a device. Also at the dispensing station, for the convenience of the worker, are placed two or more lead containers to hold spent syringes and needles. Similarly, shielded containers are also maintained in the area where patients are injected. When full, the contents of these containers can be easily transferred to a larger waste container.

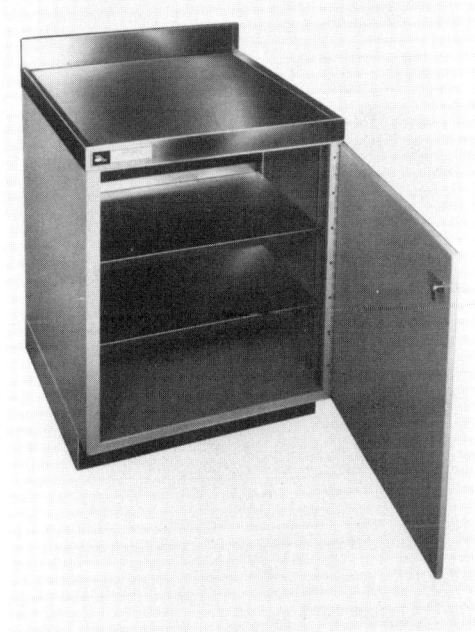

Figure 5-2. B. Lead-lined storage cabinet for radioactive sources.

of lead. By contrast the same thickness of lead will only reduce the radiation intensity from iodine-131 (HVL = 3 mm Pb) by a factor of about 2. This aspect of shielding is most important when therapy doses of I-131 are handled and transported from the pharmacy to a hospital ward.

Syringe shields made of lead or other material such as tantalum can be purchased to shield patient doses during preparation and administration. They should be used for personal protection, particularly when one considers the number of injections made each day by the technologist or physician.

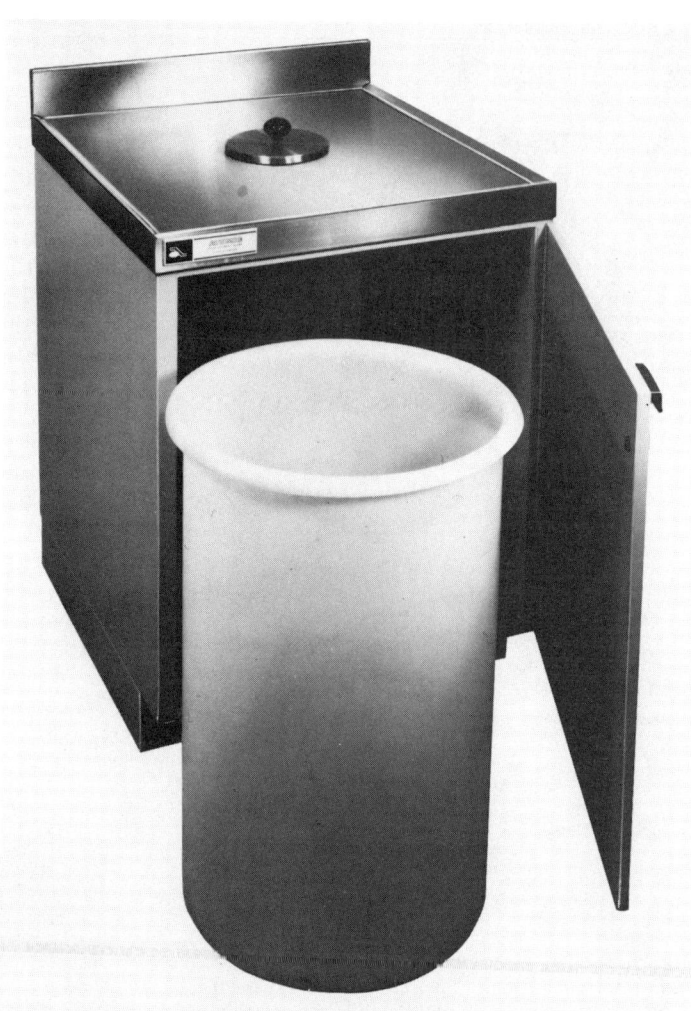

Figure 5-2. C. Lead-lined storage cabinet for radioactive waste.

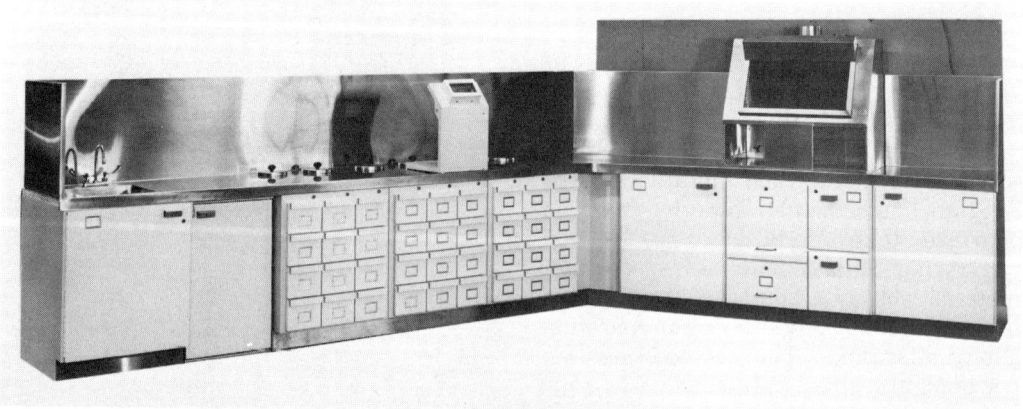

Figure 5-2. D. Workbench and storage layout suitable for a nuclear pharmacy.

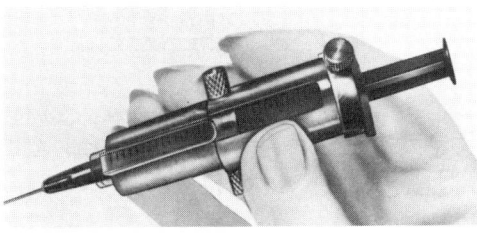

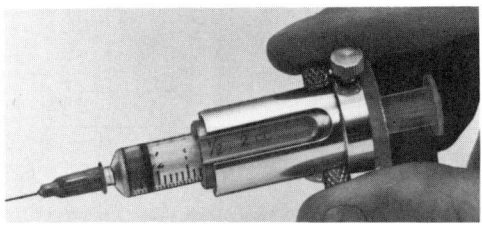

Figure 5-3. Radiopharmaceutical syringe shield. *(From Nuclear Associates, Division of Victoreen, Inc, with permission.)*

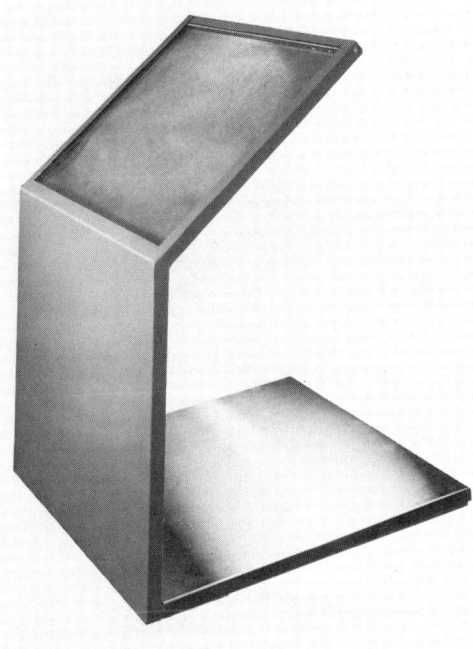

Figure 5-4. Lead L-block for preparation and dispensing of radiopharmaceuticals. *(From ADC Medical, Farmingdale, NY, with permission.)*

Countertops and Sinks

Workbench tops should be constructed of stainless steel with flanged edges to confine accidental spills and permit easy decontamination. Work surfaces should be covered with a plastic-backed absorbent sheeting to protect the surface. This material can be easily removed in the event of contamination. In some instances it may be useful to place open beakers and vials of radioactive solutions in plastic or metal trays that can be easily transported and will contain any spilled liquid.

Sinks are necessary for washing contaminated glassware and for disposal of small quantities of radioactive solutions. One must be certain that disposal of liquid radioactive waste does not exceed the regulatory codes.[7] Radioactive warning signs should be used to mark "hotsinks" to identify them as being potentially contaminated. Ideally, these sinks should be of the deep-well type to minimize splashing of surrounding areas.

Hoods

It is desirable to have some type of exhaust hood in the radiopharmacy to contain volatile radiopharmaceuticals such as iodine and radioactive gases. The type of hood will depend upon the nature of the work to be performed. The traditional chemical exhaust hood (fume hood) is useful if the work does not require a sterile air environment. It is also necessary to have such a hood if iodine radiolabeling is carried out. The exhaust rate for such hoods should be about 700 cubic feet per minute to ensure adequate outflow from the room.

Certain labeling procedures, such as blood cell and protein labeling, may require a sterile air environment. Laminar air flow hoods are most suitable for such applications because the room air is filtered before it enters the work space of the hood. Under normal circumstances room air is in a turbulent state and contains thousands of suspended particles per cubic foot. Some of these particles contain microorganisms. A laminar air flow hood filters ambient room

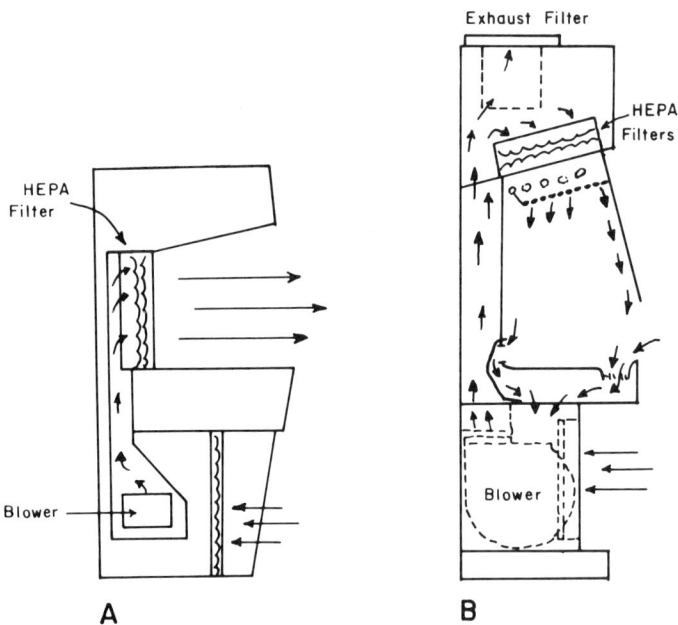

Figure 5-5. Diagram of laminar air flow hoods. **A.** Horizontal flow. **B.** Vertical flow.

air by removing these particles and places the air in a directional movement at a velocity that produces a work area free of particles and microorganisms. Air entering the hood is forced through high-efficiency particulate air (HEPA) filters so that the quality of air in the hood is 99.9 percent free of particles less than 0.3 μm. The direction of air flow in laminar air flow hoods is usually horizontal or vertical to the work surface (Fig. 5-5). Only the vertical flow hood is suitable for radioactive materials. Additionally, the hood should be an exhausting type hood to ensure protection to the worker and the environment. Figure 5-6 illustrates a totally exhausting laminar air flow hood that is well suited for use in the nuclear pharmacy.

Exhaust fans for all hoods should be located at the terminus of the exhaust duct to provide negative pressure throughout the length of duct work. Ideally, the hood should be connected to its own separate exhaust system. The exhaust terminus should be located at least 30 feet from the nearest air intake to the building. Exhausted air

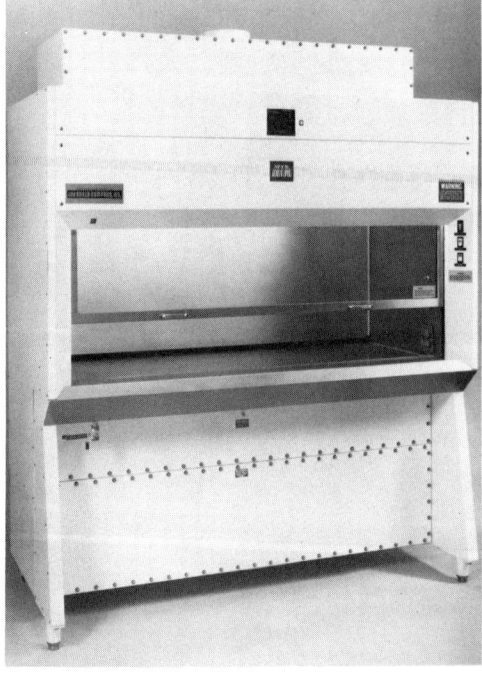

Figure 5-6. Exhausting laminar air flow hood, Baker NCB-B6. *(From The Baker Co, Sanford, ME, with permission.)*

should be appropriately filtered to restrict environmental contamination.

RADIATION DETECTION INSTRUMENTATION IN THE NUCLEAR PHARMACY

The essential pieces of equipment necessary for radiation measurement in the nuclear pharmacy include a dose calibrator, a portable Geiger–Müller (GM) survey meter, a Geiger–Müller radiation monitor, and a scintillation well counter. Their principles of operation were discussed in Chapter 2.

Dose Calibrator

This instrument is an ionization chamber that is calibrated to measure the radioactivity of radiopharmaceutical doses (Fig. 5-7). It is capable of measuring activities ranging from a few microcuries to several curies. It is quite simple to operate. Typically the instrument is adjusted for the radionuclide to be measured either by pushing a preset nuclide button or turning a potentiometer dial to a specific calibration number. The dose that is contained in a vial or syringe is then placed into the well of the ionization chamber, and the activity is displayed on a digital meter readout. Calibration number settings for each radionuclide are provided by the instrument manufacturer for all of the commonly used radionuclides; however, calibration numbers can be established by the user. This is accomplished by obtaining a standard reference source of the radionuclide, placing it into the ionization chamber well, and adjusting the calibration dial until the true activity is displayed on the meter. Standard radionuclide sources are usually supplied in 5-ml glass ampules available from either the National Bureau of Standards or a commercial supplier such as New England Nuclear Corporation or Amersham Corporation.

When establishing a calibration number in the aforementioned manner, one

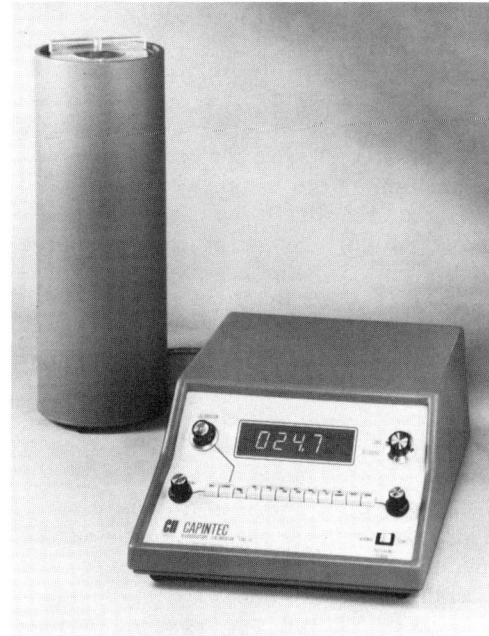

Figure 5-7. Radionuclide dose calibrator. *(From Capintec, Inc, Ramsey, NJ, with permission.)*

should be aware of photon absorption by the nuclide container. Generally, for radionuclides with photon energies above 100 keV there is less than a 10 percent difference between measurements made in glass serum vials, ampules, or plastic syringes.[8] Photon energies below 100 keV, however, may exhibit substantial differences in readings, depending on the container configuration. For example, activity measurements of iodine-125 ($\sim$ 30 keV) in glass ampules will be about 50 percent lower than in plastic syringes. For such weak gamma emitters calibration numbers should be established for the container actually used to make dose measurements, e.g., plastic syringes.

Dose calibrators are quite durable and usually operate satisfactorily for several years. Daily and periodic quality control measures are required to document good operating order and will be discussed in Chapter 6.

Geiger–Müller Survey Meter

This is a portable device for measuring radiation exposure in counts per minute or milliroentgens per hour. It is a very sensitive detection device and is used primarily to monitor work areas for radioactive contamination and to establish exposure rate. For example, the Geiger–Müller survey meter is useful when setting up a work area to determine whether adequate shielding is being used. Additionally, it can be used to monitor hospitalized patients treated with I-131 to determine exposure rate at the bedside and to determine when the patient can be released from the hospital. A typical instrument is shown in Figure 5–8.

Geiger–Müller Radiation Monitor

This instrument is similar to the survey meter except that it is stationary and operates on regular line current although it may be transported and operated on battery power. It is usually positioned strategically in the nuclear pharmacy to detect the presence of unshielded radiation sources. It provides an audible ticking sound characteristically associated with Geiger counters. The device is also very useful for monitoring the hands to detect any radioactive contamination. For this purpose it is useful to have the instrument placed near the door of the nuclear pharmacy so that monitoring can be done just before one exits from the room. A typical monitor is shown in Figure 5–9.

Scintillation Well Counter

This instrument is primarily used for measuring radioactive samples in test tubes. It is a very sensitive detector and should be used to measure samples whose activity is less than 1 μCi. Larger activities may exceed the resolving time of the detector and yield inaccurate results. This instrument should be located in a low-level counting area to reduce background radiation levels. In laboratories where only a few in vitro studies are performed each week, samples can usually be counted manually. For a large number of samples, however, a multiple sample holder with an automatic sample changer may be purchased. The well counter is coupled to a spectrometer system so that photon energy discrimination is possible and samples containing more than one radionuclide may be counted. A typical well counter is shown in Figure 5–10.

MISCELLANEOUS INSTRUMENTS AND SUPPLIES

A number of other items are necessary in the nuclear pharmacy. A microscope and hemacytometer slide are useful for quality control of particulate agents such as radio-

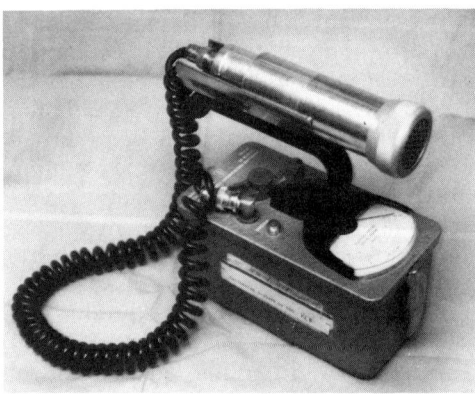

Figure 5-8. A Geiger–Müller survey meter. *(From Eberline Instrument Corp, Santa Fe, NM, with permission.)*

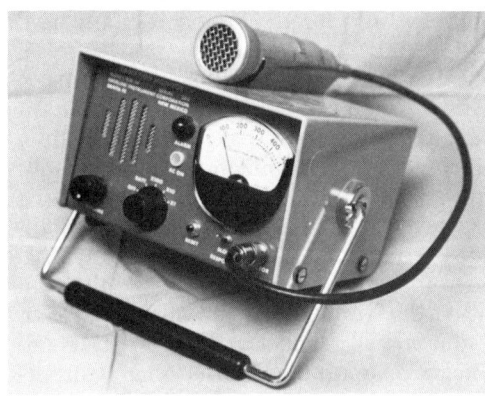

Figure 5-9. A Geiger–Müller radiation monitor. *(From Eberline Instrument Corp, Santa Fe, NM, with permission.)*

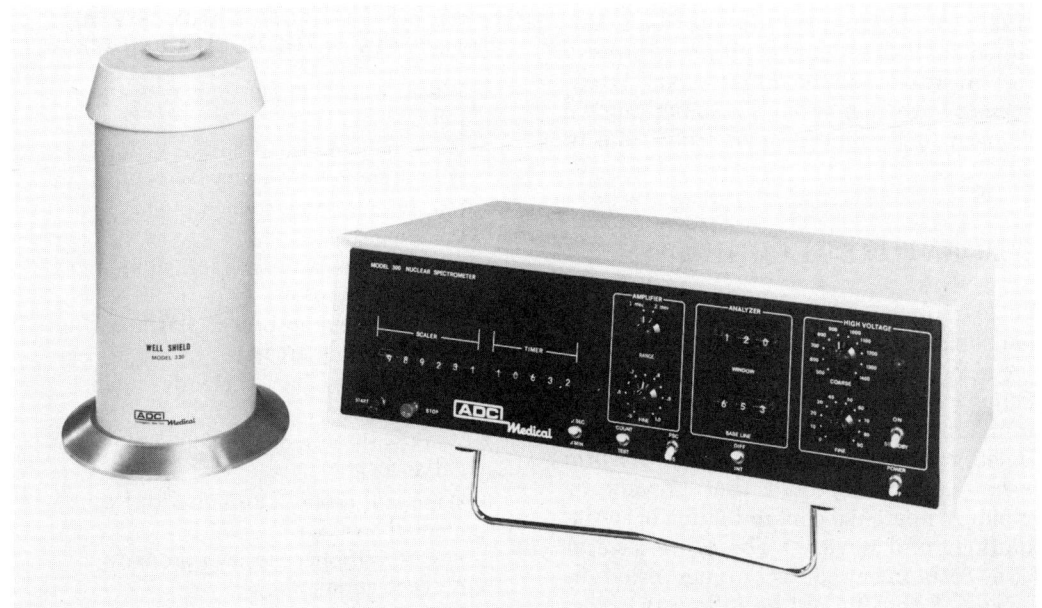

Figure 5-10. A scintillation well counter. *(From ADC Medical, Farmingdale, NY, with permission.)*

colloids, albumin macroaggregates and microspheres, and labeled cells. A centrifuge is needed for separating plasma from blood cells in various in vivo and in vitro studies. Balances are needed for weighing materials such as chemicals and balancing centrifuge tubes. A wide variety of glassware including beakers, flasks, bottles, graduated cylinders, and pipettes are required for conducting experiments and in vitro studies. A hot plate with a magnetic stirrer is necessary for procedures that require heat and mixing. A calculator is needed for making dose calculations. A refrigerator with a freezer is necessary for various types of agents that require below room temperature storage such as labeled biologic products. The refrigerator need not be lead lined because adequate shielding can be provided with vial shields. A pH meter is useful for preparing buffered solutions and for quality control measures. Various types of chromatography materials and reagents are needed for quality control of radiopharmaceuticals. Of course, if research functions are carried out in the nuclear medicine department, a much more extensive list of more sophisticated equipment and supplies would be needed.

PERSONNEL

One of the cardinal rules of pharmacy is to get the right dose to the right patient at the right time. Patients deserve the best possible care, and we must always strive to serve their needs as if we were serving members of our own families. The best equipment and facilities alone will not guarantee that the patient is best served. That job is the responsibility of the professional staff who conduct the nuclear medicine studies. Nuclear pharmacy labs are operated by radiopharmacists and nuclear medicine technologists who are competent practitioners. This requires that they be well trained, informed, and properly motivated. A strong knowledge base is foremost to competent nuclear pharmacy practice. Additionally, however, one must use good techniques while applying this knowledge.

Finally, a vigilant attitude must be maintained at all times during all procedures so that mistakes can be minimized. Attentiveness to the job at hand is something we all need to be reminded of from time to time.

LABORATORY TECHNIQUES

Nuclear pharmacy laboratory techniques can be divided into two categories: protective techniques and aseptic techniques. *Protective techniques* are methods that prevent or minimize radioactive contamination and unnecessary radiation exposure. *Aseptic techniques* are methods that prevent or minimize microbial contamination of sterile solutions and devices. There are several basic recommended techniques listed in Table 5-2 that should be followed.

When handling radioactive solutions one can expect occasional inadvertent contact contamination, especially of the hands. Disposable plastic gloves are the best protective measure because they can be readily removed and discarded. This very simple measure can prevent skin contamination, which often is quite difficult to remove. It is important to prevent hand contamination not only from a radiation safety standpoint but also to minimize transferring the contamination to equipment and to test tube samples that are to be counted in scintillation well counters. One should remember that a small drop of a radiopharmaceutical solution may contain several hundred microcuries. Contaminated perspiration from the hand that is transferred to the surface of a test tube could easily invalidate the results of an in vitro study. A lab coat or apron would protect the clothing from accidental splashing.

Effective protection from external exposure from unshielded sources is provided by the lead L-block with a protective glass viewscreen. This device will shield the head, torso, and gonadal areas and limit exposure only to the less critical arms and hands.

Syringe shields are an important factor for protecting the hands and fingertips. It was pointed out earlier that a one-eighth inch thick lead shield will reduce the radiation exposure from Tc-99m by a factor of 1000 as shown in Figure 5-11. One should also keep in mind the utility of the inverse square law in reducing exposure. Figure 5-12 illustrates the radiation dose rate to the fingers as a function of the finger position on a syringe containing Tc-99m. It is evident that the highest dose rate is received by the finger placed directly over the radioactive volume in the syringe (position A).

TABLE 5-2. PROTECTIVE AND ASEPTIC TECHNIQUES IN THE NUCLEAR PHARMACY

1. Wear disposable plastic gloves and a lab coat.
2. Work behind a lead barrier L-block with a leaded glass view screen.
3. Use syringe shields when preparing and injecting doses.
4. Use the inverse square law to reduce radiation exposure.
5. Use trays and absorbent plastic-backed paper at work areas.
6. Work quickly and efficiently—plan ahead.
7. Work with only one radiopharmaceutical at a time.
8. Wipe vial rubber closures with fresh alcohol swabs.
9. Puncture rubber closures properly to prevent coring.
10. Remove solution from ampules properly.
11. Don't force air into vials and create pressure.
12. Enter vials only with a new syringe and needle.
13. Use fresh needles on syringes before injecting patients.
14. Keep all openings in sterile set-ups protected before use.
15. Inspect all materials, devices, and solutions carefully—be observant at all times.
16. No eating, drinking, smoking, or pipetting by mouth.

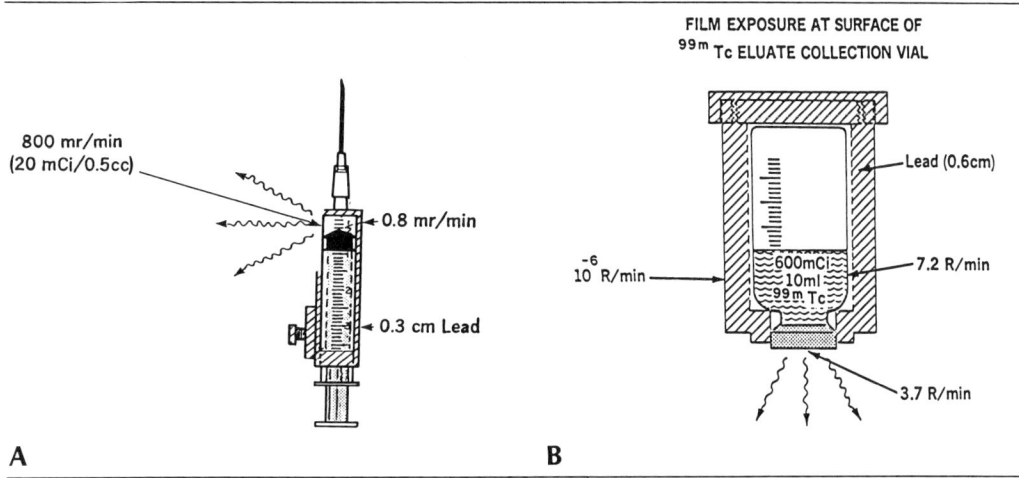

Figure 5-11. Exposure rate from a Tc-99m source. **A.** Syringe, shielded and unshielded. **B.** Vial, shielded and unshielded. (Courtesy of Dr. John R. Howley, Radiation Safety Branch, National Institutes of Health, Bethesda, MD.)

If the average dose administered is 0.5 ml in a 2-ml syringe, the dose rate is 55 mrem/mCi/min. Considering that finger contact time to the syringe during injection averages 15 seconds,[9] a 20-mCi dose would deliver 275 mrem to the finger at position A. When the fingers are placed at position B, this dose is reduced significantly to 6.25 mrem. According to the *Radiation Protection Guides* the average dose to the hands

SYRINGE SIZE	VOLUME	POSITION mREM/min/mCi Tc-99m *		
		A	B	C
	0.5 ml	55	1.25	0.30
2 ml	1.0	40	1.75	0.25
	2.0	25	5.95	0.20

* From Ref. 3

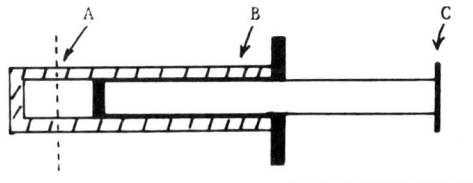

Figure 5-12. Exposure rate to fingers at various positions on an unshielded plastic syringe containing Tc-99m. (Data from Henson PW, 1973, p 972.[3])

should not exceed 1500 mrem per week. In the example just cited it is clear that one could easily exceed this limit after administration of only six unshielded doses with the fingers held at position A and over 250 doses at position B. It is obvious then that finger position on the syringe is an important factor in reducing exposure to the hands. Additionally, it should be kept in mind that radiation badges used to monitor hand exposure are typically worn on the ring finger and do not give a true estimate of radiation exposure to the fingertips. In summary, some simple rules should be followed: (1) use syringe shields, (2) hold syringes at a position farthest away from the volume of activity, and (3) handle the syringe for only that length of time required to complete the injection.

Although most doses administered in nuclear medicine are gamma emitters, occasionally a dose of phosphorus-32 as sodium or chromic phosphate is dispensed. Although P-32 is a pure beta emitter, the beta particles are quite energetic (E_{max} = 1.7 MeV), and a significant number of these beta particles will penetrate the walls of a plastic syringe. One should therefore refrain from holding such doses over the volume in the syringe for even a short length of time. It has been estimated that a dose of 4.5 rad will be delivered to the finger held for 30 seconds in contact with a syringe containing 10 mCi of P-32 in a 5-ml volume.[3]

When doses are dispensed at the lead L-block, it is a good habit to place the radiopharmaceutical vial in a small plastic tray or on a plastic-backed absorbent paper. In this way if contamination occurs, the tray or paper can be readily replaced. Additionally, during the dispensing operation one should have only one radiopharmaceutical vial present at a time to prevent cross-contamination between vials during dose preparation. Each vial rubber closure should be cleaned with a fresh alcohol swab. Reuse of the same swab on other vials only serves to spread any contamination from vial to vial and increases the chances of contaminating the fingers.

Solutions should be removed from vials and ampules properly. The heel of large-gauge needles can easily core the rubber closure during puncture. To minimize coring use smaller-gauge needles, enter the vial with the needle bevel toward you, and give it slight pressure away from you as the needle is inserted into the stopper as shown in Figure 5-13. When ampules are opened by

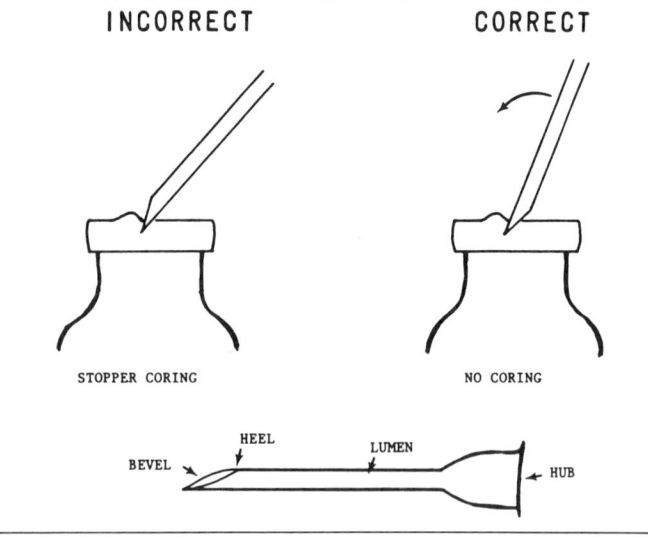

Figure 5-13. Technique for needle puncturing of rubber closures on serum vials. Correct technique lessens chances of coring.

snapping off the top, small pieces of glass may fall into the ampule and settle to the bottom. To minimize removal of these particles the solution should be withdrawn in a decanting position while tipping the ampule forward as if pouring the liquid out and at the same time withdrawing the volume with the syringe. The needle bevel should rest against the side of the ampule to exclude any glass particles as shown in Figure 5-14.

When removing solutions from vials containing nonradioactive drugs, it is common practice to inject into the vial a volume of air equal to the volume of solution required. In this way the pressure created in the vial will facilitate removal of the solution into the syringe. This is *not* good practice, however, for radioactive solutions because increased vial pressure may cause the solution to drip out as the needle is removed. A slightly negative pressure is desirable in radiopharmaceutical vials to minimize the chance of radioactive contamination.

When preparing Tc-99m radiopharmaceuticals, it is mandatory that a new syringe and needle be used to obtain the Tc-99m pertechnetate to prevent contamination of the pertechnetate stock solution with radiopharmaceutical. For example, the preparation of Tc-99m DMSA requires that a stannous DMSA reagent solution be mixed with Tc-99m pertechnetate. If the DMSA reagent is obtained first and the same syringe is used to obtain the Tc-99m pertechnetate, the entire pertechnetate solution will become contaminated with Tc-99m DMSA.

Before injecting a patient with a radiopharmaceutical it is good practice to replace the needle that was used to obtain the dose with a new needle. Multiple punctures of a needle into a rubber closure causes the point to dull and the silicone lubricant to be rubbed off. A sharp lubricated needle greatly facilitates nontraumatic venipuncture.

To prevent bacterial contamination of infusion setups one should be careful to keep stopcock and tubing ports capped with sterile closures. One should carefully inspect all materials used. Syringes are sometimes cracked or deformed, needle tips may be bent, and foreign material such as dirt particles or insects can be found in sterile tubing, stopcocks, etc. Additionally, foreign matter such as lint particles or precipitates are sometimes present in drug solutions.

Finally, one should not bring food into the nuclear pharmacy, and all pipetting should be performed using mechanical pipetting devices.

NUCLEAR PHARMACY FUNCTIONS

Numerous functions are performed in the nuclear pharmacy, but the primary activities are as follows:

1. Procurement and receipt of radiopharmaceuticals
2. Compounding radiopharmaceuticals
3. Dispensing radiopharmaceuticals
4. Quality control of radiopharmaceuticals and instruments
5. Control of radioactive waste
6. Record keeping

Procurement and Receipt of Radiopharmaceuticals

The purchase of radioactive material can only be carried out with proper authorization granted to the user through a radio-

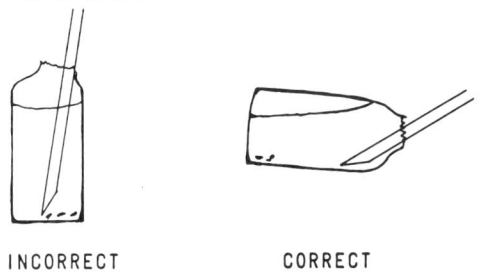

Figure 5-14. Technique for removing solutions from ampules using a syringe and needle. Correct technique minimizes chances of removing glass particles.

active materials license. The radiopharmaceutical supplier cannot ship radioactive material to a user unless it obtains written documentation assuring that the user is duly licensed to receive the types and quantities of radioactive material requested. The licensee may then submit purchase orders for radiopharmaceuticals. It is sometimes desirable to submit bids to various radiopharmaceutical suppliers to obtain the most economic contract of price and service. Because many radiopharmaceuticals are used routinely in nuclear medicine, it is also convenient to establish standing orders with a supplier to have certain radiopharmaceuticals shipped automatically on a regular basis. Otherwise, radiopharmaceuticals may be ordered on an as-needed basis. Shipping and transportation arrangements are usually such that materials can be received within 24 hours of order placement. Purchase orders typically contain specifications regarding the type and quantity of radioactive material, price, dates and time of delivery, calibration time, and specific delivery instructions.

Arrangements should be made for delivery of radiopharmaceuticals into the nuclear medicine department. Frequently, deliveries are made after normal working hours, and arrangements should be made with hospital security to receive and secure packages at those times, usually in the nuclear medicine department.

Upon receipt, packages of radioactive material should be inspected for damage and leakage of solutions. They should be located in an isolated part of the lab for a survey of radiation levels and wipetest monitoring for external surface contamination as specified in the *Code of Federal Regulations* (10 CFR 20.205). A survey of each package with an appropriate survey meter is generally the first procedure. No package shall exceed 200 mR/hr at the package surface or 10 mR/hr at 1 m.

Monitoring for external contamination shall be performed no later than 3 hours after receipt during normal working hours or 18 hours if received after normal working hours. For these surveys, a wipe of the entire package surface using an absorbant paper is conducted, and the wipe is counted in a scintillation counter calibrated for the particular radionuclide. If removable radioactive contamination in excess of 0.01 μCi (22,000 dpm) per 100 cm^2 is found on the external surface, the licensee shall immediately notify the final delivery carrier and by telephone and telegraph the appropriate Nuclear Regulatory Commission (NRC) regional office. Most radionuclides used in nuclear medicine are exempted from wipetest monitoring according to 10 CFR 20.205. Those radionuclides that must be monitored are items in liquid form (except Mo–Tc generators) and items with half-lives greater than or equal to 30 days and containing more than 100 mCi. Specific items requiring monitoring in nuclear medicine are more than 100 mCi of I-131 and Tc-99m (instant only), 10 mCi of I-125 and 1 mCi of ytterbium-169 and selenium-75. The reader is referred to Chapter 18 for more detailed discussion involving regulatory control of radioactive packages.

It is also useful to radioassay each vial in the dose calibrator to compare the labeled amount of activity with that actually received. Values should agree within ±10 percent. In some instances it may be desirable to perform gamma spectrometry on a shipment to confirm radionuclide identity. This procedure is most useful for radiochemicals used in research-type radiolabeling procedures. Figure 5–15 illustrates examples of receiving reports for documenting information.

Compounding of Radiopharmaceuticals

When handling radioactive material one should keep in mind the parameters of time, distance, and shielding for minimizing radiation exposure. Working quickly and efficiently will decrease exposure time. The use of remote handling devices such as long-handled tongs are useful for handling unshielded sources. Of course, shielding is the most effective method for protection but is not always readily possible.

NORTH CAROLINA MEMORIAL HOSPITAL   DIVISION OF NUCLEAR MEDICINE
ISOTOPE SOURCE CONTROL RECORD

ISOTOPE-CHEMICAL FORM	MFR.	LOT NO.	NUMBER OF UNITS	TOTAL VOL.	DATE REC	CAL. DATE	ACTIVITY THEORETICAL	ACTIVITY MEASURED	SURFACE mr/hr	REC' BY
Mo-99 (generator)	UC	B80A05Z	1	--	1-9-84	1-5-84	1417 mCi	--	27	RK
I-131 Hippuran	Mall.	1154041	3 vials	13.2 mL	10-15-84	10-19-84	4.65 mCi	4.8 mCi	8	RH

1. Shipment Identification: Supplier
   Radionuclide _____ Lot # _____ Carrier _____

2. Radiation level measured at 1 meter from package ___ mR/h

3. Surface wipe of external package (area 100 cm^2 or greater) End-Window GM _____ C/M Gamma Spectrometer-Scaler _____ C/M NOTE: If the levels are above "reportable" take necessary precautions: Call carrier and NRC and/or State Health Department (circle as appropriate).

4. Open package and wipe internal package or container (surface area 100 cm^2 or as near as possible), measured end-window GM _____ C/M, Gamma Spectrometer-Scaler C/M

   NOTE: If levels above 1/2 "reportable," take contamination control action: call supplier.

5. Gamma Spectrometer Assay
   Radionuclide _____ (Supplier Provided)
   Radionuclide _____ (By Our Assay)
   Contaminants _____ (By Our Assay)

6. Approximate quantity by assay _____ mCi on / /
   Supplier's assay _____ mCi on / /

Report Completed By

Figure 5-15. Receiving reports for radiopharmaceuticals. *(From Branson BM: In Sodd VJ (ed): Radiation Safety in Nuclear Medicine: A Practical Guide. Rockville, MD, US Department of HHS, 1981, p 24.)*

Preparation of volatile materials such as I-131 therapy solutions or radioactive gases should be conducted in an exhausting hood. It is preferable if solution preparations are conducted in trays with absorbent paper. Gloves and aprons or lab coats should be worn.

All radioactive solutions and other preparations such as flood sources, standards, etc., should be labeled as to radionuclide identity, chemical form, activity, time, date, control number, expiration time, and date and contain a radioactive symbol and the words *Caution: Radioactive Material.*

Tc-99m Kit Preparation. Radiopharmaceutical preparation in the nuclear pharmacy involves primarily that of Tc-99m agents. This is most commonly accomplished by reconstituting a particular kit with the appropriate quantity of Tc-99m-pertechnetate activity. Frequently, sterile normal saline injection is added to the kit for volume adjustment. For this purpose one should use saline without preservatives. Manufacturers' instructions should be followed for the preparation of Tc-99m agents. Within the manufacturer's guideline an amount of activity is selected that will yield the required number of doses from the vial within the desired time period of use and a sufficient excess to allow for radioactive decay. The following example will illustrate one method of preparing a bone imaging agent, Tc-99m oxidronate.

Example:

Four bone scans are scheduled to be performed in nuclear medicine. Two inpatients will be injected immediately after radiopharmaceutical preparation; one outpatient will be injected 2 hours later and another outpatient 4 hours later. The usual dose of Tc-99m oxidronate for bone imaging is 15 mCi. How much activity should be used to prepare the pharmaceutical?

Radiopharmaceutical preparation: The two inpatient doses will require 30 mCi. The outpatients will require doses adjusted for decay. With a Tc-99m decay factor for 2 and 4 hours, the first outpatient dose will require 19 mCi (15 mCi ÷ 0.794), and the second outpatient will require 24 mCi (15mCi ÷ 0.630). The total amount of activity needed for patient doses at radiopharmaceutical preparation time is therefore 73 mCi. About 10 percent extra is needed for vial residual, thus increasing the requirement to 80 mCi. Frequently, it is also wise to add sufficient activity for one additional dose that may be scheduled later in the day. One may thus add an additional 25 mCi to make a grand total of 105 mCi at the time of initial radiopharmaceutical preparation. Finally, enough saline is added to achieve the final desired volume.

Each radiopharmaceutical has either a formulation worksheet that describes how to prepare it with space to record activities, volumes, etc., used or a master formulation card describing step-by-step preparation and a separate sheet to record information. Usually a control number is assigned to each product made. There are several methods to establish a control number system, but one simple method is to use a seven-digit number; the first two digits identify the month, the next two digits the year, and the last three digits the number of the product made in that month. For example, if the Tc-99m oxidronate prepared above was the 27th product made in January 1984, its control number would be 0184027. Figure 5–16 illustrates a simple continuously running formulation control record for recording information regarding Tc-99m kit preparations. Details and precautions regarding technetium chemistry and the preparation of Tc-99m compounds were discussed in Chapter 4.

After initial preparation each Tc-99m radiopharmaceutical must be labeled to indicate the name of the radiopharmaceutical, activity, concentration, time, date, control number, and expiration time and date. Figure 5–17 illustrates a typical label that relates to the Tc-99m oxidronate prepared in the previous example.

THE NUCLEAR PHARMACY

NORTH CAROLINA MEMORIAL HOSPITAL DIVISION OF NUCLEAR MEDICINE

TECHNETIUM-99m RADIOPHARMACEUTICAL CONTROL RECORD

DATE	NUCLEAR MED CONTROL NO.	Tc-99m PERTECHNETATE				TIME	RADIO Rx KIT				SALINE			TOT VOL	PREP BY	uCi Mo-99	uGm Al+3
		SOURCE	LOT NO.	ACT	VOL.		TYPE	VOL	SOURCE	LOT NO.	SOURCE	LOT NO	VOL				
1-10-84	0184027	UC	B801057	867	16 ML	7:00	—	—	—	—	Trav.	8C94452	—	16 ML	SWC	27	<10
"	0184028	NM	0184027	105	2 ML	7:10	HDP	--	P & G	DL83048	"	"	3 ML	5 ML	SWC	—	—

Figure 5-16. Tc-99m radiopharmaceutical control record.

Dispensing Radiopharmaceuticals

An authorized prescription should be obtained by the nuclear pharmacy before dispensing any radiopharmaceutical dose for a patient. It should contain the patient's full name, identification number, date, age or date of birth, radiopharmaceutical dosage form, activity, route of administration, type of study to be performed, and signature of a licensed nuclear medicine physician. Frequently in hospitals, radiopharmaceuticals are ordered on a hospital requisition that lists only the patient's name, date of birth, date, identification number, type of study requested, and physician's signature. Radiopharmaceutical information is omitted. Most routine nuclear medicine studies are performed, however, using a particular radiopharmaceutical, activity, and route of administration, and the dispenser selects the appropriate agent and dose. In these situations, however, it is necessary that a written authorization be established by the nuclear medicine physicians identifying which radiopharmaceuticals and activities are to be dispensed for each type of study. Exceptional cases should be noted in writing on the requisition. Figure 5-18 illustrates a hospital requisition and a prescription form for requesting a bone scan with Tc-99m oxidronate.

Before obtaining a patient dose, a calculation must be made to determine what volume of solution is needed for the desired activity. This must take into consideration the time of decay from initial

```
CAUTION  ☢ RADIOACTIVE
                MATERIAL
NAME
Rx    Tc-99m Oxidronate (HDP)
ACTIVITY  21 mCi   PER   1   ML
TIME  7:10 AM   DATE  1-9-84
CONTROL NO.  0184027   VOL  5 ML
North Carolina Memorial Hosp. Division of Nuclear Medicine
```

Figure 5-17. Label for radioactive material.

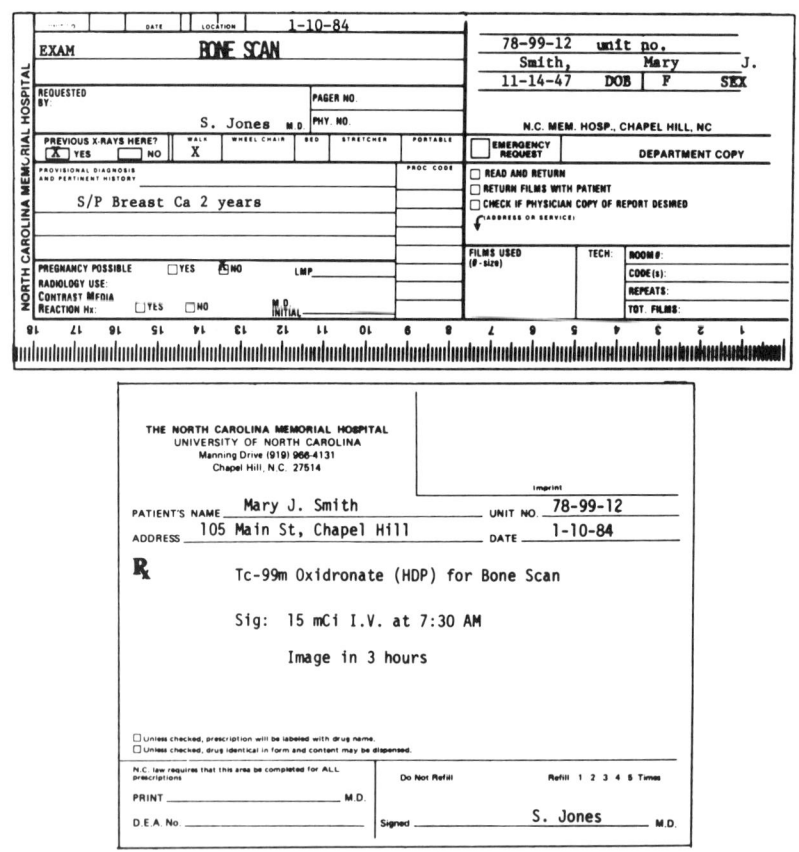

Figure 5-18. Examples of a hospital requisition and a prescription for a radiopharmaceutical order.

preparation. From the previous example, the volume required for the outpatient bone scan to be injected at 11:00 AM from the Tc-99m oxidronate prepared at 7:00 AM is calculated as follows:

1. $\begin{pmatrix} \text{Concentration} \\ \text{at 7 AM} \end{pmatrix} \begin{pmatrix} \text{Decay} \\ \text{factor} \end{pmatrix} = \begin{pmatrix} \text{Concentration} \\ \text{at 11 AM} \end{pmatrix}$

   21 mCi/ml × 0.631 = 13.25 mCi/ml

2. Volume required for a 15 mCi dose and 11 AM

   $$\frac{15 \text{ mCi}}{13.25 \text{ mCi/ml}} = 1.13 \text{ ml}$$

The dose is drawn up into a prelabeled syringe using aseptic and safety techniques. It is radioassayed in the dose calibrator to make certain that the activity drawn up does not deviate by more than ± 10 percent of that required. The syringe is then placed into a lead shield. The syringe label should contain the name of the patient and radiopharmaceutical, the activity, volume, date, time, and control number. This information should also be recorded in the dispensing record.

Pediatric Doses. There are several methods that can be used to calculate doses of drugs for children, but experience has shown that calculations based upon body surface area are more accurate in achieving the correct dose–response relationship. One reason for this is that organ growth and physiologic function conform more nearly to body surface area than to body weight. Most notably, hepatic and renal function is immature in young infants so that many drugs exhibit slowed metabolism and excretion compared with that in adults. An additional factor is that the total body water (TBW) and extracellular water (ECW), where most drugs distribute, are higher in children. TBW may range from 78 percent of a newborn's body weight to 60 percent in the adult. ECW occupies approximately 45 percent of a newborn's body weight compared with only 20 percent in the adult. Consequently, pediatric doses calculated as a fraction of the adult dose based upon body weight frequently leads to underdosage in children. Fortunately, body surface area is proportional to the 0.7 power of body weight, and a nomogram is available that allows surface area determinations from body weight.[10] The average adult is considered to have a body surface area of 1.7 m^2. Using this nomogram, Bell[11] developed a nomogram for calculating pediatric radiopharmaceutical doses (Fig. 5–19). For example, if the adult dose of a radiopharmaceutical is 15 mCi, the dose for a 10-kg child is calculated as follows: construct a line from the adult dose, in this case 15,000 μCi on the nomogram, to the average adult weight of 70 kg. This crosses the reference line at point X. Next, construct a line from the child's weight (10 kg) through point X on the reference line to the total-dose line where it intersects at the child's dose of 3850 μCi. Predetermined cross points for routine adult doses can be placed on the reference line to facilitate pediatric dose estimation.

Quality Control in the Nuclear Pharmacy

The principal considerations for quality control in the nuclear pharmacy are instrumentation and radiopharmaceuticals. A more detailed discussion on this topic will

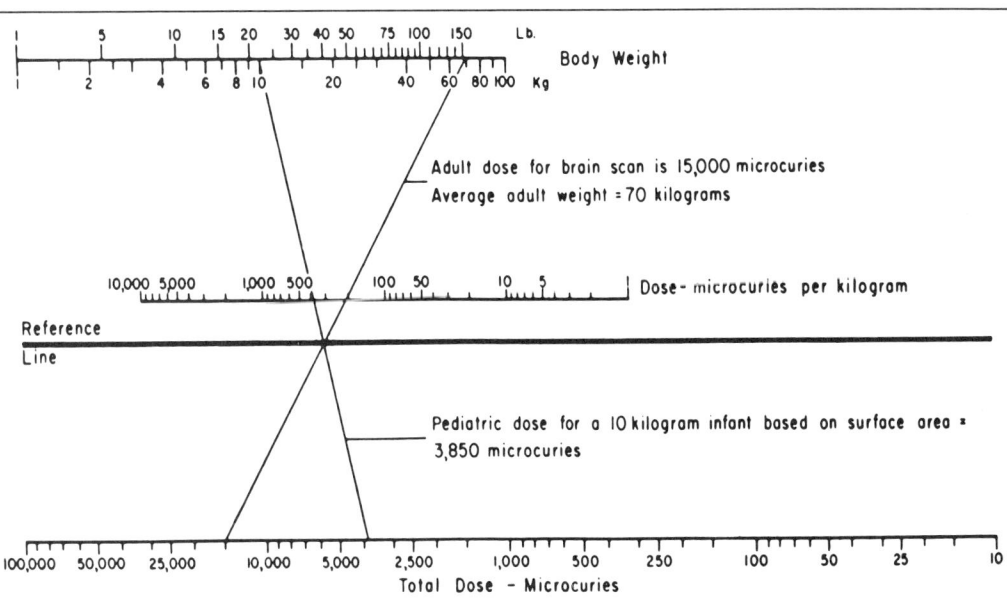

Figure 5-19. Nomogram for determining pediatric radiopharmaceutical doses. *(From Bell EG, et al, 1974, p 92, with permission.[11])*

be presented in Chapter 6 and therefore it will not be considered further at this time.

Radionuclide Waste Disposal in the Nuclear Pharmacy

Details regarding the disposal of radioactive waste can be found in the *Code of Federal Regulations*, Title 10 (10 CFR), Part 10.301, and *Regulatory Guide 10.8*, *Guide for the Preparation of Applications for Medical Programs, 1980*. The following methods are considered suitable for the disposal of radioactive waste in the hospital:

1. Transfer to an authorized recipient
2. Release into a sanitary sewer system
3. Burial in the soil
4. Other methods approved by the NRC
5. Storage for decay to negligible radiation and disposal in regular trash

Radiopharmaceutical waste generated in nuclear medicine is usually disposed of by methods 1, 2, or 5.

Transfer to an Authorized Recipient. Material may be transferred to an authorized commercial facility that will bury the waste on authorized property. All waste must be packaged and shipped according to the NRC's Title 10 and the Department of Transportation's Title 49, *Code of Federal Regulations* (CFR 1980). With the cost of burial rising dramatically and the reduction in the number of available burial sites, this method is becoming less frequently used by nuclear medicine departments. One viable route of disposal, however, is the return of spent Mo-99/Tc-99m generators to the manufacturer for disposal. This is accomplished by placing the spent generator into the shipping container of the newly received generator. The package is then sealed and labeled appropriately according to the instructions received with the generator. A bill of lading is filled out and the package returned to the manufacturer by the authorized delivery carrier for the hospital. Typically, the old generator is picked up at the time a new generator is delivered.

Release of Waste into Sanitary Sewer. It is not the usual practice to dispose of all radioactive waste into the sewer system; however, there are occasions when radionuclide waste is disposed of in this manner, and one should be aware of the allowable limits for disposal. Radioactive material may be released into a sanitary sewer under the condition that the material is readily soluble and dispersible in water (this excludes liquid scintillation samples in organic solvents) and the amounts do not exceed the following limits[12]:

1. Daily: Ten times the limits specified in Appendix C, 10 CFR 20, or the quantity of radioactive material that when diluted by the average daily amount of liquid released into the sewer system results in an average concentration not greater than the amount specified in Appendix B, Table I, column 2, of 10 CFR 20. The greater of the two values previously determined is permitted. For calculation purposes, the volume of sewage in a hospital is approximately 1000 liters per bed per day and 500 liters per person in other institutions.
2. Monthly: The quantity of radioactive material that when diluted by the average monthly amount of liquid released into the sewer system results in an average concentration not greater than the amount specified in Appendix B, Table I, column 2, of 10 CFR 20.
3. Yearly: A total of not more than 1 Ci of NRC licensed and other radioactive materials such as accelerator-produced material.

Note that excreta from persons administered radioactive materials for medical diagnosis or therapy are exempt from the three limitations just mentioned.

The following example calculation involving soluble I-131 disposal will illustrate the working of these disposal limits.[12] The volume of sewage generated by an institution must be known; *National Bureau of Standards Handbook 80* (1961) states that hospitals release 1×10^6 ml per bed per day. This example assumes a 200-bed hospital; i.e., one that would release 2×10^8 ml per day and 6×10^9 ml per month into the sewer system. The daily limit is the greater of the following two calculations: ten times the value for I-131 listed in Appendix C, 10 CFR 20, which is 1 µCi, i.e., (10) (1 µCi) = 10 µCi; or the sewage released per day times the soluble value listed in Appendix B, Table I, column 2, 10 CFR 20, i.e., (6×10^{-5} µCi/ml) (2×10^8 ml) = 12,000 µCi. The calculations in this case show that the daily upper limit is 12,000 µCi. The monthly limit for soluble I-131 for this 200-bed hospital is the value listed in Appendix B, Table I, column 2, times the monthly sewage volume or (6×10^{-5} µCi/ml) (6×10^9 ml) = 360,000 µCi. The yearly limit for disposal of all radionuclides is 1 Ci. In summary, then for each 100 beds in a hospital the following limits exist for I-131 disposal: daily, 6 mCi; monthly, 180 mCi; yearly, 1 Ci. The reader is referred to the example and rules of Appendix B, 10 CFR 20, for disposal of mixtures and unknown radionuclides.

Storage for Decay. The storage of radioactive material for decay and disposal in normal trash is not specified in 10 CFR 20 but is an acceptable method by the NRC.[12] The licensee must have a "storage for decay" condition in the license to be allowed to use this option.[13] The recommended procedure used to determine what material can be thrown away is to remove all shielding from the decayed material and monitor gamma-emitting waste with a low-level survey instrument such as a GM counter. If background levels are indicated on the meter, the material can be discarded after all radioactive labels are removed. This method is particularly useful for disposal of Tc-99m or other short-lived radionuclides. In such instances it is wise to separate Tc-99m waste from other waste that will require longer decay times.

Records in the Nuclear Pharmacy

The primary records one should maintain in the nuclear pharmacy are those for receipt, disposition, waste disposal, and compounding of radioactive material. Receipt records were discussed previously, and examples of forms to be used are shown in Figure 5-15. Disposition records include dispensing sheets for radiopharmaceutical doses and forms for the transfer of radioactive material to another authorized user within the hospital or institution. Examples of these records are shown in Figures 5-20

DRUG LOT NUMBER	DATE	PATIENT NAME (or use)	AGE (or CHILD'S WEIGHT)	HOSPITAL NUMBER	ACTIVITY mCi	VOLUME ml	TYPE STUDY	TIME	DISP BY
0184028	1-10-84	Doe, Joe	37	12-34-56	15.4	0.73	Bone	7:30	DS
"	"	Smith, Mary	46	78-99-12	15.4	0.73	"	"	DS
"	"	Jones, John	42	65-43-21	15.6	0.94	"	9:30	RK
"	"	Duke, Jane	25	10-20-30	15.3	1.16	"	11:30	NM

N.C. MEMORIAL HOSPITAL — RADIOPHARMACEUTICAL DISPENSING SHEET — Tc-99m Oxidronate (HDP) — IMAGING DIVISION

Figure 5-20. Radiopharmaceutical dispensing record.

Figure 5-21. Transfer record for radioactive material.

TRANSFER OF RADIOACTIVE MATERIAL

Under the rules of the University, it is permissible to transfer radioactive material from one authorized user to another. In quantity above exempt amounts, the following information should be given:

Radioisotope & Chemical form - _____ Activity _____

Transferred from - _____
    Staff member in charge   Room No.   Building

Transferred to - _____
    Staff member in charge   Room No.   Building

Copies to: Transferer
          Transferee   Date Transferred _____
          R.S.O.

Signature of Responsible Person _____

and 5-21. The dispensing record as illustrated is of the continuously running type. This format provides continuity and quick reference back to previous studies and conserves space. Essential information includes drug lot number, date, patient name, age or child's weight for calculating pediatric doses, patient hospital number (or prescription number could be entered here), activity dispensed, volume of the dose, type of study performed, time, and initials of the person dispensing the dose. The name of the radiopharmaceutical appears at the bottom of the sheet.

The radionuclide waste disposal record is shown in Figure 5-22 and lists the date of disposal, the radionuclide and chemical form, the drug lot number, and the activity disposed. If radioactivity is disposed of through different means, a column could also be included on the record to indicate how the material was disposed. A copy of

NORTH CAROLINA MEMORIAL HOSPITAL -- DIVISION OF NUCLEAR MEDICINE

RADIONUCLIDE WASTE DISPOSAL SHEET

DATE	RADIONUCLIDE	CHEMICAL FORM	LOT NUMBER	ACTIVITY DISPOSED
1-10-84	Tc-99m	HDP (oxidronate)	0184027	9.65 mCi (4:30 pm)

Figure 5-22. Radionuclide waste disposal record.

this record must accompany the waste drum when it is removed for burial.

The compounding record for radiopharmaceuticals can be of the simple continuously running type as illustrated previously in Figure 5–16 for Tc-99m radiopharmaceuticals prepared from sterile kits. The compounding record for special or extemporaneous preparation of radiopharmaceuticals should be more elaborate and include more detailed information regarding the particulars for preparing the radiopharmaceutical. The record should include the name of the radiopharmaceutical, date, control number, formula with chemical amounts, manufacturer and lot numbers, compounding procedure, quality control tests, and results.

RADIATION EMERGENCIES

A radiation emergency may exist if unplanned exposure to radioactive material is possible because of loss of a source, misplaced material, or an accident. In the case of a lost or misplaced source the radiation safety office should be notified. The primary radiation emergency in the nuclear pharmacy and nuclear medicine laboratory occurs from accidental spills of radioactive material. This may range from simple spills of small amounts of radioactive solution where no serious contamination problem results to major spills where large amounts of radioactive contamination presents a serious threat of harmful exposure. Each situation will undoubtedly be unique and be handled differently; however, there are a few general guidelines that should be followed. In any emergency situation the primary concern must be the protection of laboratory personnel from radiation hazard. Second, there should be confinement of the contamination to the local area of the spill. Because an emergency requires immediate action to minimize harmful effects, accidents involving a large number of millicuries should be considered a major emergency and microcurie quantities a minor emergency.

Major Emergency Procedures

This situation involves a spill on the order of 1 to 1000 mCi.

1. Notify all persons not involved to vacate the room.
2. Cover the material with absorbent pads to contain the spill.
3. Shield the source if possible without contaminating yourself.
4. Notify supervisory personnel and the radiation safety officer immediately.
5. Survey all personnel involved for contamination. Remove contaminated clothing, and wash exposed skin areas with soap and water.
6. Consult with the radiation safety officer regarding decontamination procedures to be followed.

Minor Emergency Procedures

This situation involves a spill on the order of 1 to 1000 μCi.

1. Notify persons in the area that a spill has occurred. Restrict others from the area.
2. Cover the material with absorbent pads to contain the spill.
3. Clean up the spill using protective clothing and disposable plastic gloves. Use decontamination solutions to remove radioactivity and clean from the perimeter toward the center of the spill. Place contaminated materials into a plastic bag for disposal.
4. Survey the area with a Geiger–Müller survey meter. Decontaminate the area until background radiation levels are obtained.
5. Survey for personal contamination and remove contaminated clothing for isolation and decay.
6. Notify the radiation safety officer.

The responsibilities of the radiation safety officer are as follows:

1. Supervise cleanup or restriction of the area until an emergency situation no longer exists.
2. Determine that available personnel have cleaned the area or have the emergency in hand.
3. Determine whether a report must be made to regulatory agencies in case of loss of material or exposure of personnel and make the necessary report.

MISADMINISTRATION OF RADIOPHARMACEUTICALS

Even the most well intentioned and competent practitioner will occasionally make a mistake. Errors are bound to occur in the busy nuclear medicine department, and sometimes a patient receives the wrong amount of activity or the wrong radiopharmaceutical agent. The handling of such misadministrations has been clearly described and can be found in the *Code of Federal Regulations*, Part 35. Under this ruling a misadministration means the administration of the following:

1. A radiopharmaceutical or radiation from a sealed source other than the one intended
2. A radiopharmaceutical or radiation to the wrong patient
3. A radiopharmaceutical or radiation by a route of administration other than that intended by the prescribing physician
4. A diagnostic dose of a radiopharmaceutical differing from the prescribed dose by more than 50 percent
5. A therapeutic dose of a radiopharmaceutical differing from the prescribed dose by more than 10 percent or
6. A therapeutic radiation dose from a sealed source such that errors in the source calibration, time of exposure, and treatment geometry result in a calculated total treatment dose differing from the final prescribed total treatment dose by more than 10 percent

Therapy Misadministration Reports

In the event of therapy misadministration the licensee shall notify, within 24 hours (or as soon as practicable) of the event by telephone only, the appropriate NRC regional office, the referring physician of the affected patient, and the patient or a responsible relative or guardian, unless the referring physician personally informs the licensee either that he will inform the patient or that, in his medical judgement, telling the patient or the patient's responsible relative or guardian would be harmful to one or the other, respectively. Within 15 days after the initial report to the NRC, the licensee shall report in writing to the NRC regional office initially telephoned and to the referring physician and furnish a copy of the report to the patient or the patient's responsible relative or guardian if either was previously notified. The written report shall include the licensee's name; the referring physician's name; a brief description of the event; the effect on the patient; the action taken to prevent recurrence; and whether the licensee informed the patient or the patient's responsible relative or guardian, and if not, why not. The report shall not include the patient's name or other identifying information.

Diagnostic Misadministration Reports

The Radiation Safety Officer is required to investigate the cause of all diagnostic misadministrations and record the event for NRC review. If the misadministration involves the use of byproduct material not intended for medical use, administration of a dosage five-fold different from that intended, or administration of byproduct material such that the patient is likely to receive an organ dose greater than 2 rem or a whole body dose greater than 0.5 rem, the licensee shall also notify the referring physician and the appropriate NRC office in writing within 15 days of the misadministration. Licensees may use dosimetry tables in package inserts, corrected only for amount of radioactivity administered, to determine whether a report is required. A sample report form can be found in Draft Regulatory Guide 10.8, 1985, as exhibit 1.14.

Misadministration Records

Records of all misadministrations shall be maintained for NRC inspection for 10 years. These records shall contain the names of all individuals involved in the event (including the physician, allied health personnel, the patient, and the patient's referring physician), the patient's social security number, a brief description of the event, the effect on the patient, and the action taken to prevent recurrence.

REFERENCES

1. Porter WC, Ice RD, Hetzel KR: Establishment of a nuclear pharmacy. Am J Hosp Pharm 32:1023, 1975
2. Kawada T, Wolf W, Seibert S: Planning a radiopharmacy. Am J Hosp Pharm 31:153, 1974
3. Henson PW: Radiation dose to the skin in contact with unshielded syringes containing radioactive substances. Br J Radiol 46:972, 1973
4. Clayton RS, White JE, Brieden M, et al: Skin exposure from handling syringes containing radioactive isotopes. Am J Roentgenol 105:897, 1969
5. Neil CM: The question of radiation exposure to the hand from handling Tc-99m. J Nucl Med 10:732, 1969
6. Branson BM, Sodd VJ, Nishiyama H, et al: Use of syringe shields in clinical practice. Clin Nucl Med 1:56, 1976
7. Code of Federal Regulations, Title 10, Part 20, Standards for Protection Against Radiation, Section 20.303, 1983
8. Kowalsky RJ, Johnston RE, Chan FH: Dose calibrator performance and quality control. J Nucl Med Tech 5:35, 1977
9. Anderson DW, Richter CW, Ficken VJ, et al: Use of TLD for measurement of dose to the hands of nuclear medicine technicians. J Nucl Med 13:627, 1972
10. Glazka AJ: Simplified procedures for calculating drug dosage from body weight in infancy and childhood. Pediatrics 27:503, 1961
11. Bell EG, McAfee JG, Subramanian G: Radiopharmaceuticals in pediatrics. In James AE, Wagner HN Jr, Cooke RE (eds): Pediatric Nuclear Medicine. Philadelphia, Saunders, 1974, p 84
12. Scholz KL: Waste disposal regulations. In Sodd VJ (ed): Radiation Safety in Nuclear Medicine: A practical Guide. HHS Publication FDA 82-8180. US Department of Health and Human Services, Rockville, Md, 1981
13. Regulatory Guide 10.8: Guide for the Preparation of Applications for Medical Institutions. US Nuclear Regulatory Commission, Washington, DC, October 1980

CHAPTER 6

Quality Control of Radiopharmaceuticals

There is an old saying that "a chain is only as strong as its weakest link." This saying can be applied to many aspects of life and to nuclear medicine practice as well. In the final analysis the nuclear medicine physician must be assured that the information obtained from a radiodiagnostic procedure is a true representation of the patient's condition. The strength and conviction of a physician's diagnostic impression is based not only on his or her knowledge and experience but also on a trustworthiness in a nuclear diagnostic system where all measures have been taken to rule out errors. In such a system there are several areas where problems can occur to weaken the system. The main areas of concern include competency of personnel, data collection, data processing and display systems, instrumentation, and radiopharmaceuticals. In this chapter we will focus attention on practical methods used in the nuclear pharmacy to assure high-quality radiopharmaceuticals and the proper operation of instrumentation used in preparing them.

RADIOPHARMACEUTICAL QUALITY CONTROL

Quality control of radiopharmaceuticals has been defined as "a series of tests, observations, and analyses that will indicate beyond reasonable doubt the identity, quality and quantity of all ingredients present in a product and which will demonstrate that the technology employed in its formulation or manufacture will yield a dosage form of the highest possible safety, purity, and efficacy.[1] This statement implies that the quality control program be in operation continuously throughout the radiopharmaceutical production process. An ongoing quality control program is an imperative requirement for the radiopharmaceutical manufacturer who prepares drugs from raw materials and ultimately sells and distributes them to a very large population of users. Because many radiopharmaceuticals used in hospitals require daily preparation and assay, some form of quality control program must also be in operation, albeit more limited in scope than that of the pharmaceutical manufacturer. In the hospital nuclear pharmacy, quality control procedures for radiopharmaceuticals may be identified within three groups: radiation considerations, pharmaceutical considerations, and biologic considerations.

Radiation Considerations

The safe and efficacious use of radiopharmaceuticals requires that they be of the highest purity with regard to their radionuclide and chemical composition. Any nuclear medicine procedure requires the administration of a particular radionuclide in a particular chemical form. The presence of other radionuclides or different chemical forms of the desired radionuclide would constitute impurities that may produce undesirable information from the diagnostic procedure. It is therefore important to conduct before-the-fact purity tests on all radiopharmaceuticals.

Radionuclidic Purity. Radionuclidic purity is defined as the fraction of the total radioactivity in a source that is present in the form of the desired radionuclide and is expressed as a percentage. For example, a 100 μCi source of sodium pertechnetate containing 99.5 μCi as Tc-99m and 0.5 μCi Mo-99 would have a radionuclidic purity of 99.5 percent with respect to Tc-99m. In this example, the Mo-99 activity would represent a 0.5 percent radionuclidic impurity.

Radionuclidic impurities in radiopharmaceuticals usually arise from the method of radionuclide production or from incomplete radionuclide separation during radiochemical processing. During radionuclide production in a cyclotron or nuclear reactor, undesirable nuclear reactions may occur because of target impurities producing unwanted radionuclides. Sometimes changing the target material and type of nuclear reaction will improve the system. For example, the production of iodine-123 by the (p,2n) reaction on a tellurium-124 target produces significantly more radionuclidic impurities (I-124, I-126, I-130, I-131) than the (p,5n) reaction on an iodine-127 target, which only produces an I-125 impurity. Of course, commercially produced radiopharmaceuticals are carefully monitored by the manufacturer for such impurities, and it is not imperative that all such agents be checked rigorously by the nuclear pharmacy. It is important, however, that the daily generator eluate be checked for Mo-99 contamination. Detailed methods for performing this test were discussed in Chapter 3. Additionally, careful attention to radionuclidic purity should be paid to radionuclide sources obtained as radiochemicals for certain radiolabeling procedures because these sources are not sold in a final-use form.

Radionuclidic impurities are significant in that they may contribute to an increased radiation dose without adding to the diagnostic information. Of greatest significance are those impurities with half-lives longer than the desired nuclide because the percent impurity will increase with time. Some examples of this situation are the presence of 67-hour Mo-99 impurity in 6-hour Tc-99m, the presence of 4-day I-124 impurity in 13-hour I-123, and the presence of 12-day thallium-202 impurity in 73-hour thallium-201.

Measurement of radionuclidic purity is usually made with a calibrated sodium iodide scintillation detector or preferably with the higher-resolution germanium lithium compensated, Ge (Li), detector coupled to a multichannel spectrometer. The gamma ray spectrum and corresponding half-lives are used to identify the radionuclides present. The limits of radionuclidic purity and extent of allowable impurities may be found in the US Pharmacopeia (USP).

Radiochemical Purity. Radiochemical purity is defined as the fraction of the total radioactivity in a source that is present in the desired chemical form and is expressed as a percentage. For example, a 100-μCi sample of Tc-99m sulfur colloid, of which 95 μCi is present as Tc-99m bound to sulfur particles and 5 μCi is Tc-99m pertechnetate, would have a radiochemical purity of 95 percent. The product in this case contains a 5 percent pertechnetate radiochemical impurity.

Radiochemical impurities may be formed as a result of competing chemical reactions during the radiolabeling process or from chemical or radiolytic decomposition of the final product. In the production of Tc-99m radiopharmaceuticals from kits it was shown in Chapter 4 that Tc-99m pertechnetate and hydrolyzed–reduced impurities may be produced as a result of inadequate reaction conditions or radiolysis. Orthoiodohippuric acid I-131 (hippuran I-131) may contain the radiochemical impurities o-iodobenzoic acid I-131 and iodide I-131 as shown in Figure 6-1.

Radiochemical impurities are significant because they have biodistribution patterns different from the desired radiopharmaceutical. This may degrade image quality, increase the absorbed radiation dose, and cause problems with diagnostic interpretation. For example, in the hippuran renogram study the presence of radioiodide impurity in excess of 3 percent may prolong renal transit time because of tubular reabsorption of iodide. When cardiac blood pool imaging is performed with Tc-99-labeled red blood cells, excess pertechnetate localizing in the stomach may interfere with study interpretation because of the proximity of the heart and stomach. Technetium pertechnetate present in bone imaging radiopharmaceuticals at 5 percent or greater impurity is readily seen as stomach and thyroid uptake on the scan as shown in Figure 6-2.

Radiochemical purity is usually determined by in vitro analytic methods and by in vivo biodistribution in animals. Details of test methods and purity limits may be

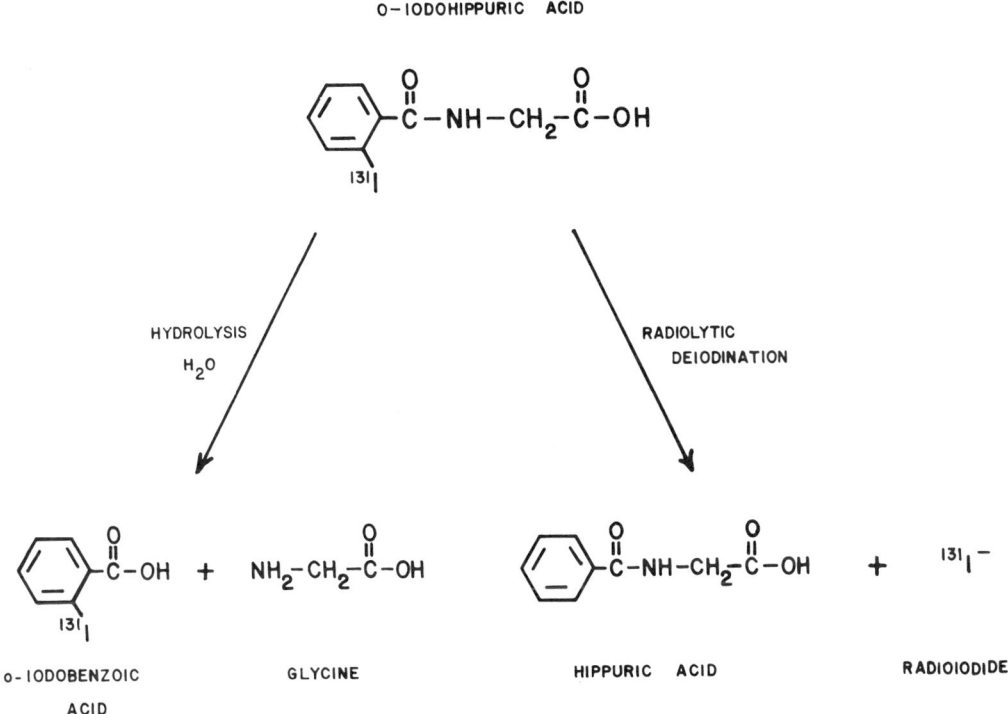

Figure 6-1. Degradation of I-131-orthoiodohippuric acid.

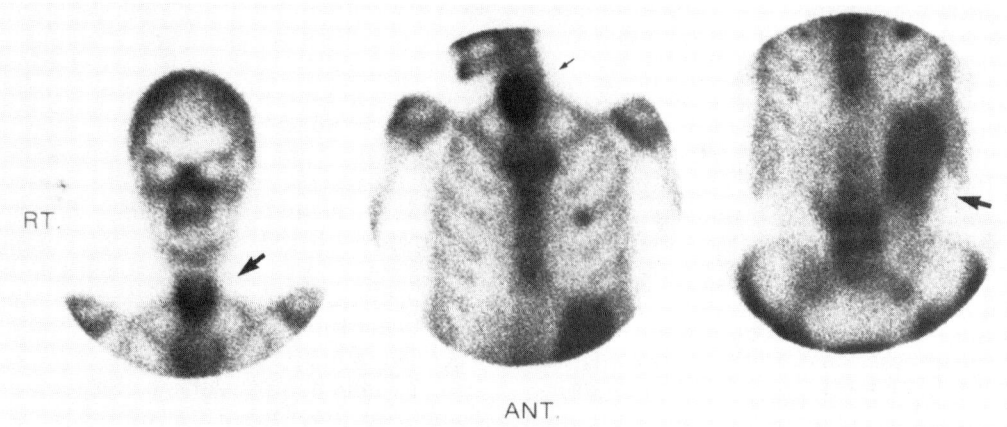

Figure 6-2. Bone scan with Tc-99m-medronate demonstrating Tc-99m-pertechnetate impurity localized in the thyroid gland and stomach.

found in several reference works[2-5] and in Table 6-1; however, a concise discussion will be presented to illustrate the various in vitro techniques.

In vitro analytic methods usually involve thin-layer and paper chromatography methods or some form of column chromatography such as ion exchange or gel filtration techniques.

Thin-Layer and Paper Chromatography. Thin-layer and paper chromatography are the simplest and most rapid methods for routine quality control of radiopharmaceuticals. In each of these techniques a sample of the radiopharmaceutical is spotted on a solid support (the stationary phase), which is then placed into an appropriate solvent (the mobile phase). The stationary phase may be paper, such as Whatman No. 1 or 3MM paper, or a thin-layer support, usually silica gel layered on glass or plastic. A modified thin-layer support is also used called instant thin-layer chromatography (ITLC). This is a glass microfiber mesh impregnated with silica gel (ITLC-SG) or silicic acid (ITLC-SA), resulting in a support resembling paper. The solvent, which is usually aqueous or organic, transports the radiopharmaceutical over the stationary phase by adsorption and capillary action.

The mobile and stationary phases compete for the various radiochemical species present in the radiopharmaceutical sample as they are carried along. The electrostatic attractive forces of the stationary phase retard movement of the various radiochemical species while their solvent solubility moves them along. Through the selection of appropriate support and solvent systems the different chemical species in the radiopharmaceutical may be separated. After chromatogram development the strip is removed, dried, and analyzed by using a radiochromatogram scanner or some other method of counting the radioactivity distribution on the strip.

The standard method of analysis is to determine the Rf (relative front) values for the various species on the strip and compare them to Rf values of known substances in the same system. The Rf value is the ratio of the distance a species travels to the distance the solvent travels from the origin on the strip as shown in Figure 6-3. The Rf values are determined by one of several methods:

1. Scanning the strip with a radiochromatogram scanner that traces out various activity peaks. Peak position is indicative of the particular species present, and

TABLE 6-1. RADIOCHEMICAL PURITY LIMITS OF COMMONLY USED RADIOPHARMACEUTICALS FROM THE USP XXI

Chemical Form	Minimum Percent Radioactivity as the Desired (Stated) Chemical Form	Principal Impurity
Chromic phosphate P-32 suspension	95	Ortho phosphate
Cyanocobalamin Co-57 oral capsules and solution	95	Cobalt ion
Gallium citrate Ga-67 injection	85	Gallate, gallium hydroxide
Indium In-111 pentetate injection	90	Indium hydroxide
Iodinated I-125 albumin injection	97	Iodide
Iodohippurate sodium I-131 injection	97	Iodide
Sodium chromate Cr-51 injection	90	Chromic ion
Sodium iodide I-123 capsules and solution	95	Iodate, iodine
Sodium iodide I-125 capsules and solution	95	Iodate, iodine
Sodium iodide I-131 capsules and solution	95	Iodate, iodine
Sodium pertechnetate Tc-99m injection	95	Reduced technetium
Sodium phosphate P-32 solution	100	Pyro- and meta-phosphate
Technetium Tc-99m albumin aggregated injection (MAA)	90	Pertechnetate
Technetium Tc-99m albumin injection (HSA)	90	Pertechnetate, colloidal-Tc
Technetium Tc-99m etidronate injection (EHDP)	90	Pertechnetate, colloidal-Tc
Technetium Tc-99m gluceptate injection (GH)	90	Pertechnetate, colloidal-Tc
Technetium Tc-99m medronate injection (MDP)	90	Pertechnetate, colloidal-Tc
Technetium Tc-99m oxidronate injection (HDP)	90	Pertechnetate, colloidal-Tc
Technetium Tc-99m pentetate injection (DTPA)	90	Pertechnetate, colloidal-Tc
Technetium Tc-99m pyrophosphate injection (PPi)	90	Pertechnetate, colloidal-Tc
Technetium Tc-99m succimer injection (DMSA)	85	Pertechnetate, colloidal-Tc
Technetium Tc-99m sulfur colloid injection (SC)	92	Pertechnetate
Thallous chloride Tl-201 injection	95	Trivalent thallium
Ytterbium Yb-169 pentetate injection	96	Ytterbium hydroxide

peak area corresponds to the respective amount of activity for each species.
2. Cutting the chromatogram into centimeter segments that are individually counted. Subsequently, a histogram plot of the activity distribution is made and the amount of activity in each species determined.
3. Using a miniaturized chromatography system that uses only a 6-cm strip. This

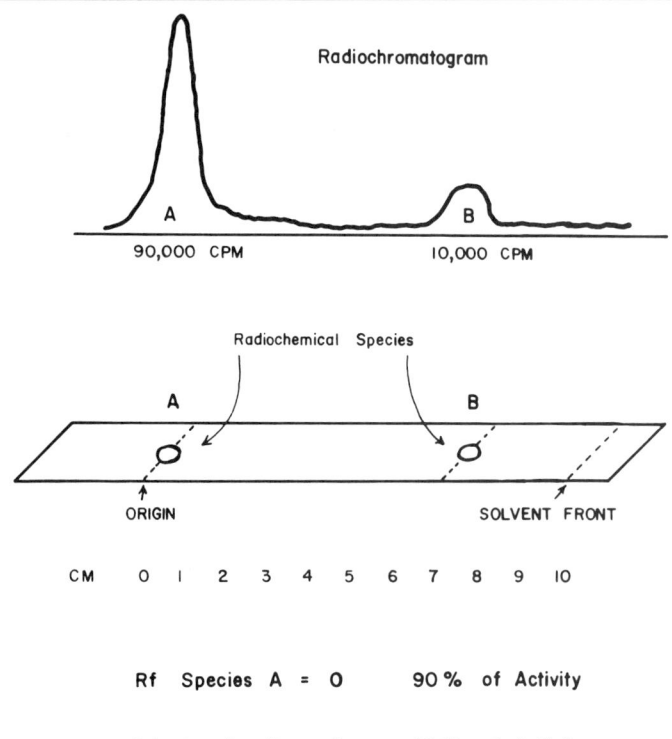

Figure 6-3. Analysis of a radiochromatogram: species A represents the desired radiopharmaceutical, species B represents radiochemical impurity. See the text for an explanation of Rf.

method is used when the species are well separated on the strip so that it can be cut into two pieces and counted for analysis.

The third method is used routinely for Tc-99m radiopharmaceuticals because it is rapid and easy to perform on a daily basis.

Figure 6-4 illustrates the single-strip radiochemical purity analysis procedure for labeled particles such as Tc-99m sulfur colloid, macroaggregates of albumin (MAA), and microspheres. The stationary phase is ITLC-SG, and the mobile phase is either acetone, saline, or water. In this system the particles remain at the origin because they are insoluble and exhibit an Rf of 0, whereas any pertechnetate impurity travels with the solvent front with an Rf of 1. The developed strip is then cut into two pieces and counted. Analysis of Tc-99m pertechnetate and DMSA is also shown.

For soluble Tc-99m radiopharmaceuticals such as Tc-99m-labeled DTPA, glucoheptonate (GH), diphosphonates, and hepatobiliary agents, three radiochemical species may be present. One of these species is the desired chemical form, the Tc-99m complex, and the other two species are the radiochemical impurities, hydrolyzed-reduced technetium colloid (Tc-HR) and Tc-99m pertechnetate. Analysis of these agents requires a two-solvent dual-strip system shown in Figure 6-5. Because the Tc complex is always associated with one of the impurities and cannot be isolated by itself, its radiochemical purity is determined indirectly. This is accomplished by subtracting the percentage of each impurity from 100 percent. For example, if for Tc-99m DTPA the Tc-HR impurity is 2 percent and the pertechnetate impurity is 3 percent, then the radiochemical purity of Tc-99m DTPA is 95 percent.

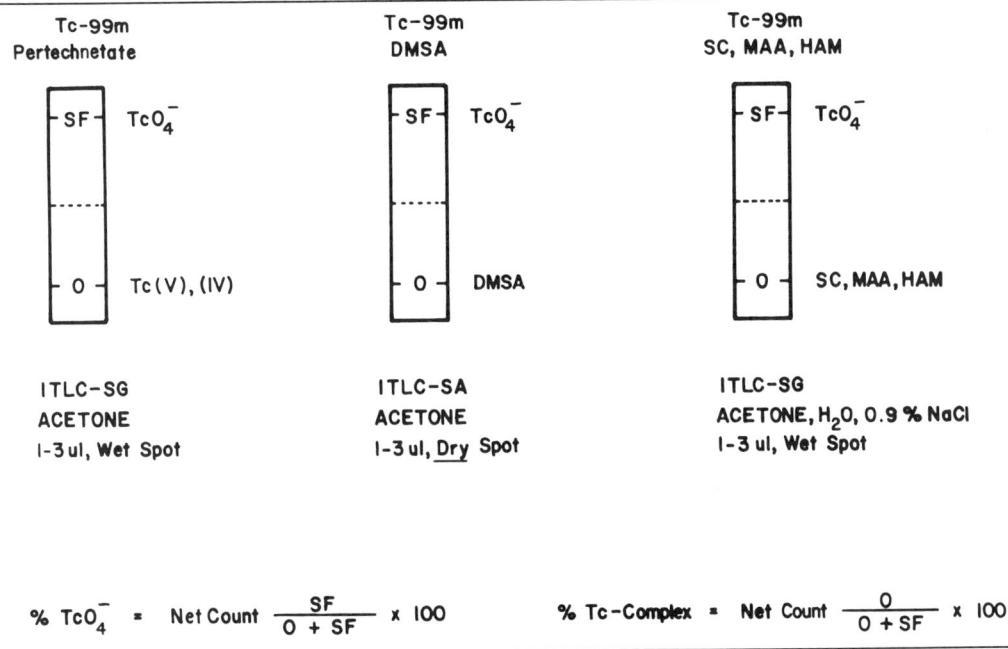

Figure 6-4. Single-strip miniaturized chromatography systems for Tc-99m radiopharmaceuticals.

CHROMATOGRAPHY TECHNIQUES AND PITFALLS. The procedure involves spotting a 1- to 5-μL sample of the radiopharmaceutical on a chromatography strip of 5 to 10 cm in length. The spot should not be too large and is either dried or left wet depending on the solvent used. The strip length depends on the extent of peak separation and is determined by trial and error. The spotted strip is placed into the solvent and developed for several minutes until the solvent reaches the top. The strip is then removed, dried, cut in half, and the origin and solvent front pieces counted in a dose calibrator or scintillation well counter. Strips counted in a dose calibrator should contain at least 100 μCi of activity to keep the counting error to 1 percent or less. This assumes a dose calibrator sensitivity of 1 μCi and, at minimum, a 1 percent impurity in the 100-μCi sample. If the scintillation well counter is used for counting, the strips should be counted far enough away from the detector so that the counting rate does not exceed the dead time of the detector.[5,6] This is not a problem with the dose calibrator or radiochromatogram scanner. The radiochromatogram scanner can be used if the strips are long enough (at least 10 cm); however, it is more time consuming.

Some pitfalls may be encountered in radiochromatography by the uninitiated technician. First, the spot should be placed at least 1 cm from the bottom of the strip so that the spot itself does not enter the solvent but is well above its level. In this way the solvent will pass through the spot and cause soluble species to migrate in a normal manner. If the spot is submerged in the solvent, even partly, these species will be retarded from migration, and erroneous results will occur.[7] Second, it is important that the spot be dried before development in organic solvents such as acetone, especially if the spot size is 5 μL or larger. Acetone is miscible with water, and radiochemical species that are soluble in water but not soluble in acetone, such as the Tc-99m com-

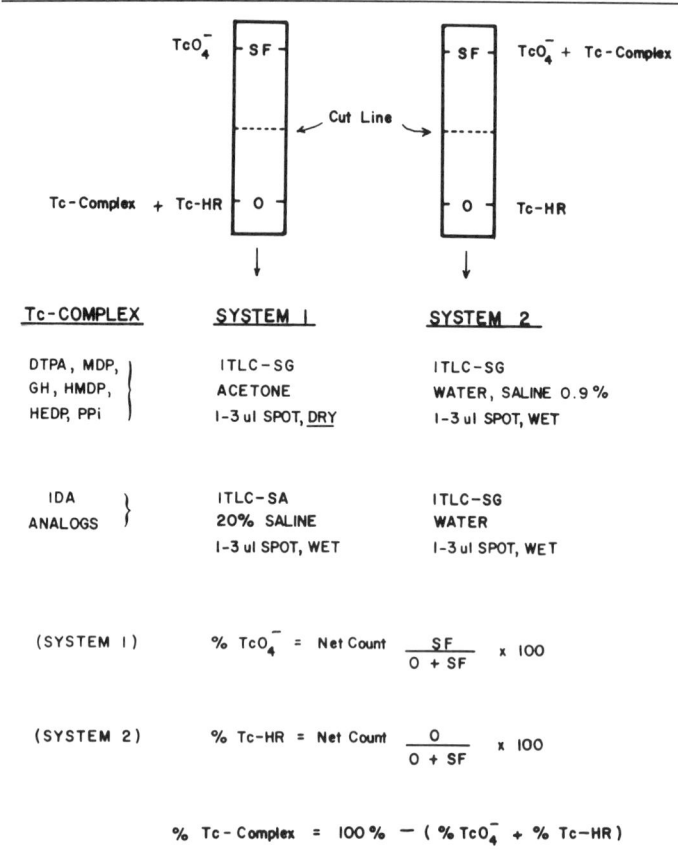

Figure 6-5. Dual-strip miniaturized chromatography systems for Tc-99m radiopharmaceuticals.

plexes, will streak up the strip from the origin if the spot is wet. If streaking extends into the top half of the strip, erroneous results will be obtained. This is more likely to occur with the 5-cm ministrips than if 10-cm strips are used. Figure 6-6 illustrates that the extent of streaking depends on spot size, and Table 6-2 lists the results obtained with several Tc-99m complexes developed on 5-cm ITLC-SG strips in acetone after application of a 5-μL wet or dried spot. It is evident from these data that significant migration (i.e., streaking) of the Tc-99m complex occurs into the solvent-front half of the strip if a wet spot is developed in acetone. During analysis this would be interpreted as a Tc-99m pertechnetate impurity but in fact would be an artifact created by improper technique.[7]

A number of other technical parameters may contribute to artifacts on the radiochromatogram.[5] Some of these include, among others, the following: (1) prolonged air drying of the applied spot on the chromatogram before development may cause oxidation of the Tc-99m complex on the chromatogram and produce false information regarding the actual condition of the complex in the vial,[7] (2) spattering of solution on the strip during the spotting operation, (3) use of contaminated forceps or scissors when handling chromatograms, and (4) using the wrong solvents or strips for a particular radiopharmaceutical.

Column Chromatography. Column chromatography with radiopharmaceuticals is usually accomplished by ion exchange or gel

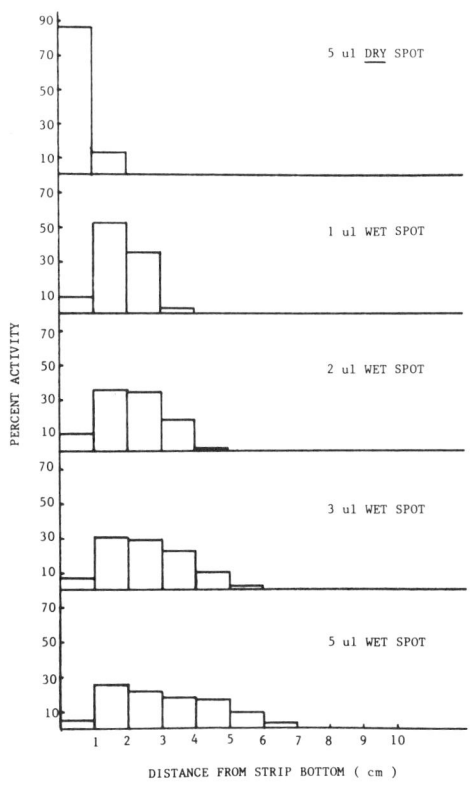

Figure 6-6. Demonstration of chromatogram streaking of Tc-99m DTPA in the ITLC-SG/acetone system as a function of wet spot size.

these systems can also be used preparatively to purify radiopharmaceuticals because the original sample is fractionated and resolved into its individual components.

The general technique requires that the dry beads of ion exchange resin or gel are soaked in water or electrolyte for a time to hydrate and produce the appropriate ionic character to the material. The excess solution is poured off, and the slurry is then poured into a glass column stoppered at the bottom with glass wool that serves to retain the beads but allows fluid to pass. During analysis the radiopharmaceutical sample is applied to the top of the column and washed through with an eluting fluid. Samples of fluid emerging from the column are collected for counting purposes as shown in Figure 6-7.

Ion exchange resins are used to separate electrically charged species. For example, an Amberlite IRA 400 anion exchange resin is used to separate unbound radioiodide from that bound to molecules such as labeled proteins or drugs like orthoiodohippurate. In these instances the iodide is bound to the resin (iodide exchanging with less tightly bound chloride), and the iodinated drug is eluted.

Gel filtration is based on the principle of molecular sieving. The material used is either a cross-linked dextran gel available commercially as Sephadex or a polyacrylamide gel marketed under the trade name Bio-Gel. Both Sephadex and Bio-Gel are available in forms with different degrees of cross-linking to control the size of molecules

filtration techniques. This is a more sophisticated method of analysis and requires more time and technical expertise but can accommodate larger samples; therefore,

TABLE 6-2. EFFECT OF WET VERSUS DRY SPOT ON MINICHROMATOGRAPHY RESULTS OF Tc COMPOUNDS IN THE ITLC-SG-ACETONE SYSTEM (PERCENT ACTIVITY)

Agent	Wet Spot		Dry Spot	
	Origin	Solvent Front	Origin	Solvent Front
Tc-GH	74.01	25.99	99.81	0.19
Tc-DTPA	60.04	39.96	99.70	0.30
Tc-PPi	85.37	14.63	99.39	0.61
Tc-MDP	82.60	17.40	99.82	0.18

The results are means of five determinations on 5-cm ITLC strips.

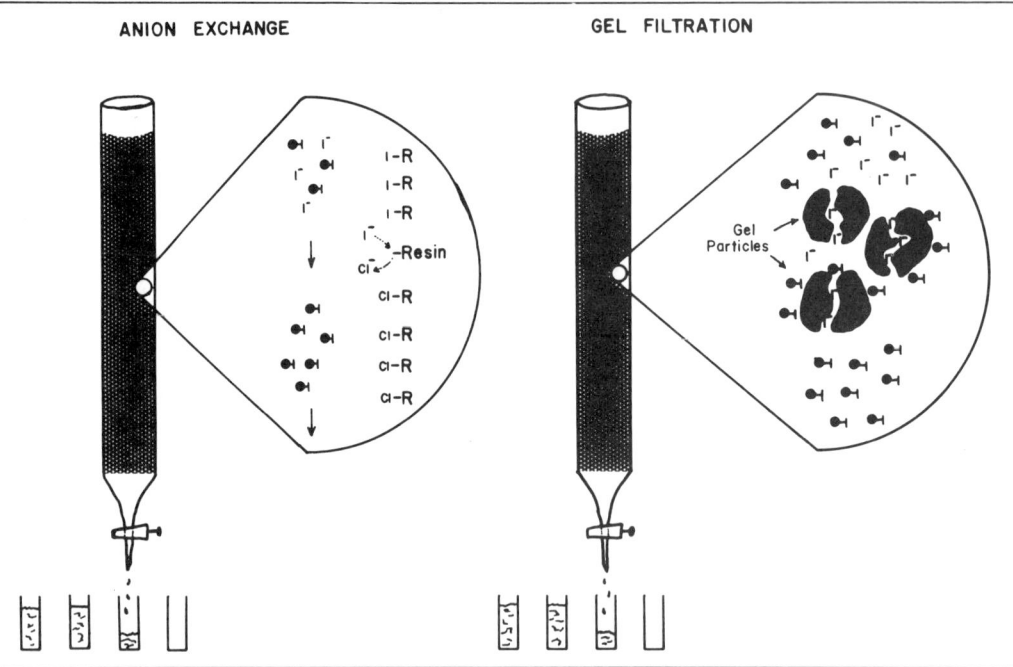

Figure 6-7. Separation mechanism involved in anion exchange and gel filtration column chromatography.

that will be excluded from the gel particles. The dry beads of gel are allowed to hydrate and swell, after which they are poured into a glass column to serve as the stationary phase. A solution containing the components (radiochemical species) to be fractionated is applied to the top of the column, and the development process is started by washing a solvent through the column. As the species pass through the column, molecules larger than the largest pores of the swollen gel cannot penetrate the gel particles and therefore pass through the bed in the liquid phase outside the beads. Larger molecules are therefore eluted first. Smaller molecules, however, penetrate into the gel particles to varying degree depending on their size and shape. Their migration rate through the column is therefore retarded. Molecules are thus eluted from the column in the order of decreasing molecular size, and this provides a method of separating different molecular weight solutes. In the example of radio-iodinated albumin contaminated with unbound radioiodide, the albumin would be eluted first from a gel column, usually in the void volume, and the radioiodide eluted later because of its detainment by the gel.

An interesting application of column chromatography in radiopharmaceutical quality control is gel column scanning.[8] With this method the radiopharmaceutical is applied to a 25-cm Sephadex column, and a predetermined volume of eluent is washed through the column. This results in a separation of the radiochemical species on the column, which is then scanned with a collimated detector to identify the peaks. The scanning method saves time in the analysis because samples are not collected and counted.

Although the theory of separation in gel filtration is based on a physical principle and it is generally assumed that there is no interaction between the solute and the gel, there are some instances where chemical interaction does occur. Such interaction has been identified between certain weak chelates of Tc-99m, such as Tc-99m gluconate and Tc-99m mannitol, and Sephadex. What apparently occurs is that during analysis the Sephadex competes with the weak chelate for the reduced technetium.[9] This causes a dissociation of the complex and a binding of technetium to the column. This suggests, in the final analysis, the presence of reduced unbound forms of technetium in the product, which, in fact, is an artifact caused by the effect of the chromatographic system on the radiopharmaceutical product. The Sephadex artifact can be avoided by using Bio-Gel P-10, which is inert to competitive interaction with technetium.[10] Alternatively, the Sephadex column can be eluted with the same concentration of chelating agent used in the preparation of the radiopharmaceutical.[11]

Assessment of Radioactivity. Measurement of the amount of radioactivity in a radiopharmaceutical is usually determined by whole-vial assay in a dose calibrator or by counting an aliquot of a known dilution with a calibrated scintillation counter. Radioactive concentration is usually expressed in terms of specific concentration, which is activity per unit volume (μCi or mCi per ml), and specific activity, which is the activity per unit weight of compound (μCi or mCi per mg). These values are usually listed on the vial label along with the calibration date. Each vial should be radioassayed to confirm that it contains ± 10 percent of the labeled amount of activity after decay correction.

Pharmaceutical Considerations

The basic points to consider within the realm of nuclear pharmacy practice are visual inspection of the product, pH determination, and chemical purity.

Visual Inspection. One should be thoroughly familiar with the normal appearance of every radiopharmaceutical. Liquid formulations used in nuclear medicine may be true solutions, colloidal dispersions, or suspensions. One should perform gross macroscopic inspection of solutions to identify any foreign material or change in appearance such as color change. For example, sodium iodide I-131 solution is clear and colorless when freshly prepared but turns light amber with time because of radiolysis effects. One should note that this color change is not deleterious. Also one should note the distinction between sodium phosphate P-32 which is a clear colorless solution, and chromic phosphate P-32 which is a greenish-colored insoluble suspension.

Particulate pharmaceuticals such as Tc-99m sulfur colloid and Tc-99m MAA or microspheres normally appear cloudy. Microscopic inspection may be performed to confirm that particles are uniformly dispersed and of proper size. The use of a light microscope and hemacytometer grid provides a ready means of estimating particle size and number as shown in Figure 6–8.

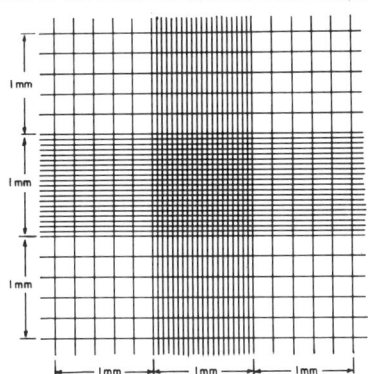

NOTE – ruled surface is 0.1mm below the cover glass on the slide, therefore the volume under the central square is 0.1 mm³

QUESTION – If the central square contains 110 MAA particles seen under a microscope, calculate the total number in a vial containing 5 ml of MAA suspension.

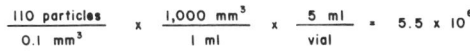

Figure 6–8. Estimating size and number of MAA particles with the hemacytometer grid.

pH. All radiopharmaceuticals have an optimum pH range for stability. Although pH determinations may not be made routinely, it is important to recognize potential problem areas. For example, radioiodide solution should be kept at an alkaline pH to prevent volatilization of iodine. Indium chloride solution must be kept quite acid (pH 1 to 3) to remain in solution and prevent insoluble indium hydroxides from forming, whereas In-DTPA is very soluble at neutral pH values because the indium is chelated. Most products are within the pH range of 4 to 8 with a few exceptions.

Chemical Purity. Chemical purity is a measure of the presence of undesirable chemical species in radiopharmaceuticals. Two examples will be considered. The first is the assessment of aluminum ion concentration in the Tc-99m generator eluate. This is usually performed as a spot test and should be done on a daily basis. Details regarding this test are discussed in Chapter 3. Excess aluminum ion may induce flocculation of Tc-99m sulfur colloid because of the formation of insoluble aluminum phosphate from the phosphate buffers in the product.

A second area where chemical purity is important is with radiolabeling procedures. We have already discussed the effect of carrier iodide in suppressing the labeling yield with radioiodides. In another example the contamination with trace metals such as iron in solvents can significantly reduce labeling yields with indium, especially in platelet labeling with indium oxine.[12]

Biologic Considerations

This area includes producing and maintaining parenteral radiopharmaceuticals in a sterile and pyrogen-free condition.

Sterility. A sterile solution is one that contains no living organisms, pathogenic or nonpathogenic. All parenteral products are required to be sterile. There are two ways to render radiopharmaceuticals sterile: autoclaving and membrane filtration. Autoclaving uses steam under pressure and is useful only for those products that can withstand the severe physical conditions of 121 °C under pressure at 15 pounds per square inch gauge (psig). These conditions obviously exclude protein and biologic products. For heat labile products, filtration using sterile membranes (Millipore or Gelman) is the method of choice. Membrane porocity should be at least 0.45 μm, and blood products should be filtered with 0.22-μm membranes capable of removing pleomorphic forms of *Pseudomonas* bacteria (0.3 μm in size) that may be present in such products.

If radiopharmaceuticals are formulated from raw materials, one should use sterile glassware, syringes, etc., to lessen the chance of introducing microorganisms and pyrogenic material into the product. Such products should be subjected to the USP sterility test either before use or afterward if the half-life places a limit on the test. The official sterility test[13] uses fluid thioglycolate medium to test for bacterial contamination and soybean casein digest medium to test for fungi. Sterility tests can usually be conducted in the hospital's epidemiology laboratory. Of course, proper precaution must be taken if the product is radioactive.

Pyrogens. Pyrogens are metabolic products (endotoxins) of living microorganisms, or the dead organisms themselves, that cause a pyretic response upon injection. The pyretic response in humans is characterized by the sudden onset of chills and fever within 45 to 90 minutes after injection of pyrogenic material. There is also general malaise and headache. The response may last for 3 to 4 hours but is not fatal.

All parenteral products are required to be pyrogen free. Although pyrogens are filterable, they will not be removed by routine membrane filtration methods used to sterilize solutions; therefore, a pyrogen-contaminated solution could be rendered sterile but still be pyrogenic. The most likely source of pyrogens is contaminated water and chemicals used to prepare parenterals. The best method for preventing pyrogen contamination, therefore, is to use high-quality chemicals and water for injection that have been tested for pyrogens. Glassware can be rendered pyrogen free by dry heat at 250 °C for 45 minutes. These conditions will incinerate pyrogens. Autoclaving will not destroy pyrogens.

The official test for the presence of pyrogens in parenterals has been the USP rabbit test. Although this has been a reliable test for pyrogens, it has limitations for use with radiopharmaceuticals, particularly those containing short-lived radionuclides. Additionally, the rabbit test appears to lack the sensitivity required to detect endotoxin in radiopharmaceuticals intended for intrathecal use.[14] Fortunately, an in vitro test has been developed that is far more sensitive to bacterial endotoxin than the rabbit test. This test is the limulus amebocyte lysate (LAL) test. The LAL test contains a purified protein obtained from the blood cells of the horseshoe crab *(Limulus polyphemus)* that clots in the presence of bacterial endotoxin (pyrogens). The LAL test as it was first called is now officially known as the bacterial endotoxin test (BET) introduced in the USP XX and assigned official status by the USP Committee of Revision. One major requirement for acceptance of the BET as an official end product test for pyrogens is the assignment of endotoxin limits for the drug in question. To date not all drugs have been assigned endotoxin limits, and for those that have not, the manufacturer must validate the BET for such drugs before Food and Drug Administration approval to use the BET. Fortunately, endotoxin limits have been assigned for radiopharmaceuticals.

The USP rabbit pyrogen test requires the intravenous administration of the drug to be tested into the marginal ear vein of three rabbits whose body temperature is monitored. The temperature is recorded each hour for 3 hours and compared with the baseline temperature before injection. The product passes the test if no rabbit shows an individual rise in temperature of 0.6 °C or more above its respective control temperature and if the sum of the three individual maximum temperature rises does not exceed 1.4 °C. Other details of the test may be found in the USP. An example of a pyrogen test report is shown in Figure 6–9. The rabbit test requires special care and facilities to house the rabbits so that the test will be valid. Sham testing must be performed to assure reliability. Commercial laboratories located throughout the country are available for pyrogen testing.

The LAL test is much easier to perform because it is an in vitro test. It involves mixing a solution of the drug with the freeze-dried lysate and incubating it for 60 minutes, during which time the lysate either causes gelation of the solution (positive test) or no gelation (negative test). The test drug is compared with control solutions of known endotoxin concentration. Extensive testing has demonstrated the LAL test's simplicity, sensitivity, and reproducibility. An additional advantage of the LAL test is that it can be used to test drugs not amenable to the rabbit test such as anesthetics, cancer chemotherapeutic agents, sedatives, narcotics, intrathecal drugs, and drugs that exert potent pharmacologic effects on animal systems.[15]

INSTRUMENT QUALITY CONTROL

The routine nuclear pharmacy laboratory will usually have a dose calibrator, a scintillation well counter, and a Geiger–Müller survey meter as standard equipment for measuring radioactivity. Each instrument has a defined purpose, and the principles of operation of each were discussed in Chapter 2. This section will describe the routine considerations of quality control on these instruments with particular emphasis on the dose calibrator.

Dose Calibrator Quality Control

The dose calibrator is the most extensively used instrument in the nuclear pharmacy. It is used several times each day to measure the activity of radiopharmaceuticals. To assure that the dose calibrator is operating properly a number of quality control tests are required. These tests and the time in-

PYROGEN TEST FOR:	UNIVERSITY OF NORTH CAROLINA of Chapel Hill, N.C.	QUALITY CONTROL REPORT
PRODUCT: Stannous PYP	LOT NO. 061002	DILUTION: Dilute with 5 ML TS
TEST NO. PS 14581	TEST DATE: 7-7-81	

RABBIT NO. 37-81			RABBIT NO. 38-81			RABBIT NO. 39-81		
WEIGHT: 2.9 K GMS.			WEIGHT: 2.9 K GMS.			WEIGHT: 3.0 K GMS.		
39.6 C CONTROL			39.6 C CONTROL			39.8 C CONTROL		
TIME: 10:00			TIME: 10:00			TIME: 10:00		
0.71 Ml/Kg			0.71 Ml/Kg			0.71 Ml/Kg		
TIME	TEMP.	VAR.	TIME	TEMP.	VAR.	TIME	TEMP.	VAR.
11:00	39.6 C	C	11:00	39.6 C	C	11:00	39.8 C	C
12:00	39.7 C	C	12:00	39.6 C	C	12:00	39.7 C	C
1:00	39.8 C	C	1:00	39.8 C	C	1:00	39.7 C	C
TOTAL TEMP.VAR.	0.2 C		TOTAL TEMP.VAR.	0.2 C		TOTAL TEMP.VAR.	--- C	

RESULTS: FAIL: _____   RERUN: _____   PASS: X

Figure 6-9. Example of a pyrogen test report for a pharmaceutical tested by the USP rabbit test.

terval required for each is summarized as follows[16,17]:

1. Accuracy (at installation and annually)
2. Precision (daily)
3. Linearity (at installation and quarterly)
4. Geometric variation (at installation)

After instrument repair or adjustment these tests should be repeated to assure proper operation.

Accuracy. The purpose for using a dose calibrator is to measure the activity of a radiopharmaceutical with a high degree of accuracy. Accuracy may be defined as the closeness of a measurement to the true magnitude. Dose calibrator accuracy is established by measuring a radionuclide standard reference source certified to contain a given number of disintegrations per second. A variety of different standard sources can be obtained from the National Bureau of Standards. The overall uncertainty of these sources is 1 to 3 percent. The following steps are usually performed in the accuracy test.

1. Adjust the instrument for the radionuclide to be measured.
2. Zero the background activity and assay the source to allow a stable reading to be obtained.
3. Repeat step 2 for three independent determinations and average the net activity measured.
4. The average activity measured should agree with the certified activity of the standard within ±5 percent after decay corrections.
5. Perform steps 1 to 4 for other commonly used radionuclides for which reference standards are available.
6. At the same time that each accuracy check is made, also measure a long-lived source such as cesium-137 or radium-226 in the calibrator at the various radio-

National Bureau of Standards Certificate

Standard Reference Material 4417L

Radioactivity Standard

Indium-111

This Standard Reference Material consists of indium-111, as indium chloride in 5.2091 grams of approximately 3 molar hydrochloric acid in a flame-sealed borosilicate-glass ampoule. The density of this solution is 1.049 ± 0.001 g/mL at 20.0 °C.

The radioactivity concentration of the indium-111 as of 1200 EST August 16, 1977, was

$$3.247 \times 10^6 \text{ s}^{-1}\text{g}^{-1} \pm 1.33\%*.$$

This Standard Reference Material was measured, relative to a radium-226 reference source, in the National Bureau of Standards "4π"γ pressure ionization chamber which had previously been calibrated, in terms of a radium-226 reference source, with indium-111 solutions from which quantitative sources had been prepared and 4π(A,x)-γ coincidence-counted using the efficiency-extrapolation method.

Figure 6-10. Example of a certificate supplied with an In-111 reference standard supplied by the National Bureau of Standards.

nuclide settings used. This cross-calibration with a long-lived source allows a check on instrument calibration at subsequent times without requiring more reference standards.*

7. Record the reference standard readings and the respective cross-calibrated readings of the long-lived source.

Example:

A standard of indium-111 is obtained from the National Bureau of Standards with the specifications shown in Figure 6–10. Determine the accuracy of your dose calibrator for this radionuclide.

1. The activity of the standard is expressed in SI units (International System of Units) for which the unit of activity is the becquerel (Bq). One Bq is equal to one nuclear transformation (disintegration) per second and is given in units of reciprocal seconds, s^{-1}. The activity of the In-111 standard in microcuries is thus determined as follows:

$$\frac{(3.247 \times 10^6 \text{ dps/g})(5.2091 \text{ g})}{3.7 \times 10^4 \text{ dps/}\mu\text{Ci}} =$$

457.13 µCi at noon 8-16-77

2. The activity present at the time of dose calibrator assay at noon on 8-19-77 is as follows:

$$A = 457.13 \, \mu\text{Ci } e^{\frac{-0.693}{2.83 \text{ d}}(3 \text{ d})}$$

$$A = 219.28 \, \mu\text{Ci}$$

3. The actual activity measured in the dose calibrator expressed as a mean of three independent measurements is 213.10 µCi.

4. The error between measured activity and the true activity is as follows:

$$\frac{213.10 \, \mu\text{Ci} - 219.28 \, \mu\text{Ci} \times 100}{219.28 \, \mu\text{Ci}} = -2.8\%$$

Since the error between the measured and true activity is less than 5 percent the dose calibrator is capable of assaying In-111 with

---

* It is quite expensive to perform the accuracy test using newly purchased radionuclide references standards each year; however, it is acceptable practice to use a set of long-lived sources that span the low, medium, and high photon energy range. Typical sources are cobalt-57, 1 mCi or more; barium-133, 100 µCi or more; and cesium-137, 100 µCi or more; they must have a calibration accuracy within ± 5 percent.

acceptable accuracy. If the error is greater than 5 percent, a new radionuclide calibration factor should be established for In-111 to bring measured readings within acceptable limits.

Precision. The precision test is a test of the instrument's ability to measure a source of constant activity repeatedly within a stated degree of reproducibility. Satisfactory performance of this test will assure that the dose calibrator is operating consistently from day to day. Usually a long-lived source such as the one used as a cross-reference in the accuracy test is used. This source is measured once daily at its own radionuclide setting and ideally at several other settings. After decay corrections the measured activity should not vary by more than ±5 percent of the calculated activity. Measurements made at several radionuclide settings are more useful than one measurement alone. Thus, if one of the readings is out of bounds, the fault is probably an incorrect calibration setting; if all readings are out of bounds by the same percentage the instrument is out of calibration and needs repair.

A useful method to document precision is to prepare a table of the source's activity over time corrected for decay. The calibrated activity is multiplied by 1.05 and 0.95 to determine the upper and lower limits of ±5 percent. Daily measurements are then compared with these limits to establish whether the instrument's precision is within acceptable limits. This is illustrated in Figure 6–11.

Linearity. Linearity is a measure of the dose calibrator's ability to measure activity accurately within a ±5 percent error over a wide range of activity. Generally, ion chambers demonstrate a linear response below 100-mCi activities. That is, the instrument will read out the true activity present. At very high activities, however, a nonlinear response may result, which can be observed as a lower reading than is expected. This falsely low reading at high activity is most likely due to recombination of ion pairs in the chamber before they can be collected at the chamber electrodes.[18] The linearity test should be done over the entire range of activities used for measuring radiopharmaceuticals. There are several methods for checking the linearity of the dose calibrator. Two methods will be described: the decay method and the shielding method.

DOSE CALIBRATOR DAILY PRECISION TEST

Source Cs-137 Serial No. 3560884A-08 NEN -- NES 356
Calibration Date 8-14-84   212 uCi   Dose Calibrator--Capintec CRC-10
                                      Calibration Factor 220

DATE	Cs-137 Activity Theoretical	Cs-137 Activity Assayed	Theoretical Activity x 0.95	Theoretical Activity x 1.05	Readings at Pushbuttons Tc-99m	Readings at Pushbuttons I-131	Readings at Pushbuttons In-111
9-20-84	212	210	201	223	386	270	164

Figure 6–11. Record used to document the daily dose calibrator precision test using a Cs-137 standard.

Decay Method. In this method the largest source of activity expected to be measured is obtained and assayed over a prolonged time interval. The following steps are to be observed:

1. Obtain a Tc-99m source, e.g., the first elution from a new generator.
2. Measure the net activity of the source in the dose calibrator initially and at 6, 24, 30, and 48 hours thereafter.
3. Using the 30-hour activity measurement as a reference point, calculate the predicted activity at 0, 6, 24, and 48 hours using the following table. Note: assume $T_{1/2}$ for Tc-99m = 6.02 hours.

Assay Time (hr)	Correction Factor
0	31.611
6	15.844
24	1.995
30	1.000
48	0.126

Example: The net measured and calculated activities for a Tc-99m source at various times are given below. Note that the calculated activities are determined by multiplying the 30-hour measured activity (assumed to be an accurate value) by the respective correction factor. The 6-hour calculated activity is thus 20 mCi × 15.844 = 316.88 mCi.

Time (hr)	Measured Activity (mCi)	Calculated Activity (mCi)
0	472.59	632.22
6	250.00	316.88
24	38.57	39.90
30	20.00	20.00
48	2.52	2.52

4. On log–log coordinate paper, plot the net measured activity for each time interval versus the calculated activity for the same time interval. See Figure 6–12 for a plot of the given data.

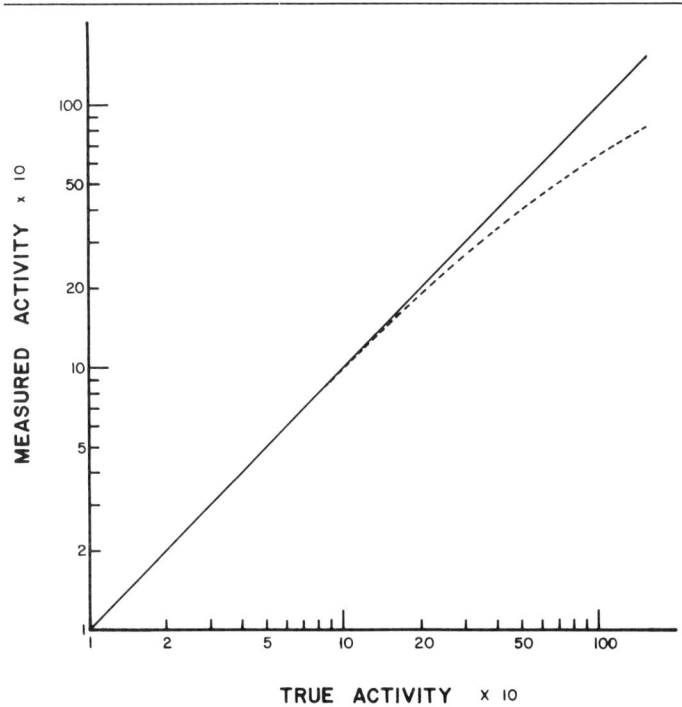

Figure 6-12. Log-log plot of dose calibrator linearity using the decay method linearity test. See the text for details.

5. The activities plotted should be within ±5 percent of the calculated activity if the instrument is linear. If nonlinearity is found, the instrument should be repaired.
6. If linearity cannot be corrected, it will be necessary in routine assays to either (1) measure activities within the range of acceptable linearity (below 300 mCi in the previous example) or (2) determine correction factors that apply to the non-linear region.

Shielding Method. This method is quite simple and takes only a few minutes to perform once the initial calibration procedure is established. It is significantly less time-consuming than the decay method and greatly reduces radiation exposure. The method involves the use of a commercially available kit.* The kit consists of seven cylindrical tubes, six of which are lead lined to attenuate gamma radiation and a seventh is an unlined tube. Each lead-lined tube varies in lead thickness so as to simulate various times of radioactive decay. These tubes are sequentially placed over the source of radioactivity in the dose calibrator, and within minutes, seven successive measurements are obtained representing values that would have been obtained at approximately 0, 6, 12, 20, 30, 40, and 50 hours after the initial assay of Tc-99m. It is important to use the largest activity source expected to be assayed with the dose calibrator and to establish a defined geometry of measurement. That is, the vial size and solution volume should be the same for the tube calibration procedure and all subsequent linearity tests. The initial tube calibration procedure is as follows:

1. The Tc-99m source is placed into the black unlined tube, assayed in the dose calibrator, and recorded.
2. Next the first lead-lined tube (thinnest lining and colored red) is placed over the unlined tube and the reading recorded, which will be less than the first reading because of absorption by the lead.
3. The red tube is removed and replaced by the next thicker tube colored orange and the reading recorded.
4. This process is repeated until all the tubes are used. The configuration is shown in Figure 6–13.
5. Attenuation (calibration) factors are then determined for each lead-lined tube. See the example in Table 6–3.

After the initial calibration procedure the dose calibrator linearity test is con-

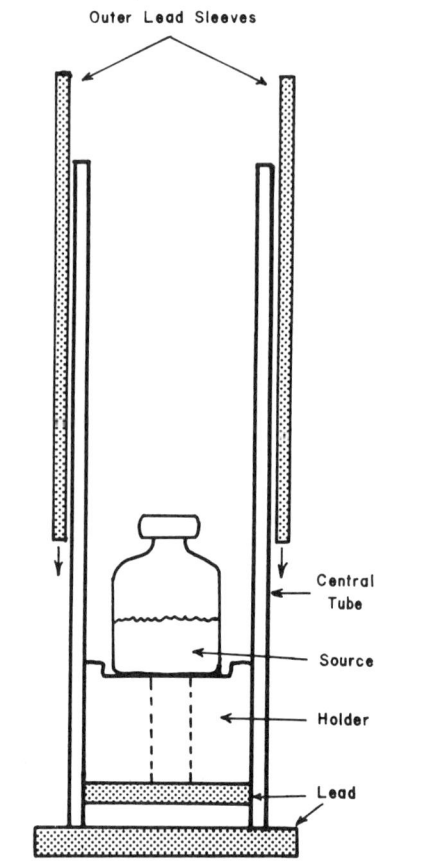

Figure 6–13. A. Diagram illustrating the shielding method for measuring dose calibrator linearity. *(From Calcorp, Inc, Cleveland, Ohio, with permission.)*

---

*Calicheck, Calcorp, Inc, Cleveland, OH.

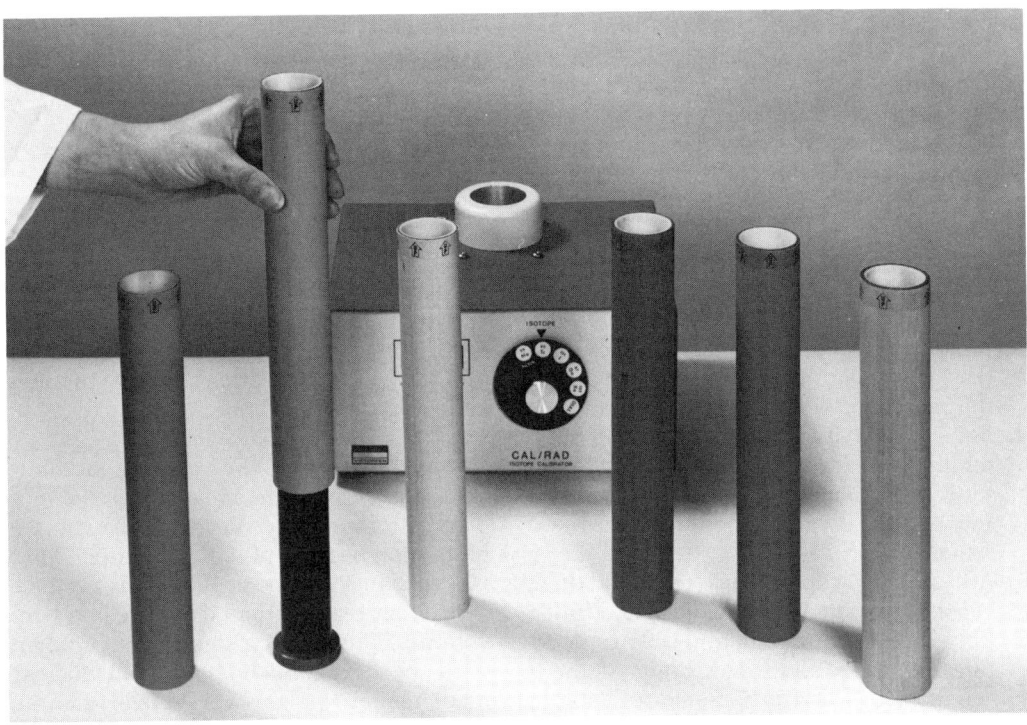

Figure 6-13. B. Illustration of the lead sleeve shielding system for the dose calibrator linearity test. *(From Nuclear Associates, division of Victoreen, Inc, with permission.)*

TABLE 6-3. CALIBRATION FACTORS FOR THE CALICHECK KIT[a]

Shielding Tubes		Measured[b] Activity			Calibration Factor
Black only	=	29.6	mCi	=	1.00
Black only		29.6	mCi		
Black only	=	29.6	mCi	=	1.79
Black + red		16.5	mCi		
Black only	=	29.6	mCi	=	3.35
Black + orange		8.84	mCi		
Black only	=	29.6	mCi	=	12.46
Black + yellow		2.38	mCi		
Black only	=	29.6	mCi	=	45.82
Black + green		0.646	mCi		
Black only	=	29.6	mCi	=	143.46
Black + blue		0.2063	mCi		
Black only	=	29.6	mCi	=	543.79
Black + purple		0.0544	mCi		

[a]Note: Factors are for a particular kit and dose calibrator.
[b]Mean of three determinations.

ducted as follows on a quarterly basis:

1. Obtain a similar-size source of Tc-99m activity in the identical geometry (vial size and volume) used for calibration. Adjust the dose calibrator to measure the Tc-99m activity.
2. Place the source into the unlined central black tube and assay in the dose calibrator. Record the results.
3. In a similar manner to the calibration procedure, take readings with each of the colored lead-lined tubes in place over the source.
4. For each activity measured, multiply the result by the appropriate calibration factor from Table 6–3. Record the results. Ideally, these values should all be the same.
5. Add all the products from step 4 and divide by 7 to obtain the mean value. Multiply the mean by 1.05 and 0.95 to define the upper and lower limits of the ±5 percent variation. Refer to Table 6–4. If the individual tube values fall within these two limits the dose calibrator has acceptable linearity.

It is important to note that this method will only measure a change in dose calibrator linearity from the initial calibration. It will not make the dose calibrator linear; therefore, before using the shielding method, the dose calibrator linearity must be established initially using the decay method linearity test described earlier.

Geometry Considerations. There are three considerations regarding dose calibrator geometry. There may be variation in activity measured because of (1) source volume, (2) source container configuration, and (3) source position within the ion chamber well.

Volume Variations. For a given radionuclide and activity the measured value in a dose calibrator may vary with the volume of solution because of self-absorption. That is, 1 mCi in a volume of 10 ml may produce a different reading than if it were in a 1-ml volume. This is not a significant problem with most radionuclides used in nuclear medicine except for very weak gamma emitters such as I-125. One can easily test for volume variation by placing 1 mCi of the radionuclide in a 1-ml volume into a 30-ml vial. An initial reading and subsequent readings after 2-ml increments of water are added will indicate whether cor-

TABLE 6-4. EXAMPLE OF A QUARTERLY LINEARITY TEST OF THE DOSE CALIBRATOR

Tube Color	Measured Activity (mCi)		Calibration Factor		Product
Black only	1503	×	1.00	=	1503
Black and red	838	×	1.79	=	1500
Black and orange	449	×	3.35	=	1504
Black and yellow	121.1	×	12.44	=	1506
Black and green	32.9	×	45.82	=	1507
Black and blue	10.52	×	143.46	=	1509
Black and purple	2.78	×	543.79	=	1509
			Sum	=	10538

$$\text{Mean} = \frac{\text{Sum}}{7} = 1505$$

Mean × 1.05 = 1580 = Upper limit

Mean × 0.95 = 1430 = Lower limit

rection factors need to be applied for different volumes.

Container Configuration. The type of container can have a significant effect on the accuracy of radionuclide measurements. This will be most significant with weak gamma emitters. It is important to be aware that dose calibrator isotope calibration factors are established for a particular instrument by the manufacturer using reference standards in a particular container configuration. Typically, this is 5 ml of reference solution in a glass ampule. Naturally, one would expect other containers such as glass serum vials or plastic syringes to yield somewhat different values because of variations in photon absorption by the container. Fortunately, this is not a significant problem with most radionuclides used in nuclear medicine, but a few exceptions exist such as Xe-133 and I-125. Table 6-5 demonstrates the difference in the assay of Tc-99m, I-131, and I-125 in standard containers[18] and indicates the significant influence of container configuration on I-125 measurements. For such weak gamma emitters it would be more appropriate to determine dose calibrator calibration factors for the specific container used to assay radiopharmaceutical doses. For example, one may determine a calibration factor for I-125 in plastic syringes by transferring a known weight of I-125 reference solution into the syringe. This can be accomplished by weighing the syringe empty and then full of the reference solution. The difference will be the weight of reference solution. The true activity in the syringe is calculated from the known activity per unit weight of the reference solution. Subsequently, the filled syringe is assayed in the dose calibrator, and the calibration factor dial is adjusted to display the true activity on the readout meter. From that point on all doses of I-125 solution measured at that calibration factor in a similar syringe will be accurate. This same procedure can be performed for other radionuclides as well, such as P-32.

Ion Chamber Well Geometry. The position of the source in the ion chamber well will affect the accuracy of measurement. Each chamber well has a position where the sensitivity for detecting radiation is greatest. Ideally, this position will extend over a reasonably wide range to minimize variation in measurements. Figure 6-14 illustrates typical variations in dose calibrator activity measurements of a 1.0-mCi source in a 10-ml serum vial at different distances from the bottom of the ion chamber well. Note that accurate readings are obtained only between 4 and 8 cm from the well bottom. Readings near the bottom and top of the well are lower because a significant number of photons escape from the detection volume of the chamber in these positions. Well geometry characteristics vary and should be determined for each dose calibrator.

Scintillation Counters and Geiger–Müller Survey Meters

Scintillation counters and survey instruments require routine quality control to as-

TABLE 6-5. EFFECT OF CONTAINER CONFIGURATION ON DOSE CALIBRATOR MEASUREMENTS OF Tc-99m, I-131, AND I-125

	Activity Concentration (μCi/g of Solution)[a]		
Radionuclide	*Ampule*	*Serum Vial*	*Plastic Syringe*
Tc-99m	44.5	44.0 (−1.1%)	45.2 (+1.4%)
I-131	37.1	35.8 (−3.5%)	38.6 (+4.0%)
I-125	39.6	20.4 (−48.4%)	57.8 (+45.9%)

[a]Percent deviations relative to ampule activity.
(Data from Kowalsky RJ, et al, 1977, p. 35.[18])

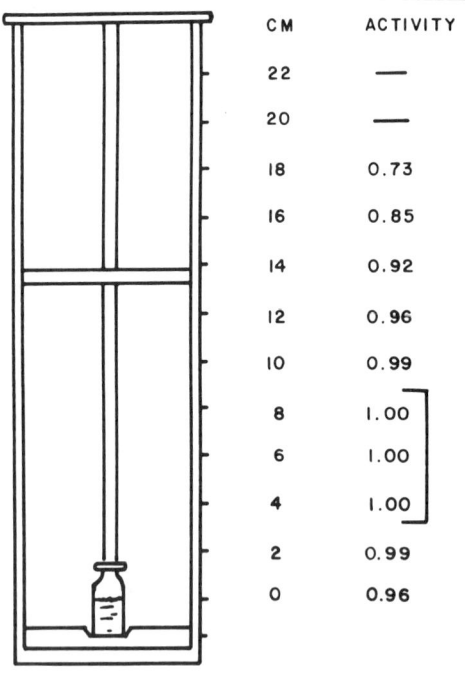

CM	ACTIVITY
22	—
20	—
18	0.73
16	0.85
14	0.92
12	0.96
10	0.99
8	1.00
6	1.00
4	1.00
2	0.99
0	0.96

Figure 6-14. Ion chamber well geometry effect on activity measurements in a dose calibrator.

sure that they are operating correctly. More detailed procedures can be found in standard nuclear medicine instrumentation texts. Only a brief discussion will be made in this chapter.

Scintillation counters should be calibrated with a long-lived monoenergetic source such as Cs-137 each time the instrument is used to establish consistent operating characteristics. Usually a 0.1-μCi source is placed into the detector well and the net counts per minute obtained at defined instrument settings. The counting rate from day to day should not vary more than a few percent after adjustment for radioactivity decay. Other tests that should be made at instrument installation and at regular intervals are a check on amplifier linearity and crystal resolution.

Geiger–Müller survey meters need to be calibrated initially, annually, and after repair using an approximate point source of a standard radionuclide source. The source should be certified within a 5 percent accuracy and be traceable to the US National Bureau of Standards.[16] Each scale of the instrument should be calibrated at least at two points located at approximately one-third and two-thirds full scale. The exposure rate measured by the instrument should differ from the true exposure rate by less than 20 percent at the two points on each scale. Sources of Cs-137, Ra-226, or Co-60 are appropriate for use in calibrations. These are high-energy sources, and therefore the Geiger–Müller survey instrument will be calibrated as such but will not be suitable for accurate measurements from a lower-energy source such as Tc-99m. The instrument should be calibrated using appropriate standards of low-energy nuclides if accurate measurements of such nuclides are to be made. In any case the activity of the calibration standard used should be sufficient to calibrate scales up to 1 R/hr. Typically, sources are in the range of 10 to 20 mCi, but this would depend upon the type of survey meter and the geometry of the calibration setup. Figure 6–15 demonstrates a typical setup for the calibration of a survey meter. A long-lived reference check source such as Cs-137 of nominal activity should also be measured at the time of meter calibration. The measurement should be taken with the check source placed in a specified geometry relative to the detector. Check source readings should be made as follows: (1) before each use and after each survey to ensure that the instrument is operating properly, (2) after instrument repair and battery change, and (3) at least annually.[16] If deviations of more than 120 percent from the initial reading occur, the instrument should be recalibrated. Survey instruments should be calibrated either at the local hospital or at an outside firm by qualified health physicists. A record of survey instrument calibration shall be retained for 2 years and must include a description of the calibration procedure, date of calibration, description of the source used

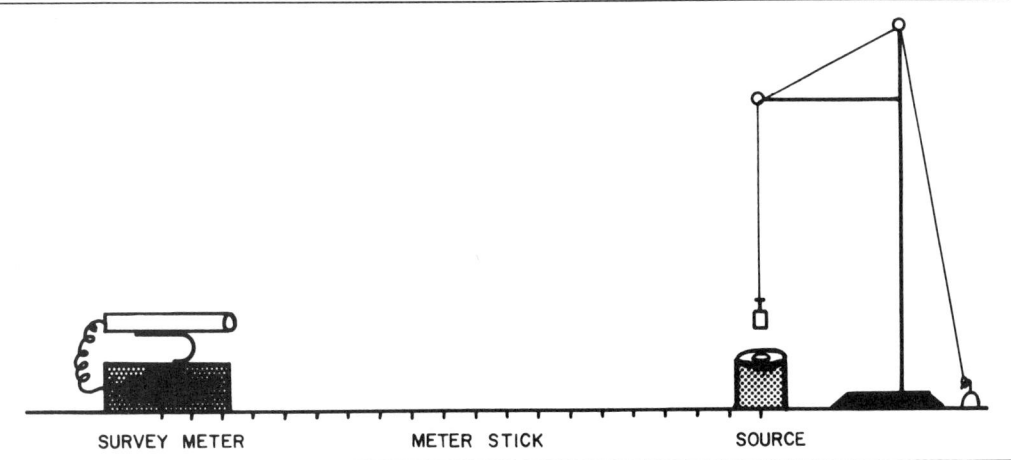

Figure 6-15. Setup for calibration of a survey meter.

and its certified exposure rates, exposure rates indicated by the instrument being calibrated, any correction factors deduced from the calibration, and signature of the individual who performed the calibration.

REFERENCES

1. Briner WH: Sterile kits for the preparation of radiopharmaceuticals: Some basic quality control considerations. In Subramanian G, Rhodes B, Cooper J, Sodd V (eds): New York, Radiopharmaceuticals. Society of Nuclear Medicine, 1975, p 246
2. Cohen Y, Besnard M: Analytical methods of radiopharmaceutical quality control. In Subramanian G, Rhodes BA, Cooper JF, Sodd VJ (eds): Radiopharmaceuticals. New York, Society of Nuclear Medicine, 1975, p 207
3. Persson BRR: Gel chromatography column scanning: A method for identification and quality control of Tc-99m radiopharmaceuticals. In Subramanian G, Rhodes B, Cooper J, Sodd V (eds): Radiopharmaceuticals, New York, Society of Nuclear Medicine, 1975, p 228
4. Krohn KA, Jansholt AL: Radiopharmaceutical quality control of short-lived radiopharmaceuticals. Int J Appl Radiat Isot 28:213, 1977
5. Robbins PJ: Chromatography of Technetium-99m Radiopharmaceuticals—A Practical Guide. New York, Society of Nuclear Medicine, 1984
6. Taukulis RA, Zimmer AM, Pavel DG, et al: Technical parameters associated with miniaturized chromatographic systems. J Nucl Med Tech 7:19, 1979
7. Kowalsky RJ, Creekmore JR: Technical artifacts in chromatographic analysis of Tc-99m radiopharmaceuticals. J Nucl Med Tech 10:15, 1982
8. Persson BRR: Gel chromatography column scanning: A method for identification and quality control of Tc-99m radiopharmaceuticals. In Subramanian G, Rhodes BA, Cooper JF, Sodd VJ (eds): Radiopharmaceuticals. New York, Society of Nuclear Medicine, 1975, p 228
9. Valk PE, Dilts CA, McRae J: A possible artifact in gel chromatography of some Tc-99m chelates. J Nucl Med 14:235, 1973
10. Billinghurst MW, Palser RF: Gel chromatography as an analytical tool for Tc-99m radiopharmaceuticals. J Nucl Med 15:722, 1974
11. Steigman J, Williams HP: Gel chromatography in the analysis of Tc-99m radiopharmaceuticals. (Letter to Editor.) J Nucl Med 15:318, 1974
12. Goodwin DA, Bushberg JT, Doherty PW, et al: Indium-111 labeled autologous plate-

lets for location of vascular thrombi in humans. J Nucl Med 19:626, 1978
13. United States Pharmacopeia XXI: Sterility Tests. Easton, Pa, Mack Publishing, 1985, p 1156
14. Cooper JF, Harbert JC: Endotoxin as a cause of aseptic meningitis after radionuclide cisternography. J Nucl Med 16:809, 1975
15. Cooper JF: Official status imminent for LAL test. Particulate Microbial Control 2: 1983, 22
16. Regulatory Guide 10.8: Draft Guide for the Preparation of Application for Medical Institutions, Washington, DC, US Nuclear Regulatory Commission, 1985
17. American National Standard Calibration and Usage of Dose Calibrator Ionization Chambers for the Assay of Radionuclides, ANSI 42.13-1978. New York, Institute of Electrical and Electronics Engineers, 1978
18. Kowalsky RJ, Johnston RE, Chan FH: Dose calibrator performance and quality control. J Nucl Med Tech 5:35, 1977

CHAPTER 7

Brain and Cerebrospinal Fluid

Radiopharmaceuticals for evaluation of the central nervous system (CNS) can be classified into two main categories: brain imaging agents and cisternography agents. These agents have unique properties and will be discussed separately.

Brain imaging radiopharmaceuticals can be divided further into three groups. The first group includes the conventional hydrophilic compounds that undergo nonspecific mechanisms of localization. They are excluded from entering the normal brain by an intact blood–brain barrier (BBB). Under pathologic conditions, however, the barrier is disrupted, and radiotracer concentrates in the lesion for positive identification. In such brain studies, lesions appear as hot spots against a cold background. Typical lesions include tumors, abscesses, and subdural hematomas to name a few. The next two groups are the newer-type agents that are not yet in routine clinical use. One of these groups of agents measures biochemical changes in glucose metabolism occurring in the brain by imaging the distribution of radiolabeled glucose analogues under various conditions. The agents in this group include the positron emitters carbon-11 and fluorine-18 labeled deoxyglucose. Studies of this type require highly sophisticated equipment and personnel and are limited to major research centers. The final group includes agents that enter the normal brain through an intact BBB. Studies with these agents are still in the investigational stages but offer the promise of measuring cerebral perfusion in the normal and diseased brain.

Radiopharmaceuticals for cisternography are administered by lumbar puncture into the cerebrospinal fluid (CSF) and are used to evaluate the dynamics and distribution of CSF.

PHYSIOLOGIC ANATOMY OF CEREBRAL BLOOD FLOW AND THE BLOOD–BRAIN BARRIER

This discussion will focus on the normal cerebral perfusion of the brain and the concept of the BBB.

Blood is supplied to the brain by the carotid and vertebral arteries as shown in Figure 7–1. Only the major vessels are shown, the minor arteries being omitted for clarity. The right and left vertebral arteries join to form the single, basilar artery that supplies blood to the brain stem and the occipital cortex through the posterior cerebral

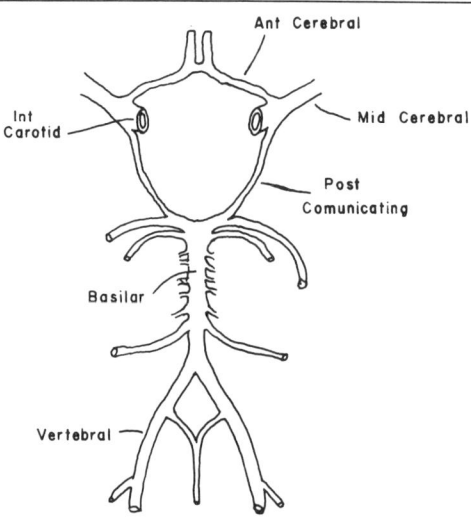

Figure 7-1. Arterial circulation at the base of the brain.

arteries. The internal carotid arteries divide into the anterior and middle cerebral arteries and contribute communicating branches that anastomose with the posterior cerebrals. The circle of Willis at the base of the brain is formed by the interconnection of the two anterior cerebrals, the two posterior cerebrals, the two internal carotids, and the anterior and posterior communicating arteries.

The right and left anterior cerebral arteries run side by side in the longitudinal fissure along the medial surface of each hemisphere and end near the terminal branches of the posterior cerebral arteries. The right and left middle cerebral arteries arise as the largest branches of the internal carotid arteries. Each runs, at first, lateralward in the sylvian fissure, then back and up where its eight discrete branches distribute blood on the lateral surface of each hemisphere.

Blood drains from the brain through large venous sinuses. The superior sagittal sinus is the large venous channel that runs posteriorly from the nasal cavity over the top of the brain between the two hemispheres to the occipital region ending in the confluence of sinuses (torcula). Other major sinuses that drain into the torcula include the straight, occipital, and inferior sagittal sinuses. From the torcula blood drains bilaterally into the right and left transverse sinuses, which run horizontally, laterally, and rostrally to terminate as the internal jugular veins, which return blood to the heart.

A routine brain imaging study is conducted in two phases: a dynamic phase and a static phase. In the *dynamic phase* the radiopharmaceutical is injected into an arm vein, and blood perfusion to the brain is monitored with a gamma camera by following the activity as it arrives and leaves the head (Fig. 7-2). The major vessels seen during the arterial phases are the internal carotids, the circle of Willis, the anterior cerebral arteries, and the middle cerebral arteries. After this there is a blush of activity throughout the head as the radiopharmaceutical distributes into the capillaries. Subsequently, venous drainage is seen by visualization of the superior sagittal sinus, the lateral (transverse) venous sinuses, and the jugular veins, which return blood to the heart. Obstructions to blood flow are seen as activity deficits in those areas. In the *static phase* images of the brain are taken 3 or more hours later to identify any lesions that concentrate activity significantly above background.

Unlike other body tissues, the CNS is highly discriminating as to which solutes are transported into its tissues from the blood. The so-called BBB, which protects the brain, is actually a hypothetic physiologic concept rather than some microanatomic structure, although certain structural differences exist in the brain vasculature that contribute to the barrier. The mechanism by which the barrier functions is not entirely clear but has been related to the anatomic uniqueness of brain capillaries and to the physicochemical properties of drug molecules. These properties include ionic charge, molecular size, and lipophilicity.[1]

Studies have demonstrated that endothelial cells of the brain capillaries differ from their counterparts in most other tissues by the absence of intercellular pores and pinocytotic vesicles.[1] This is shown dia-

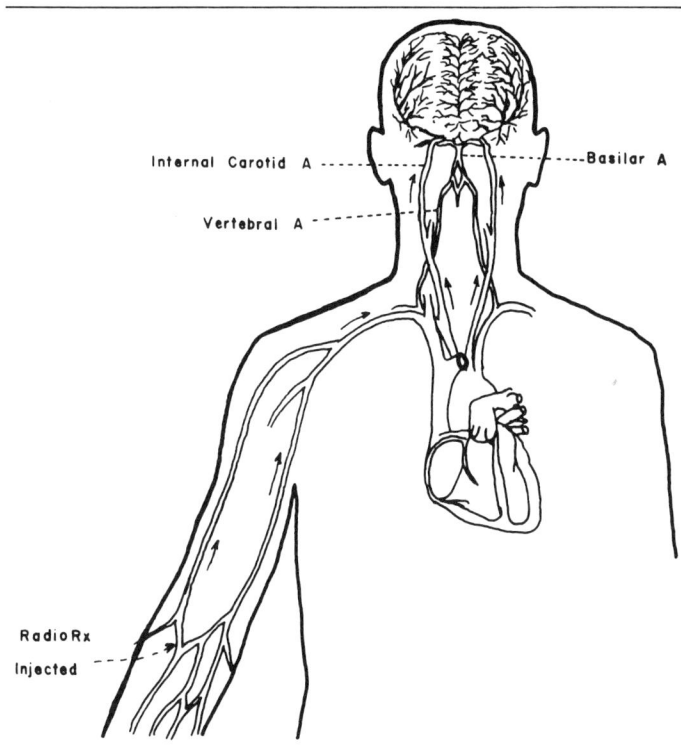

Figure 7-2. Activity distribution route to the brain after intravenous injection of a radiopharmaceutical into an antecubital vein.

grammatically in Figure 7-3.[2] Tight endothelial cell junctions (clefts) predominate, restricting the passage of large-molecular weight substances into the brain. In addition to the tight endothelial cell junctions is a diffusional barrier that is defined, in part, by a drug's lipid solubility and ionic character. In general, un-ionized lipophilic species readily diffuse into the brain through the endothelial cells, whereas ionized, hydrophilic molecules are generally restricted from doing so unless they are actively transported.[3] Further discussion concerning these properties will be made later in the chapter.

DEVELOPMENT OF BRAIN IMAGING AGENTS

Brain imaging was initially conceived to localize intracranial tumors. George Moore, a neurosurgeon at the University of Minnesota, attempted to visualize brain tumors at an operation first by using UV light to detect previously injected fluorescein, which concentrated in tumors.[4] This was followed by use of I-131 diiodofluorescein[5] and eventually I-131-labeled human serum albumin (HSA).[6] Although I-131 HSA demonstrated high tumor-to-brain ratios, blood clearance was too slow.

In 1959 Blau and Bender[7] introduced Hg-203 chlormerodrin for brain imaging because it cleared quickly from the blood and had better physical properties for imaging. This was followed soon by the Hg-197 label introduced by Sodee.[8] Both products had shortcomings. The Hg-203 agent produced a high kidney radiation dose because of beta radiation and long effective half-life, and the 77-keV gamma of Hg-197 was easily attenuated in brain tissue.

In the 1960s Tc-99m was introduced. The Mo-99/Tc-99m generator was developed at Brookhaven National Laboratories[9] and refined for medical use by

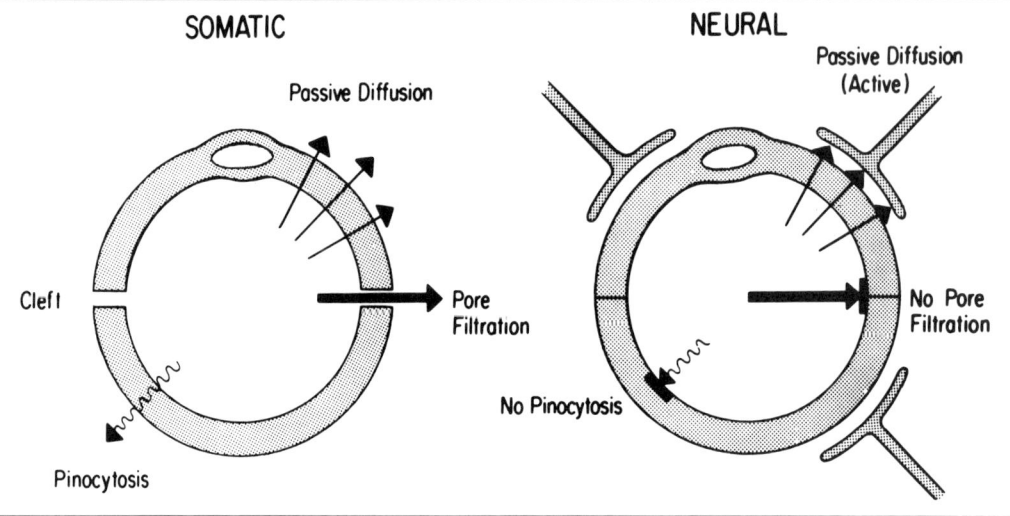

Figure 7-3. Differences between neural and somatic capillaries contributing to the concept of the blood–brain barrier; neural capillaries demonstrate closed endothelial clefts, absence of pore filtration and pinocytosis, and energy-dependent active transport of glucose and electrolytes into the nerve cells after passive diffusion. (From Holmes RA, et al, 1975, p. 252, with permission.[2])

Richards.[10] Harper used the first generator eluate to scan mice and found that Tc-99m pertechnetate activity was localized in the stomach, salivary glands, and thyroid gland.[11] Several other Tc-99m radiopharmaceuticals were subsequently developed for brain, liver, kidney, lung, and blood pool scanning.[11]

Tc-99m produced high-quality images because large amounts of activity could be administered yielding 12 to 15 times higher count rates than previous agents.[12] Its physical properties were also more suitable for the gamma camera. Tc-99m pertechnetate became the agent of choice for brain scanning for several years, requiring only prior administration of potassium perchlorate to retard concentration in by the choroid plexus.

The desire to shorten the time between Tc-99m administration and imaging (3 hours) stimulated investigation into the use of other Tc-99m agents that had faster blood clearance.[13] Tc-99m-labeled DTPA and glucoheptonate (GH) were compared with pertechnetate in several studies.[13-16] Although faster blood clearance was obtained with the technetium complexes, images obtained at early times with DTPA and pertechnetate (1.5 hours) after dose administration were less accurate than at delayed times (3 hours). The GH complex yielded the same accuracy at early and delayed imaging times and became the agent of choice for brain imaging.

After the development and refinement of transmission computed tomography (TCT) techniques, interest in and usefulness of conventional planar brain imaging studies with the gamma camera declined significantly. Only those studies that gave dynamic or physiologic information were of interest, and these were in limited number, primarily because of a limited arsenal of radiopharmaceuticals. The desire for physiologic information from brain imaging studies led to the development of compounds labeled with carbon, nitrogen, and oxygen isotopes by necessity; however, the only practical radionuclide choices of these elements are the short-lived positron emitters C-11, N-13, and O-15, which require positron emission tomography (PET). A great deal of effort is being made at major research centers to develop useful physiologic tracers. Much of this research focuses on radiolabeled glucose analogues as tracers of brain metabolism. The principal agents used are 2-deoxy-D-glucose labeled with C-14 for animal work and C-11 and F-18 for clinical studies. These agents have been shown to be accurate markers of glucose utilization in the brain and provide useful tools to study the brain's response under normal, pathologic, and interventional stimuli.[17] PET studies, however, are highly technical and are not expected to achieve practical usefulness in routine nuclear medicine practice soon.

The development of single-photon emission computed tomography (SPECT) coupled with new radiopharmaceuticals has caused a renewed interest in brain imaging studies. SPECT offers the advantage of potentially using all of the currently available radiopharmaceuticals in imaging as well as newly developed chemical tracers. The new brain imaging radiopharmaceuticals that show promise with SPECT include the radioiodinated amine compounds such as N-isopropyl I-123 p-iodoamphetamine (IMP), N,N,N'-trimethyl-N'-(2-hydroxy-3-methyl-5(I-123) iodobenzyl)-1,3- propanediamine (HIPDM),[18,19] and Tc-99m hexamethylpropyleneamineoxime (Tc-99m HMPAO). These lipophilic species enter normal brain parenchyma, and functional tomographic images can be obtained that reflect blood flow distribution within brain structures. These agents can thus be used to locate and evaluate perfusion derangements in neurologic disorders. Several other applications are also expected to be found.

HYDROPHILIC BRAIN IMAGING AGENTS

Table 7–1 lists the properties of Tc-99m and several other radiopharmaceuticals that have been used for brain imaging. Although Tc-99m pertechnetate is no longer the agent of choice for routine brain studies, it still finds useful application in certain studies of the CNS. Additionally, it is used as the primary radionuclide label for many other

TABLE 7-1. RADIOPHARMACEUTICALS FOR BRAIN IMAGING

Radiopharmaceutical	mCi Administered Activity	Decay Mode	$T_{1/2}$	Gamma Energy (keV)	Radiation Dose[a] (rad Administered Activity)		Pretreatment Required
I-131 RISA	0.4	Beta	8 d	364	5.2	Bladder wall	Potassium iodide
Hg-203 chlormerodrin	0.7	Beta	47.9 d	279	70	Kidney cortex	1 ml "cold" chlormerodrin
Hg-197 chlormerodrin	1.0	EC	2.7 d	77	12	Kidney cortex	1 ml "cold" chlormerodrin
Tc-99m pertechnetate	20.0	IT	6 hr	140	2.4	ULI	200–500 mg Potassium perchlorate
					2.2	LLI	
					2.8	Kidney	
Tc-99m DTPA	20.0	IT	6 hr	140	9.0	Bladder	None
					5.6	Kidney	
Tc-99m GH	20.0	IT	6 hr	140	4.8	Bladder	None

[a]From Kereiakes JG, et al, 1976, p 101, and National Council of Radiation Protection and Measurements, 1982, p 116.[20,21]

compounds in which it may be present as an impurity and therefore warrants a detailed discussion of its properties.

Production and General Properties of Tc-99m Pertechnetate

Tc-99m sodium pertechnetate is most readily obtained as a sterile, pyrogen-free solution from the Mo-99/Tc-99m generator as described in Chapter 3. As the anion, $[TcO_4]^{-1}$, technetium is in its highest and most stable valence state. When combined with suitable reducing agents it can assume lower valences and bind avidly to many substances. Tc-99m decays by isomeric transition and emits a gamma ray of 140 keV energy with 88 percent photon abundance. Its physical half-life is 6.02 hours, its specific gamma dose constant is 0.80 R/hr/mCi at 1 cm, and its half-value layer in lead is 0.3 mm. The decay scheme for Tc-99 is shown in Figure 7–4.

Biologic Distribution of Tc-99m Pertechnetate

The clinical use of Tc-99m as pertechnetate anion began in 1961 at the University of Chicago. Several comprehensive investigations have been made with this agent and its biologic behavior has been reviewed by Lathrop and Harper.[22] Tc-99m pertechnetate is usually administered by intravenous injection; however, oral, subcutaneous, and intramuscular administration are

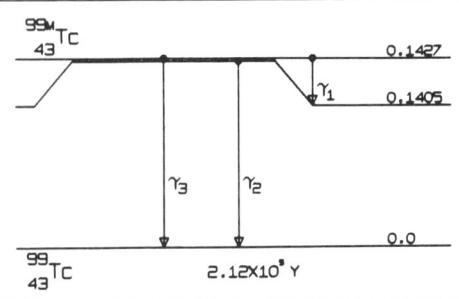

Figure 7-4. Decay scheme of Tc-99m. (From Dillman LT, Von der Lage FC: MIRD Pamphlet No. 10. New York, Society of Nuclear Medicine, 1975, with permission.)

also used. Of the total pertechnetate activity circulating in the blood stream 1 hour after injection, an average of 30 percent is contained in the red cell fraction and 70 percent in the plasma.[23] The activity is freely diffusible into and out of the red cells and can be removed by serial washing of cells in saline. Approximately 75 percent of plasma activity is protein bound, with one third of this very loosely bound. The disappearance of activity in blood after intravenous (IV) injection is multicxponential and of wide variation in individuals, with half-lives ranging from 1 to 2 minutes (50 to 60 percent), 5 to 20 minutes (15 percent), and 100 to 300 minutes (20 to 30 percent) without the coadministration of potassium perchlorate. These times are significantly prolonged if perchlorate is given.[22]

One hour after IV administration, Tc-99m pertechnetate has the following organ distribution: 30 percent in gastric mucosa and juice, 2 percent in the thyroid gland, and 5 percent in salivary glands and saliva.[22] Similar to iodide, pertechnetate is concentrated and secreted by the mucoid cells of the gastric glands and not by the peptic (chief) cells or oxyntic (parietal) cells.[23,24] In the thyroid gland pertechnetate is not metabolized as is iodide, and its accumulation is limited to the ion-concentrating mechanism of thyroid epithelial cells, i.e., it is trapped but not organified. The striated epithelial cells of the salivary glands have concentrating mechanisms for the group VII anions, including iodide, and its analogues, including pertechnetate, thiocyanate, and perchlorate.

Tissue distribution and blood clearance of pertechnetate are similar to iodide, but its excretion from the body is somewhat different. The renal clearance of pertechnetate (17 ml/min) is about half that of iodide.[25] This represents about 14 percent of the inulin clearance, and thus about 86 percent of pertechnetate is reabsorbed by the renal tubule, assuming the filtration fractions for pertechnetate and inulin are similar. This explains why plasma clearance is so slow after intravenous administration of pertechnetate. Another important difference between pertechnetate and iodide occurs in the bowel. Although iodide is completely absorbed by the intestine, pertechnetate is partly bound to fecal material after its secretion into the intestinal lumen and is excreted with a half-time dependent upon the movement of material out of the intestine.[26] For these reasons, by 72 hours only 50 percent of pertechnetate is completely eliminated from the body by urinary and fecal routes whereas iodide excretion exclusive of thyroid activity is greater than 98 percent by this time.

The long-term retention of technetium in humans after pertechnetate administration has been measured using the longer-lived isotopes Tc-95m ($T_{1/2}$ = 60 days) and Tc-96 ($T_{1/2}$ = 43 days).[27] After oral or IV administration, urinary excretion of pertechnetate is rapid within the first 24 hours but drops dramatically on days 2 and 3, with less than 1 percent excreted per day thereafter. Fecal excretion begins more slowly but is the principal route of elimination 1 day after administration; it reaches a maximum by 4 to 5 days and decreases thereafter. Cumulative urinary and fecal excretion is 30 percent in 1 day (27 percent urine, 3 percent fecal), 72 percent in 4 days (31 percent urine, 41 percent fecal), and 90 percent in 8 days (34 percent urine, 56 percent fecal).[27] Long-term retention studies estimate that 77 percent of the dose is eliminated with a biologic half-life of 1.6 days, 19 percent with a half-life of 3.7 days, and 4 percent with a half-life of 22 days.[27]

Pertechnetate has been reported to concentrate in the choroid plexus of the brain.[28] It has been shown previously that radioiodide also concentrates in the choroid plexus by a process of active transport from spinal fluid into the blood.[29] This process can be retarded significantly by the administration of carrier iodide or perchlorate.[29] Pertechnetate is also believed to be transported by the same mechanism as iodide. Oral administration of perchlorate prevents accumulation of pertechnetate in the choroid plexus and readily displaces what has already accumulated. This technique has been used in conventional brain imaging with pertechnetate to prevent or identify choroid plexus accumulation during brain scans.[28] To block the uptake of pertechnetate activity by the choroid plexus effectively, perchlorate may be given orally at any time before or after the injection of pertechnetate provided that perchlorate administration precedes imaging by at least 60 minutes.[30] The usual oral dose of sodium or potassium perchlorate is 200 to 1000 mg. Up to 450 mg of sodium perchlorate has also been given intravenously.[31] Uptake in the thyroid and stomach is also retarded by perchlorate.

Perchlorate anion also influences the distribution and clearance of pertechnetate from the blood. In patients pretreated with 200 mg of sodium perchlorate 30 minutes before IV pertechnetate, blood clearance was slower during the first 2 hours when compared with nonpretreated patients but became faster after this time.[32] Apparently perchlorate causes higher early blood concentrations of pertechnetate by decreasing tissue binding[32] and a more rapid later clearance by displacement from plasma protein-binding sites.[33] This effect was one reason for delayed (3 hours) imaging in the days of pertechnetate brain scanning.[34]

Pertechnetate is secreted in human milk, and it is recommended that breast feeding be suspended for 48 hours subsequent to radionuclide studies.[35,36]

Pertechnetate also undergoes placental transfer, which is reduced by perchlorate; however, posttreatment with perchlorate does not release Tc-99m from the fetus.[22] Pertechnetate is thus contraindicated in pregnancy.

Radiation Dose from Tc-99m Pertechnetate

Table 7–2 lists the radiation dose to various organs from Tc-99m pertechnetate. The major dose is to the thyroid and intestine, which concentrate and maintain radioactivity for prolonged periods of time. Note the reciprocol relationship in the stomach wall and intestinal dose between resting and nonresting populations. Apparently, the

TABLE 7-2. RADIATION ABSORBED DOSE FROM TC-99M PERTECHNETATE

Organ	rad/20 mCi Administered Activity[a]	
	A	B
Bladder wall	1.06	1.70
Stomach wall	5.00	1.02
Upper large intestine wall	1.36	2.40
Lower large intestine wall	1.22	2.20
Ovaries	0.44	0.60
Red marrow	0.38	0.34
Testes	0.02	0.02
Thyroid	2.60	2.60

Abbreviations: A, resting population; B, Nonresting population.
[a]From National Council of Radiation Protection and Measurements, 1982, p 116.[21]

more active nonresting population has a greater rate of gastric secretion that lowers their stomach wall dose but increases the intestinal dose from Tc-99m bound to feces.

Tc-99m Complexes for Brain Imaging

The complexes of Tc-99m with DTPA and GH have replaced pertechnetate for routine brain imaging. These agents have demonstrated higher target-to-nontarget ratios and do not require perchlorate pretreatment. The reader is referred to Chapter 12 for details of their production and properties.

New lipophilic Tc-99m complexes that enter normal brain parenchyma are currently being developed, and it is hoped that they will open a new dimension in brain imaging in nuclear medicine.

MECHANISMS OF LOCALIZATION OF BRAIN IMAGING AGENTS

This discussion will be divided into the three groups of brain-imaging agents previously mentioned: (1) hydrophilic compounds, (2) radiolabeled glucose analogues, and (3) lipophilic amine compounds.

Hydrophilic Compounds

This group includes the traditional brain imaging compounds such as I-131 HSA, chlormerodrin, and Tc-99m pertechnetate and its complexes. In general these agents are excluded from the normal brain by the intact BBB. The diversity of compounds used in brain imaging indicates that they localize in brain lesions by nonspecific mechanisms secondary to the disrupted barrier and perhaps the unique properties associated with the brain pathology. Some of the basic mechanisms for the localization of radiopharmaceuticals in brain tumors have been summarized by Tator[37] and are illustrated in Figure 7-5.

Vascularity. Many tumors are highly vascularized, and a large fraction of their radioactive content is due to their intravascular activity. Examples include hemangioblastomas, vascular meningiomas, arteriovenous (A-V) malformations, and certain malignant gliomas.

Interstitial Fluid. Almost all brain tumors contain more interstitial fluid than normal brain tissue. Many substances have a tendency to accumulate in this space including I-131 HSA and Tc-99m pertechnetate.

Capillary Permeability. In many tumors the endothelial cell junctions widen, and larger molecules can readily diffuse through the open pores into the brain. Additionally, pinocytosis, not widely present in normal endothelial cells, has been demonstrated to be present to a greater extent in brain tumors.

Intracellular Uptake in Tumor Cells. There must also be other mechanisms besides increased vascularity and diffusion that are operative to bind the radiotracer in tumors, otherwise the same processes could readily wash the tracer out of the tumor as well. The mechanisms of uptake directly within

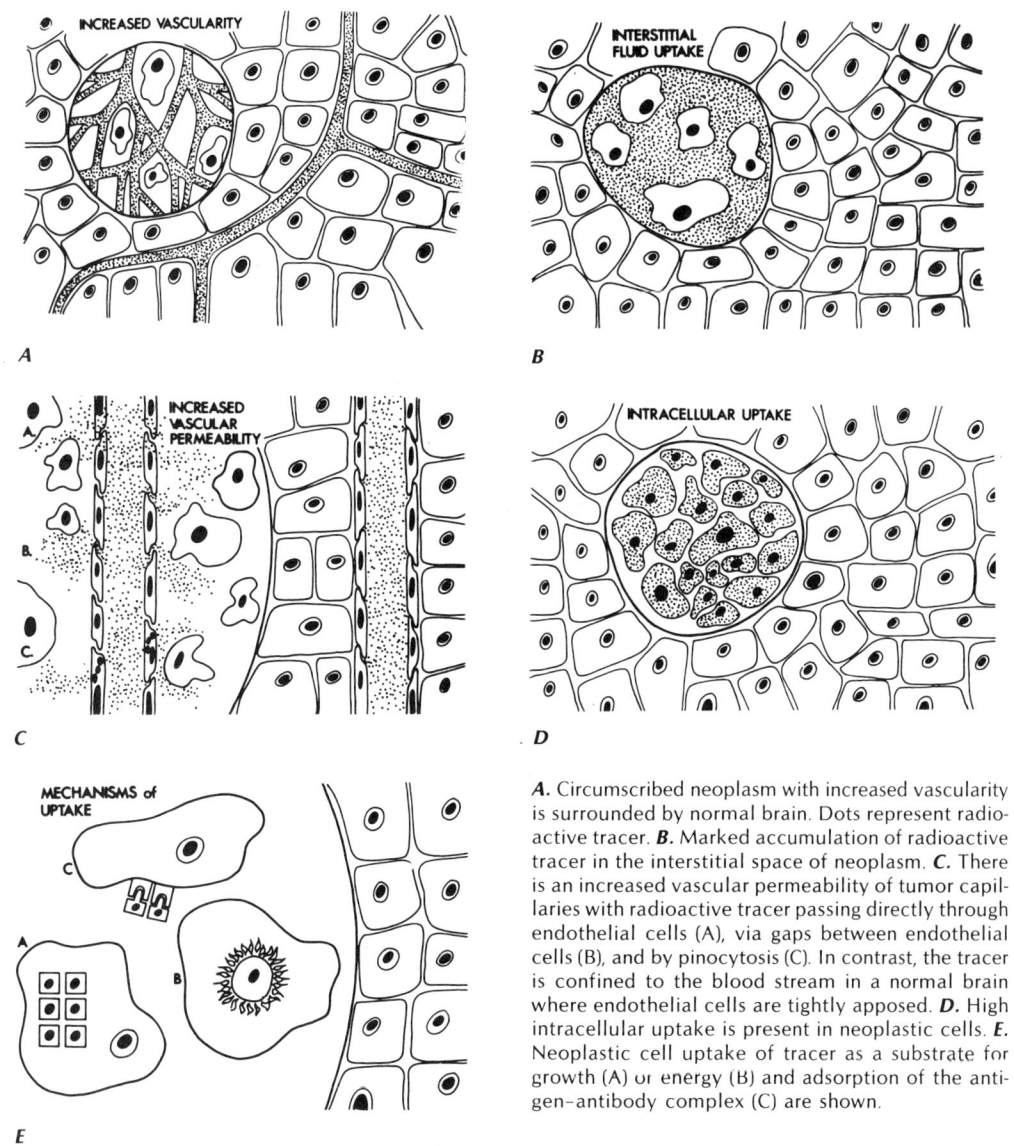

Figure 7-5. Basic mechanisms for the localization of radiopharmaceuticals in brain tumors. (*From Tator CH, 1975, pp 476-478, with permission.*[37])

neoplastic cells are not well defined but may involve uptake of substances as substrates for energy requirement (glucose and phosphates) and for growth (amino acids) and uptake by immunologic reaction (tumor antibody). Although these are theoretic considerations, they form a rational basis upon which future development of agents rests. Perhaps, as has been noted with gallium-67 uptake in tumors, there is some intracellular protein that binds tracer that is not present in normal cells.

Glucose Analogues

The need for a method of measuring rates of energy metabolism in specific regions of the brain in normal and altered states of brain functional activity has led to the development of radiolabeled glucose analogues. To do such measurements one must study the normal substrates of energy metabolism, namely, oxygen and glucose. A problem arises, however, when radioisotopic tracers of these substrates are used. Oxygen isotopes are too short-lived, and additionally, oxygen and glucose are too rapidly converted to carbon dioxide, which is rapidly cleared from cerebral tissues. For example, C-14 carbon dioxide is lost from the brain within 2 minutes after administration of C-14 glucose, which presents great difficulty in making quantitative measurements.[17]

Quantitative autoradiographic studies have shown that the glucose analogue 2-deoxy-D-glucose (DG) labeled with C-14 is metabolized through part of the pathway of glucose metabolism at a definite rate relative to that of glucose[17] as illustrated in Figure 7-6. Under normal conditions glucose is actively transported into the brain where it is converted to glucose-6-phosphate (G-6-P) and subsequently metabolized to CO_2 and H_2O. DG, similarly, is transported into the brain and converted to deoxyglucose-6-phosphate (DG-6-P) but cannot be metabolized further because it lacks the oxygen atom necessary for the conversion. DG-6-P, once formed, is therefore essentially trapped in the cerebral tissues long enough for quantitative measurements.

The combined results of research

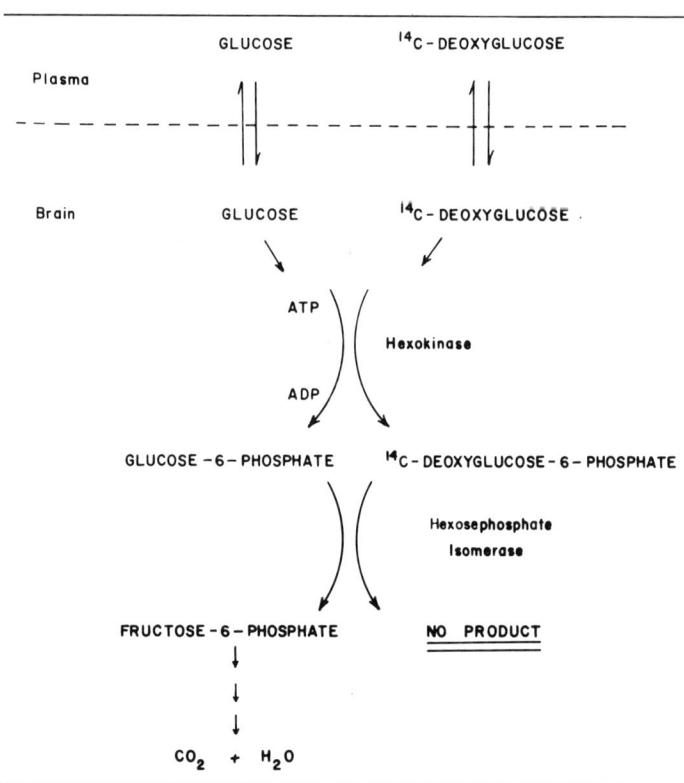

Figure 7-6. Metabolic scheme of glucose and DG in the brain.

studies comparing the measurement of local cerebral blood flow by using C-14 iodoantipyrine[17] and glucose metabolism by using C-14 DG have shown that energy metabolism and functional activity are closely coupled in the nervous system and that local blood flow is distributed and adjusted in cerebral tissues according to local metabolic demands and local functional activity.

Recent developments in PET have made it possible to extend these in vivo/in vitro animal studies to in vivo studies in humans. For this purpose the radiolabeled gamma-emitting analogues 2-F-18-fluoro-2-deoxy-D-glucose,[38] which has been found to retain the biochemical properties of DG, and C-11-2-deoxy-D-glucose[39] have been used. The advantages of these analogues for imaging is their prolonged concentration of activity in the affected areas of the brain because of the trapping of the DG-6-P activity. They thus provide a useful tool for external mapping of brain glucose utilization under various normal, pathologic, and interventional conditions.

Lipophilic Compounds

This group of radiopharmaceuticals include the radioiodinated amines, namely, iodoamphetamine, HIPDM, and perhaps in the near future newly developed Tc-99m compounds. These agents were developed after the initial development of the so-called pH shift compounds by Kung and Blau.[40] Because these agents enter normal brain, they must possess special properties.

Diffusion of any drug from the blood into the brain through an intact endothelial cell membrane requires that it be un-ionized and lipid soluble. The concentration of the un-ionized species depends on the blood pH, the type of drug, and its dissociation constant (K) usually expressed as its negative log, pKa. For drugs that are weak bases such as the amines, a pH value below the drug's pKa will promote drug ionization, and pH values above it will favor the un-ionized species. The opposite effects are produced with drugs that are weak organic acids.

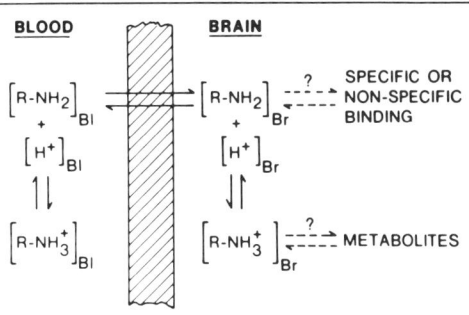

Figure 7-7. Partitioning of weak bases across the BBB. *(From Loberg MD, 1980, p 183, with permission.[42])*

The driving force causing a lipophilic drug to diffuse from the blood into the brain is controlled by a difference in pH between the blood and the brain. This is termed the pH gradient hypothesis.[41] According to this hypothesis a lipid-soluble drug can freely diffuse into the brain if it is more highly un-ionized in the blood than in the brain. Under normal conditions blood pH is 7.4, and brain intracellular pH is 7.0 to 7.1;[40] thus, with weak bases such as amines, the un-ionized species in blood readily diffuses into the brain where it becomes more highly ionized because of a lower pH. This results in a species less likely to diffuse back out. This process is shown diagramatically in Figure 7-7 for a weak base.

It should also be noted that the pH gradient hypothesis influences the transport of drugs in other tissues as well and is not unique to the brain. This is one of the fundamental processes influencing drug absorption in the gastrointestinal (GI) tract.

RADIOPHARMACEUTICALS FOR CISTERNOGRAPHY

Physiologic Anatomy of the Cerebrospinal Fluid Space

The entire cavity enclosing the brain and spinal cord has a volume of approximately 1650 ml.[3] The major structures are shown in Figure 7-8. Normally about 800 ml of

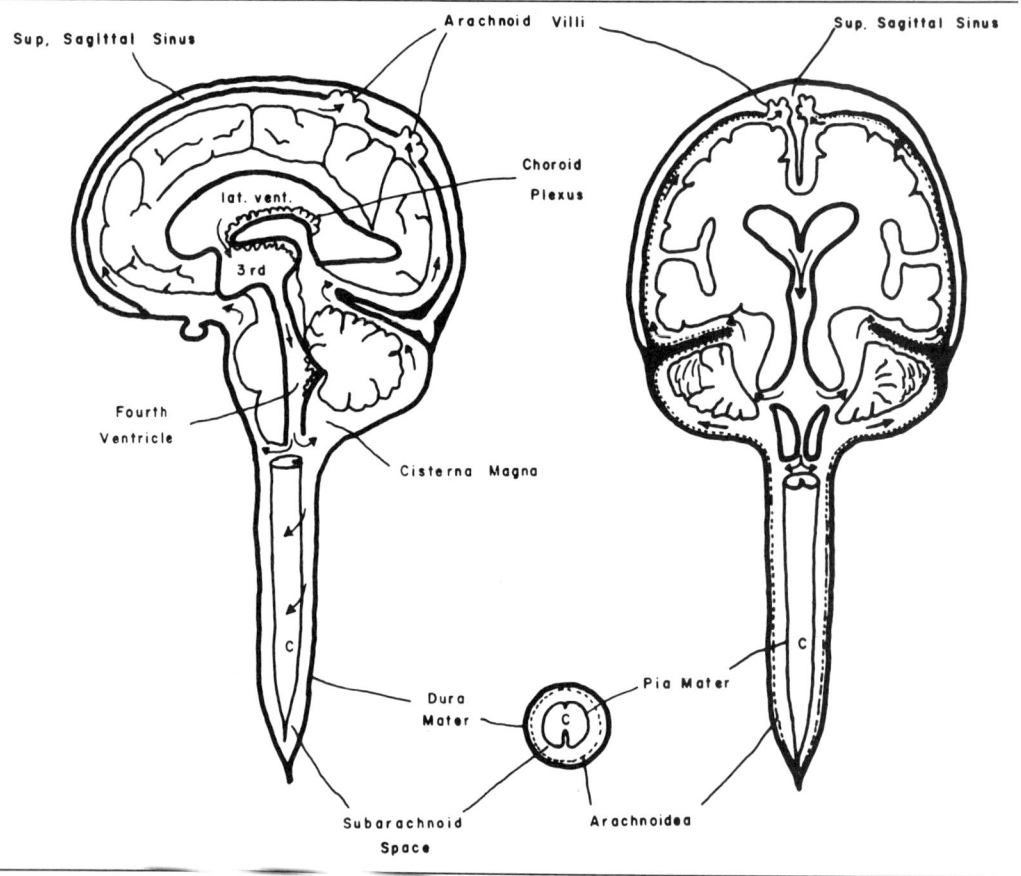

Figure 7-8. The CSF space demonstrating CSF production in the lateral, third, and fourth ventricles, with flow proceeding out of the ventricles in a caudad direction around the spinal cord and cephalad over the cerebral hemispheres and being absorbed at the arachnoid villi into the superior sagittal sinus. The cord cross section demonstrates the meninges and subarachnoid space.

CSF is produced each day. In humans its total volume is about 150 ml, 30 ml of which is in the spinal canal. Its rate of formation is about 30 to 35 ml per hour, chiefly by secretion through the choroid plexus. CSF composition is different from interstitial fluid in that its concentration of sodium is 7 percent greater, glucose is 30 percent less, and potassium is 40 percent less. Protein concentration is extremely low, being only about 0.025 g/100 ml, and is similar to brain interstitial fluid. Normal CSF pressure is 10 mm Hg (135 mm H_2O), ranging from 6 to 14 mm Hg.

The choroid plexuses are cauliflower-like tufts of capillaries covered by a thin coat of epithelial cells. These plexuses project into the temporal horns of the lateral ventricles, the posterior portions of the third ventricle, and the roof of the fourth ventricle.

Fluid normally passes from the lateral ventricles through the foramen of Monro into the third ventricle and through the aquaduct of Sylvius into the fourth ventricle. Fluid escapes from the fourth ventricle through the median foramen of Magendie and two lateral foramina of Luschka to enter the cisterna magna. From the cisterna it flows in the subarachnoid space through the tentorial opening and out over the cerebrum where it is absorbed by the arachnoid granulations and passes into the venous sinuses of the brain. Flow through the arachnoid granulation membrane has minimal resistance, and large molecules such as proteins and substances up to 1 μm in size readily pass through the membrane into the blood.

A small quantity of the CSF is formed by the blood vessels of the brain and spinal cord parenchyma and meninges. This fluid combines with that from the choroid plexus to flow through the subarachnoid space of higher levels. Most of the CSF bathing the spinal cord comes from this source.

Development of Cisternography Agents

The technique of radioisotope cisternography was first decribed by DiChiro et al.[43] In his method 100 μCi of high specific activity I-131 HSA was injected into the lumbar subarachnoid space. This agent was used for several years but suffered from the disadvantages of I-131, namely, a high radiation dose from beta radiation, which restricted the amount of activity that could be administered. The radiation dose was particularly high if the patient had a spinal fluid block. Additionally, there were isolated reports of aseptic meningitis associated with the procedure that were ascribed to the amount of albumin administered.[44-46]

The desire for a higher photon yield and lower radiation dose led to the development of other radiopharmaceuticals. Tc-99m albumin was introduced for CSF rhinorrhea studies in 1968.[47] The technique of preparation was somewhat involved but allowed the administration of 2-mCi doses; however, the use of Tc-99m in cisternography was limited to short-term studies such as CSF leaks because of the 6-hour half-life. Routine cisternography for hydrocephalus evaluation requires imaging periods ranging from 6 to 72 hours after isotope administration and necessitates a longer half-life than 6 hours.

In 1970 Yb-169 DTPA was introduced for cisternography.[48] Its advantages were a highly stable complex and a 32-day half-life that permitted strict quality control before human use. Additionally, it had a biologic half-life in the CSF compartment of about 10 hours, which was long enough for cisternography but short enough to keep the radiation dose low. A disadvantage of this isotope was the higher radiation dose in the event of reduced renal clearance because of the long physical half-life of Yb-169.

In 1971 In-111 was introduced for CSF scanning as a complex with transferrin and as a colloid.[49] It was noted that In-111 was well suited for such studies because of its ideal physical properties, namely, 2.8-day half-life, no beta emission, and emission of two gamma photons per disintegration. The In-111 colloid preparation was unsatisfactory, however, because it collected at the region of the basal cisterns. The In-111 transferrin complex gave satisfactory images but required in-house labeling using the patients own serum. When In-111 chelated to transferrin, DTPA and EDTA were compared, the transferrin complex exhibited a slower rate of clearance from the CSF space and the blood.[50] This was due apparently to a slower rate of absorption of the larger molecular weight transferrin molecule (88,000 daltons) from the CSF space. The close correlation between the appearance of peak activity of In-111 transferrin in the head at 24 hours with its appearance in the blood at this time suggested that most of its absorption from the CSF is through the arachnoid granulations. By contrast the In-111 chelates with EDTA, and DTPA demonstrated peak plasma levels at 2 to 6 hours after intrathecal injection, thus suggesting that these smaller molecules are absorbed into the blood throughout the spinal subarachnoid space as well as from the intracranial sites. Similar results have been reported in a comparison of I-131 HSA and Yb-169 DTPA for cisternography.[51] In this comparison the cisternogram patterns were all nearly identical with the two radiopharmaceuticals during the first 12 hours after intrathecal injection. Better anatomic detail was observed with Yb-169-DTPA because of the superior decay properties of Yb-169; however, by 24 hours there was a striking difference between the images obtained with Yb-169 DTPA and I-131 HSA. Cisternal detail was preserved in the I-131 HSA images, but the Yb-169 DTPA images were obscured because of the presence of cerebral cortical activity. The cortical activity was attributed to a greater extent of transependymal diffusion of Yb-169 DTPA into the cerebral extracellular space. A similar pattern was observed also with In-111 DTPA by these investigators. It thus appears that the faster clearance of DTPA chelates from the CSF may be caused by transependymal absorption in addition to that occurring at the arachnoid granulations.

For short-term studies such as the localization of CSF leaks, Tc-99m agents have been used. Tc-99m inulin was one of the earlier agents used, and a kit was developed for its preparation.[52] Additionally, Tc-99m DTPA was also reported to be satisfactory for cisternography,[53] and because of the commercial availability of a DTPA kit, it may be selected for use instead of Tc-99m inulin, although use of Tc-99m DTPA in cisternography has not been officially recognized by the Food and Drug Administration (FDA). In-111 DTPA is also satisfactory for leak studies but is not routinely stocked in most nuclear medicine labs and is relatively expensive. Table 7-3 lists the properties of several agents used in cisternography. In 1982 the FDA granted a new drug application for In-111 DTPA that released it from investigational status. It is now available to all nuclear medicine practitioners for routine use and is considered the agent of choice for cisternography.

DISTRIBUTION OF IN-111 DTPA IN THE CEREBROSPINAL FLUID

The production and physical properties of In-111 DTPA have been well described[54] and are discussed in Chapter 14. After intrathecal injection into the lumbar subarachnoid space, In-111 DTPA moves slowly, with the natural flow of spinal fluid away from the injection site toward the head. Leakage at the injection site can be minimized by administering the radiopharmaceutical in two to three times its volume of sterile 10 percent dextrose solution.[55] This also improves the rate of transport of activity toward the head. In normal human subjects the tracer migrates first to the basal

TABLE 7-3. RADIOPHARMACEUTICALS FOR CISTERNOGRAPHY

Agent	Decay Mode	Physical $T_{1/2}$	Effective $T_{1/2}{}^a$	Photon Energy keV	%	Administered Activity (mCi)	rad/Administered Activity[b] (Spinal Cord)	Study Beyond 24 hr
I-131 HSA	Beta-	8 d	26 hr	364	83	0.1	7.1	Yes
Yb-169 DTPA	EC	32 d	12 hr	177	22	0.5	8.0	Yes
				198	35			
In-111 DTPA	EC	2.8 d	10 hr	171	91	0.5	1.9	Yes
				245	94			
Tc-99m inulin	IT	6 hr	5 hr	140	88	2.0	5.0	No
Tc-99m DTPA	IT	6 hr	5 hr	140	88	2.0	5.0	No

[a]From Rapoport SI, 1976, p 154.[41]
[b]From Bell EG, et al, 1975, p 399.[52]

cisterns then flows over the cerebral convexities to the parasagittal regions where it exits through the arachnoid granulations into the blood. Activity does not normally enter the ventricular system; however, in certain types of hydrocephalus, activity may reflux into the ventricles. Activity reaches the basal cisterns in about 1 hour, achieving peak concentration at 4 hours.[56] The first activity appears in the parasagittal region at 4 hours, reaching a peak at about 14 to 17 hours. The activity in this region falls rapidly, decreasing to half the peak values in 10 to 14 hours[56] by being absorbed into the blood through the arachnoid membrane. In the blood, In-111 DTPA follows a route of excretion similar to Tc-99m DTPA by being rapidly excreted through renal glomerular filtration. About 65 percent of the DTPA chelate is eliminated in the urine in 1 day and increases to 85 percent in 3 days.[50] The systemic distribution of In-111 DTPA is described in Chapters 12 and 14.

Mechanisms of Drug Transport in the Cerebrospinal Fluid

To remain in the CSF a radiopharmaceutical must have certain properties as outlined by Bell et al.[52] First, it must not be lipid soluble, or it will diffuse through the pia mater into the underlying nervous tissue. It must not be metabolized by CSF enzymes. Proteins can be metabolized, but the chelates of DTPA are not. Substances of molecular weights less than 200 daltons can readily diffuse through the meninges out of the spinal fluid. The DTPA chelates have molecular weights between 500 and 600 daltons and remain, for the most part, in the spinal fluid during the cisternography procedure.

Transport of tracer molecules in the spinal fluid occurs either by bulk flow or diffusion. Smaller molecules would favor diffusion, and larger molecules such as albumin and inulin have been noted to move by bulk flow with the spinal fluid. Opinion appears to be mixed on DTPA chelates, which suggests that bulk flow[57] and diffusion mechanisms[52] are both operational.

Egress of radiopharmaceutical from the CSF space into the blood occurs, regardless of molecular weight, primarily with the flow of CSF through the arachnoid granulations into the superior sagittal sinus. Flow through the arachnoid membrane is facilitated by the numerous pores and by the difference in pressure between the dural venous blood (about 90 mm H_2O) and the mean CSF pressure (about 135 mm H_2O).[57] Some agents such as the DTPA chelates may also undergo transependymal diffusion because nearly normal clearance has been shown to occur with Yb-169 DTPA during spinal canal obstruction.[57] Large molecular weight molecules such as I-131 HSA have been shown to exhibit a clearance rate ten times slower than normal in the case of obstruction which leads to an excessive radiation dose.[58] For this reason radiolabeled chelates are valid choices for cisternography.

Some agents are cleared rapidly from the CSF space by active transport through the choroid plexus. These substances include iodide, bromide, thiocyanate, phenol red, phenolsulphonphthalein, and Diodrast. Notably, Tc-99m pertechnetate clears rapidly by this mechanism also, but its rate of clearance can be significantly reduced by administering oral perchlorate.[59,60] The mechanisms for tracer clearance from the CSF space are summarized in Figure 7–9.

SAFETY AND SPECIAL PRECAUTIONS IN CISTERNOGRAPHY

Injection of foreign material into the spinal fluid where it comes into intimate contact with the spinal nerves and the brain deserves special attention regarding the potential for adverse reactions. The integrity of nerve function is closely related to proper control of fluid pH, electrolyte balance, and osmolarity.[61] Additionally, drug substances present may have a direct effect on nerve function.[62,63] In particular, depletion of calcium ion readily causes tetany,[63] and low pH causes dilation of pial blood vessels.[61]

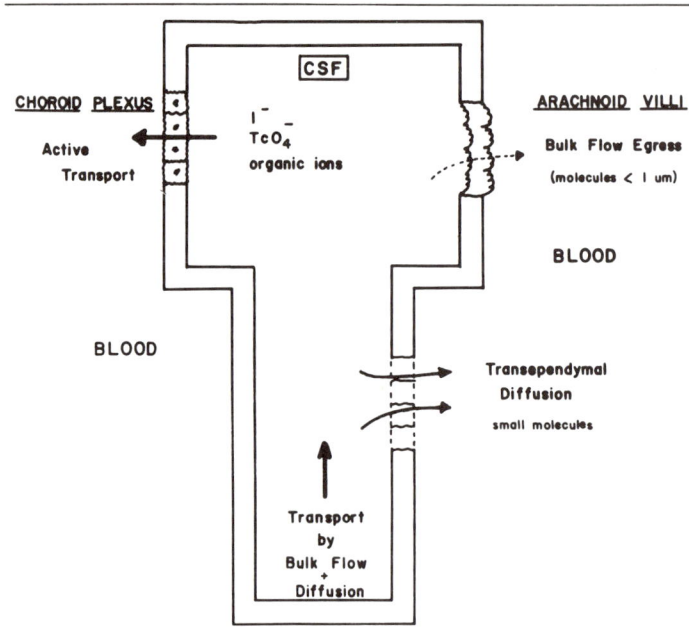

Figure 7-9. Mechanisms of drug transport within and out of the CSF space.

The first documented cases of aseptic meningitis after radioisotope cisternography with I-131 HSA were reported by Detmer and Blockner in 1965[44] who administered 28 mg of albumin and by Nicol in 1967[45] who used 100 to 130 mg of albumin. The reactions were believed to be related to the amount of albumin injected. This prompted the use of high specific activity I-131 HSA containing less than 2 mg of albumin per dose. In spite of this precaution, however, reactions still occurred.[46] Cooper and Harbert suspected a pyrogenic chemical contaminant rather than the concentration of albumin as the cause for the frequency of aseptic meningitis.[64] They tested different lots of commercial radiopharmaceuticals using the limulus test specific for bacterial endotoxin (pyrogen). Every lot of I-131 HSA and In-111 DTPA implicated in cases of aseptic meningitis yielded a strongly positive result by the limulus test. In one of the lots of I-131 HSA the cause of pyrogenic contamination was traced to a contaminated anion exchange resin used to remove non-protein-bound radioiodine. With some of the In-111 DTPA lots the source of pyrogen was traced to the phosphate buffer used during its preparation. Probably a more significant finding was that the radiopharmaceutical lots that were positive for endotoxin by the limulus test had passed the supplier's pyrogen and sterility tests. Endotoxin is much more potent in producing a febrile response when administered by the intrathecal route than by the IV route. Furthermore, the limulus test is more sensitive, by a factor of five to ten times, for detecting bacterial endotoxin than the US Pharmacopeia (USP) pyrogen test. The authors concluded, therefore, that the limulus test should be required for intrathecal drugs to provide a more sensitive test.[64] One should note that the bacterial endotoxins test for pyrogens is now officially recognized by the USP for use with radiopharmaceuticals. Greater detail regarding this test is covered in Chapter 6.

The decline in use of I-131 HSA and improvement in methods of preparing and testing intrathecal radiopharmaceuticals has diminished the incidence of adverse reactions significantly. The chelates of DTPA have the ability to sequester calcium ion and potentially produce a tetany reaction; however, the small amounts of DTPA present in commercial In-111 DTPA (20 to 50 μg) are not likely to present problems. If larger amounts are to be administered, a calcium salt of DTPA should be used.

OVERPRESSURE CISTERNOGRAPHY

In 1977 a new procedure, controlled overpressure cisternography, was developed by Magnaes and Solheim[65] to localize CSF rhinorrhea. The advantage of this procedure was to increase the detection rate in patients with intermittent CSF leaks by raising the CSF pressure four to six times normal for a short period of time to induce the leak. This technique also reduced the time required to complete a study to less than 1 hour. Patient candidates for the overpressure study should have no symptoms or signs of elevated intracranial pressure, no intracranial expanding lesion such as a hematoma or tumor, and the test should not be performed in the early stage of a head injury with brain edema.[65] An upper limit of CSF pressure at 800 mm H_2O is recommended so as not to reduce cerebral blood flow, although most studies are successful at a range of 400 to 600 mm H_2O. Procedural side effects are usually limited to headaches that occur toward the end of the procedure and subside on termination of the study.

An important consideration in conducting the overpressure cisternography study is the composition of the fluid that is pumped into the intrathecal space to elevate the pressure. A typical study requires infusion of 90 to 120 ml of fluid that essentially displaces most of the natural spinal fluid. Consequently, only artificial CSF[66] or

TABLE 7-4. ARTIFICIAL CSF (ELLIOTT'S B SOLUTION)

Formula

1. NaCl	5.608 g	Dissolve ingredients (1-5) in 970 ml SWFI. Add drop-wise (with glass pipette) the acid salt solution (~2 ml) with stirring to pH 7.4 and qs to 1000 ml. Sterile filter through a 0.22 u sterile membrane into vials or syringes for immediate use.
2. $Na_2CO_3 \cdot H_2O$	2.557 g	
3. KCl	0.285 g	
4. Na_2HPO_4	0.076 g	
5. Glucose	0.758 g	
6. Acid salt solution qs	pH 7.4	
7. Sterile water for injection qs	1000 ml	

Acid Salt Solution

$CaCl_2$	2.0 g	Dissolve salts in 20 ml of HCl with heating. Cool and qs to 25 ml. Pass through a membrane filter to remove particles.
$MgCl_2 \cdot 6 H_2O$	1.0 g	
HCl 12 M qs	25.0 ml	

Final preparation contains the following:

Substance	mg/100 ml
Na^+	318.0
Cl^-	450.0
K^+	14.9
Ca^{++}	5.5
Mg^{++}	0.9
P	1.7
HCO_3^-	126.0
Glucose	76.0

(Data from Elliott KAC, et al, 1949, p 140.[61])

similar fluid having the necessary electrolytes, osmolality, and proper pH should be used to prevent adverse reactions. The use of saline alone is not recommended because tetanic reactions are likely to occur.[67] Several patient studies have been performed using the overpressure–artificial CSF technique with no untoward effects from the procedure.[65,68] Table 7–4 summarizes the preparation of artificial CSF.

Clinical Evaluation of the Brain and Cerebrospinal Fluid

INTRODUCTION

The ancient Egyptian and Aztec civilizations have left us with evidence in their art of humans' delving into the mysteries of the abnormally functioning brain. The aura has continued into this century with the cascading development of more neurologic and surgical techniques. In the early years of nuclear medicine much information was gained in diagnosing CNS disease with a wide variety of tracer materials. With the advent of the superb anatomic detail of the CNS portrayed by TCT studies in the late 1970s, the number of brain scans performed diminished precipitously. Brain scans, however, continued to be performed even in centers with excellent TCT facilities because indications were found for which the brain scan answered the question better that the TCT study. Interest was renewed in the 1980s for the development of brain imaging radiopharmaceuticals that answered more specific questions about brain chemistry than TCT or magnetic resonance imaging procedures.

RATIONALE

The earliest indications for brain scanning included the diagnosis and workup of cerebrovascular accidents (CVA), primary and metastatic malignancy, and arteriosclerotic carotid or vertebral artery disease manifested as transient ischemia attacks. Inflammatory lesions such as brain abscesses, viral (herpes) encephalitis, and subdural empyema were distinguishable by their pattern of concentration and A-V malformations by the sequence of image abnormalities. Some brain scans have been performed after the lesion has been well localized on TCT studies, with the reason for the brain scan being to give neurosurgeons better three-dimensional localization of the abnormal process to afford them a more precise approach through the skull to the lesion. Dementia and the effects of trauma have been investigated with techniques studying the flow patterns of tracer material in the CSF.

PROCEDURES

Flow and *blood pool* studies are an integral part of the majority of brain scans. This part of the study is a series of 2- to 10-second duration sequential frames that are obtained in the anterior projection (with the exception of children under 10 where they are obtained in the posterior projection because of the greater likelihood of a posterior lesion) (Fig. 7–10). Care should be exercised by the technologist to align the patient's head such that the floor of the cranial vault extends at as nearly a 90-degree angle from the collimator as possible. The blood pool image is made during the first 5

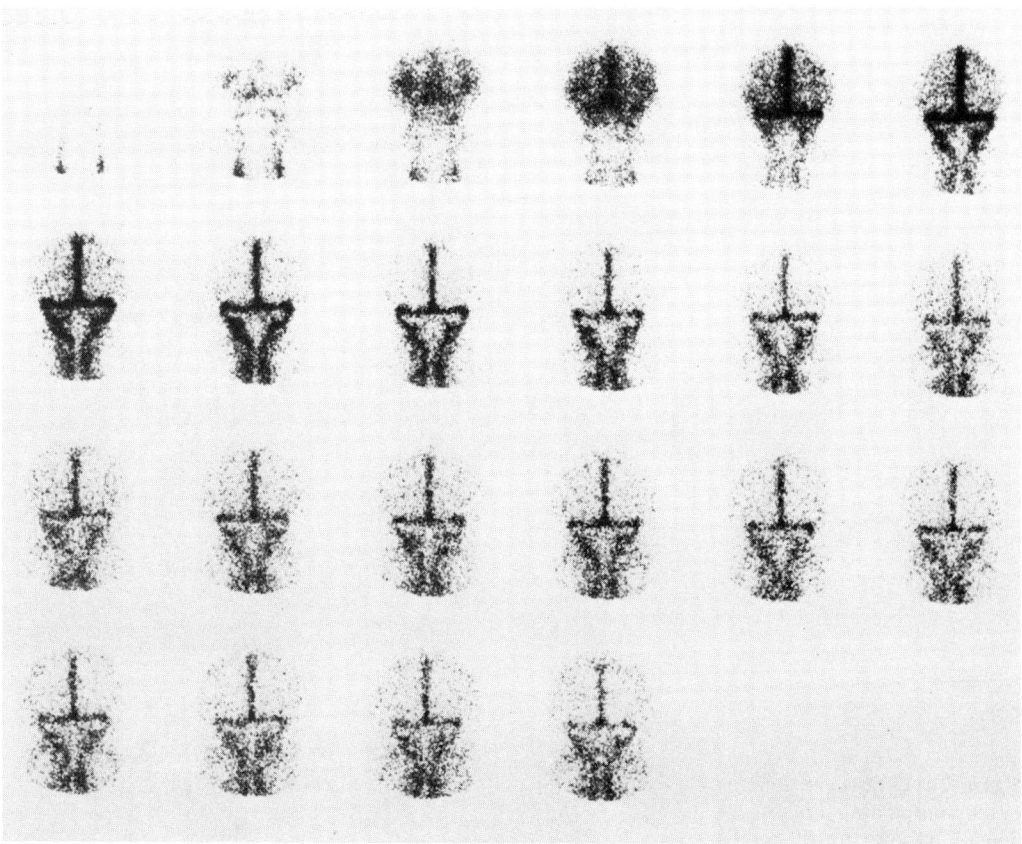

Figure 7-10. Normal posterior radionuclide cerebral angiogram (flow study). Images shown are made at 2-second intervals after IV injection of 20 mCi of Tc-99m glucoheptonate. The arterial phase (first 2 to 6 seconds) is characterized by visualization of the two internal carotid, the two middle cerebral, and the paramedial posterior cerebral arteries. This is followed by a capillary "blush" phase leading quickly to the venous phase, which is recognized by the appearance of activity in the superior sagittal sinus (midline). Subsequent images show venous drainage through the lateral (transverse) venous sinuses and the jugular veins, which return blood to the heart.

minutes after injection of the bolus.

Delayed images are obtained from 1 to 24 hours after injection. The earliest brain scans were obtained at approximately 1 hour after injection of the tracer material; however, the optimal time for nearly all of the tracers has since been found to be with as much delay as possible. The generally recommended delay is 3 to 4 hours after injection (Fig. 7-11). Even though the apparent degradation in image quality, i.e., difficulty in seeing normal anatomic structures, has seemed to make extended imaging (mistakenly) unacceptable, it should be noted that sensitivity with most of the brain-scanning agents improves up to 24 hours after injection. Emission computed tomographic (ECT) imaging with both positron- and single photon-imaging agents has added greatly to anatomic localization of abnormal concentrations of tracer material inside the skull. ECT imaging is a virtual necessity

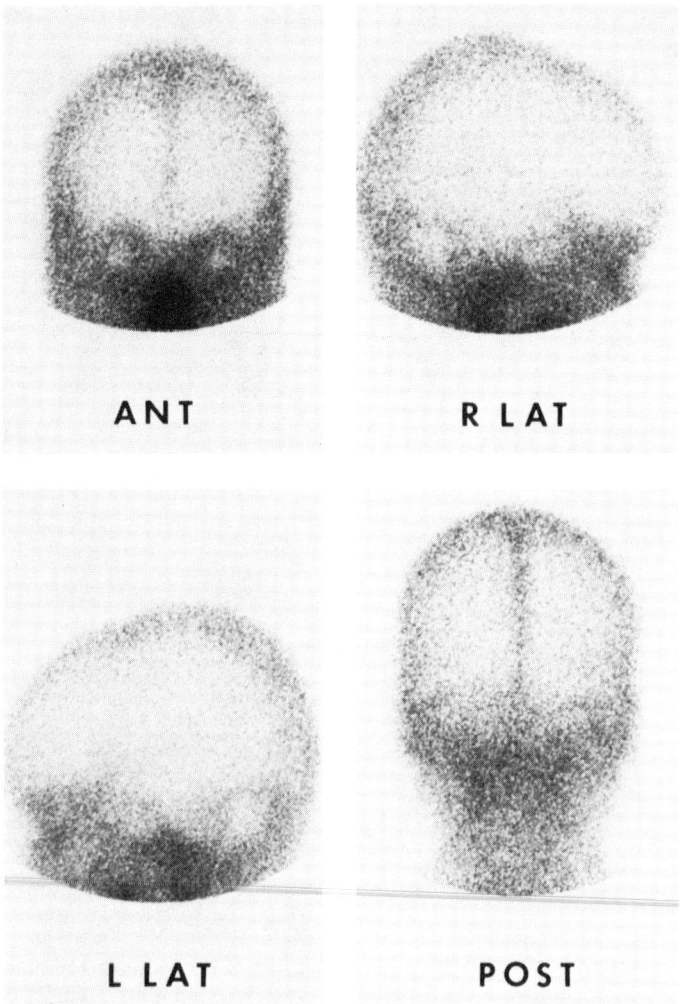

Figure 7-11. Delayed images of the normal brain obtained 4 hours after injection of 20 mCi of Tc-99m glucoheptonate. The four standard views are shown. Other viewing angles may be chosen (such as vertex or orbital views) to acquire additional information.

for imaging agents that bind to specific receptor sites in the brain.

CSF flow has been studied by the injection of tracer material into the CSF of the lumbar space (or C-1 dural space in some instances) to demonstrate the flow dynamics of the CSF in normal and disease processes and to pinpoint the location of CSF leaks caused by cranial trauma. The more commonly performed CSF flow studies for dementia are done with images obtained immediately postinjection to determine the accuracy of subarachnoid placement of the tracer material in the CSF and at 4, 24, and 48 hours to observe the flow kinetics in the cranial vault. Various techniques have been used to augment the flow of CSF and tracer material through a leak. Having the patient's head lower than the lumbar spine and having the part of the head suspected of having the leak in the dependent-most position are thought to augment leakage. Infusion of artificial CSF resulting in a sustained elevation of CSF pressure after the injection of tracer material has been used with success.

PHARMACEUTICALS

Tc-99m pertechnetate was the first widely used brain-scanning agent. It still offers some at least theoretic advantage for abnormalities that are usually hard to demonstrate such as herpes encephalitis and inflammatory lesions of the brain because of its slower blood clearance. Pertechnetate was replaced by DTPA and GH because the latter significantly improved sensitivity for the detection of brain lesions. Some of this may be due to the difference in clearance rates; however, in the case of GH there was speculation that the material might be being metabolized by some tumors. Ga-67-citrate- and In-111-labeled white blood cells have been used to localize a variety of abnormal intracranial processes and to try to improve the specificity for the lesion being due to inflammation.

In-111 DTPA is the usual choice for CSF flow studies that last 48 hours. The CSF rhinorrhea–otorrhea leak studies may be easily accomplished with Tc-99m DTPA because flow augmentation is an inherent part of the technique, and the study will usually be completed within 4 hours. Additionally, the high photon flux of Tc-99m is extremely helpful in pinpointing the source of the leak. It should be noted, however, that general use of Tc-99m DTPA

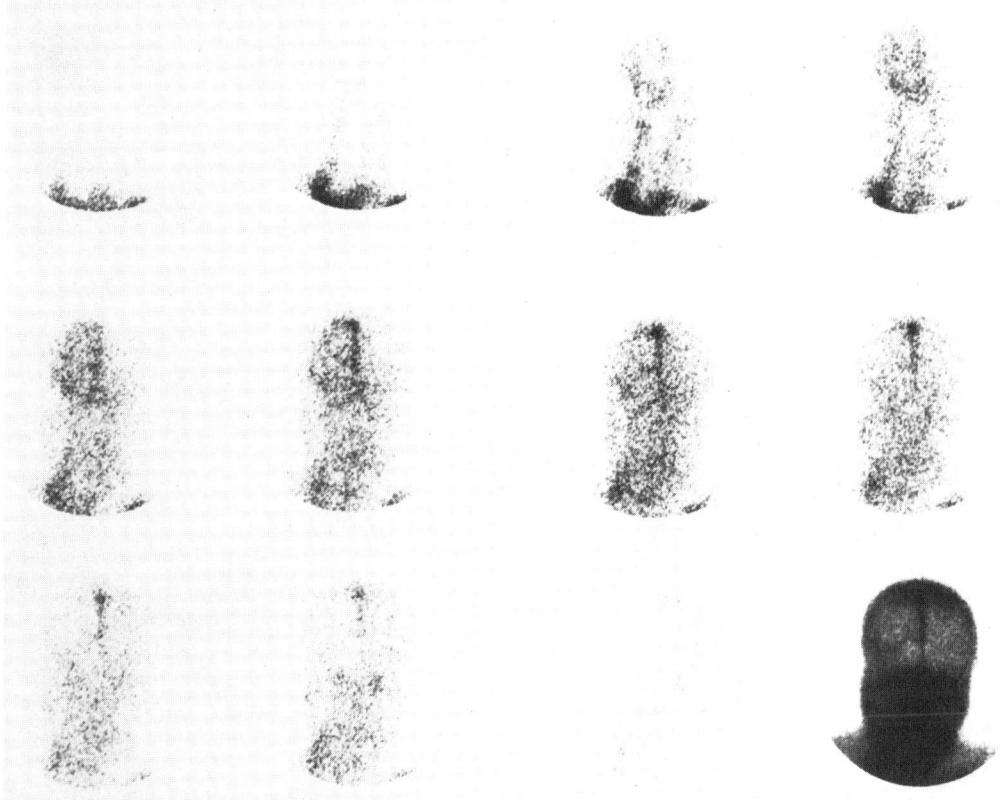

Figure 7-12. CVA. **A.** Abnormal anterior cerebral blood flow study demonstrating diminished middle cerebral perfusion on the left side during the arterial phase with relative hyperperfusion during the venous phase (flip–flop phenomenon).

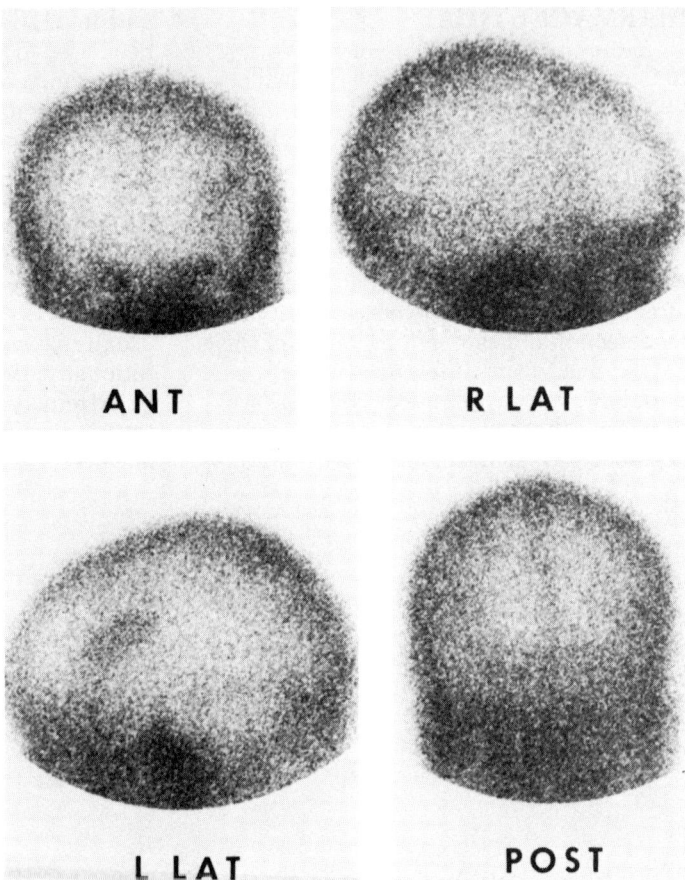

Figure 7-12. CVA. **B.** Delayed images reveal an infarcted area in the left hemisphere.

for radionuclide cisternography by group medical licensees is not allowable unless the individual physician files an IND with the FDA.

An unusual group of imaging agents that are taken up by nearly all of the CNS tissue in the first pass are the lipophilic amine class of compounds. These drugs, HIPDM and IMP, are being investigated for their ability to demonstrate differences in CNS vascular perfusion not readily detectable with TCT studies or with other tracer materials. The newest agents are those used in ECT studies that bind to specific receptor sites because of their biochemical product nature or because they are factors in an antigen–antibody reaction. Lastly, there is Tc-99m hexamethylpropyleneamineoxime (HM-PAO), which has the ability to pass through the BBB to measure regional cerebral blood flow.[69,70]

INTERPRETATION

Timing, configuration, and precise location are the key observable findings on brain scanning. Brain tumors and CVAs may have a similar abnormal appearance on delayed images. Timing is important, however, in that delayed images in patients with CVAs show no abnormality for 3 days after the event, show the greatest concentration at 3 weeks, and show no concentration after 3 months—the so-called "rule of threes." When flow studies are included with the brain scan, CVAs illustrate another abnormality known as the "flip-flop" phenome-

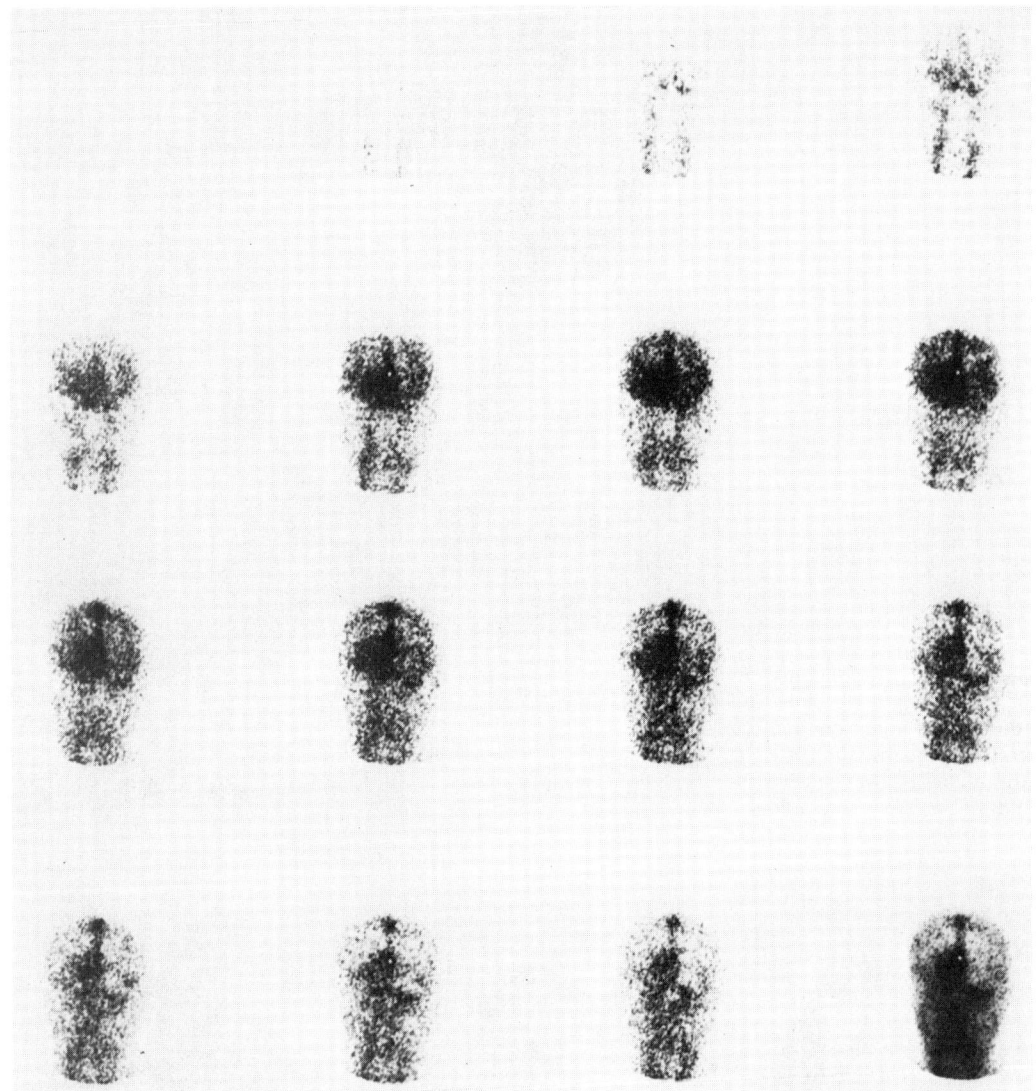

Figure 7-13. Meningioma. **A.** Abnormal anterior cerebral blood flow study demonstrating a hypervascular region in the right paramedial area after an injection of 20 mCi of Tc-99m glucoheptonate.

non wherein there is diminished perfusion to the side of the CVA during the arterial phase of perfusion, and relative hyperperfusion during the venous phase (Fig. 7-12). A-V malformations show increased vascularity on the flow and blood pool images but no abnormal concentration on the delayed images. Meningiomas, on the other hand, are hyperconcentrated in all three phases (Fig. 7-13). The glioblastoma multiforme tumor has a distinctive configuration when it spreads interhemispherically; it has a multilobulated or "peanut shell" shape. Herpes encephalitis has a characteristic serpentine bitemporal concentration on the delayed images (Fig. 7-14). Brain death is characterized by lack of cerebral perfusion (Fig. 7-15). Quantitation of impaired blood

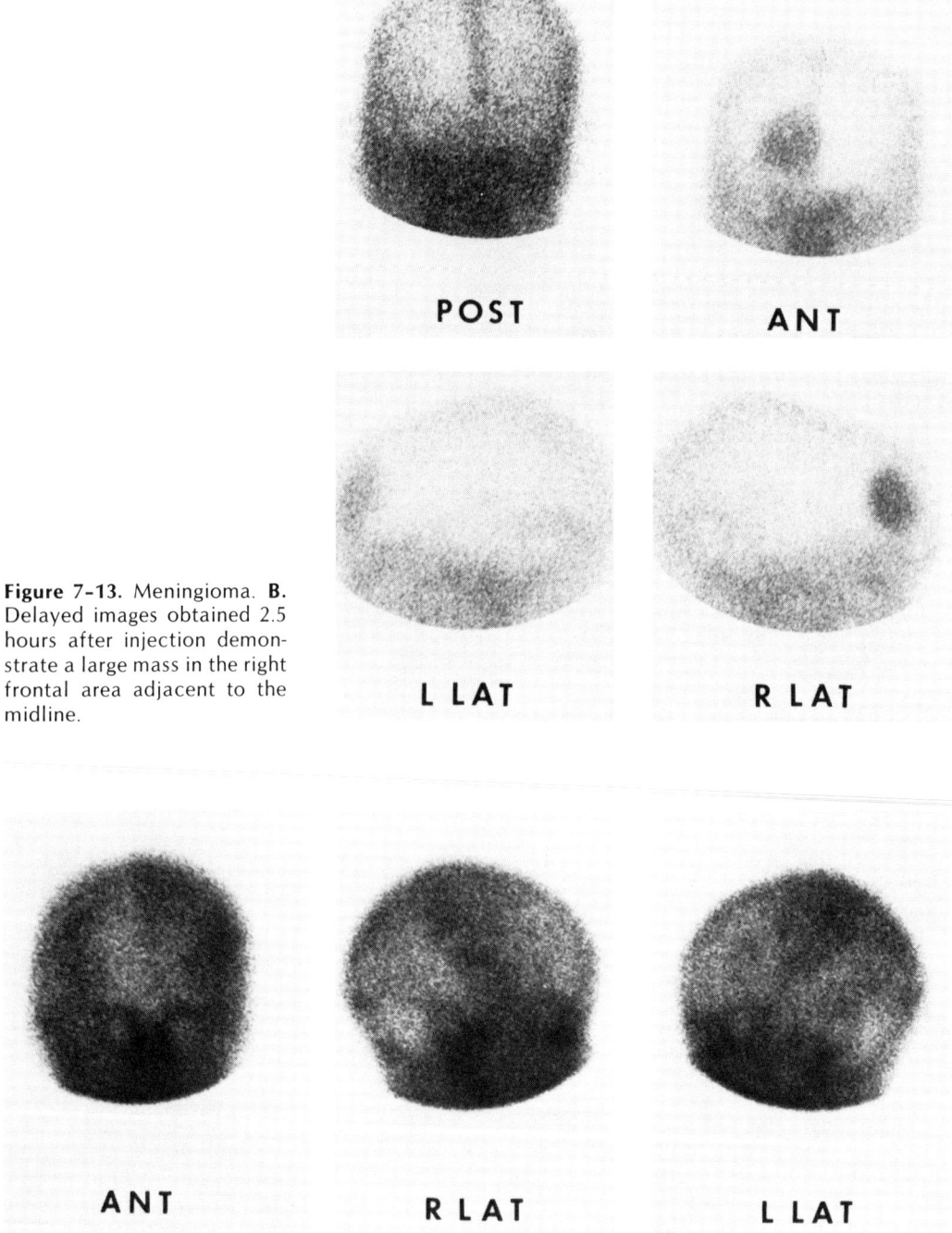

Figure 7-13. Meningioma. **B.** Delayed images obtained 2.5 hours after injection demonstrate a large mass in the right frontal area adjacent to the midline.

Figure 7-14. Herpes encephalitis with serpiginous concentration of tracer material in temporal lobe fissures bilaterally.

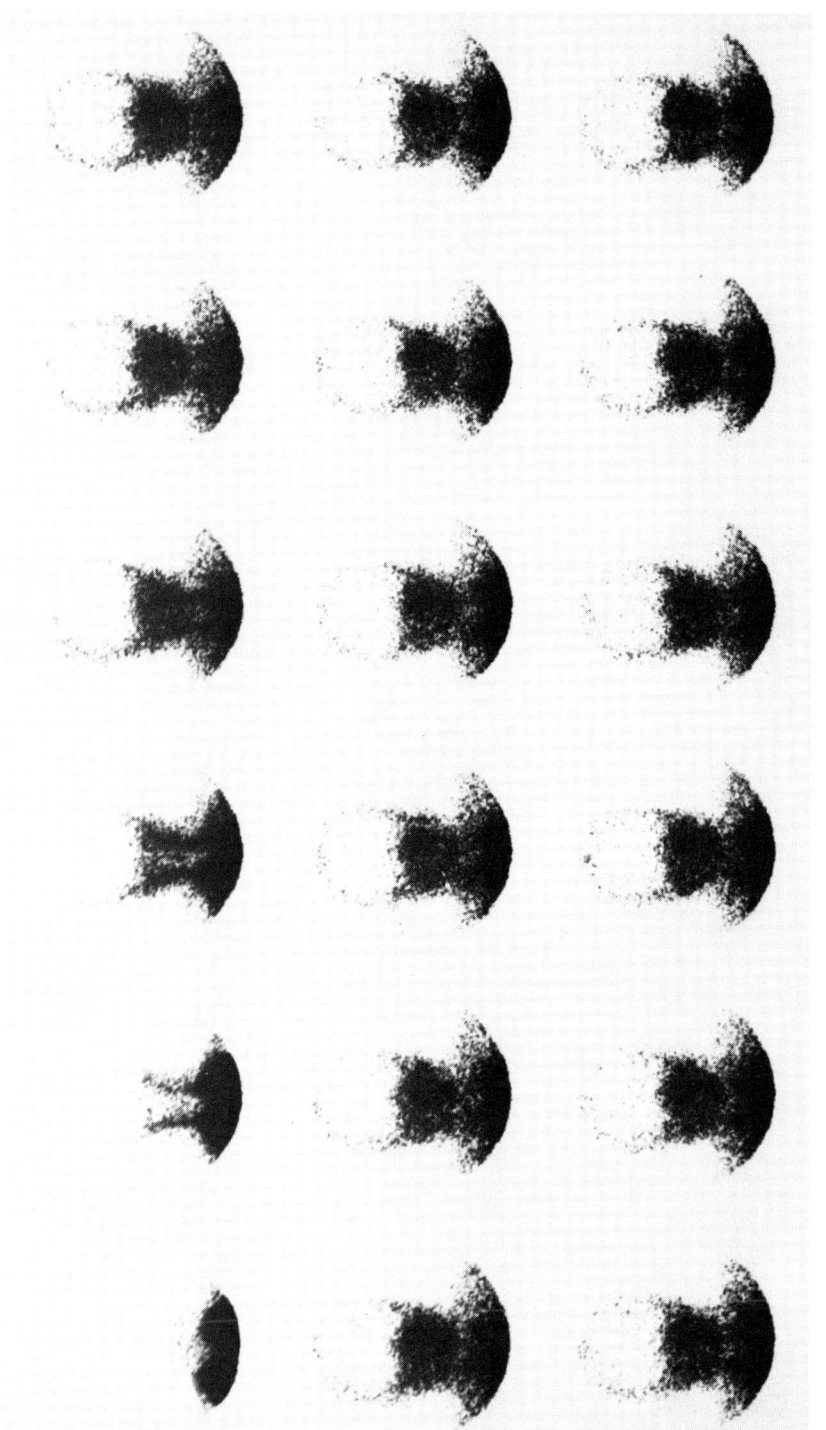

Figure 7-15. Brain death. Absence of cerebral perfusion after IV injection of Tc-99m gluceptate is seen in this 11-month-old child, a victim of smoke inhalation in a house fire.

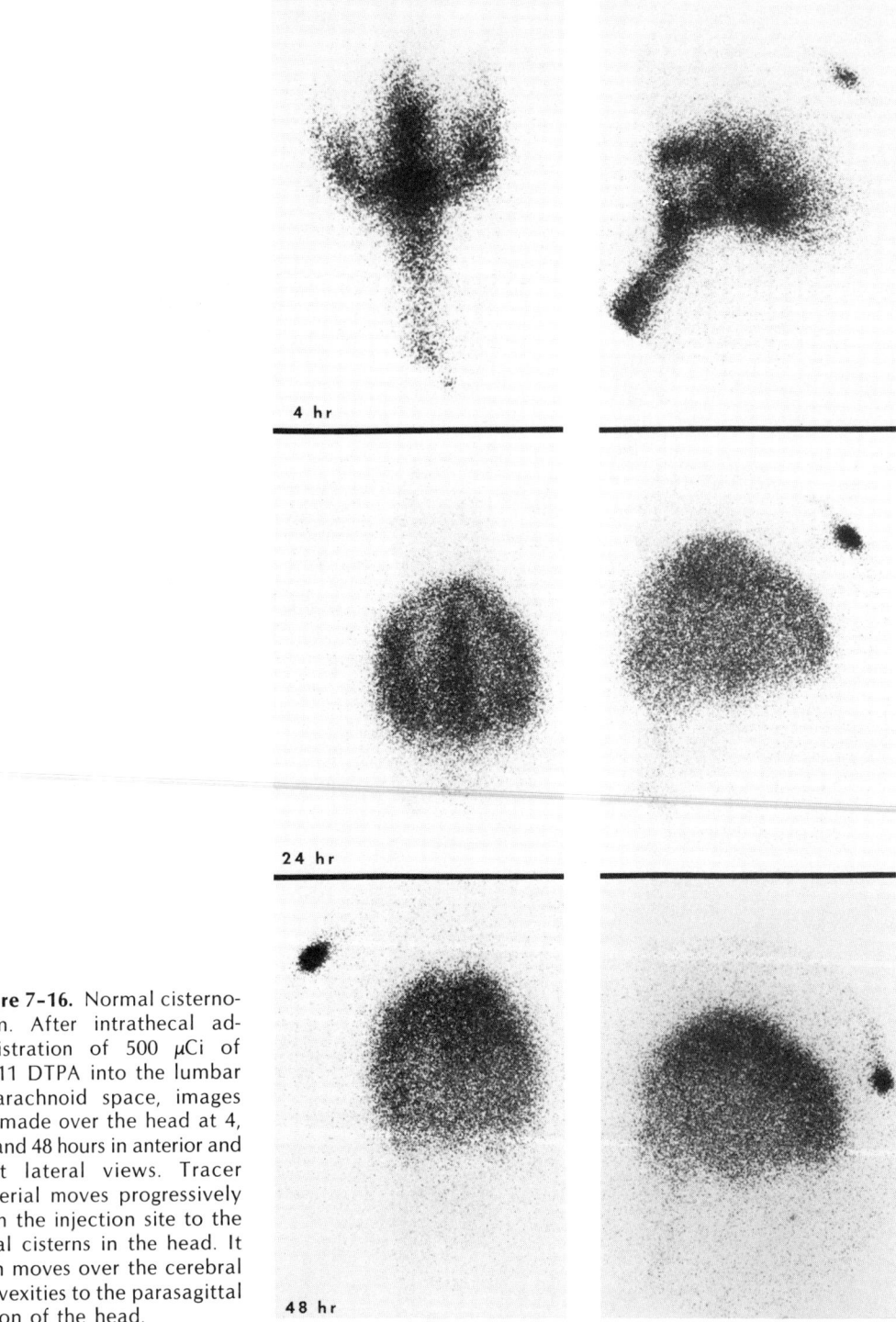

Figure 7-16. Normal cisternogram. After intrathecal administration of 500 μCi of In-111 DTPA into the lumbar subarachnoid space, images are made over the head at 4, 24, and 48 hours in anterior and right lateral views. Tracer material moves progressively from the injection site to the basal cisterns in the head. It then moves over the cerebral convexities to the parasagittal region of the head.

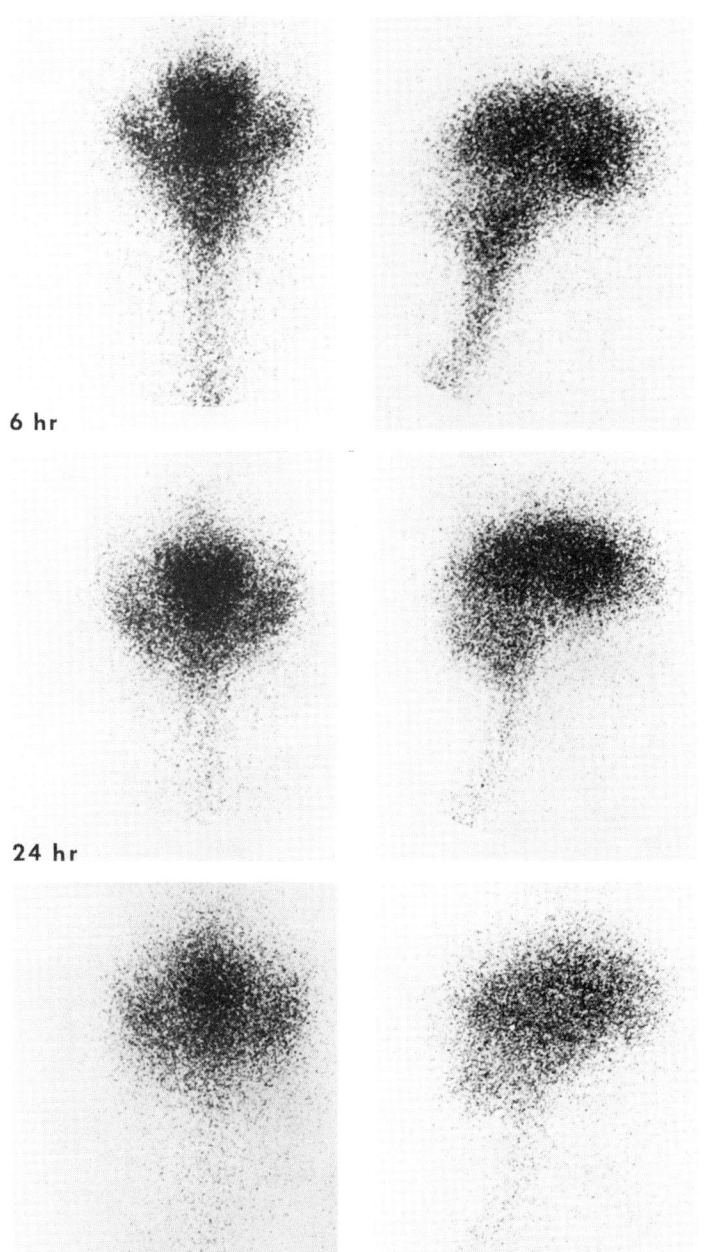

Figure 7-17. NPH. In the 6-hour images In-111 DTPA activity is seen in the spinal subarachnoid space, basal cisterns, and lateral ventricles. At 24 hours the activity persists in the lateral ventricles and in this patient there is very slow progression over the hemispheres. This pattern is essentially the same at 48 hours and indicates extraventricular obstruction and NPH.

flow may be obtained by using one of the amine group of agents and the ECT technique to integrate the volume of tissue involved or to compare the uptake of the tracer on one side versus the other.

CSF flow studies are most commonly done to aid in making the diagnosis of normal pressure hydrocephalus (NPH). In this disease there is an abnormal reflux of the CSF-containing tracer into enlarged lateral ventricles that persists at 24 and 48 hours after injection of the tracer into the lumbar

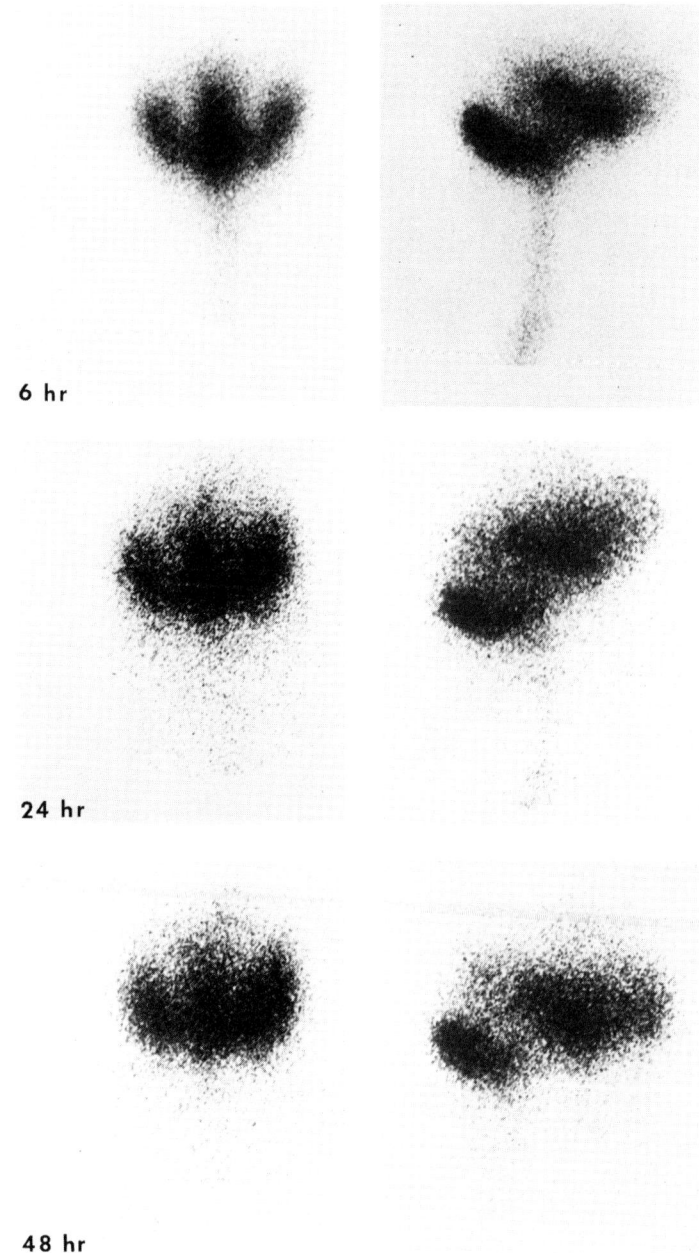

Figure 7-18. CNS atrophy. No ventricular penetration of the In-111 DTPA activity is seen; however, there is a slow flow of tracer around the convexities at 24 and 48 hours.

CSF space. CNS atrophy, otherwise described as "involutional change," causes slowing of flow over the cerebral hemispheres at 24 and 48 hours. At times the findings of these two disease processes are concurrent (Fig. 7-16 to 7-18). ECT techniques yield transaxial slice images similar to TCT but display better functional information than anatomic detail. In addition, the ECT images are easily re-sorted into

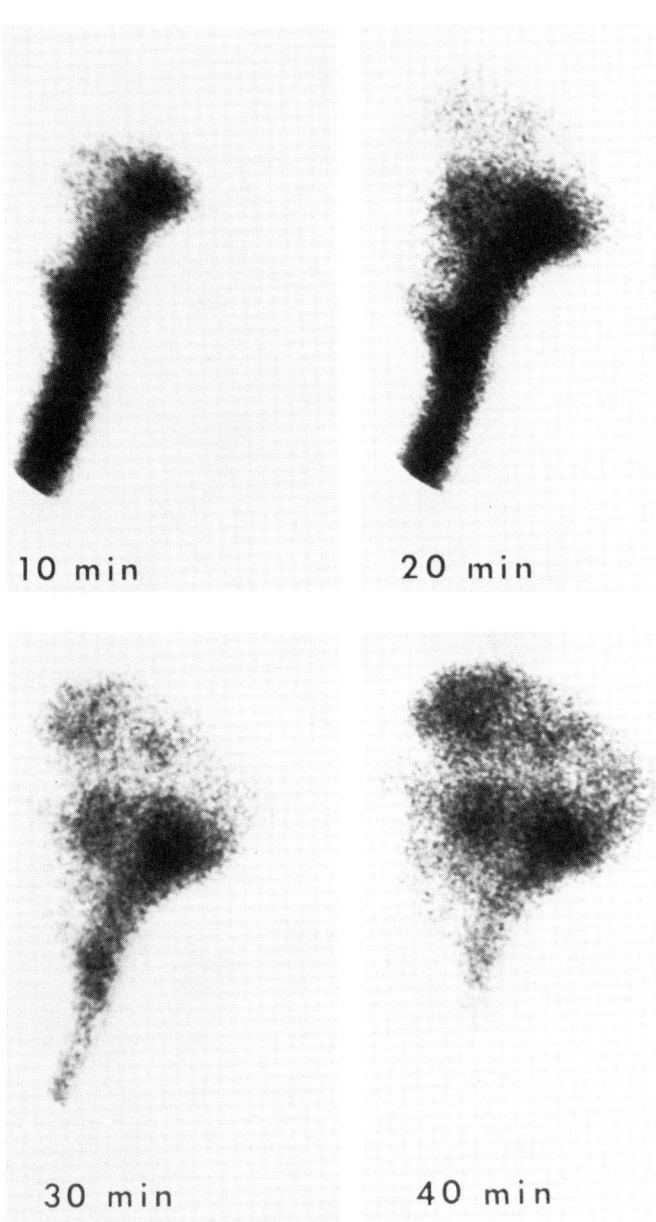

Figure 7-19. Normal overpressure CSF rhinorrhea study. One millicurie of Tc-99m DTPA is injected intrathecally after lumbar puncture. With a routine overpressure technique the radiopharmaceutical is rapidly delivered to the brain with artificial CSF. Right lateral images are obtained at 10, 20, 30, and 40 minutes. Pressures are routinely increased to 400 mm of water. Under these controlled conditions no CSF leak is evident.

sagittal and coronal slices, which oftentimes aid greatly in defining the exact location of an abnormality. With CSF leakage the primary information sought is the exact site of the leak. Because this is usually a very small volume and therefore difficult to detect visually, the technologist usually overexposes the normal part of the image in order to see the activity from the area of the leak. As an additional safeguard, in case the leak is not detected, pledgets are placed in the nose to be removed at the end of the study and counted in a well counter to determine whether an unvisualized leakage was present during the study (Fig. 7-19 and 7-20).

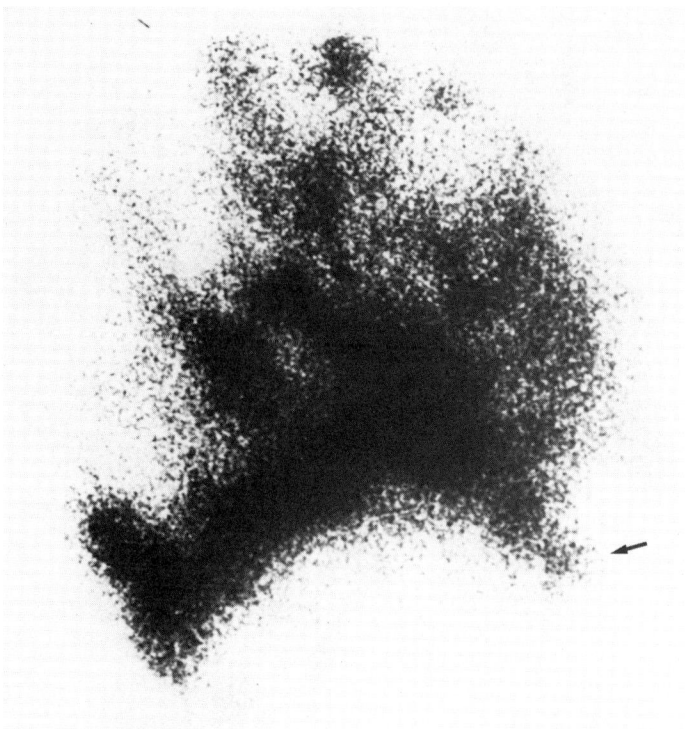

Figure 7-20. CSF leak. Right lateral view in a 35-year-old male 8 months after undergoing ethmoidectomy demonstrating rhinorrhea (arrow). Pledgets from the right middle meatus were positive. (From Curnes JT, et al, 1985, p 795, with permission.[68])

REFERENCES

1. Gilman AG, Goodman LS, Gilman A: The pharmacological basis of therapeutics, 6th ed. New York, Macmillan, 1980, pp 10, 244
2. Holmes RA, Staab EV: The central nervous system. In Freeman LM, Johnson PM (eds): Clinical Scintillation Imaging, 2nd ed. New York, Grune & Stratton, 1975, p 252
3. Guyton AC: Textbook of Medical Physiology; 6th ed. Philadelphia, Saunders, 1981, p 383
4. Moore GE: Fluorescein as an agent in the differentiation of normal and malignant tissues. Science 106:130, 1947
5. Moore GE: Use of radioactive diiodofluorescein in the diagnosis and localization of brain tumors. Science 107:569, 1948
6. Chou SN, Aust JB, Moore GE, et al: Radioactive iodinated human serum albumin as a tracer agent for diagnosing and localizing intracranial lesions. Proc Soc Exp Biol Med 77:193, 1951
7. Blau M, Bender Ma: Radiomercury (Hg-203) labeled Neohydrin: A new agent for brain tumor localization. J Nucl Med 3:83, 1962
8. Sodee DB: A new scanning isotope, mercury-197: A preliminary report. J Nucl Med 4:335, 1963
9. Lindeman JF, Quinn JL III: The recent history of clinical procedures in nuclear medicine. In Gottschalk A, Potchen EJ (eds): Diagnostic Nuclear Imaging. Baltimore, Williams & Wilkins, 1976 p 8
10. Richards P: A survey of the production at the Brookhaven National Laboratory of radioisotopes for medical research. In 5 Congresso Nucleare, Rome, Comitato Nazionale Ricerche Nucleare, Rome, 1960, Vol 2, p 225
11. Harper PV, Lathrop KA, Gottschalk A: Pharmacodynamics of some technetium-99m preparations. In Andrews GA, Kniseley RM, Wagner HN Jr (eds): Radioactive Pharmaceuticals. USAEC, Symposium 6, 1966, p 335
12. McAfee JG, Fueger CF, Stern HS, et al: Tc-99m pertechnetate for brain scanning. J Nucl Med 5:811, 1964

13. Eckelman W, Richards P: Instant Tc-99m DTPA. J Nucl Med 11:761, 1970
14. Wolfstein RS, Tanasescu D, Sakimura IT, et al: Brain imaging with Tc-99m DTPA: A clinical comparison of early and delayed studies. J Nucl Med 15:1135, 1974
15. Waxman A. Tanasescu DT, Siemsen J, et al: Tc-99m glucoheptonate as a brain scanning agent: Critical comparison with pertechnetate. J Nucl Med 17:345, 1976
16. Rollo DF, Cavalieri RR, Born M, et al: Comparative evaluation of Tc-99m GH, TcO_4, and Tc-99m DTPA as brain imaging agents. Radiology 123:379, 1977
17. Sokoloff L: Localization of functional activity in the central nervous system by measurement of glucose utilization with radioactive deoxyglucose. J Cereb Blood Flow Metab, 1:7, 1981
18. Fazio F, Gerundini P, Gilardi MC, et al: Single photon emission computerized tomography (SPECT) evaluation of the brain imaging agent, (I-123), HIPDM in man with rotating gamma camera. J Nucl Med 24:5, 1983
19. Holman BL, Lee RG, Hill TC, et al: A comparison of two cerebral blood flow tracers, N-isopropyl I-123 p-iodoamphetamine and I-123 HIPDM. J Nucl Med 24:P6, 1983
20. Kereiakes JG, Simmons GH, Feller PA: Whole body and critical organ dosimetry for technetium-99m labeled pharmaceuticals. In Kereiakes JG, Carey KR (eds): Biophysical Aspects of the Medical Use of Technetium-99m. AAPM Monograph No. 1, 1976, p 101
21. NCRP Report No. 70: Nuclear Medicine—Factors Influencing the Choice and Use of Radionuclides in Diagnosis and Therapy. Bethesda, Md, National Council of Radiation Protection and Measurements, 1982, p 116
22. Lathrop KA, Harper PV: Biologic behavior of Tc99m from Tc-99m pertechnetate ion. Prog Nucl Med 1:145, 1972
23. McAfee JG, Fueger CF, Stern HS, et al: Tc-99m pertechnetate for brain scanning. J Nucl Med 5:811, 1964
24. Brown-Grant K: Extrathyroidal iodide concentrating mechanisms. Physiol Rev 41:189, 1961
25. Dayton DA, Maher FT, Elveback LR: Renal clearance of technetium (Tc-99m) as pertechnetate. Mayo Clin Proc 44:549, 1969
26. Andros G, Harper PV, Lathrop KA, et al: Pertechnetate-99m localization in man with application to thyroid scanning and the study of thyroid physiology. J Clin Endocrinol 25:1067, 1965
27. Beasley TM, Palmer HE, Nelp WB: Distribution and excretion of technetium in humans. Health Phys 12:1425, 1966
28. Witcofski RL, Janeway R, Maynard CD, et al: Visualization of the choroid plexus on the technetium-99m brain scan. Clinical significance and blocking by potassium perchlorate. Arch Neurol 16:286, 1967
29. Coben LA, Loeffler JD, Elsasser JC: Spinal fluid iodide transport in the dog. Am J Physiol 206:1373, 1964
30. Alazraki N, Littenberg RL, Hurwitz S, et al: Differences in choroid plexus concentration of pertechnetate produced by varying time of perchlorate administration and brain imaging. J Nucl Med 15:884, 1974
31. Scheu JD, Tetalman MR, Araujo O, et al: The efficacy of intravenous sodium perchlorate in choroid plexus blocking. J Nucl Med 17:528, 1976
32. Welch MJ, Adatepe M, Potchen EJ: An analysis of technetium pertechnetate kinetics: The effect of perchlorate and iodide pretreatment. Int J Appl Radiat Isot 20:437, 1969
33. Oldendorf WH, Sisson WB, Iisaka Y: Compartmental redistribution of Tc-99m pertechnetate in the presence of perchlorate ion and its relation to plasma protein binding. J Nucl Med 11:85, 1970
34. Welch M, Adatepe M, Potchen EJ: Technetium kinetics in humans—The effect of heavy-ion pretreatment on optimal time for brain imaging. J Nucl Med 9:359, 1968
35. Rumble WF, Aamodt RL, Jones AE, et al: Accidental ingestion of Tc-99m in breast milk by a 10 week-old child. J Nucl Med 19:913, 1978
36. Vagenakis AG: Duration of radioactivity in the milk of a nursing mother following Tc-99m administration. J Nucl Med 12:188, 1971
37. Tator CH: Radiopharmaceuticals for tumor localization with special emphasis on brain tumors. In Subramanian G, Rhodes BA, Cooper JF, Sodd VS (eds): Radiopharmaceuticals. New York, Society of Nuclear Medicine, 1975, p 474
38. Padgett HC, Barrio JR, MacDonald NS, et al: The unit operations approach applied to the synthesis of (1-C-11) 2-deoxy-D-glucose

for routine clinical application. J Nucl Med 23:739, 1982
39. Phelps ME, Huang SC, Hoffman EJ, et al: Tomographic measurement of local cerebral glucose metabolic rate in humans with (F-18) 2-fluoro-2-deoxy-d-glucose: Validation of method. Ann Neurol 6:371, 1979
40. Kung HF, Blau M: Regional intracellular pH shift: A new mechanism for radiopharmaceutical uptake in brain and other tissues. J Nucl Med 21:147, 1980
41. Rapoport SI: Blood–Brain Barrier in Physiology and Medicine. New York, Raven Press, 1976, p 154
42. Loberg MD: Radiotracers for cerebral functional imaging—A new class. J Nucl Med 21:183, 1980
43. DiChiro G, Reames PM, Matthews WB Jr: RISA–ventriculography and RISA–cisternography. Neurology 14:105, 1964
44. Detmer DE, Blockner HM: A case of aseptic meningitis secondary to intrathecal injection of I-131 human serum albumin. Neurology 15:642, 1965
45. Nicol CP: A second case of aseptic meningitis following isotope cisternography using I-131 human serum albumin. Neurology 17:199, 1967
46. Oldham RK, Staab EV: Aseptic meningitis following the intrathecal injection of radioiodinated serum albumin. Radiology 97:317, 1970
47. Ashburn WL, Harbert JC, Briner WH, et al: Cerebrospinal fluid rhinorrhea studied with the gamma scintillation camera. J Nucl Med 9:523, 1968
48. Wagner HN Jr, Hosain F, DeLand FH, et al: A new radiopharmaceutical for cisternography: Chelated ytterbium 169. Radiology 95:121, 1970
49. Matin P, Goodwin DA: Cerebrospinal fluid scanning with In-111. J Nucl Med 12:668, 1971
50. Goodwin DA, Song CH, Finston R, et al: Preparation, physiology, and dosimetry of In-111 labeled radiopharmaceuticals for cisternography. Radiology 108:91, 1973
51. Harbert JC, Reed VR, McCullough DC: Comparison between I-131 HSA and Yb-169 DTPA for cisternography. J Nucl Med 14:765, 1973
52. Bell EG, Maher B, McAfee JG, et al: Radiopharmaceuticals for gamma cisternography. In Subramanian G, Rhodes BA, Cooper JF, Sodd VJ (eds): Radiopharmaceuticals. New York, Society of Nuclear Medicine, 1975, p 399
53. Som P. Hosain F, Wagner HN Jr, et al: Cisternography with chelated complex of Tc-99m. J Nucl Med 13:551, 1972
54. Welch MJ, Welch TJ: Solution chemistry of carrier-free indium. In Subramanian G, Rhodes BA, Cooper JF, Sodd VJ (eds): Radiopharmaceuticals. New York, Society of Nuclear Medicine, 1975, p 73
55. Alazraki NP, Halpern SE, Ashburn WL, et al: Hyperbaric cisternography: Experience in humans. J Nucl Med 14:226, 1973
56. Partain CL, Alderson PO, Donovan RL, et al: Regional kinetics of indium-111 DTPA in CSF imaging of normal volunteers. In Cloutier RJ, Coffey JL, Snyder WS, Watson EE (eds): Radiopharmaceutical Dosimetry Symposium. Oakridge, Tenn, HEW Publication (FDA) 76-8044, 1976, p 404
57. DeLand FH, Simmons GH: Spinal cord and cerebrospinal fluid. In Cloutier RJ, Coffey JL, Snyder WS, Watson EE (eds): Radiopharmaceutical Dosimetry Symposium. Oakridge, Tenn, HEW Publication (FDA) 76-8044, 1976, p 390
58. Harbert JC, McCullough D, Zeiger LS, et al: Spinal cord dosimetry in I-131 HSA cisternography. J Nucl Med 11:534, 1970
59. McAfee JG, Subramanian G: Radioactive agents for imaging. In Freeman LM, Johnson PM (eds): Clinical Scintillation Imaging, 2nd ed. New York, Grune & Stratton, 1975, p 13
60. Harper PV, Lathrop KA, Jiminez F, et al: Technetium-99m as a scanning agent. Radiology 85:101, 1965
61. Elliott KAC, Jasper HH: Physiological salt solutions for brain surgery. J Neurosurg 6:140, 1949
62. Mahaley MS Jr, Odom GL: Complication following intrathecal injection of fluorescein. J Neurosurg 25:298, 1966
63. Huggins CB, Hastings AB: Effect of calcium and citrate injections into cerebrospinal fluid. Proc Soc Exp Biol Med 30:459, 1933
64. Cooper JF, Harbert JC: Endotoxin as a cause of aseptic meningitis after radionuclide cisternography. J Nucl Med 16:809, 1975
65. Magnaes B, Solheim D: Controlled overpressure cisternography to localize cerebrospinal fluid rhinorrhea. J Nucl Med 18:109, 1977
66. Lewis RC, Elliott KAC: Clinical uses of ar-

tificial cerebrospinal fluid. J Neurosurg 7:256, 1950
67. Nelson JR, Goodman SJ: An evaluation of the cerebrospinal fluid infusion test for hydrocephalus. Neurology 21:1037, 1971
68. Curnes JT, Vincent LM, Kowalsky RJ, et al: CSF rhinorrhea: Detection and localization using overpressure cisternography with Tc-99m DTPA. Radiology 154:795, 1985
69. Sharp PF, Smith FW, Gemmell HG, et al: Technetium-99m HM-PAO sterioisomers as potential agents for imaging regional cerebral blood flow: Human volunteer studies. J Nucl Med 27:171, 1986
70. Leonard JP, Nowotnik DP, Neirinckx RD: Technetium-99m-d,l-HM-PAO: A new radiopharmaceutical for imaging regional brain perfusion using SPECT—A comparison with iodine-123 HIPDM. J Nucl Med 27:1819, 1986

CHAPTER 8

Thyroid

Radionuclide studies of the thyroid gland and its function span the entire gamut of the types of procedures performed in nuclear medicine. These include (1) an in vivo function study, namely, the radioactive iodine uptake (RAIU) study to assess thyroid function where the patient receives a small (5 μCi) dose of iodide I-131 and the gland activity is counted after a defined period of time to determine the percent dose taken up by the gland; (2) thyroid therapy whereby a larger dose (usually 5 to 30 mCi for hyperthyroidism or 150 to 200 mCi for thyroid carcinoma) is given to destroy diseased thyroid tissue; (3) thyroid imaging studies where diagnostic images of the thyroid gland or metastatic lesions are obtained with a gamma camera following pertechnetate or radioiodine administration to the patient; and (4) in vitro tests where no radioactive material is given to the patient but a sample of the patient's blood is subjected to one of several radioassay tests such as the T_3 and T_4 radioimmunoassays to assess thyroid function.

The application of radiopharmaceuticals either as radioiodine or technetium-99m pertechnetate to conduct the first three thyroid procedures mentioned will be the subject of this chapter. A more detailed discussion of radioimmunoassay in vitro tests will be covered in Chapter 16.

PHYSIOLOGIC ANATOMY

The thyroid gland is composed of a large number of follicles, each lined with epithelial cells and filled with a substance called colloid as shown in Figure 8–1.[1] The major constituent of the colloid is thyroglobulin, which is the base for production and storage of the thyroid hormones thyroxine (T_4) and triiodothyronine (T_3). Ingested iodide is removed from the blood by the thyroid epithelial cells. Once inside the cells the iodide is very rapidly oxidized by peroxidase enzymes and hydrogen peroxide to an oxidized form of iodine of undefined nature.[2] For simplicity it will be called iodine. The iodine then reacts with tyrosine residues on thyroglobulin and is stored outside the cell in the colloid. This trapping of iodide by the epithelial cell is the rate-limiting step in hormone production. It is an active transport process, and the thyroid

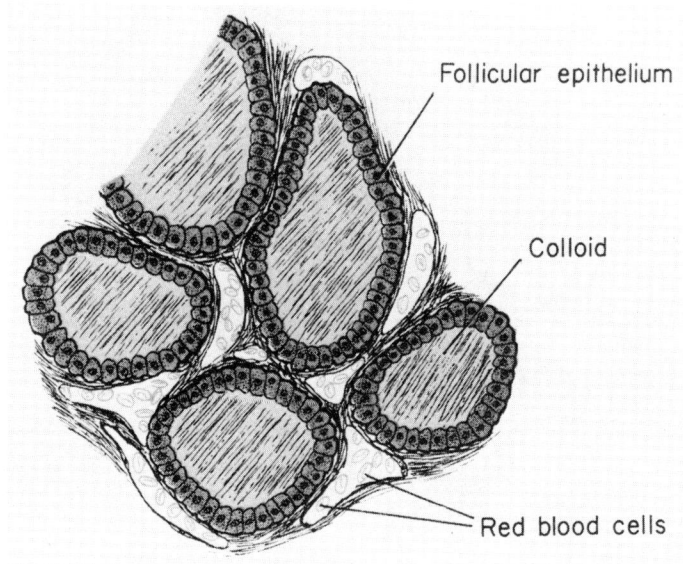

Figure 8-1. Microscopic appearance of the thyroid gland. (From Guyton AC, 1981, p 931, with permission.[1])

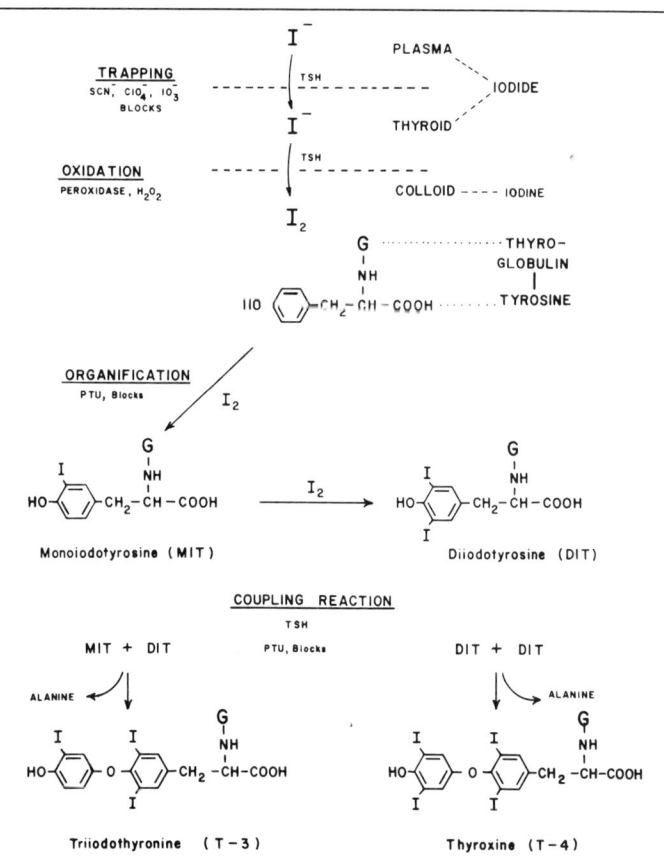

Figure 8-2. Schematic representation of iodine metabolism in the thyroid gland.

cell is capable of concentrating iodide 40 times the plasma concentration under normal circumstances but may increase tenfold in hyperthyroid states. Iodine binds to tyrosine to form monoiodotyrosine (MIT) and diiodotyrosine (DIT), which then undergo coupling reactions to form the final hormones triiodothyronine and thyroxine as shown by the scheme in Figure 8-2.

Figure 8-3 illustrates the daily turnover of iodine in the body.[3] In a review of thyroid physiology Rapoport and DeGroot[4] discuss the kinetics of iodine metabolism as a three-compartment model: compartment I, the extrathyroidal iodide pool (75 μg iodine); compartment II, the thyroid iodine pool (6000 μg iodine); and compartment III, the extrathyroidal iodine hormone pool (500 μg iodine). With this model an average daily intake of iodide is 300 μg. This value can vary widely according to geographic location and dietary habits. This intake is balanced by a urinary loss of 285 μg and a fecal loss of 15 μg. About 75 μg of iodide is made into thyroid hormone and released into the blood. Of this amount 15 μg is metabolized in the liver and excreted in the feces. The remaining hormone undergoes enzymatic deiodination in the tissues with recycling of 60 μg of iodide back into compartment I for reuse or renal excretion. During an average day about 20 percent of the ingested iodide is organified into hormone, and 80 percent is excreted.

A number of substances either promote or block the synthesis of thyroid hormone. Thyroid-stimulating hormone (TSH) from the anterior pituitary gland controls several of these functions including iodide trapping, the coupling reactions between MIT and DIT, and hormone release from the colloid into the blood. Excess plasma iodide suppresses thyroid plasma clearance of iodide.

The drugs methimazole and propyl-

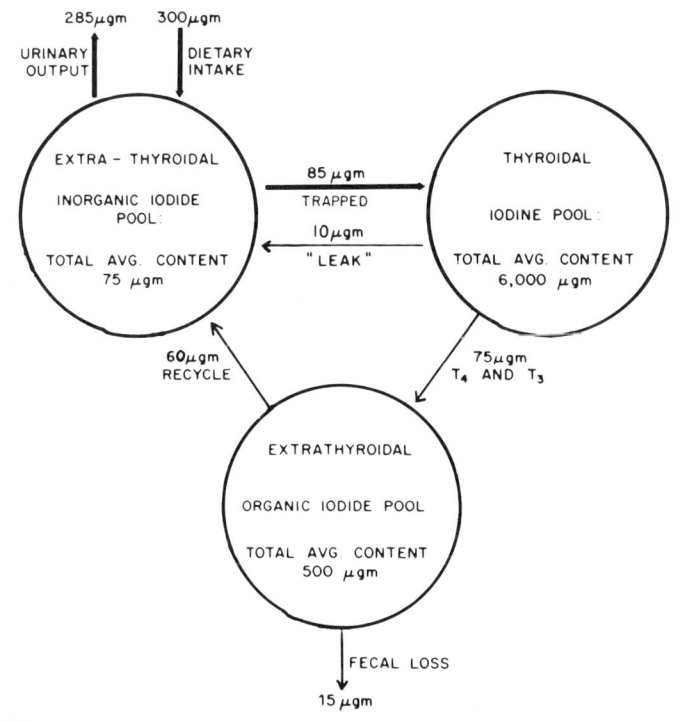

Figure 8-3. Daily turnover of iodine in the body. *(From Hoffer PB, et al, 1976, p 255, with permission.[3])*

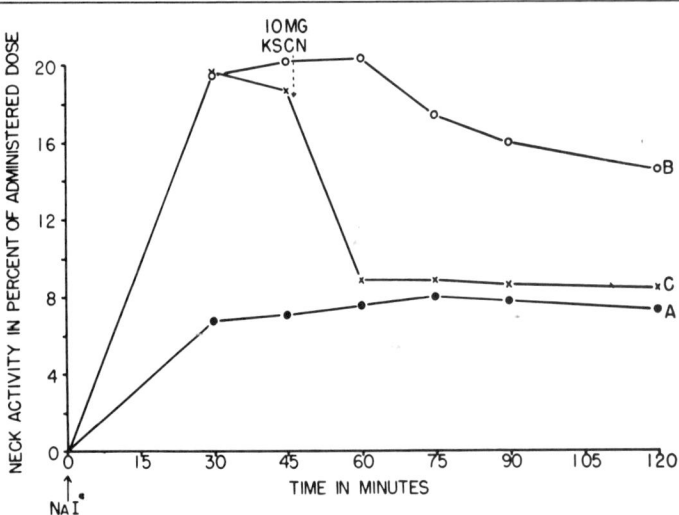

Figure 8-4. Accumulation of radioiodide in thyroid glands of rats (A) pretreated with thiocyanate to block trapping, (B) pretreated with PTU to block organification, and (C) pretreated with PTU but administered thiocyanate after the radioiodide dose. See the text for details. (From Wyngaarden JB, et al, 1952, p 537, with permission.[5])

thiouracil (PTU) block the organification of iodine with tyrosine as well as the coupling reactions of MIT and DIT. Several halogen oxyanions and thiocyanate are capable of inhibiting the iodide-trapping mechanism and also cause discharge of iodide from the PTU-blocked thyroid. These effects are shown in Figure 8-4, which demonstrates iodide trap kinetics in the treated rat.[5] Curve A represents thyroidal radioiodide in rats previously treated with thiocyanate to block the iodide-trapping mechanism. Curve B represents the thyroidal radioiodide in rats treated with PTU 1 hour before radioiodide administration and illustrates that iodide is trapped but is not organified as evidenced by the slow decline in curve B as iodide is cleared from the plasma by the kidney. Curve C demonstrates the effect of 0.1 mM of thiocyanate in promptly discharging the trapped iodide from the PTU-blocked thyroid gland.

Of the halogenated oxyanions, perchlorate (ClO_4^-) is the most effective agent in discharging trapped iodide and is ten times more potent than thiocynanate.[5] Periodate (IO_4^-) and iodate (IO_3^-) are equally effective as perchlorate, but their rate of response is slower than perchlorate.[5]

HISTORIC PERSPECTIVES IN THE DEVELOPMENT OF RADIOPHARMACEUTICALS FOR THYROID STUDIES

The first production of radioiodine for clinical application was made by Robley Evans at the Massachusetts Institute of Technology in 1937.[6] He produced I-128 by the neutron irradiation of ethyl iodide. Evans administered the I-128 to rabbits and clearly demonstrated for the first time the rapid accumulation of radioiodide in the thyroid gland after intravenous injection.[7]

Following the discovery of artificial radioactivity in 1934, cyclotrons were built at several research centers in the United States to produce radionuclides, mainly for medical research. Collaboration between institutions led to the rapid discovery of several iodine isotopes. Large quantities of I-128 were produced at Berkeley, but its short half-life (25 minutes) was unsatisfactory for extended metabolic studies. In 1938 at Michigan, Tape and Cork produced 13.3-day I-126,[8] and Livingood and Seaborg at Berkeley made 8-day I-131.[9] At that time mostly I-126 was used until I-131 could be produced in larger yields. In 1940 MIT produced 12-hour I-130 and I-131 in larger quantities. Hamilton and Soley reported on the first use of I-131 in human subjects with thyroid diseases.[10] Keston et al first reported on the uptake of radioiodine in thyroid metastasis in 1942,[11] but probably the most significant application of I-131, which led to its notoriety and heralded the value of radioisotopes in medicine, was the report by Seidlin et al in 1946[12] on the use of the I-131 "atomic cocktail," as the press called it, in the treatment of metastatic thyroid cancer. Before this, I-131 had been used to treat Graves' disease,[13] but a "cancer cure" had much more dramatic impact than a treatment for hyperthyroidism. Thus began a strong public and monetary support for the fledgling discipline of nuclear medicine.

PRODUCTION AND PROPERTIES OF RADIOIODINES

Iodine-131

This isotope of iodine is currently obtained by chemical separation as a by-product of uranium fission but may also be produced by the neutron activation of tellurium. Both methods produce tellurium-131, which decays to I-131 according to the following reactions:

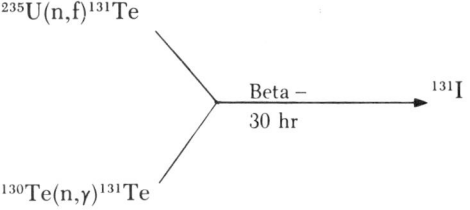

The nuclear material is processed to yield sodium iodide as the final chemical form.

The I-131 nucleus is characterized by 53 protons and 78 neutrons, four neutrons more than the stable isotope iodine-127. The neutron-rich I-131 thus undergoes negatron (beta minus) decay to stable xenon-131 according to the following decay equation. The nuclear transformation is given under the arrow.

$$^{131}_{53}I_{78} \xrightarrow[n \to p^+ + e^- + \bar{\nu}]{8.04 \text{ d}} {}^{131}_{54}Xe_{77} + 971 \text{ keV} (\beta, \gamma, \nu)$$

130.906117 AMU   130.905075 AMU

The transition energy between I-131 and the Xe-131 ground state is 971 keV. Several beta transitions are possible in I-131 decay as shown in Figure 8–5. In the most frequent transition (beta-5) about 607 keV goes to the beta alone or is split between the beta and neutrino (ν), and the remaining 364 keV is emitted as a gamma ray (gamma-9) from the excited Xe-131 nucleus in its transition to the ground state. Other beta transitions produce minor abundances of other gamma rays, which are listed in Table 8–1 along with other properties of I-131. The higher-energy gammas are the principal reason for using heavy detector collimation with I-131 imaging. The 364-keV gamma has good abundance and penetrates tissue efficiently, but it is inefficiently stopped (23 percent) by a half-inch sodium iodide crystal. This makes I-131 less than ideal for imaging with the gamma camera. The half-value layer (HVL) in lead is quite high requiring thick lead shielding of vials for adequate protection.

Iodine-125

This isotope of iodine was discovered in 1946 by Reid and Keston[14] as a long-lived "contaminant" in a mixture of radioiodines produced by deuteron irradiation of tellurium. An alternate method of producing pure I-125[15] involves the neutron irradiation of a xenon target producing short-lived Xe-125, which then decays to I-125 according to the following scheme:

$$^{124}Xe(n,\gamma)^{125}Xe \xrightarrow[17 \text{ hr}]{EC} {}^{125}I$$

The I-125 is separated from any residual Xe-125 by cooling to liquid nitrogen temperature and fractional vaporization (Xe boiling point (BP), 107°C; I BP, 183°C).

I-125 is characterized by 53 protons and 72 neutrons in its nucleus, two neutrons less than I-127. This neutron-deficient

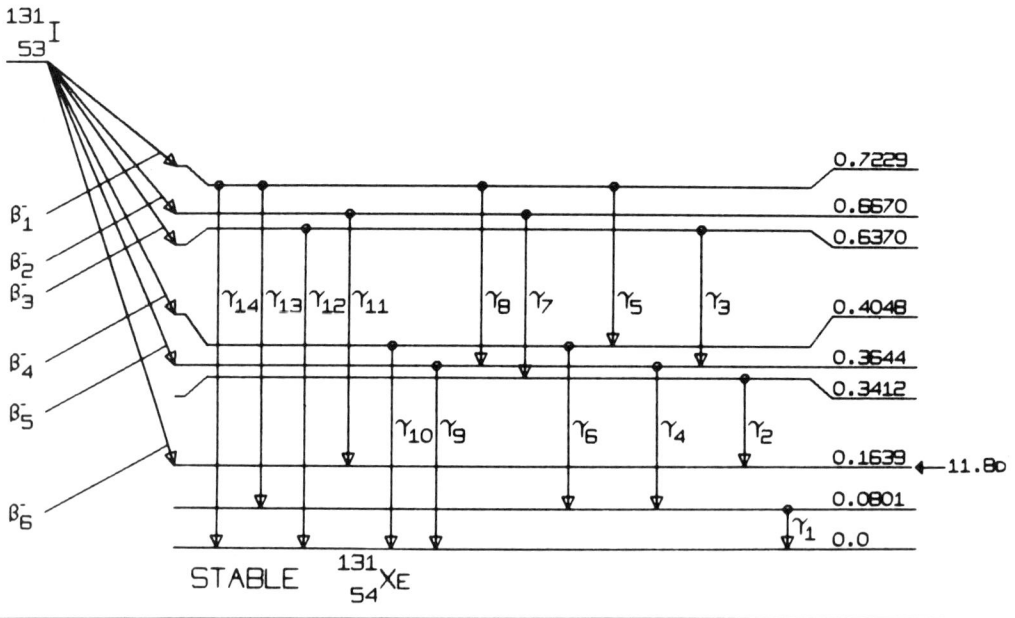

Figure 8-5. Decay scheme of I-131. *(From Dillman LT, Von der Lage FC: MIRD Pamphlet No. 10. New York, Society of Nuclear Medicine, 1975, with permission.)*

nucleus undergoes electron capture (EC) decay to stable Te-125 according to the following decay equation:

$$^{125}_{53}I_{72} \xrightarrow[p^+ + e^- \rightarrow n + \nu]{59.9d} {}^{125}_{52}Te_{73} + 178 \text{ keV } (\nu, \gamma)$$

124.904624 AMU   124.904433 AMU

The transition energy for this decay is 178 keV. The decay scheme is shown in Figure 8–6. Of this 178 keV, the neutrino carries away 143 keV in the transition to the excited state of Te-125, and 35 keV is emitted as a gamma ray when Te-125 deexcites to its ground state. For every 100 atoms of I-125 that decay, 93 of the 35-keV gammas undergo electron conversion (K, L, and M-shell electrons) so that only seven gamma

TABLE 8-1. PROPERTIES OF IODINE RADIOISOTOPES

Nuclide	$T_{1/2}$	Decay Mode/Products	Photons	keV	Abundance (%)	R/hr/mCi at 1 cm	HVL (mm Pb)
I-123	13.1 hr	EC/Te-123	Gamma	159	83	1.5	0.37
			Te x-rays	28	87		
I-125	59.9 d	EC/Te-125	Gamma	35	7	0.7	0.015
			Te x-rays	27	115		
				31	21		
				32	4		
I-131	8.04 d	β^-/Xe-131	Gamma	364	82	2.2	3.0
				284	6		
				637	7		
				723	2		

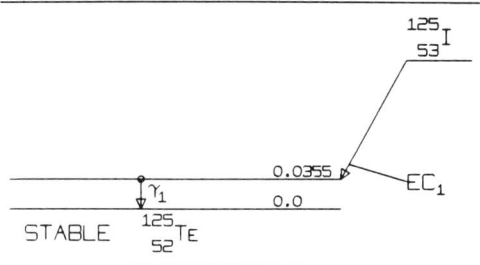

Figure 8-6. Decay scheme of I-125. *(From Dillman LT, Van der Lage FC: MIRD Pamphlet No. 10. New York, Society of Nuclear Medicine, 1975, with permission.)*

rays are detectable (7 percent abundance). A high percentage of Te-125 characteristic x-rays (115%), however, are emitted that can be used for detection. Table 8-1 lists the properties of I-125. The HVL in lead is quite small, which allows easy shielding of I-125. In fact, the weak gamma photons are so easily stopped that about 50 percent will be absorbed by the glass vials containing the I-125 source. Therefore, container geometry must be considered for accurate measurement of I-125 sources. The reader is referred to Chapter 6 for more details on I-125 assay.

Soon after its discovery I-125 was suggested for use as a replacement for I-131 because of the potential for a reduced radiation dose; however, the reduction in the radiation dose to the thyroid is not that significant (about one-third less than I-131). Additionally, the weak I-125 photons present problems with in vivo quantitative thyroid counting and with imaging deep-seated thyroid tissue such as substernal thyroid because of significant absorption by thicker tissues and bone. Its long half-life, however, makes I-125 an economically useful radiolabel for many compounds. In this regard I-125 is favored over I-131 for radiolabeling also because its lack of beta emission minimizes radiolytic decomposition of the labeled molecule.

Iodine-123

This iodine isotope has nearly ideal properties for thyroid studies.[16] It is produced in a cyclotron by several methods.[17] A significant problem with earlier methods of production was the simultaneous production of radioiodine contaminants, namely, I-124, I-125, I-130, and I-131. The percent impurity of the longer-lived contaminants relative to I-123 increase with the time of decay after cyclotron production. They thus contribute to an increase in the radiation dose, and the higher-energy photons from contaminants significantly decrease image resolution when camera images are obtained with low-energy collimators[17] (Fig. 8-7).

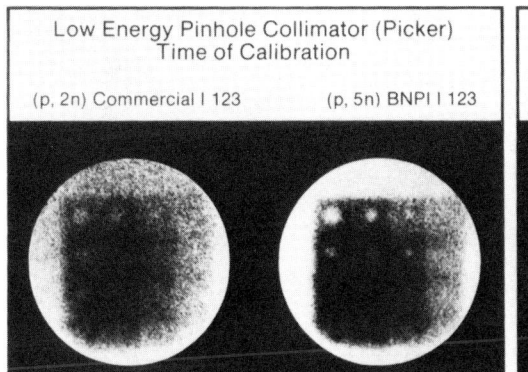
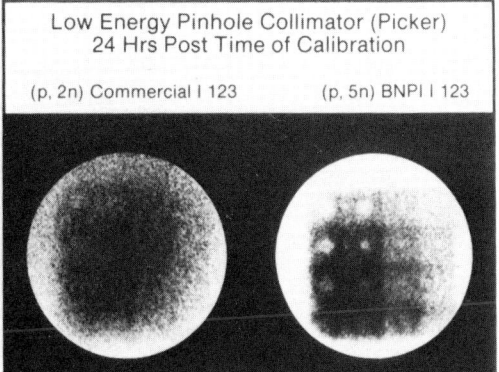

Figure 8-7. Comparison of scintillation camera images for I-123 produced by (p, 2n) and (p, 5n) reactions. *(From Hines HH, Lagunas-Solar M: Comparison of scintillation camera images for I-123 produced by (p, 2n) and (p, 5n) reactions. J Nucl Med 23:121, 1982, with permission.)*

TABLE 8-2. IODINE-123 PRODUCTION

Nuclear Reaction	Impurities, $T_{1/2}$, Energy
1.[a] $^{127}I(p, 5n)^{123}Xe \xrightarrow{EC, 2\ hr} {}^{123}I$	I-125 (59.9 d; 27–35 keV)
2.[a] $^{124}Te(p,2n)^{123}I$	I-124 (4.2 d; 603 keV)
3.[a] $^{122}Te(d,n)^{123}I$	I-124
	I-126 (13d; 389, 66 keV)
	I-130 (12.5 hr; 740, 1150 keV)
	I-131 (8d; 364 keV)
4.[b] $^{124}Xe(p,2n)^{123}Cs \longrightarrow {}^{123}Xe \longrightarrow {}^{123}I$	Te-121m (150 d; 212 keV)

[a]From Baker GA, et al, 1976, p 740.[17]
[b]From Atomic Energy of Canada, Ltd.

The production method of choice is the (p,5n) reaction on I-127 or the (p,2n) reaction on Xe-124 (Table 8–2).

The I-123 nucleus is characterized by 53 protons and 70 neutrons, making it four neutrons less than I-127. It decays by electron capture to Te-123, which is essentially stable $T_{1/2} = 1.2 \times 10^{13}$ yr).

$$^{123}_{53}I_{70} \xrightarrow[p^+ + e^- \rightarrow n + \nu]{13.1\ hr} {}^{123}_{52}Te_{71} + 1230\ keV(\nu, \gamma)$$

122.905596 AMU   122.904276 AMU

The transition energy for the decay is 1230 keV. This energy is dissipated by several EC transitions shown in the decay scheme of Figure 8–8. In 98 out of 100 decays it oc-

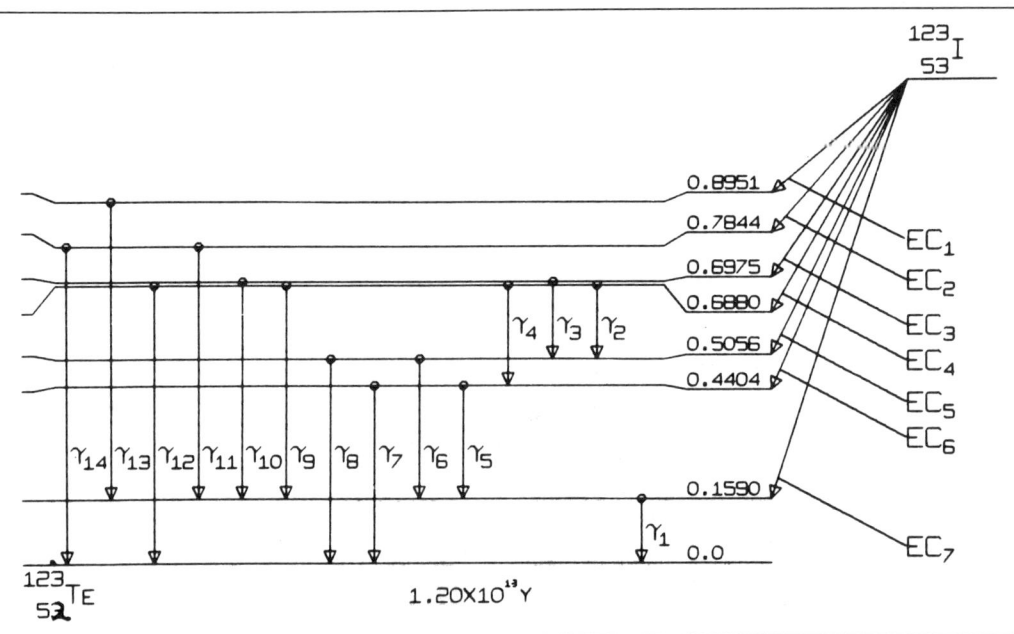

Figure 8-8. Decay scheme of I-123. *(From Dillman LT, Von der Lage FC: MIRD Pamphlet No. 10. New York, Society of Nuclear Medicine, 1975, with permission.)*

curs with a 1071-keV neutrino emitted (EC-7) to the excited state of Te-123, which subsequently de-excites, emitting 159-keV gamma rays (gamma-1). Loss of gamma-1 to conversion electrons yields a photon abundance of 83 percent.

I-123 is easily collimated and shielded, and its gamma energy is efficiently detected by the gamma camera. Its short half-life and lack of beta radiation significantly lessen the radiation dose to the thyroid gland to one 100th that of I-131. The main disadvantages of I-123 are availability and cost because of cyclotron production and the short half-life necessitating daily delivery.

CHEMISTRY, HANDLING PROCEDURES, AND PRECAUTIONS OF RADIOIODINE

Chemically, the iodide anion is quite reactive. It will readily oxidize under favorable conditions to produce volatile forms such as elemental iodine and hydrogen iodide. Both of these forms present a potential health hazard to personnel handling radioiodine solutions. There are two main routes of oxidative degradation: chemical and radiochemical. Iodide may be oxidized in acidic medium by atmospheric and dissolved oxygen or by any iodate contaminant present according to the following reactions:

$$4\,I^- + O_2 + 4\,H^+ \longrightarrow 2\,I_2 + 2\,H_2O$$

$$5\,I^- + IO_3^- + 6\,H^+ \longrightarrow 3\,I_2 + 3\,H_2O$$

Oxidation reactions can be minimized in several ways[18]: (1) buffering the solution to maintain an alkaline pH (7.5 to 9.0), thereby reducing the formation of volatile forms of iodine; (2) use of antioxidants such as sodium thiosulfate to retard oxidation of iodide to iodine according to the following reaction:

$$I_2 + 2\,S_2O_3^{2-} \longrightarrow 2\,I^- + S_4O_6^{2-}$$

and (3) use of chelating agents such as EDTA salts to retard catalytic oxidation induced by metal ions. Additionally, because oxidative reactions are accelerated by heat and light, storage in a dark cool environment will help. Because iodine has a low solubility in water (0.03 percent at 20°C), refrigerated storage will lower its vapor pressure. A number of papers discuss the hazards of radioiodine and techniques used to minimize them.[18-22]

Indirect oxidation of iodide in aqueous solution can also occur by radiolytic effects. The radiation-induced free radicals and peroxides in I-131 solutions oxidize iodide to iodine (I_2) and iodate (IO_3^-). These reactions are accelerated by a high radioactive concentration and the presence of oxygen.[23,24] Radiolytic effects are most significant with an I-131 solution because of its beta radiation. These effects can be reduced primarily by lowering the radioactive concentration and use of antioxidants. Dilutions of radioiodide I-131 solutions should be made with an antioxidant such as 0.2 percent sodium thiosulfate in distilled water. Tap water should not be used because it contains sufficient chlorine to spontaneously oxidize iodide.[25]

Despite preventative measures by manufacturers, some degree of iodide oxidation still occurs, and the user is cautioned to open vials in an exhaust hood to vent the head space over the solution before use.

Upon receipt into the nuclear medicine lab, bottles of I-131 solutions should be wipetested with a cotton-tipped applicator to detect any external contamination. This can be readily detected by a Geiger–Müller or scintillation counter. In some instances broken bottles, bottles with loose caps, and even bottles with tight caps having a grossly contaminated external surface have been discovered upon receipt from the supplier. Wearing disposable rubber or plastic gloves is necessary. Inadvertant skin contamination with I-131 is best removed by first rinsing with water followed by soap and water lather and a final rinse. A mild scrubbing with a soft brush may be needed. Table 8–3 lists some recommendations for handling radioiodine solutions.

TABLE 8-3. RECOMMENDATIONS FOR HANDLING RADIOIODIDE SOLUTIONS

1. Wear disposable rubber or plastic gloves.
2. Wipe test solution vials for removable contamination upon receipt.
3. Open vials in an exhaust hood.
4. Store solutions at a cool temperature.
5. Dilute solutions with distilled water for immediate use and with 0.2 percent sodium thiosulfate for prolonged storage.
6. Make solution transfers only with a syringe or pipette and pipette bulb. Do not pipette by mouth.
7. Perform regular thyroid bioassay exams on personnel who handle radioiodine frequently.

RADIOIODIDE DOSAGE FORMS

I-131 is the standard radionuclide used for routine thyroid studies because it is inexpensive and available when needed. Sodium iodide I-131 is available from commercial suppliers in hard gelatin capsules and in aqueous solution for oral administration. Capsules used for diagnostic studies are generally available in 15-, 25-, 50-, and 100-μCi sizes. These capsules may contain sodium radioiodide mixed with polyethylene glycol and thiosulfate[26] as a thin film on the inside surface of the capsule, or the radioiodide may be mixed with a granulated powder mixture.

Therapeutic capsules for use in hyperthyroidism and thyroid carcinoma are also available and made to order on a 24-hour notice. These may contain sodium iodide mixed with semisolid polyethylene glycol appearing as a small blob inside the capsule or adsorbed on anhydrous sodium phosphate.

It is very important that the activity between diagnostic capsules of a given lot not vary by more than a few percent to minimize error in thyroid uptake measurements. The US Pharmacopeia (USP) XXI requires manufacturers to assure that at least 19 of 20 capsules in a lot contain activity within 96.5 percent and 103.5 percent of the mean capsule activity. It is recommended that all capsules received in the nuclear medicine lab be counted and statistically analyzed to assure these limits. A method for performing this analysis is shown in Figure 8-9.

The usual dose for a thyroid uptake study is 5 μCi of sodium iodide I-131. A convenient way to assure a ready supply of usable capsules is to have higher-activity capsules delivered a few weeks before they are needed to allow for decay to the desired activity range.

Oral solutions of sodium iodide I-131 are manufactured to maintain their stability against oxidation. One product contains disodium phosphate to maintain the pH at 7.5 to 9.0, sodium bisulfite as an antioxidant, and disodium EDTA. Another product is stabilized with 0.1 percent disodium EDTA and is buffered to pH 8. It is important to note that stabilizers will not interfere with the clinical use of radioiodide but that such solutions are not satisfactory for radiolabeling procedures because the antioxidants prevent iodide oxidation, which is necessary in iodination reactions.

The expiration date for diagnostic capsules is 1 month and for solutions 2 months from the date of manufacture to limit the amount of radiation-induced impurities in the dose (mainly iodate). Radiochemical purity, determined by radiochromatography, must be at least 95 percent of the total radioactivity as iodide.

Iodide I-131 solutions may turn an amber color with age because of radiation-induced chromophores. This is a normal process and does not affect the quality of the radiopharmaceutical.

Sodium iodide I-125 is not routinely used in nuclear medicine for thyroid studies, and no pharmaceutical dosage forms are marketed for human use. A radiochemical solution usually in 0.1 M sodium hydroxide is available for radiolabeling proteins and other molecules. It is sold in various specific activities. Radiolytic decomposition reactions do not occur as readily with I-125 because of its lack of beta radiation. Proteins, antibodies, and other compounds of

DIVISION OF NUCLEAR MEDICINE   NORTH CAROLINA MEMORIAL HOSPITAL

RADIONUCLIDE CAPSULE COUNTING WORKSHEET

RADIONUCLIDE   I-131 Sodium Iodide   DATE COUNTED   1-19-78
LOT NUMBER   3007032F   DATE ASSAYED   1-16-78
ACTIVITY   22 uCi/Capsule   COLOR   Yellow

NET CAPSULE COUNTS

1. 112,919	11. 117,510	21.
2. 115,374	12. 113,388	22.
3. 113,590	13. 112,316	23.
4. 112,782	14. 114,124	24.
5. 111,568	15. 115,102	25.
6. 111,546	16. 110,983	26.
7. 110,635	17. 114,949	27.
8. 114,117	18. 115,342	28.
9. 113,380	19. 116,830	29.
10. 114,417	20. 115,182	30.

BACKGROUND: PRE-COUNT   54 CPM   POST-COUNT   57 CPM

Procedure: Count each capsule over the scintillation crystal well counter using the specially designed capsule counting holder so that the counting rate does not exceed 10^6 CPM. Collect at least 100,000 counts per capsule. Subtract background count and determine the mean net count. Discard any capsule whose counts do not fall within 96.5% to 103.5% of the mean count. Select and save as a standard the capsule whose count is closest to the mean count.

Mean Net Count 113,802   { x 0.965 = 109,820 (lower limit)
                          { x 1.035 = 117,786 (upper limit)

Figure 8-9. Capsule-counting work sheet for statistical analysis of sodium iodide I-131 capsules.

biologic interest are thus frequently labeled with I-125. Additionally, its 60-day half-life provides a long shelf life that is especially useful for radioimmunoassay and other in vitro tests.

Sodium iodide I-123 is commercially available in capsule and solution form for oral administration. Gelatin capsules are produced in various activities, usually 100, 200, and 400 μCi. These may contain an adsorbant filler such as sucrose to which an accurately measured volume of sodium iodide I-123 solution is added. Oral solutions contain sodium iodide in purified water adjusted to pH 8 with sodium bicarbonate. The specific concentration is about 2 mCi/ml at calibration. Radiolytic decomposition of I-123 solutions is not significant because of its short half-life and lack of beta emission.

BIOLOGIC DISTRIBUTION AND EXCRETION OF IODIDE

A diagrammatic representation of iodine metabolism is shown in Figure 8–10.[27] After oral administration the rate of gastrointestinal (GI) absorption of radioiodide is rapid, on the order of 5 percent per minute,

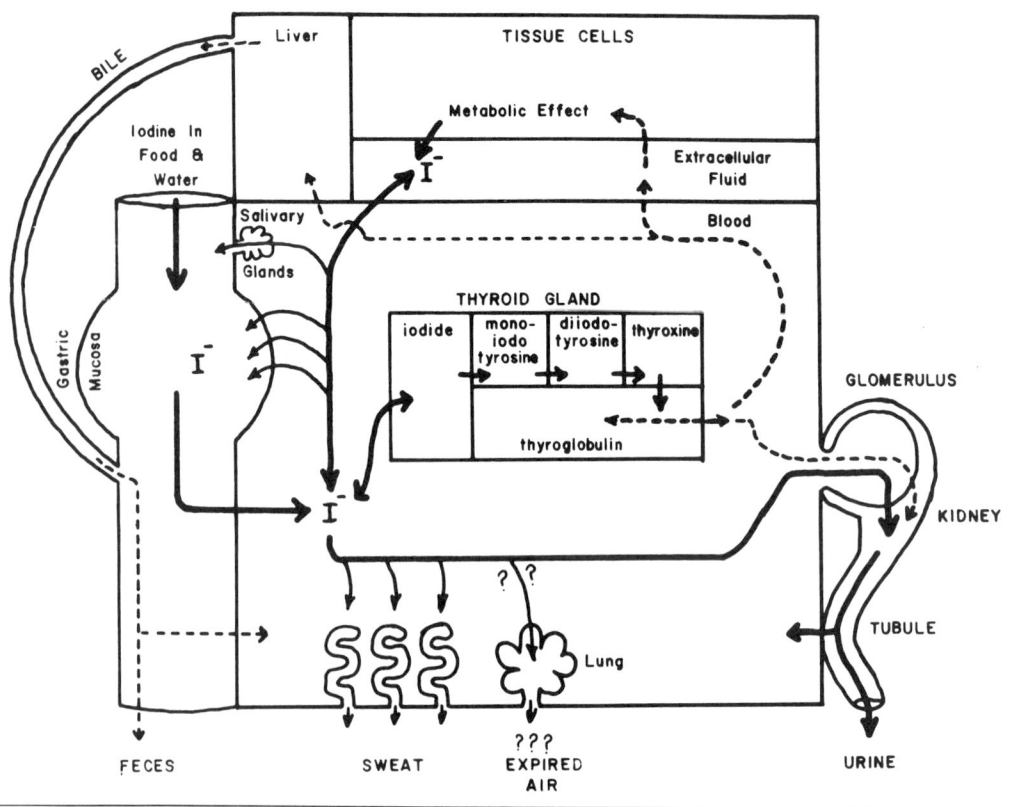

Figure 8-10. Scheme of iodine metabolism in the body. Major pathways are represented by thick arrows and minor pathways by thin arrows. Solid lines designate inorganic, and broken lines, organic iodine. *(From Riggs DS, 1952, p 284, with permission.[27])*

and is nearly complete within 1 to 2 hours.[28] The absorption rate may be delayed if food is present and is directly influenced by thyroid function, being increased in hyperthyroidism and decreased in hypothyroidism.[28]

Iodide is cleared from the plasma primarily by the thyroid gland, other organs, and renal excretion. Table 8–4 lists the normal plasma clearance of iodide by various organs in euthyroid subjects.

Renal Clearance

Renal clearance of iodide is by glomerular filtration. Because the clearance value (34 ml/min) is only 27 percent of the normal glomerular filtration rate (GFR), about 73 percent of filtered iodide is reabsorbed by the tubule. Iodide is not bound by the kidney. Renal clearance of iodide is fairly con-

TABLE 8-4. PLASMA IODIDE CLEARANCE IN EUTHYROID SUBJECTS

Organ	Clearance (ml/min)	Literature Reference
Thyroid	16.4	30
	17.7	31
Kidneys	34.0	27
Salivary glands	17.5	32
Gastric mucosa	24.5	32
Mammary glands	12.1	32

stant over a wide range of plasma concentrations. After doses of 10 μCi of iodide I-131 and carrier doses of 0.001, 0.1, 1.0, and 10.0 mg of stable iodide in exophthalmic goiter patients, no difference in the renal clearance of iodide is found, but a significant reduction of thyroid uptake occurs.[29] The low doses of stable iodide produce no apparent effect on thyroid uptake, but the 1.0- and 10.0-mg doses produce uptakes similar to euthyroidism and the athyrotic state, respectively.[29] The ability of the kidney to maintain a constant renal clearance of iodide in the face of high plasma levels makes possible the practical technique of administering stable carrier iodide to protect the thyroid gland from unnecessary radiation exposure from either metabolized radiopharmaceuticals or from accidental ingestion of radioiodide. The latter is an important consideration in the event of a nuclear power plant disaster.

The thyroid-blocking dose of potassium iodide recommended by the Food and Drug Administration (FDA) is 130 mg per day for adults and children more than 1 year old and 65 mg per day for children less than 1 year old. These doses can block 90 percent of radioiodine absorption if the first dose is given a few hours before or immediately after intake of radioiodine. The drug can still block 50 percent of radioiodine absorption if the first dose is administered within 4 hours after exposure. Potassium iodide (KI) is supplied in tablets of 130 mg and 650 mg and as a saturated solution (SSKI). The lower strength tablet and SSKI may be purchased over the counter (without prescription). A single tablet containing 130 mg of KI will provide a dose of 100 mg of iodine. The tablet should be dissolved in 4 ounces of water or fruit juice before ingestion to reduce gastric irritation. A dose of 100 mg of iodine is contained in 0.13 ml of SSKI.

Occasionally, one sees reference to Lugol's solution as an iodine supplement. This solution contains one sixth of the iodine in SSKI, and therefore a 100-mg iodine dose will be contained in 0.8 ml of Lugol's solution. These dosages can be summarized as follows:

100 mg of iodine is contained in:

1. One potassium iodide tablet (130 mg)
2. 0.8 ml of Lugol's solution
3. 0.13 ml of SSKI (about six drops, depending on dropper calibration)

The fraction of an administered dose of radioiodide excreted by the kidney is inversely related to thyroid function as shown in Table 8-5. This follows directly from the fact that renal clearance of iodide is a function of plasma iodide concentration. In the hyperthyroid state, the clearance of plasma iodide by the thyroid gland is thus significantly increased, leaving less for excretion by the kidney. The reverse is true in hypothyroidism.

Thyroid Uptake of Radioiodide

Measurement of thyroid function with radioiodide is predicated on the use of a

TABLE 8-5. CUMULATIVE URINARY EXCRETION OF RADIOIODIDE IN VARIOUS THYROID CONDITIONS

Condition	Percentage Excreted	
	24 hr	48 hr
Euthyroidism	60.3 (48.3–71.5)	66.6 (52.7–84.1)
Myxedema	64.2 (57.2–76.0)	83.1 (72.4–91.7)
Thyrotoxicosis	17.4 (5.5–30.8)	19.2 (6.2–32.3)
Thyroidectomy	>75	>95

(From Skanse B, 1948, p 251,[33] and Skanse B, 1949, pp 1–186.[34])

radiotracer that is physiologic, i.e., will not alter the normal function of the gland. The average daily dietary intake of iodide is 300 µg.[4] A 10-µCi diagnostic dose of I-131 is equivalent to 8×10^{-5} µg of iodine and represents only one one-millionth of the extrathyroidal iodide pool (80 µg I) and one eighty-millionth of total body iodine. Radioiodide will thus act as a true tracer of thyroid physiology. The largest radioiodide dose administered to a patient is 200 mCi for thyroid carcinoma and is equivalent to 1.6 µg of iodine but represents only 0.25 percent of the total body iodine (6500 µg). Consequently, radioiodide doses should not pose a threat to patients who have demonstrated hypersensitivity reactions to iodine.

The RAIU study is one of the oldest in vivo function studies performed in nuclear medicine. It is based upon the physiologic incorporation of radioiodine into the thyroid gland as a tracer of stable iodide. A measure of thyroid function can be determined by this study because the amount of administered radioactivity concentrated in the gland is directly related to gland function. The RAIU study is quite simple. A capsule containing 5 to 10 µCi of sodium iodide I-131 is administered to the patient by mouth. A period of time (usually 4 and 24 hours) after administration the radioactivity concentrated in the gland is measured by counting the activity over the neck region with a stationary scintillation detector. The percentage of the administered dose that is taken up by the gland is determined from the following equation:

$$\% \text{ Thyroid uptake} = \frac{\text{Net cpm in thyroid gland}}{\text{Net cpm in administered dose}} \times 100$$

The net counts per minute of the administered dose is determined by counting a mean standard capsule of sodium iodide I-131 from the same lot of capsules used for the patient dose. The method of selecting the standard capsule is illustrated in Figure 8-9. The standard capsule is counted in a Lucite container (thyroid phantom) that simulates the geometric configuration of the patient's neck. When the patient counts and standard counts are made on the same day, no decay correction is necessary.

The measurement of thyroid function with time after a radioiodide dose is a measure of the sum total of iodide trapping, hormone production, and release into the blood. The theoretic uptake of radioiodide

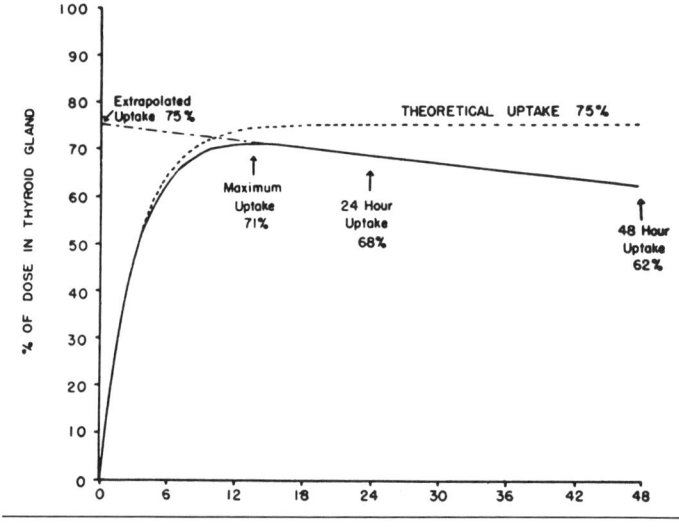

Figure 8-11. The relationship between various estimates of the uptake of radioactive iodine. The solid line represents the theoretic curve for the uptake and early decay of radioactive iodine in the thyroid gland after intravenous administration of a tracer dose at time 0 to a thyrotoxic subject. The broken line represents the manner in which radioactive iodine would accumulate were there no loss of labeled hormone from the gland. The line of long and short dashes represents an extrapolation of the decay curve to time 0. (From Riggs DS, 1952, p 284, with permission.[27])

TABLE 8-6. COMMON DRUGS AND CHEMICAL SUBSTANCES THAT DECREASE THE 24-HOUR THYROID UPTAKE OF I-131

Substance	Average Duration of Effect
Competing anions	
TcO_4^-, ClO_4^-, SCN^-	1 wk
Iodides	
SSKI, Lugol's solution	1-4 wk
Certain vitamin–mineral products (Micebrin and Unicap)	
Antitussive medicines (Organidin preparations, pima syrup)	
Topical iodide products	
Vioform, Betadine, Iodex, Isodine	1-9 mo
Iodine tincture	2 wk
X-ray contrast media	
Hypaque, Renografin	1-2 wk
Diodrast	1-3 mo
Lipiodol, Ethiodol (oily agents)	1 yr or more
Cholografin	3 mo
Telepaque	2 mo
Antithyroid drugs	
PTU, Methimazole (Tapazole)	2-8 d
Thyroid medication	
Thyroid hormone, thyroxine, Triiodothyronine	1-2 wk
Other drugs	
Phenylbutazone	1 wk
Meprobamate, morphine	Unknown
Sodium nitroprusside	Unknown
Sulfonamides	1 wk
Salicylates	Unknown
Adrenal and Gonadal Steroids	8 d
Adrenocorticotropic hormone	8 d

(From Magalotti MF, et al, 1959, p 47,[35] and Hladik WB III, et al, 1982, p 184.[36])

may be defined as the proportion of a tracer dose that would be accumulated by the thyroid at infinite time if there were no secretion of labeled hormone from the gland.[27] In the euthyroid state labeled hormone secretion begins 2 hours after dose administration so that at subsequent times the proportion of a tracer dose actually present in the gland is less than the theoretic value. This concept is illustrated in Figure 8–11. The ideal time for measurement of thyroid function in the uptake study would be the time of maximum tracer uptake, but this time is different in hypo-, hyper-, and euthyroid states.[27] It is thus routine practice to obtain early measurements at 4 hours to detect increased thyroid function and late measurements at 24 hours to detect normal and decreased function. The normal range for 24-hour thyroid uptake is between 5 and 35 percent. An accurate and reliable uptake determination is predicated on the following considerations: (1) a normal body iodide pool, (2) normal renal function, and (3) lack of interference from medications and other substances. Several exogenous factors may affect the RAIU. Most importantly is the presence of excessive stable plasma iodide from drugs or x-ray contrast material. Table 8–6 lists several agents that decrease uptake and the approximate duration of their effects on the 24-hour thyroid uptake study.[35]

Other Iodide-Concentrating Organs

Salivary Glands. A significant amount of iodide is secreted by the salivary glands, but most of this is eventually swallowed and reabsorbed again from the GI tract. However, expectoration of saliva containing radioiodide may inadvertently lead to clothing contamination as a source of scan artifact with patients undergoing total-body scans. Similar artifacts are more likely with urinary contamination, and therefore it is wise to use clean hospital gowns just before imaging. Concentration and secretion of iodide in salivary glands may produce a metallic taste in the mouth within a few hours after administration of a treatment dose of I-131.[37] After large therapeutic doses radiation sialadenitis may also occur, producing dry mouth and swelling and tenderness of the submaxillary glands.[37]

Gastric Glands. Radioiodide is highly concentrated in the gastric mucosa. Plasma clearance of iodide by the gastric glands is on the order of 25 ml per minute, and gastric juice-to-plasma ratios may be as high as 40.[38] This concentration is inhibited by stable iodide and by perchlorate, thus suggesting an active transport process also by the gastric cells. Studies have shown that iodide transport and concentration occur primarily with the mucoid cells rather than the chief cells or the parietal cells.[38] The significance of the gastric-concentrating mechanism is not known. Secretion of iodide into the gastric juice at high concentration increases the apparent iodide space of the body, but the iodide is normally rapidly reabsorbed after passing into the small intestine.[38]

Mammary Glands. Clearance of iodide by mammary glands may achieve milk-to-plasma ratios as high as 33:1.[32] The milk of a suspected thyrotoxic woman who discontinued breast feeding after a 29.5-μCi dose of sodium iodide I-131 was analyzed.[39] Inorganic iodide was the principal form present in milk, with small amounts in protein form. A total of 4.5 percent of the administered dose was excreted in 2 days.

Sweat. Some evidence of iodide excretion in sweat has been reported. In a rough iodine balance study in men who received milligram quantities of iodine while performing physically stressful work in a hot environment it was found that the sweat concentration of iodide was 35 percent of the plasma concentration and equaled 4 to 8 percent of the total iodide ingested.[40] Although normally active patients receiving therapeutic amounts of radioiodine may excrete significantly less than this amount in sweat, this route of excretion should not be ignored because it presents a potential source of contamination to clothing and objects handled by the patient.

Placental Transport of Iodide. Several studies reviewed by Brown-Grant[38] indicate that placental transport of iodide occurs and high fetal-to-maternal thyroid ratios are achieved in many instances near term. Human studies have also demonstrated that the human fetal thyroid has the ability to accumulate iodide I-131 by the 12th to 14th week of gestation.[41,42] Consequently, the use of radioiodine in pregnancy is contraindicated.

Biliary Excretion. Experimental studies in animals have demonstrated that thyroid hormone undergoes excretion as a glucuronide conjugate which is poorly absorbed back into the blood, although small amounts of hormone can be hydrolyzed in the cecum, thus enabling absorption of free hormone by the large intestine.[43,44] These amounts, however, are very small so that essentially all hormone excreted in the bile is eliminated in the feces.

In summary, radioiodide is widely distributed in the body within the first 24 hours after administration, with the majority of it excreted after 24 hours and the remainder mostly localized in the thyroid gland. The bodily distribution of radioiodide between 1 hour and 80 days is summarized in Figure 8–12.[45]

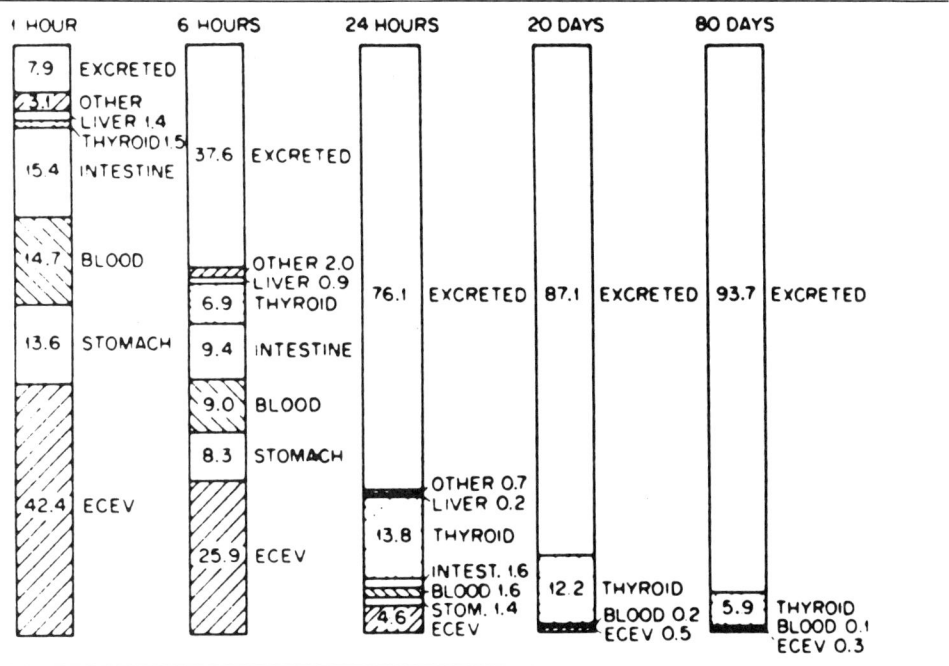

Figure 8-12. Estimated percentage of administered radioiodine in tissues of the body at various times after a single oral administration of radioiodide corrected for radioactive decay. The maximum thyroid uptake is assumed to be 15 percent. *(From MIRD Report No. 5, 1975, p 857, with permission.*[45]*)*

RADIATION DOSE FROM RADIOIODINES

The critical organ for radioiodine is the thyroid gland. The magnitude of the radiation dose to the gland and other body organs depends on the radionuclide administered and the uptake by the gland. The radiation dose estimates to various body organs from I-123, I-125, and I-131, assuming a 25 percent uptake by the thyroid, are provided in Table 8-7.

TABLE 8-7. RADIATION-ABSORBED DOSE FROM RADIOIODINES
(rad/mCi of Radioiodine Administered)

Target Organ	I-123	I-125	I-131
Thyroid	13.0	790.0	1300.0
Liver	0.027	0.36	0.48
Stomach wall	0.21	0.26	1.40
Red marrow	0.030	0.12	0.26
Ovaries	0.031	0.039	0.14
Testes	0.021	0.024	0.09

The values assume a 25 percent maximum uptake by the thyroid.
(Data from MIRD Report No. 5, 1975, p 857.[45]*)*

TABLE 8-8. RADIOPHARMACEUTICALS FOR THYROID IMAGING

Radiopharmaceutical	Administered Activity (μCi)	Route	Dose-to-Image Time	Thyroid Dose[a] (rad/μCi Administered)
Sodium iodide I-131	50–100	Oral	24 hr	1.30
Sodium iodide I-125	50–100	Oral	24 hr	0.79
Sodium iodide I-123	300	Oral	24 hr	0.013
Sodium pertechnetate-Tc99m	1000–5000	IV, SQ (oral)	20–30 min (1 hr)	0.0002

[a]Based upon a 25 percent thyroid uptake. I-123 dose does not include any contribution from I-125 or I-124 radiocontaminants present.[55]
(Data from MIRD Report No. 5, 1975, p 857.[45])

TC-99M-PERTECHNETATE FOR THYROID IMAGING

In the thyroid gland pertechnetate is not metabolized as is iodide, and its accumulation is limited to the ion-concentrating mechanism. It is trapped because the pertechnetate anion has a charge and ionic volume similar to iodide. The normal thyroid gland handles pertechnetate in the same manner that the PTU-blocked thyroid handles iodide, i.e., pertechnetate is discharged from the gland by perchlorate.[46] This is demonstrated in Figure 8-13. Uptake of pertechnetate by the thyroid gland is between 1 and 2 percent in euthyroid subjects but may be ten times greater in thyrotoxicosis.[46] Even though uptake in the normal gland is low, multimillicurie amounts may be administered because the radiation dose to the gland is only 0.2 rad/mCi. Pertechnetate is useful for thyroid imaging. The usual intravenous dose is 1 to 5 mCi, and imaging is performed between 20 and 30 minutes because maximal uptake is achieved by this time.[47] If necessary, subcutaneous rather than intravenous injection may be used with little effect on the time of maximum uptake.[47] Additionally, oral administration may be used with imaging done at 1 hour. Table 8-8 compares pertechnetate with the radioiodines for thyroid imaging.

More complete biologic data on Tc-99m pertechnetate can be found in Chapter 7.

Clinical Evaluation of the Thyroid Gland

INTRODUCTION

There are three activities that nuclear medicine personnel may be involved with in the care of patients with thyroid disease. They are the RAIU, the thyroid scan, and radioiodine therapy. These activities have been performed for nearly as long as nuclear medicine has been in existence and are considered relatively stable in their application.

RADIOACTIVE IODINE UPTAKE

Rationale
Radioactive iodine is the main substance used for measuring the biological turnover by the thyroid gland. The uptake test gives a direct measure of the thyroid's metabolism of the substance with which it may be treated therapeutically. The RAIU test is indicated for assessment of hypothyroidism, thyroiditis,

and hyperthyroidism. The latter is its most common indication. More specifically, it is used for calculating the dose in radioactive iodine therapy.

Procedure

It is best to perform the RAIU with the patient in a fasting state for at least 3 hours before administration of capsulated or liquid iodine to insure uninhibited absorption from the GI tract. The administration of antithyroid drugs such as PTU or methimazole (Tapazole) should have been stopped 4 days before the radioiodine uptake. Five to 10 µCi of I-131 (NaI) given orally is sufficient for an uptake test. The range provides good counting statistics while maintaining a very low radiation burden. The patient should be asked to avoid ingestion of food for 45 minutes after dosing. The uptake of iodine by the thyroid should be measured at approximately 4 and 24 hours after ingestion.

The *perchlorate washout test* is a variation on the RAIU wherein a nonradioactive substance is given to compete with the uptake of radioactive iodine by the thyroid. The reader will recall that several substances may be trapped by the thyroid and that these substances include iodine, Tc-99m pertechnetate, sodium or potassium perchlorate ($NaClO_4$ or $KClO_4$), and thiocyanate (SCN). Iodine, however, is the only one of this group that is normally metabolized by the thyroid, i.e., goes through a process called organification by which iodine molecules are incorporated into thyroid hormones. If the process for organification is intact within the thyroid gland, then the level of radioactive iodine contained by the patient's thyroid will not be changed after the administration of 1 g (adult dose) of sodium or potassium perchlorate, which competitively blocks further uptake, i.e., the uptake will remain fairly constant when measured by the probe. An abnormal response is indicated by a 20 percent or more fall in the amount of retained radioiodine 1 hour after the administration of sodium or potassium perchlorate (Fig. 8-13).

Pharmaceuticals

The isotope of choice for the RAIU is I-131 (NaI). I-123 may be used but is more expensive, may be contaminated with other iodine isotopes, and has a much shorter effective half-life. Tc-99m pertechnetate has been used in uptake tests for diagnostic purposes, primarily in an effort to make things more convenient for the patient since most of this testing has usually been done in conjunction with a thyroid scan with pertechnetate. The reader is referred to the section on scanning for what is considered a more practical test of thyroid functional activity with pertechnetate.

Interpretation

Normal individuals generally demonstrate one fourth to half of the 24-hour radioiodine uptake at the 4-hour time period. The 24-hour uptake in the United States varies from 5 to 35 percent. This range variation reflects the amount of iodine in the diet.

The RAIU is seldom ordered as the primary lab test for determining thyroid function because of the greater ease with which other thyroidal blood tests may be obtained. The most common indication for the RAIU is in the calculation of a therapeutic dose of radioiodine for the treatment of hyperthyroidism. The 24-hour uptake is the value generally used in calculating the therapy dose. Occasionally the 4-hour uptake will be considerably higher than the 24-hour uptake in hyperthyroid patients, indicating a more rapid than usual biologic turnover of iodine by the thyroid and the likely need for increasing the dose of I-131 to provide effective and timely treatment.

The uptake of radioiodine will be influenced by the prior administration of iodinated contrast materials to a varying degree depending on the pharmaceutical base and the location of the contrast material. The oily myelographic contrast materials have the greatest influence, extending for years. Bronchogram and biliary contrast agents may exert an influence for 6 months. Water-soluble intravenous con-

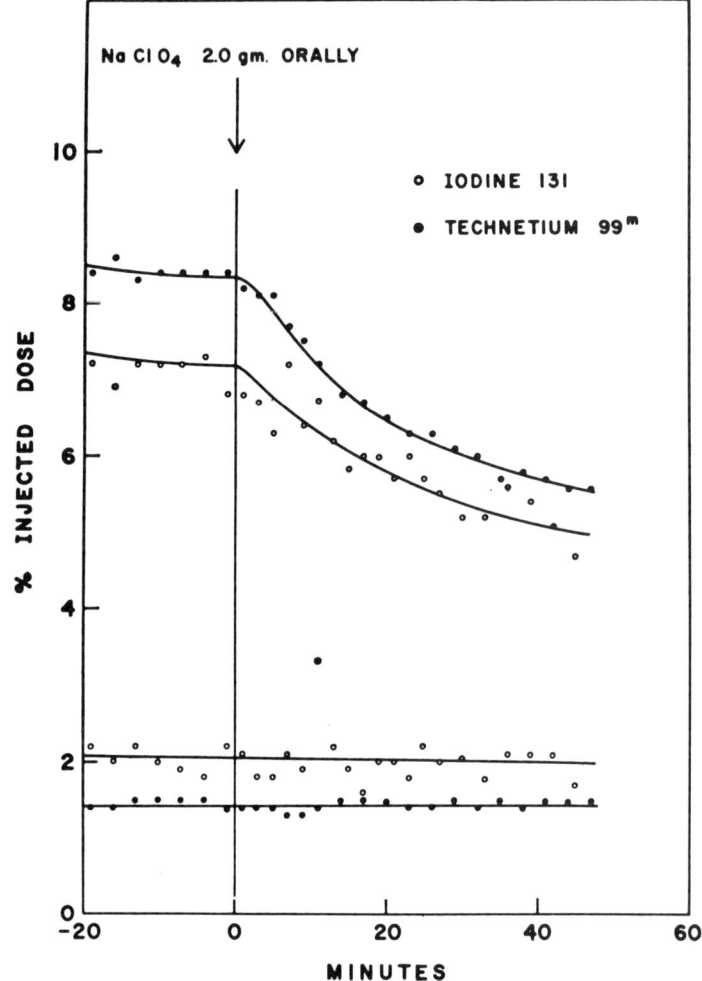

Figure 8-13. Discharge by NaClO$_4$ of iodide I-131 and pertechnetate-99m from the thyroid gland in a euthyroid subject. Methimazole (50 mg) was administered orally 60 minutes before intravenous iodide I-131 injection. Two grams of NaClO$_4$ was administered orally 1 hour after the isotope injection. The curves in the lower portion represent measurements over the thigh. *(From Andros G, et al, 1965, p 1072, with permission.[46])*

trast used for intravenous pyelography or computed tomographic studies will have an influence duration of 4 to 6 weeks. Lugol's iodine, SSKI, steroids, expectorants, vitamin preparations, and numerous other medications will effect the RAIU for several weeks. Administration of thyroid hormone will have an influence in normals for 1 to 3 weeks depending on the biologic half-life of the major ingredient. T_3 has a biologic half-life of 1 day, and T_4, 6 days. Thyroid hormone will not suppress the RAIU in patients with Graves' disease hyperthyroidism.

If the RAIU is being done in preparation for radioiodine therapy, then these waiting periods may be shortened because the purpose is not so much diagnostic as therapeutic. Abrupt cessation of antithyroid drugs may cause a rebound effect with elevation of the RAIU. Occasionally one will find a seemingly low or normal 24-hour RAIU in a patient who is obviously hyperthyroid. This occurrence should be a clue to ask again when the last dose of antithyroid drug was taken or to look for a toxic multinodular goiter, toxic adenoma, thyroiditis, or factitious hyperthyroidism.

The perchlorate washout test is used to

confirm disorders affecting the organification process, e.g., hereditary diseases of the thyroid, Hashimoto's thyroiditis, previous I-131 therapy, and early thyroid failure.

SCANNING

Rationale

Indications for thyroid scanning include the evaluation of palpable nodules, mediastinal masses (substernal goiter), hyperthyroidism, thyroglossal duct cysts, subglottic thyroid, hyperparathyroidism (displacement), and patients with a history of neck area irradiation. Total-body scanning with iodine is a procedure performed in patients who are being evaluated for metastatic thyroid cancer.

Procedures

Dynamic studies of the thyroid with Tc-99m pertechnetate have been used diagnostically to confirm hyperthyroidism. Normal thyroids are visualized on a dynamic study between 2.5 and 7.5 seconds after the appearance of the common carotids.[48] Hyperthyroids will be visualized earlier than this, hypothyroids later. The rectilinear thyroid scan offers an advantage over Anger type gamma camera imaging in that it is a method by which the image made is a one-to-one reproduction of the thyroid in size; however, not many rectilinear scanners are still being maintained. The rectilinear thyroid scan has been replaced with the pinhole collimated gamma camera image, which shows greater (functional) anatomic detail of the thyroid but gives no indication of size because of geometric considerations in using a pinhole collimated camera technique. The resolution of standard gamma cameras has improved to the point now where good anatomic detail may be obtained with a high-resolution, parallel-hole collimator, particularly in a situation where the operator can use electronic zooming. Whole-body scanning with iodine is most commonly performed with a large-field-of-view gamma camera or scanning table.

Whole-body imaging for thyroid cancer metastases must be done with the patient in a prolonged (6 weeks) hypothyroid state to induce iodine uptake in the metastases.[49]

Pharmaceuticals

Tc-99m pertechnetate is the agent of choice for thyroid scanning because it yields good detail of functional anatomy within 15 minutes of injection. A 1- to 5-mCi dose is sufficient for a good dynamic study and scan. When a patient is being evaluated for a superior mediastinal mass, iodine is the radiopharmaceutical of choice because of its affinity for the thyroid. In the past, I-131 was used in a 50- to 100-μCi amount given by mouth, with imaging at 24 hours. The photon flux with I-123, however, is higher and may yield better functional anatomic detail as well as lower radiation dose. A scanning dose with I-123 is 100 to 400 μCi given orally. One to 2 mCi of I-123 or I-131 is used for whole-body imaging. I-123 gives the best images at 24 hours, whereas I-131 may allow improved lesion detection with delayed imaging beyond 24 hours.

The second most common indication for using iodine to scan the thyroid is in the further investigation of a nonautonomous hypertrapping nodule seen on a pertechnetate scan or an isoconcentrating nodule on a normal pertechnetate scan. The iodine scan is done to assess the function of the nodule in the organification phase. Thallium-201 has been used for the evaluation of cold nodules seen on pertechnetate studies because it has been shown to be taken up by a high percentage of tumors, but it is also taken up in thyroiditis and parathyroid adenomas. The specificity of studies with pertechnetate and Tl-201 seems to be similar to that of studies combining pertechnetate thyroid scans and ultrasound.

Interpretation

Most thyroid scanning is done to assess the function of a *solitary nodule*. If the nodule is cold, it is presumed to be a cyst, a nonfunctioning adenoma, or a malignancy.

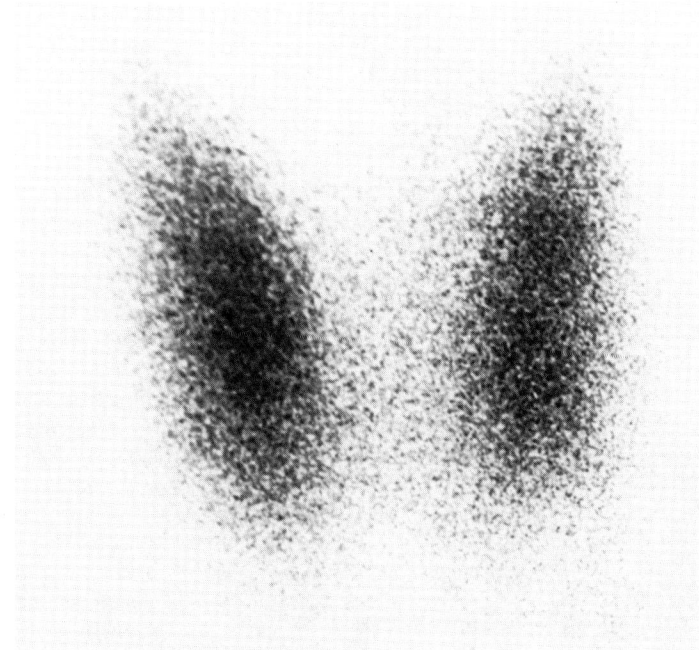

Figure 8-14. Normal anterior image of the thyroid gland in a 13-year-old male obtained 30 minutes after an injection of 7 mCi of Tc-99m sodium pertechnetate.

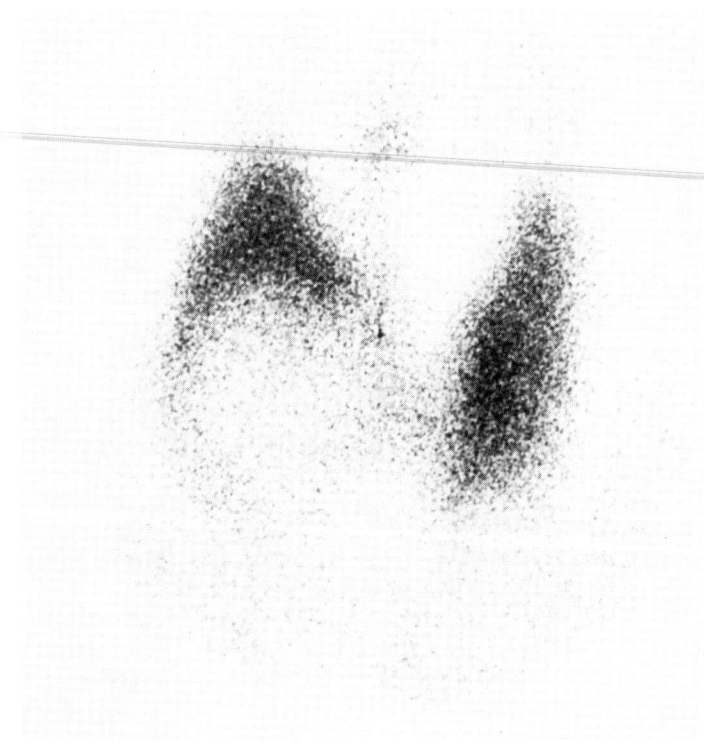

Figure 8-15. Cold nodule. Anterior image of the thyroid gland 30 minutes after an intravenous injection of Tc-99m sodium pertechnetate demonstrates a large photon-deficient area in the right lobe.

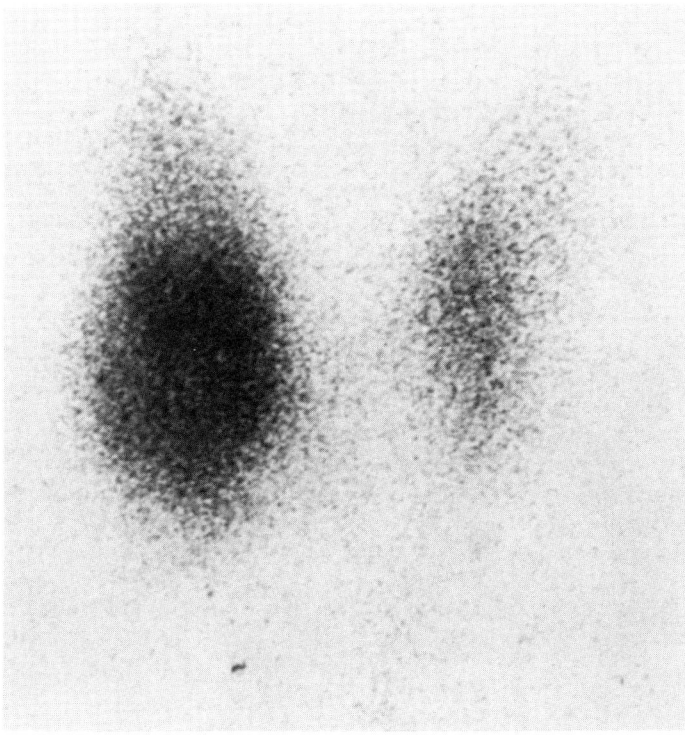

Figure 8-16. Hot nodule. Anterior image of the thyroid gland 30 minutes after an intravenous injection of Tc-99m sodium pertechnetate demonstrates a hyperfunctioning nodule in the right lobe.

Sometimes parathyroid adenomas may be seen indenting the surface of the normal thyroid gland. Cysts can be ruled out easily with ultrasound. A strong argument can be made for fine-needle aspiration of thyroid nodules as a combined or solitary procedure on the basis of cost-effectiveness, but the procedure is invasive and should be done by experienced personnel.[50] The incidence of malignancy in cold nodules is approximately 20 percent. Occasionally a solitary nodule in an otherwise normal thyroid will demonstrate normal or hypertrapping with Tc-99m pertechnetate. Three percent of these will be cold when examined in the organification phase of an iodine scan and may be malignant. Figure 8-14, 8-15, and 8-16 illustrate a normal thyroid gland, a cold nodule, and a hot nodule, respectively.

The incidence of malignancy in *multinodular goiter* is very low and scans are usually not indicated; however, patients with multinodular goiter will need thyroid scans to determine the function of nodules that the patient or physician has noticed recently or that are rock hard on palpation. The normally low incidence of malignancy is increased under these conditions.

As the thyroid gland migrates in embryonic life from the branchial cleft pouches 3 and 4, remnants may be left in the path that it follows. Sometimes these become symptomatic as bits of thyroid tissue in association with thyroglossal duct cysts, sometimes as pyramidal lobes, and rarely as a solitary subglossal thyroid. In all of these cases, the thyroid scan is useful in confirming or establishing the diagnosis.

RADIOIODINE THERAPY

Rationale
The major indications for radioiodine therapy now are the treatment of hyperthyroidism and eradication of metastatic disease from thyroid cancer. Forms of

hyperthyroidism that may be treated with radioiodine therapy are known as diffuse toxic goiter (Graves' disease), toxic multinodular goiter, and toxic adenoma.

Procedures

Graves' disease will be considered first (Fig. 8-17). The RAIU as well as the size of the thyroid and the desired result are used in calculating a therapeutic radioiodine dose. One method assumes that there will be at least 1.5 rad for every microcurie of I-131 delivered to the thyroid. The 24-hour uptake is used as an indicator of deliverable radioiodine, and the desirable dose range is from 7000 to 20,000 rad. The dosimetry also may be calculated using the 24-hour uptake for deliverable radioiodine and dividing by the estimated weight of the gland in grams. The desirable dose range is 40 to 240 μCi/g of thyroid using this method.

These dose ranges encompass what used to be known as the low and moderate therapeutic ranges. The lower end of the spectrum (1 to 8 mCi) was designed to render hyperthyroid patients euthyroid within 12 to 24 months. It became evident in follow-up that at least 50 percent of these patients were hypothyroid and needed thyroid hormone replacement therapy 10 years after being treated. Administration of thyroid hormone after radioiodine therapy is considered desirable by many thyroidologists to alleviate concern over the patient becoming gradually hypothyroid over the ensuing years and to suppress TSH stimulation of thyroid tissue that has been overactivated by the process of Graves' disease and damaged by radiation. Because of this many thyroidologists have advocated what can be categorized as a moderate dose range (9 to 29 mCi). This dose range is designed to

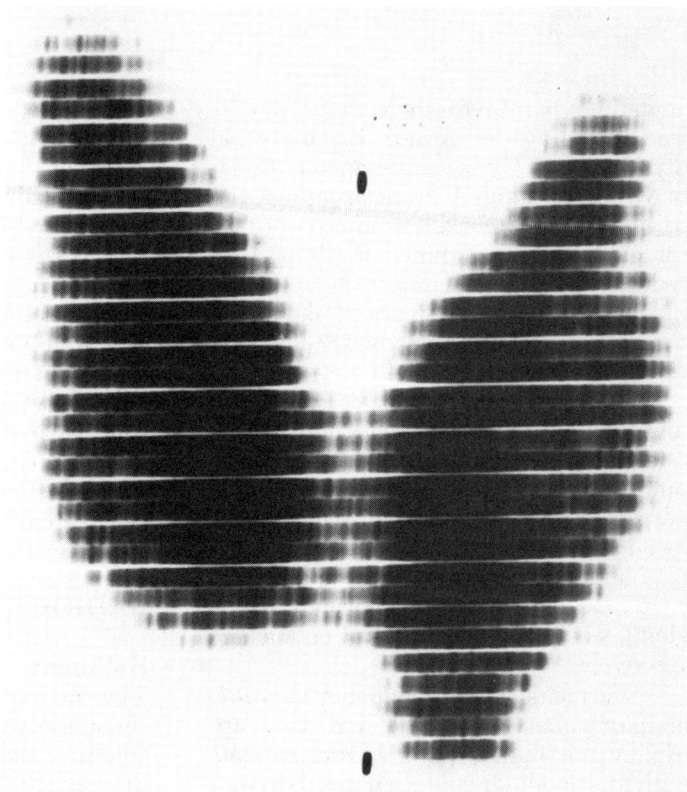

Figure 8-17. Graves' disease. Rectilinear scan of the thyroid gland after a 15-mCi injection of Tc-99m sodium pertechnetate. The scan reveals a greatly enlarged gland with diffuse uptake. The 24-hour RAIU with I-131 sodium iodide was 82 percent. The patient was subsequently treated with 10 mCi of I-131.

render the patient euthyroid or hypothyroid within 6 to 12 months. The latter group of patients will almost certainly need thyroid hormone replacement.

A single dose of radioiodine will satisfactorily treat 95 percent of patients. A small subgroup of patients who have higher RAIUs at 4 hours than at 24 hours or whose 24-hour value is less than 40 percent or greater than 70 percent seem to have a higher incidence of failure with single-dose radioiodine therapy, and for this reason these patients are often given a slightly boosted dose in an attempt to avert a more frequent need for a second treatment.

The second most commonly occurring form of hyperthyroidism for which radioiodine is used therapeutically is the toxic multinodular goiter (Plummer's disease) (Fig. 8–18). Plummer's disease patients often present with slightly elevated or normal-range iodine uptakes. The thyroid scan will reveal multiple autonomously functioning thyroid nodules, with dormant gland between nodules. These patients require two to three times the Graves' disease patient dose of radioiodine, and even with this dose usually wind up in a euthyroid state.

A less common indication for radioiodine therapy is the hyperthyroid patient with a toxic adenoma. Most of those under 40 are treated with surgery, with I-131 being reserved for the older age group.[51] In the under-40 group there is concern about the extranodular thyroid tissue and the possibility that a subtherapeutic radiation dose to it will be carcinogenic. Some nuclear medicine physicians have advocated stimulation of the suppressed normal thyroid tissue before administering a therapeutic dose of I-131 to alleviate this concern.

The administration of antithyroid drugs such as PTU or methimazole should be stopped 4 days before the RAIU and may be restarted on the fifth day after treatment with radioiodine without interfering with the effect of the radioiodine therapy.

The treatment of thyroid cancer of the

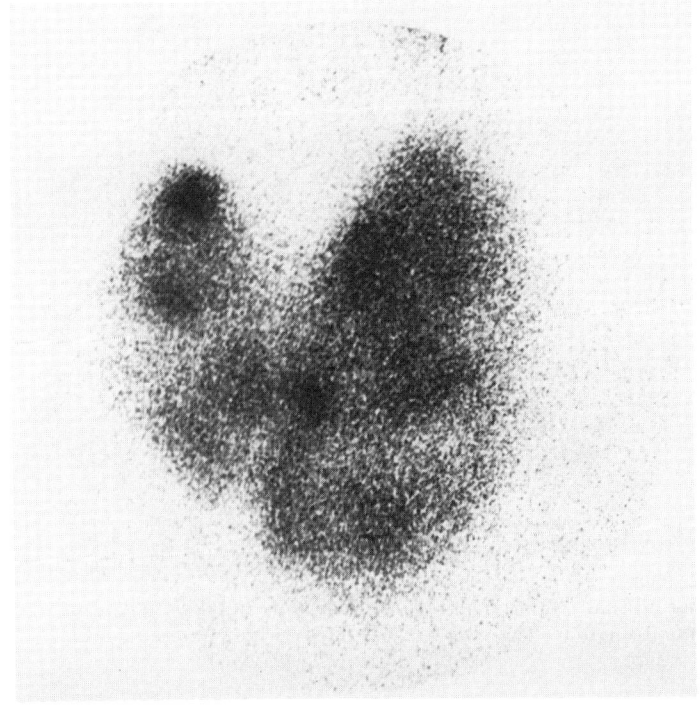

Figure 8-18. Plummer's disease. Anterior image of a multinodular goiter obtained after Tc-99m sodium pertechnetate administration.

papillary or follicular cell types is very effective and should give the patient a normal longevity if the right surgical procedure is performed initially.[52] It is important that the patient with papillary or follicular thyroid cancer have a total or near total (not subtotal) thyroidectomy when the cancer is discovered.[53] This type of operation often requires reimplantation of minced parathyroid glands in the pectoral muscles to prevent hypoparathyroidism postoperatively. Postoperatively the patient is allowed to become hypothyroid for 6 weeks. Hypothyroidism should be confirmed by checking the TSH level at 5 weeks. An adequate level of hypothyroidism will be achieved if the TSH level is ten times the upper limits of normal for the laboratory. At 6 weeks a total-body iodine scan is performed 24 hours after ingestion of I-123 or I-131 (Fig. 8-19). Any treatable evidence of metastatic disease should be manifest as iodine uptake in the metastasis. Iodine concentration in the thyroid bed warrants imaging with the neck hyper- and normally extended to determine mobility of the areas of concentration and should promote a rediscussion with the surgeon about the amount and location of residual thyroid tissue. Iodine concentration in metastases or a reasonable suspicion that concentration in the thyroid bed region may be due to metastatic disease is indication for admission of the patient to a radiation isolation room while surgically hypothyroid and

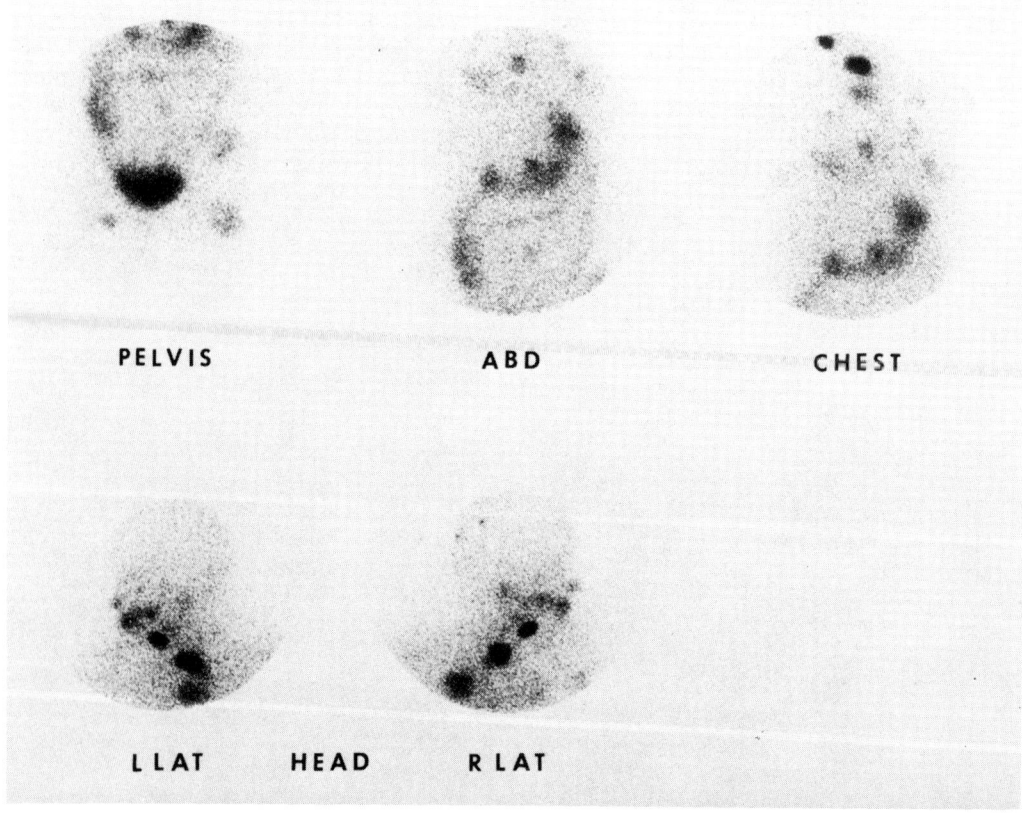

Figure 8-19. Total-body thyroid scan. Multiple areas of radioiodine uptake evident in metastatic thyroid carcinoma (follicular). The scan was obtained 24 hours after a 2-mCi oral dose of I-123 sodium iodide.

administration of 150 to 200 mCi of I-131 (NaI). Adjunctive ablation of thyroid remnants in the neck warrants a 100- to 150-mCi dose.[49] After this, when the retained body level of I-131 has dropped below 30 mCi, the patient may be discharged, and thyroid hormone replacement therapy may be started. Effectiveness of the therapy is usually checked 1 year later with a total-body iodine scan done under the same hypothyroid conditions.

Performing the total-body scan in a patient who is not in a profoundly hypothyroid state after subtotal thyroidectomy is ineffective in demonstrating iodine uptake in metastases. The administration of bovine TSH by which the patient is pulsed with a foreign biologic compound of questionable biologic activity is not nearly as effective as several weeks of endogenous TSH stimulation of the metastases. The patient whose TSH fails to reach profoundly hypothyroid levels may warrant a thyroid scan with pertechnetate to ascertain the amount of remaining tissue. A second thyroidectomy procedure is often necessary in this situation. Treatment of subtotal thyroidectomy remnants with less than 100-mCi doses of I-131 causes a delay in treatment of the metastatic disease, and there is concern that the metastatic lesions may acquire some degree of radiation resistance because the non–iodine-concentrating cells in the metastases may not be destroyed along with the iodine-concentrating cells.

Occasionally, patients are seen whose metastases produce enough thyroid-like hormones to prevent their attaining a severely hypothyroid state. If this is suspected, it is worthwhile doing a pertechnetate thyroid scan to rule out inadequate thyroid surgery. If surgery appears to be adequate, a total-body iodine scan is performed to document uptake in the metastases, and the patient is then treated with a cancer therapeutic dose of radio-iodine.

Pharmaceutical
The agent of choice is I-131 because of its particulate radiation.

Interpretation
There seems to be a paradox in the way a thyroid cancer appears to have no pertechnetate or iodine concentration on the thyroid scan, and yet, under proper conditions, the papillary and follicular forms of metastases can be shown to concentrate iodine on a total-body scan. The nonfunctioning appearance of a nodule on the thyroid scan may be due to a relatively great degree of difference in function between the normal and the neoplastic tissues.[54] Also, the metastases from papillary or follicular thyroid carcinoma most likely function quite differently under steady, intense TSH stimulation while the patient is hypothyroid.

Safety Considerations in Radioiodine Therapy
Patients who receive I-131 therapy require attention to special precautionary measures to keep contamination and exposure levels to hospital personnel and the general public as low as reasonably achievable.

Patients who receive less than 30 mCi of I-131 may be dosed in the nuclear medicine hot lab, detained for 30 minutes for precautionary observation, and released. Patients who receive greater than 30 mCi of I-131 must be hospitalized and dosed in their rooms. A private room with a private toilet is required. A patient who receives less than 30 mCi but is hospitalized will require a private room and toilet only if treated with greater than 8 mCi of I-131. The NCRP Report No. 37, Table 2, indicates that an 8-mCi dose will deliver a total integrated exposure of 0.5 rem at 1 m during complete decay. This exposure is considered safe for the general public.

Surfaces in the private room must be covered to minimize contamination. Floor walkways between the patient's bed and toilet facilities should be covered with plastic-backed absorbant paper with the absorbant side facing up. Objects handled by the patient such as telephones should be covered with plastic bags and secured with tape.

Disposable utensils, plates, and cups

must be used. A plastic bag–lined waste container must be available to receive all potentially contaminated articles. A sign must be posted on the room entrance indicating that the patient is undergoing radiation treatment.

After dosing with I-131 the room must be surveyed at the patient's bedside, 3 feet away, and at the room entrance. The radiation safety officer will then determine how long a person may remain at these positions and will post these times in the patient's chart and on the door. According to 10 CFR 20.105, nursing attendants should not be exposed to more than 100 mrem per 50-hour workweek nor more than 2 mR in any one hour. For example, if the patient is emitting 2 mR/hr at 3 feet, a nurse may work at this distance for 50 hours. If the dose rate is higher, say 20 mR/hr, the total contact time must be limited to 5 hours per workweek, but not more than 6 minutes in every one hour according to the following calculations:

$$20 \text{ mR}/60 \text{ min} = 2 \text{ mR}/x \text{ min}$$

$$x = 6 \text{ min}$$

For adjacent areas, for instance, patients in the next room, the dose rate should not exceed 0.6 mR/hr because adjacent patients may be exposed continuously for 7 consecutive days (168 hours), and this dose rate is required to keep the total weekly exposure at 100 mrem, i.e., 100 mrem/168 hr = 0.6 mR/hr.

Film badges may be worn by nursing attendants who care for patients treated with large amounts of I-131. Instructions to nurses caring for the patient must be posted on the patient's chart. The radiation safety officer should review procedures with nurses and explain the necessary precautions and the time of exposure allowed at various distances.

Visitors may be allowed but should be 18 years or older and must be instructed regarding the time of exposure. No pregnant visitors or nurses are allowed to be in the patient's room at any time.

Patient attendants are to wear disposable gloves that are to be washed before removing and discarded into the designated waste container. Hands should be washed thoroughly with soap and water after removing the gloves.

All clothing, linens, surgical dressings, and disposable items should be placed into the waste container provided. A plastic bag may be used to contain all nondisposable items.

All items must be surveyed and cleared by the radiation safety officer before they are removed from the room.

The patient must remain confined to the room and instructed to use toilet facilities with care, taking precautions to flush toilets several times and to wash hands diligently. The patient must remain hospitalized until the I-131 activity has decreased to 30 mCi. The majority of the administered dose will be excreted by 24 hours. The recommended technique for determining when a patient may be released is as follows:

1. Measure the patient with a Geiger–Müller survey meter 1 hour after dosing at a distance approximating a point source.
2. Note the meter reading and distance.
3. Release the patient when the meter reading falls to a level consistent with 30 mCi at the same distance.

Example:

Patient dosed with 100 mCi I-131 gives a survey meter reading of 6.7 mR/hr at 6 feet. What will be the meter reading when 30 mCi is present?

Solution:

30 mCi/100 mCi × 6.7 mR/hr = 2 mR/hr

Once the patient is released, the room is cleaned and decontaminated if necessary before release for use by another patient.

REFERENCES

1. Guyton AC: Textbook of Medical Physiology, 6th ed. Philadelphia, Saunders, 1981, p 931

2. DeGroot LJ: Current views on formation of thyroid hormones. N Engl J Med 272:243, 297, 355, 1965
3. Hoffer PB, Gottschalk A, Quinn J III: Thyroid in vivo studies. In Gottschalk A, Potchen EJ (eds): Diagnostic Nuclear Medicine. Baltimore, Williams & Wilkins, 1976, p 255
4. Rapoport B, DeGroot LJ: Current concepts of thyroid physiology. Semin Nucl Med 1:265, 1971
5. Wyngaarden JB, Wright BM, Ways P: The effect of certain anions upon the accumulation and retention of iodide by the thyroid gland. Endocrinology 50:537, 1952
6. Brucer M: The genesis of thyroid-iodine. In Vignettes in Nuclear Medicine, No. 90. St Louis, Mallinckrodt, 1978
7. Hertz S, Roberts A, Evans RD: Radioactive iodine as an indicator in the study of thyroid physiology. Proc Soc Exp Biol Med 38:510, 1938
8. Tape GF, Cork JM: Induced radioactivity in tellurium. Phys Rev 53:676, 1938
9. Livingood JJ, Seaborg GT: Radioactive isotopes of iodine. Phys Rev 54:775, 1938
10. Hamilton JG, Soley MH: Studies in iodine metabolism by use of a new radioactive isotope of iodine. Am J Physiol 127:557, 1939
11. Keston AS, Ball RP, Frantz VK: Storage of radioactive iodine in a metastasis from thyroid carcinoma. Science 95:362, 1942
12. Seidlin SM, Marinelli LD, Oshry E: Radioactive iodine therapy—Effect on functioning metastasis of adenocarcinoma of the thyroid. JAMA 132:838, 1946
13. Hertz S, Roberts A: Application of radioactive iodine in therapy of Graves' disease. J Clin Invest 21:624, 1942
14. Reid AF, Keston AS: Long-life radioiodine. Phys Rev 70:987, 1946
15. Harper PV, Siemans WD, Lathrop KA, et al: Production and use of iodine-125. J Nucl Med 4:277, 1963
16. Myers WG: Radioisotopes of iodine. In Andrews GA, Kniseley RM, Wagner HN Jr (eds): Radioactive Pharmaceuticals. Oak Ridge, Tenn, USAEC Symposium 6, 1966, p 217
17. Baker GA, Lum DJ, Smith EM, et al: Significance of radiocontaminants in I-123 for dosimetry and scintillation camera imaging. J Nucl Med 17:740, 1976
18. Wolfangel RL: Accumulation of radioiodine in staff members: Reply—letter to the editor. J Nucl Med 20:995, 1979
19. Howard BY: Safe handling of radioiodinated solutions. J Nucl Med Tech 4:28, 1976
20. Miller KL, Bott SM, Velkley DE, et al: Review of contamination and exposure hazards associated with therapeutic doses of radioiodine. J Nucl Med Tech 7:163, 1979
21. Pollock RW, Myser RD: Concentration of I-131 in the air during thyroid therapies. Health Phys 36:68, 1979
22. Rubin LM, Miller KL, Schadt WW: A solution to the radioiodine volatilization problem. Health Phys 32:307, 1977
23. Burgess JS, Partington EJ: Radiation decomposition effects in aqueous solutions of carrier-free sodium iodide I-131. Publication RCC/R98, The Radiochemical Center, Amersham, Bucks, England, March 1960
24. Shubnyakova LP, Kharlamov VT, Pikaev AK: Radiolysis of dilute aqueous solutions of Na^{131}I. Khimiya Vysokikh Energii 10:41, 1976
25. Maguire WJ: A precaution for minimizing radiation exposure from iodine vaporization. J Nucl Med Tech 8:90, 1980
26. Haney TA, Wedeking P, Morcos N, et al: A therapeutic and diagnostic I-131 capsule formulation with minimal volatility and maximal bioavailability. J Nucl Med 22:P74, 1981
27. Riggs DS: Quantitative aspects of iodine metabolism in man. Pharmacol Rev 4:284, 1952
28. Keating FR Jr, Albert A: The metabolism of iodine in man as disclosed with the use of radioiodine. Recent Prog Horm Res 4:429, 1948
29. Childs DS Jr, Keating FR Jr, Rall JE, et al: The effect of varying quantities of inorganic iodide (carrier) on the urinary excretion and thyroidal accumulation of radioiodine in exophthalmic goiter. J Clin Invest 29:726, 1950
30. Myant NB, Pochin EE, Goldie EAG: The plasma iodide clearance rate of the human thyroid. Clin Sci 8:109, 1949
31. Berson SA, Yallow RS, Sorrentino J, et al: The determination of thyroidal and renal plasma I-131 clearance rates as a routine diagnostic test of thyroid dysfunction. J Clin Invest 31:141, 1952
32. Honour AJ, Myant NB, Rowlands EN: Secretion of radioiodide in digestive juices and milk in man. Clin Sci 11:447, 1952
33. Skanse B: Radioactive iodine: Its use in

studying the urinary excretion of iodine by humans in various states of thyroid function. Acta Med Scand 131:251, 1948
34. Skanse B: Radioactive iodine in the diagnosis of thyroid disease. Acta Med Scand 136 (Suppl 235): 1–186, 1949
35. Magalotti MF, Hummon IF, Hierschbiel E: The effect of disease and drugs on the twenty-four hour I-131 thyroid uptake. Am J Roentgen 81:47, 1959
36. Hladik WB III, Nigg KK, Rhodes BA: Drug-induced changes in the biologic distribution of radiopharmaceuticals. Semin Nucl Med 12:184, 1982
37. Beierwaltes WH, Wagner HW Jr: Therapy of thyroid disease with radioiodine. In Wagner HN Jr (ed): Principles of Nuclear Medicine. Philadelphia, Saunders, 1968, 343
38. Brown-Grant K: Extrathyroidal iodide concentrating mechanisms. Physiol Rev 41:189, 1961
39. Miller H, Weetch RS: The excretion of radioactive iodine in human milk. Lancet 269:1013, 1955
40. Nelson N, Palmes ED, Park CR, et al: The absorption, excretion and physiological effect of iodine in normal human subjects. J Clin Invest 26:301, 1947
41. Chapman EM, Corner GW, Robinson D, et al: The collection of radioactive iodine by the human fetal thyroid. J Clin Endocrinol 8:717, 1948
42. Hodges RE, Evans TC, Brudbury JT, et al: The accumulation of radioiodine by human fetal thyroids. J Clin Endocrinol 15:661, 1955
43. Cottle WH: Biliary and fecal clearance of endogenous thyroid hormone in cold-acclimated rats. Am J Physiol 207:1063, 1964
44. Cottle WH, Veress AT: Absorption of glucuronide conjugate of triiodothyronine. Endocrinology 88:522, 1971
45. MIRD Report No. 5: Summary of current radiation dose estimates to humans from I-123, I-124, I-125, I-126, I-130, I-131 and I-132 as sodium iodide. J Nucl Med 16:857, 1975
46. Andros G, Harper PV, Lathrop KA, et al: Pertechnetate-99m localization in man with applications to thyroid scanning and the study of thyroid physiology. J Clin Endocrinol 25:1067, 1965
47. Atkins HL: The thyroid. In Freeman LM, Johnson PM (eds): Clinical Scintillation Imaging, 3rd ed. New York, Grune & Stratton, 1975, p 671
48. Ashkar FS: Thyroid imaging and function studies. Clin Nucl Med 6 (Suppl 10S): p 77, 1981
49. Beierwaltes WH, Rabbani R, Dmuchowski C, et al: An analysis of "Ablation of Thyroid Remnants" with I-131 in 511 patients from 1947–1984: Experience at University of Michigan. J Nucl Med 25:1287, 1984
50. Van Herle AJ, et al: The thyroid nodule–UCLA conference. Ann Intern Med 96:221, 1982
51. Hamburger JI: Management of Thyroid Patients. Southfield, Mich, Hamburger, pub, 1985, Vol 1, p 112
52. Beierwaltes WH: The treatment of thyroid carcinoma with radioiodine. Semin Nucl Med 8:79, 1978
53. Maxon HR, Thomas SR, Chen I: The role of nuclear medicine in the treatment of hyperthyroidism and well-differentiated thyroid adenocarcinoma. Clin Nucl Med 6 (Suppl 10S): p 87, 1981
54. Wolfman SH: Analysis of radioiodine therapy of metastatic tumors of the thyroid gland in man. J Nat Cancer Inst 13:815, 1953
55. Ziessman HA, Fahey FH, Gochoco JM: Impact of radiocontaminants in commercially available iodine-123: Dosimetric evaluation. J Nucl Med 27:428, 1986

CHAPTER 9

Heart

Radiopharmaceuticals routinely used to evaluate heart disease fall into two main categories: (1) myocardial imaging agents that localize within the heart muscle and that may be further subdivided into "cold spot" markers and "hot spot" markers, and (2) blood pool imaging agents that are used to evaluate dynamic function of the heart and include radiolabeled proteins and red blood cells.

MYOCARDIAL IMAGING AGENTS: PHYSIOLOGIC ASPECTS

The rationale for using myocardial imaging agents to detect ischemia and infarction is based on several pathophysiologic processes. Ischemic heart disease results from heart muscle oxygen deprivation secondary to insufficient regional blood perfusion.[1] In such instances the ischemia induces altered ion transport across the myocardial cell membrane. Under normal circumstances the "Na-K-ATPase pump" maintains a high extracellular Na$^+$ concentration and a high intracellular K$^+$ concentration, thus regulating cell volume. The normal exchange is two K$^+$ in and three Na$^+$ out for each molecule of adenosine triphosphate (ATP) hydrolyzed. During ischemia it is believed that the energy available for the pump is decreased so that Na$^+$ along with Cl$^-$ and H$_2$O accumulate within the cell and K$^+$ leaks out into the extracellular space. This process decreases the intracellular–extracellular K$^+$ concentration ratio and produces a marked effect on membrane polarity and heart muscle function.

The ischemic damage to the myocardial cell membrane also produces an imbalance in the intracellular/extracellular Ca^{2+} concentration. Under normal circumstances the calcium ion concentration intracellularly is about 10^{-7} M, whereas in extracellular fluid it is about 10^{-3} M. Studies in dogs have demonstrated that, after experimentally induced infarcts, calcification occurs within the injured cells.[2] The intracellular substances have the appearance of amorphous and spicular-like material that appear in mitochondrial inclusions and are primarily located in cells at the periphery of myocardial infarcts. The spicular material contains calcium and phosphorus and is believed to be an apatite-like crystal. The key factor that appears to be responsible for the intracellular concentration of calcified material is sufficient blood perfusion after the ischemic event, which allows delivery of serum calcium to damaged myocardial cells. This fact also explains why the calcified material appears to be localized in the peripheries of the infarcts rather than in the centers that have poor blood supply.

COLD SPOT MARKERS

Cold spot markers are agents that demonstrate decreased or no uptake of radioactivity in diseased myocardium and thus appear as "cold" areas outlined by radioactive or "hot" normal muscle. Several radioisotopes of potassium and its monovalent cation analogues have been investigated for myocardial perfusion studies.[3] Table 9–1 compares the properties of these agents. Potassium-43 was used early on but had the disadvantages of beta particle decay and an abundant high-energy photopeak at 619 keV that degraded image resolution. Of the potassium analogues, cesium-129 was not ideal because of slow blood clearance and poor myocardial extraction efficiency. Rubidium-81 had good blood clearance and myocardial extraction but, as a positron emitter with a short physical half-life, presented technical and logistic problems for most nuclear medicine laboratories. Thallium-201 has achieved greater clinical acceptance because it has rapid blood clearance, high myocardial extraction efficiency, and a reasonable shelf life. A more detailed discussion of Tl-201 will follow.

Production of Thallous Chloride Tl-201

Tl-201 is produced by bombarding a target of pure natural thallium metal with 31-MeV protons in a cyclotron.[4] The nuclear reaction is

$$^{203}Tl(p,3n)^{201}Pb \xrightarrow{9.4 \text{ hr}} {}^{201}Tl$$

After irradiation, the target is dissolved in mineral acid and the Pb-201 separated by ion-exchange chromatography. The Pb-201 is then allowed to decay to Tl-201. The Tl-201 is isolated by ion-exchange chromatography and the chloride salt is formed by dissolution in HCl and evaporation to dryness. The TlCl is dissolved in NaOH, adjusted to pH 7, sterilized, and tested to detect any carrier thallium present. Additionally, radiochromatography is performed to differentiate Tl^+ and Tl^{3+}. Radiochemical purity is not less than 95 percent. Gamma spectroscopy is used to identify radionuclidic impurities, mainly Tl 200 and

TABLE 9-1. PROPERTIES OF MONOVALENT CATION RADIONUCLIDES FOR MYOCARDIAL IMAGING

			Photon				Myocardial			
Radio-nuclide	Decay Mode	$T_{1/2}$ (hr)	Energy (keV)	Abundance (%)	Ionic Radius (Å)	Blood Clearance $T_{1/2}$ (min)	Extraction Efficiency (%)	Uptake (% of Dose)	Uptake Plateau (min)	Clearance $T_{1/2}$ (hr)
K-43	B^-	22.4	373, 619	85, 81	1.38	2.0	71	2–3	10–20	1
Cs-129	EC	32.1	375, 412	48, 22	1.70	9.0	22	1–2	60–120	5
Rb-81	EC, B^+	4.7	511, 190	26, 65	1.49	2.2	70	2–3	15–45	6
T1-201	EC	74.0	69, 80, 135, 167	95, 13	1.50	2.9	88	4–5	5–15	4.4

(Data from Chervu LR, 1979, p 241.[3])

Tl-202, which are usually less than 1 percent at calibration time. The US Pharmacopeia (USP) XXI states that not more than 2 percent Tl-200, 0.3 percent Pb-203, and 2.7 percent Tl-202 are present.

Tl-201 is supplied as a sterile nonpyrogenic solution for intravenous administration. It is available in a concentration of 1 mCi/ml in various activity sizes. It is made isotonic with sodium chloride and may contain benzyl alcohol as a preservative. The pH is between 4.5 and 7.5.

Physical and Biologic Properties of the Tl-201 Ion

Tl-201 decays by electron capture to stable Hg-201. It has a physical half-life of 73.1 hours. It emits gamma photons of 135 keV (2.65 percent) and 167 keV (10 percent) and Hg-201 x-rays of 68 to 80.3 keV (94.5 percent), all of which can be used for imaging. The specific gamma ray constant for Tl-201 is 4.7 R/mCi-hr at 1 cm. The half-value layer in lead is 0.0006 cm.

After intravenous (IV) administration in humans Tl-201 disappears rapidly from the blood.[5,6] In the resting stage, 90 percent of the plasma activity disappears by 20 minutes, but under stress the same percentage of activity disappears by 90 seconds. The maximum myocardial uptake occurs in 10 to 30 minutes in the resting state and at 5 minutes after exercise stress. This results in reduced background activity from the heart blood pool and a high target-to-nontarget ratio for imaging. The heart activity of Tl-201 is sustained long enough ($T_{1/2} \simeq 4$ to 7 hours) after exercise stress so that imaging can be performed. Ideally, however, it should be started and completed by 30 minutes after injection because only early after administration does regional myocardial distribution of Tl-201 reflect closely the distribution of myocardial blood flow at the time of injection. Total body elimination is slow, with a biologic half-time of 10 days. Only a small amount ($\simeq 5$ percent) is excreted in the urine by 24 hours, and insignificant fecal excretion occurs. These factors plus the long physical half-life are undesirable properties of Tl-201 from the viewpoint of multiple studies in the same patient. Kidney activity is localized primarily in the medulla. The kidneys are the critical organ, receiving 3 rad per 2-mCi dose. The remainder of Tl-201 activity is distributed throughout the body, with some concentration noted in the intestines and thyroid.

Mechanism of Localization of Tl-201 in the Heart

Tl-201, radioactive potassium, and its other analogues can be used to qualitatively assess the ischemic process in the myocardium that produces the intracellular–extracellular K^+ concentration imbalance. Some of the factors cited for the similarity of action between K^+ and its analogues include monovalent cationic charge, similarly sized hydrated ionic radii, and participation in the membrane-bound Na-K-ATPase pump.[6] Indeed, Tl^+ is known to activate Na-K-ATPase and is more firmly bound to the enzyme than K^+.[7] The thallium ion follows K^+ movement in tissue but is mobilized at a slower rate, suggesting that once it is taken up by cells the intracellular binding of Tl^+ is greater than that of K^+.[6]

There is a close relationship between Tl^+ deposition in the myocardium and myocardial blood flow. Blood flow alone, however, is not sufficient for Tl^+ uptake into myocardial cells. Adequate tissue oxygenation to support metabolism of the membrane-concentrating mechanism is required.[6] This has been demonstrated by experiments in dogs whereby myocardium perfused by venous blood demonstrated a perfusion deficit, i.e., decreased Tl-201 uptake compared with zones perfused with arterial blood. Reperfusion of the abnormal region with arterial blood restored normal Tl-201 uptake.

Thallium distribution in the myocardium is dependent on the extent of disease present (i.e., cell viability) and the level of regional blood flow. When Tl-201 is administered to a patient at rest, the myocardial cells will accumulate Tl-201 activity and appear "hot" because blood flow is adequate and Tl^+ follows K^+ into the cell. Infarcted muscle, however, will appear "cold" because of a lack of viable muscle cells. If the heart is put under stress through exercise and Tl-201 is administered, any ischemic areas produced by stress will show a decreased accumulation of Tl-201 and appear "cold" compared with normal myocardium. This is because of the disproportionate blood flow between ischemic and normal tissue after exercise. After a restful period, however, the stress-induced ischemic areas will become "hot" because of the Tl$^+$ redistribution from the blood pool into the ischemic cells. Areas that remain "cold" after rest indicate infarction because these areas are lacking in viable muscle cells and redistribution of K$^+$ and Tl$^+$ cannot occur.

HOT SPOT MARKERS

Hot spot markers are agents that demonstrate an increased concentration of activity within infarcted myocardium and appear as radioactive or "hot" areas outlined by nonradioactive or "cold" normal muscle. They are also called *infarct avid agents*.

Several agents have been studied in animal models to determine uptake in experimentally produced infarcts.[3] Table 9-2 compares some of these agents. In addition to animal studies, technetium-99m-labeled tetracycline, glucoheptonate, and pyrophosphate have also been used to detect acute myocardial infarcts in humans. Tc-99m tetracycline has slow blood clearance and requires 24 hours after intravenous administration for effective detection of the infarct, which limits its clinical utility and markedly reduces the photon flux available at the time of imaging.[8] It localizes only in irreversibly damaged infarcts, as opposed to Tc-99m phosphates, which may also localize in ischemic areas. Liver uptake is significant and may interfere with the detection of inferior wall infarcts. Tc-99m glucoheptonate gives poor target-to-background ratios and a low detection rate for acute infarcts but may be seen concentrating earlier after the infarct than Tc-99m tetracycline or pyrophosphate. Tc-99m pyrophosphate (Tc-99m PPi) has the disadvantage of bone uptake in the ribs overlying the heart, which may limit its utility in the estimation of infarct size, although clinically this has been used to grade infarct uptake in comparison with bone uptake and to help localize the infarct. The Tc-99m phosphates and phosphonates as a group have demonstrated uptake also in ischemic tissue, which may limit their specificity in the diagnosis of myocardial infarction. The high infarct-to-normal myocardium ratio and percent dose per gram of infarct for Tc-99m PPi compared with other agents are desirable properties. Additionally, Tc-99m PPi is effective in detecting acute myocardial infarcts soon after intravenous injection, and these factors make it the current drug of choice for infarct avid imaging.

TABLE 9-2. CONCENTRATION OF RADIOPHARMACEUTICALS IN DAMAGED RAT MYOCARDIUM

Agent	Percent Dose per Gram of Infarct	Infarct-Normal[a] Myocardium Ratio
Tc-PPi	2.2	25.2
Tc-EHDP	0.8	26.7
Tc-MDP	0.9	30.2
Tc-GH	0.7	20.2
Tc-tetracycline	0.9	13.9
		35.0 (at 6 and 24 hr)

[a]At 1 hour after injection.
(Data from Chervu LR, 1979, p 241.[3])

Production of Tc-99m Pyrophosphate

Tc-99m PPi is prepared as needed on a daily basis by adding Tc-99m pertechnetate to a serum vial containing a sterile, lyophilized mixture of stannous chloride or fluoride and sodium pyrophosphate. One commercial kit also contains trimetaphosphate. The latter formulation was designed with the intent of providing adequate pyrophosphate concentration over time because the trimetaphosphate will hydrolyze into orthophosphate and pyrophosphate.[9] A comparative list of pyrophosphate kits is shown in Table 9-3. The Tc-99m pertechnetate added to the kit is reduced by the stannous ion and subsequently complexed to the pyrophosphate. This reaction occurs within a few minutes. The chemical structure of Tc-99m PPi has not been determined, but it may be similar to that proposed for Tc-99m methylene diphosphonate (Chapter 13). The preparation is checked by radiochromatography for hydrolyzed reduced technetium (colloid) and free pertechnetate as radiochemical impurities. It is important that the pertechnetate impurity be less than 5 percent because excess pertechnetate may label red cells in vivo. This will prolong the clearance of blood activity and cause a high blood background that may degrade image quality. In vitro, Tc-99m PPi is a labile complex and may decompose with time and regenerate free pertechnetate. This process is accelerated by the presence of oxygen, but even in nitrogen-purged solutions, peroxides and free radicals generated by the radiolytic decomposition of water can attack the molecule and cause degradation (Chapter 13). Consequently, it is important to repeat radiochromatography on preparations that are used several hours after initial preparation.

Biologic Properties of Tc-99m Pyrophosphate

The physical properties of Tc-99m have been previously described. After intravenous injection in humans, Tc-99m PPi is cleared rapidly from the blood.[10] By 3 hours, less than 10 percent remains in the blood, and of this amount, 30 percent is in

TABLE 9-3. PYROPHOSPHATE KITS FOR INFARCT AVID IMAGING AND RED BLOOD CELL LABELING

Manu-facturer	Composition		Maximum Amount Tc-99m/Kit	Expiration Time After Tc-99m Labeling	Expiration Time After Adding Saline for Red Cell Labeling
	Formula	Amount			
A	$Na_4P_2O_7$	11.9 mg	100 mCi	6 hr	6 hr
	$SnCl_2 \cdot 2 H_2O$ (min)	3.2 mg			
	$SnCl_2 \cdot 2 H_2O$ (max)	4.4 mg			
	(Kit contains an average of about 2 mg Sn(II))				
B	$Na_4P_2O_7$	10.0 mg	200 mCi	6 hr	6 hr
	$Na_3P_3O_9$	30.0 mg			
	$SnCl_2 \cdot 2 H_2O$ (min)	0.95 mg			
	$SnCl_2 \cdot 2 H_2O$ (max)	1.8 mg			
	(Kit contains an average of about 1.2 mg Sn(II))				
C	$Na_4P_2O_7$	23.9 mg	75 mCi	6 hr	0.5 hr
	SnF_2 (min)	0.4 mg			
	SnF_2 (max)	0.9 mg			
	(Kit contains an average of about 0.75 mg Sn(II))				

Manufacturers: A, Mallinckrodt; B, Dupont-NEN; C, Squibb.

the red cells, and 43 percent is bound to plasma protein. Between 40 and 50 percent of the dose is deposited in bone, and 45 to 50 percent is excreted in the urine. The critical organ is the bladder wall, which receives a radiation dose of 3.5 rad per 15-mCi dose, assuming a 4-hour voiding interval.

During the radiolabeling process only a small fraction of the stannous ion in the kit is used to reduce the pertechnetate so that the major portion of the Tc-99m PPi dose injected is actually stannous pyrophosphate. Approximately 0.5 percent of the stannous pyrophosphate dose will become associated with the red blood cells (RBC).[11] These tinned red cells have a long biologic half-time and can bind Tc-99m pertechnetate activity to produce a substantial blood pool background. The physician should keep this fact in mind if studies involving pertechnetate injection are performed within 2 to 3 days after a dose of Tc-99m PPi.

Mechanism of Localization of Tc-99m Pyrophosphate

The mechanism of localization of Tc-99m PPi has been studied by Buja et al.[12] The extent of localization of the Tc-99m PPi dose deposited in canine myocardial infarcts is about 0.02 percent per gram of infarct that is 20 to 24 hours old. The maximal concentration occurs in peripheral zones of the infarct where there is adequate blood flow, but considerably less concentration occurs in central zones where blood flow is markedly reduced. This pattern is similar to that of Ca^{++} deposition. After fixed coronary artery occlusion in dogs, Tc-99m PPi begins to localize in the infarcted tissue within 12 to 24 hours. Scintigrams become more positive during 24 to 72 hours and re-

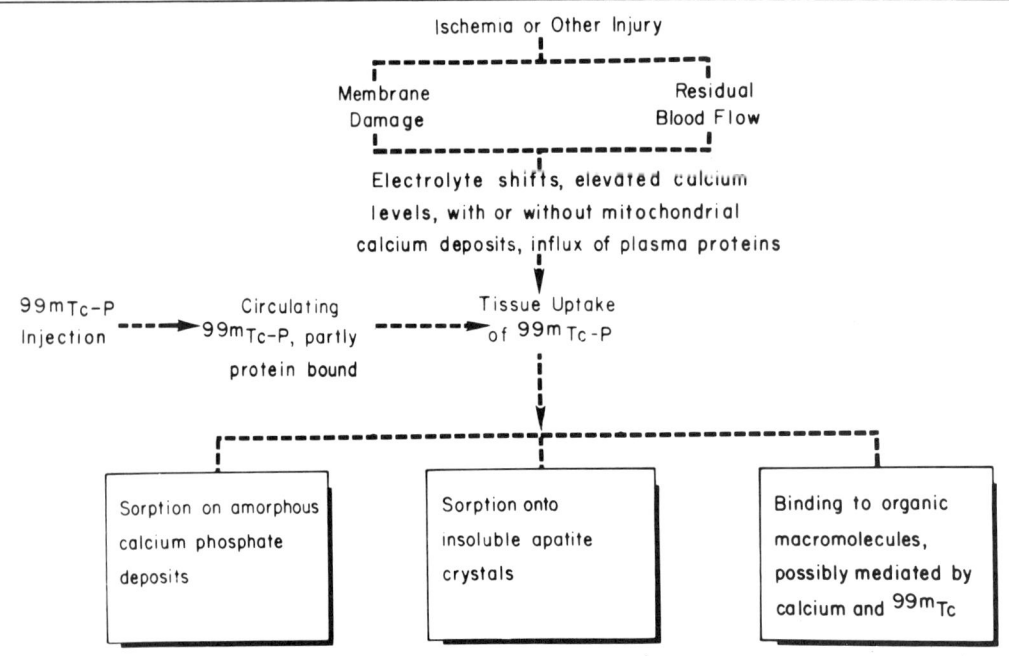

Figure 9-1. Proposed pathophysiologic basis for the scintigraphic detection of tissue damage with Tc-99m radiopharmaceuticals. *(From Buja LM, et al, 1977, p 724, copyright American Society for Clinical Investigation, with permission.[12])*

TABLE 9-4. RADIATION ABSORBED DOSE FROM Tc-99m PYROPHOSPHATE

Organ	rad/15 mCi Administered
Bone	0.59
Bone marrow	0.42
Kidneys	2.10
Bladder	
2 hr void	1.46
4.8 hr void	3.45
Testes,	
2 hr void	0.15
Ovaries,	
2 hr void	0.14
Heart	
Normal	0.11
Impaired	0.22
Total body	0.13

main abnormal for 6 days after infarction, fading thereafter and becoming negative by day 14.

Although the exact mechanism of localization has not been elucidated, the close association of tissue damage with calcium and Tc-99m PPi localization has led to the suggested mechanism that Tc-99m PPi concentrates in severely injured myocardial cells by absorption to various forms of tissue calcium stores, including amorphous calcium phosphate, crystalline hydroxyapatite, and calcium complexed with various macromolecules. This process is summarized in Figure 9-1.

Radiation Dose from Tc-99m Pyrophosphate

The radiation dose to selected organs is shown in Table 9-4. The critical organs are the kidney and bladder wall because of the high urinary excretion of Tc-99m (about 50 percent of the injected dose).

BLOOD POOL IMAGING AGENTS

The essential requirements for a blood pool imaging radiopharmaceutical for evaluating dynamic heart function include (1) slow blood clearance to provide a steady blood pool activity during the time of data collection, (2) minimal localization of radioactivity in nearby organs and the extravascular space that would interfere with measurements of the heart blood pool, and (3) high photon flux, which is necessary for high-resolution and high-sensitivity measurements of dynamic heart function with the gamma camera. The latter requirement is most easily met by Tc-99m, which is used almost exclusively for such studies. The first two requirements are met by labeling Tc-99m to either human serum albumin or red blood cells.

Tc-99m Human Serum Albumin

Several methods have been developed to prepare Tc-99m human serum albumin (Tc-99m HSA).[13] All involve the reduction of pertechnetate before its complexation with albumin. The most successful labeling is accomplished either by pertechnetate reduction at a platinum or zirconium electrode (electrolytic method) or by stannous ion (stannous chloride method) at an acid pH followed by neutralization with buffer. Both methods use presterilized kits.

Properties of Tc-99m Human Serum Albumin. When compared with radioiodinated HSA, the Tc-99m products have faster blood clearance.[14] Electrolytically prepared Tc-99m HSA clears the blood 1.5 times faster, and the tin reduced the product two to five times faster than radioiodinated HSA, which has a blood clearance rate of 1 percent per minute. In clinical studies most patients cannot be effectively imaged 1 hour after injection of Tc-99m HSA. Neither of the Tc-99m kit methods is satisfactory because various levels of impurities are produced. Reduced insoluble technetium species (primarily radiocolloids) are more common with the stannous ion kits, whereas free pertechnetate impurity is more common with electrolytic kits. In either case these impurities either concentrate in nearby organs such as the liver and stomach or diffuse into the extravascular space, thereby increasing background activity and contributing to cardiac image degradation. Such impurities may be removed by a chromatographic purification step to yield a product equivalent to radioiodinated HSA, but such techniques are not readily available to all nuclear medicine departments nor are they ideal for routine daily use. Because of these problems and the development of facile techniques to label RBC, Tc-99m HSA use for blood pool imaging has diminished.

Tc-99m Red Blood Cells

Several methods have been used to bind Tc-99m to RBC. In general, Tc-99 pertechnetate (+7 valence) must be reduced to a lower valence state for binding to occur, and this is usually accomplished with a stannous (SnII) salt. Three methods are most widely used in current practice: the in vitro method, the in vivo method, and the modified in vivo method.

In Vitro Labeling Method. This method uses a kit developed at the Brookhaven National Laboratory by Smith and Richards[15] and Srivastava and Chervu[16] and consists of a 10-ml vacutainer tube containing a freeze-dried mixture of the following ingredients:

Stannous ion	2.0 µg
Sodium citrate	3.67 mg
Dextrose	5.50 mg
Sodium chloride	0.11 mg

The citrate complexes the stannous ion to keep it soluble, and the dextrose sustains red cell metabolism, which improves cell viability. To label the cells, 4 ml of heparinized (~100 units) whole blood is added to the tube and incubated for 5 minutes, during which time the red cells become "tinned."* The cells are not damaged significantly because of the small amount of stannous ion present. One milliliter of 4.4 percent EDTA solution is then added and the tube centrifuged with the stoppered end down for 5 minutes at 1300 g. The EDTA chelates extracellular tin, which may depress labeling yields. Using a 2- to 3-ml syringe and a 20-gauge needle, 1.25 ml of packed tinned red cells are removed and transferred to a sterile vial containing 1 to 3 ml of pertechnetate. The mixture is incubated for 10 minutes and is then ready for patient administration. Labeling yields are consistently greater than 98 percent with this method but only if the number of technetium atoms used (Tc-99 and Tc-99m) do not exceed the number produced by the decay of 20 mCi of Mo-99. Details of this precaution are provided with the kit. A calculation regarding this limitation is found in Chapter 3.

The advantage of the in vitro method is a very high labeling yield that results in higher target-to-background ratios than with the in vivo labeling method.

In Vivo Labeling Method. A serendipitous event led to the discovery of this technique.[17] A pertechnetate brain scan demonstrated a positive brain lesion in a patient with right parietal metastasis from bronchogenic carcinoma. After this initial study, the patient underwent a bone scan with Tc-99m stannous pyrophosphate. Subsequently, a follow-up pertechnetate brain scan was performed, but the previously identified positive lesion was obscured because of high blood background activity. The blood background was due to an unusually high level of Tc-99m activity in the red cells. Apparently, the Tc-99m became bound to the cells because of the presence of residual stannous ion (from the bone dose) that was associated with the red cells. This event and other follow-up studies made it clear that pertechnetate studies should not be done soon after bone scans. It is important to note here, however, that red cell binding does not occur if Tc-99m labeled to DTPA or glucoheptonate is used for brain imaging the day after a bone scan because the technetium in these agents is already complexed and is therefore prevented from reacting with the red cell.

After this unusual discovery, efforts

---

* The term "tinned" is used to denote that a small fraction of administered stannous ion becomes associated with the red cells.

were made to develop a technique that would maximize Tc-99m red cell labeling in vivo for use as a blood pool imaging agent, particularly for cardiac studies.[18] Furthermore, Zimmer and Pavel demonstrated that a minimum 1.4 mg of stannous pyrophosphate (Mallinckrodt PYP) per 1000 ml of whole blood must be used to achieve the highest RBC labeling.[19] For an average 70 kg (5400-ml whole blood volume) adult this equals 7.56 mg Sn-PYP (one-half vial) per dose or 15 µg Sn(II)/kg (1.06 mg Sn(II)/70 kg). Hamilton and Alderson have shown that the maximal in vivo labeling of red cells is obtained using an IV dose of 10 µg Sn(II)/kg or greater.[20] The usual method for in vivo labeling of red cells is to add 5 ml of sterile saline to a vial of Sn-PYP. The appropriate volume of Sn-PYP, based on body weight or whole blood volume estimation, is administered IV and allowed to mix for 30 minutes, during which time the red cells become tinned. After in vivo tinning of red cells, 15 to 25 mCi of Tc-99m pertechnetate is administered IV, which produces a labeling yield of 70 to 80 percent bound to the red cells. Although these yields are less than the in vitro method, the in vivo method is more convenient and also permits first-pass dynamic cardiac studies to be performed because the volume of pertechnetate is small and may be given by rapid bolus injection. Labeling yields with this method are lower than with the in vitro method because the red cells must compete for pertechnetate with other body compartments. These include pertechnetate's rapid diffusion into the extravascular space; its concentration by the gastric mucosa, salivary glands, and thyroid glands; and its excretion by renal filtration.

Modified In Vivo Method. Labeling yields with the in vivo method can be increased to greater than 90 percent if the modified in vivo technique is used.[21] With this technique patients receive 500 µg of stannous ion as Sn-PPi IV. Twenty minutes later, 3 ml of in vivo tinned red cells are withdrawn through a heparinized (10 U/ml) butterfly infusion set into a shielded syringe containing 20 mCi of pertechnetate. The mixture is incubated for 10 minutes with gentle agitation and reinjected. Higher labeling yields are achieved because the red cells compete for pertechnetate only with the plasma in the syringe, which, in reality, is not an effective competitor because most of the tin is associated with the red cells. Because of the large volume, this technique precludes doing a first-pass bolus study.

Whole Blood Method for Labeling Red Cells with Tc-99m. An in vitro kit method for selectively labeling RBCs with Tc-99m in whole blood has been developed.[22] It eliminates the need for centrifugation and plasma separation before incubating tinned RBCs with pertechnetate. With this new technique 0.5 ml to 6 ml of heparinized whole blood is added to a vial containing 50 µg tin, 3.67 mg sodium citrate, 5.5 mg dextrose, and 1.4 mg sodium chloride. The mixture is incubated for 5 minutes to tin the cells. Subsequently, 0.6 ml of 0.1 percent sodium hypochlorite solution and 1 ml of 4.4 percent EDTA solution are added to the mixture, which is then inverted three to four times. After this, 0.5 to 3 ml of pertechnetate are added and allowed to incubate for 15 minutes to effect a 98 ± 2 percent labeling of the red cells. The hypochlorite and EDTA serve to oxidize and chelate excess stannous ion outside of the red cells so that efficient intracellular labeling can occur. This method appears promising but must await further testing and analysis before routine use.

Labeling Mechanism and Biologic Properties of Tc-99m Red Blood Cells

Red cell binding experiments conducted using a labeling method similar to the in vitro method have demonstrated that technetium ultimately becomes bound, probably by coordinate covalent bonding, to the beta chain of hemoglobin.[23] Apparently the anionic TcO_4^- readily diffuses through the cell membrane but will easily wash out unless it is reduced and bound by hemoglobin. This mechanism is similar to the labeling of red cells with chromium-51 whereby the chromate anion (CrO_4^{2-}) diffuses into the cells and becomes bound to hemoglobin in the reduced chromic (Cr^{3+}) form. Experiments on rabbits[11] administered radioactive Sn-113 PPi without technetium have indicated that the stannous ion dissociates from pyrophosphate and is localized 40 to 50 percent in bone, 15 to 20 percent in liver, and 20 to 25 percent excreted in urine. Less than 1 percent of Sn-113 activity is associated with the red cell mass. Despite this low percentage, however, tin binds to hemoglobin two to three times stronger than to albumin, which may explain why red cells can still be labeled with pertechnetate when plasma levels of stannous ion are low.[11]

Exactly where TcO_4^- is reduced is unclear. One opinion is that the small amount of stannous ion associated with the red cell is intracellular, perhaps bound to sulfhydryl groups of intracellular protein. The pertechnetate anion can readily diffuse into the cell, become reduced by the stannous ion, and subsequently bind to hemoglobin, which prevents it from diffusing back out of the cell.[23] In vitro studies have shown that within the hemoglobin molecule, approximately 20 percent of Tc-99m and 90 percent of tin are associated with heme and 80 percent of Tc-99m and 10 percent of tin are associated with globin.[24]

In humans the biologic half-life in blood of Tc-99m RBCs prepared by the in vitro technique is biexponential, with 5 percent of the activity having a 20-minute half-life and 95 percent, a 29-hour half-life.[25] With the in vivo method the labeled cells are assumed to have the normal biologic half-life of red cells, i.e., about 80 days.

Toxicity Considerations

Some concern has been addressed to the potential toxicity of IV administered phosphate compounds because of the interaction of phosphates with the plasma calcium ion.[26] Studies in rats have shown that the lethal dose for 50 percent survival of the group (LD_{50}) for pyrophosphate as the decahydrate salt ($Na_4P_2O_7 \cdot 10H_2O$) is 41 mg/kg of body weight, whereas tetany occurred at 22 mg/kg. The minimal toxic response observed was electrocardiograph (ECG) changes consistent with hypocalcemia, which occurred at 12 mg/kg and which is equivalent to 7.2 mg/kg of the anhydrous pyrophosphate salt ($Na_4P_2O_7$). The maximum recommended dose of anhydrous stannous pyrophosphate for in vivo red cell labeling, based on the administration of a whole vial (15.4 mg) of Technescan PYP per 70-kg man, is 0.2 mg/kg. This is 36 times less than the minimum toxic dose associated with electrocardiographic (ECG) changes in rats. Typical doses used clinically are half to two thirds this amount, which makes the safety factor even larger.

Radiation Dose

Effete red blood cells naturally become sequestered by the spleen. A similar fate occurs with cells damaged by radiolabeling methods. Biologic distribution studies in humans indicate that 5 percent of the administered dose of Tc-99m RBCs prepared by the in vitro method is rapidly sequestered by the spleen, which becomes the critical organ.[25] The radiation dose to the spleen is 0.16 rad/mCi administered. The critical organ for in vivo prepared Tc-99m RBCs is, however, the stomach wall because about 25 percent of the administered pertechnetate is not bound to the red cells and therefore its localization in the stomach contributes significantly to the dose of this organ.[27] The radiation dose to the stomach wall is 0.08 rad/mCi administered, whereas the spleen dose is only 0.018 rad/mCi. The radiation dose to various organs is listed in Table 9–5 and varies between resting and nonresting populations.

ALTERED BIODISTRIBUTION OF HEART-IMAGING RADIOPHARMACEUTICALS

A number of drugs have been shown to alter the biodistribution of Tl-201 chloride, Tc-99m PPi, and Tc-99m–labeled red blood

TABLE 9-5. RADIATION DOSE TO ORGANS AFTER IN VIVO LABELING OF RED BLOOD CELLS

Organ	Radiation Dose (rads/20 mCi Administered)	
	Resting Population	Nonresting Population
Bladder wall	0.54	2.40[a]
Stomach wall	1.60	0.62
Upper large intestine wall	0.64	0.90
Lower large intestine wall	0.58	0.84
Ovaries	0.42	0.46
Testes	0.24	0.24
Red marrow	0.46	0.44
Spleen[b]	0.36	0.36
Thyroid	0.82	0.82
Blood	1.06	1.04
Total body	0.34	0.32

The radiation dose assumes Tc-99m pertechnetate administered 30 minutes after Sn-PPi and 75 percent RBC labeling with 25 percent as free pertechnetate.
[a]Assumes 25 percent excreted with a biologic half-life of 1 hour.
[b]No initial splenic uptake.

cells used for imaging the heart. The reported experimental studies have been reviewed by Hladik et al.[28]

Increased uptake (1.5 to 2 times normal) of Tl-201 in the myocardium has been shown to occur after preadministration of sodium bicarbonate to dogs. Dexamethasone and isoproterenol have been found to enhance uptake of Tl-201 by the heart. In fact, isoproterenol can reverse the decrease in Tl-201 uptake induced by propranolol. The coronary vasodilator dipyridamole has produced a 60 percent increase in Tl-201 myocardial concentration in dogs. The dramatic effect of dipyridamole has led to its investigation as a pharmacologic intervention in lieu of exercise in producing regional myocardial perfusion abnormalities that can then be detected by Tl-201 imaging in patients with coronary artery disease.

Certain drugs can also decrease Tl-201 uptake by the myocardium. Animal experiments have shown that propranolol can reduce myocardial uptake of Tl-201 by 25 to 30 percent. Decreases in Tl-201 uptake can also be caused by ouabain, digitalis, and Adriamycin.

The myocardial uptake and biodistribution of Tc-99m PPi can be altered by various drugs. The known cardiotoxicity of the anthracycline antibiotics, daunorubicin (rubidomycin), and doxorubicin (Adriamycin) has stimulated the use of Tc-PPi for monitoring such toxicity during treatment with these drugs. A number of studies have demonstrated significant myocardial uptake of Tc-PPi during drug treatment. Investigations are continuing in this area to establish sensitivity of the method.

With regard to Tc-99m–labeled RBCs, there have been reports that indicate that heparin may adversely affect the distribution of activity. Consistently poor quality studies showing diminished cardiac chamber activity and increased renal uptake and excretion have been observed when Sn-PPi and pertechnetate were administered through a heparinized catheter during the in vivo labeling method.[29] Elimination of the heparin lock reversed the problem of maldistribution. Occasionally poor radiolabeling efficiency occurs with the in vivo method for labeling red cells. This usually leads to low cardiac chamber activity, high body background, and interference from activity localized in the stomach. Although there are no specific answers to why this occurs, the patient's disease, physiologic milieu, and the presence of numerous drug substances in the blood undoubtedly are contributing factors to the problem. In this regard, the disease–drug factors may stimulate the formation of the RBC antibodies that are responsible for poor labeling efficiency. Indeed, in one study,[30] RBC labeling efficiency was evaluated in 40 consecutive patients after in vivo labeling. Thirty-two patients had greater than a 90 percent label, but eight patients showed less than a 50 percent label.

These eight patients all had diseases or medications associated with RBC antibody formation; two had lupus, one had a recent transfusion reaction, and five were taking quinidine, Aldomet, or both, which are known to induce a positive direct Coombs' test in some individuals. To discover whether this same phenomenon would occur under controlled conditions in vitro, packed red cells were incubated with anti-RhD serum before labeling the cells with Tc-99m using the Brookhaven kit method. A decrease of 22 percent (95 percent control versus 73 percent postincubation) in labeling efficiency resulted.

Clinical Evaluation of the Heart with Radiopharmaceuticals

Of the four major types of cardiovascular nuclear medicine studies practiced today, the first, which was the cardiac shunt study, became widely available in the early 1970s. Infarct avid imaging became popular in the mid-1970s shortly after it was serendipitously found that Tc-99 PPi concentrated in recently infarcted myocardium. The late 1970s saw the advent of Tl-201 myocardial perfusion imaging and the simultaneous development of two cardiovascular ventriculographic techniques known as the first-pass radionuclide angiogram and the equilibrium ECG gated cardiac blood pool study (alias MUGA, etc., for multigated acquisition). Further refinement has taken place for both Tl-201 myocardial perfusion imaging and radionuclide ventriculographic techniques in regard to acquisition methods and computer techniques.

CARDIAC SHUNT STUDY

Rationale
The rationale for this study is to answer as noninvasively as possible two clinical questions: (1) is there a left-to-right intracardiac shunt present to explain a murmur heard with the stethoscope, and if present, (2) how much shunting is there.

Procedure
The procedure is angiographic, with injection of a compact bolus of the tracer material into a vein as close as possible to the heart, usually the right external jugular or a scalp vein in an infant. Data are obtained by placing the patient under a gamma camera in such a way as to visualize the central circulation and both lung fields. Data are acquired at four frames per second into a computer.

Problems come from poor bolus characteristics, i.e., not compact enough, and this can be determined by visual inspection of the time–activity curve of the bolus passing through the superior vena cava. The full width at half maximum should be less than 1.5 seconds for a good bolus injection. Repeated attempts at bolus injection of the tracer are often necessary, particularly in infants.

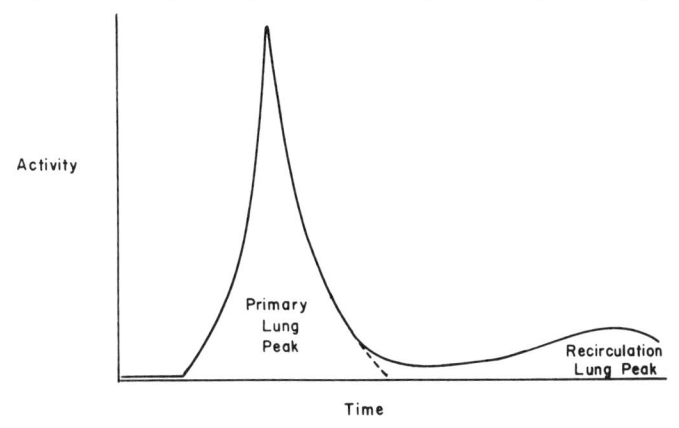

Figure 9-2. Normal patient's time–activity curve of a tracer bolus' initial passage and systemic return recirculation through the lungs.

Pharmaceuticals

Tc-99m pertechnetate is probably the most frequently used radiopharmaceutical. It's chief attribute is that it can be obtained throughout the day in high radioactive concentration for small-volume bolus injections. Because repeated injection attempts are often necessary, it makes sense to use agents that clear the bloodstream rapidly to be concentrated in organs remote from the lungs and central circulation, e.g., the kidneys. Of all the Tc-99m radiopharmaceuticals that have been used, Tc-99m pertechnetate is cleared from the central circulation most rapidly. Fifty to 60 percent of the pertechnetate dose is removed from the blood in 1 to 2 minutes, 50 percent of Tc-99m sulfur colloid in 2 to 3 minutes, and 58 percent of Tc-99m DTPA in 4 minutes. If an ultrashort half-life tracer is used, the time–activity curve must be corrected for radioactive decay and deadtime losses of the gamma camera–computer system, and special collimation may be necessary. With dynamic collimation of the gamma camera, 3- to 5-mCi doses of Tc-99m pertechnetate are sufficient.

Interpretation

Analysis of the data is carried out by drawing regions of interest over the lung fields, superior vena cava, etc., and generating time–activity curves (Fig. 9–2 and 9–3). Left-to-right shunts produce disruption of the washout phase of the bolus clearing the lungs. This is caused by the premature reap-

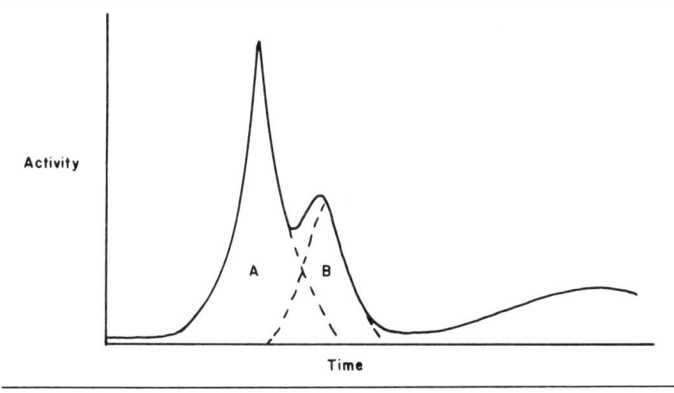

Figure 9-3. Left-to-right shunt time–activity curve. Fitting of portions of the curve result in areas representing the right heart output (A) and shunted blood (B). Normal right or left heart output can be represented as A − B.

pearance of the tracer in the lungs from blood that has completed a primary pass through the lungs and on into the left side of the heart, but that went from the high-pressure side to the low-pressure side across an atrial or ventricular septal defect back into the right side of the heart and thus reappeared prematurely in the lungs again. These time–activity curves are fitted by using a mathematical function called a gamma variate and then quantified by making a ratio of the areas under the parts of the curves that represent the total right side of the heart's output (A) and the shunted blood (B) and expressed as the quantity of pulmonic/quantity of systemic or $\dot{Q}p/\dot{Q}s = A/A - B$. The $\dot{Q}p/\dot{Q}s$ determination is most accurate for shunt ratios between 1.2/1 and 3.0/1. This method is not used for right-to-left shunts.

INFARCT IMAGING

Rationale
The rationale for the imaging of myocardial infarction lies in the ability of the technique to aid in the diagnosis of an acute infarction at times when cardiac-specific enzyme determinations cannot be made, to localize and show the extent of the infarction, and to serve as a means for prognostication regarding the patient's future course based on certain patterns of uptake. Infact imaging may be the only way of establishing the presence of a perioperative infarction that occurred during or after cardiac surgery.

Procedure
There are two methods for infarct imaging. The first, infarct avid imaging with Tc-99m PPi, is an on-demand study in which the radiopharmaceutical is most strongly concentrated between 24 and 72 hours after an acute event but that may show concentration out to 7 days or more. This study is performed by injection of 15 mCi of Tc-99m PPi followed in 2 hours by multiangled imaging of the left chest. Occasionally there is a delayed clearance of tracer from the blood pool, necessitating even later views, e.g., at 4 hours, and for this reason, some practitioners have advocated intentional early and late imaging of the central circulation blood pool for comparison purposes.

Nonavid infarct imaging with Tl-201 is the second method and has the attribute of showing abnormality virtually the instant the patient has the myocardial infarction; thus it can be used to triage patients effectively when coronary intensive care beds are in short supply. Injection of the Tl-201 tracer may be accomplished anywhere in the hospital, e.g., the emergency room or coronary care unit, and multiangled images obtained with a mobile gamma camera beginning 20 minutes later. Static image acquisition using emission computed tomography techniques is a significant aid in the localization and quantification of infarcts with Tc-99m PPi and Tl-201.

Pharmaceuticals
Several radiopharmaceuticals preceded Tc-99m PPi for infarct avid imaging. These included Hg-197 chlormerodrin, Tc-99m tetracycline, and Tc-99m glucoheptonate. Each has its own peculiarities with regard to time of peak concentration in the infarcted myocardium, etc.; however, the chief attribute of imaging with Tc-99m PPi is the presence of skeletal landmarks (ribs, sternum, etc.) in the image that aid in localizing and grading the amount of uptake in the infarct. Tl-201, on the other hand, is a myocardial perfusion agent that is concentrated best in the normal myocardium and leaves the infarcted area as a void in the concentration.

Interpretation
Pyrophosphate is attracted to hyperconcentrations of calcium such as that present during the 24- to 72-hour phase of necrosis repair after an infarction, in unstable angina patients, and sometimes at the base of a ventricular aneurysm. If the study is positive, not only is the uptake localized as to the area of myocardium involved, but the uptake is graded by comparison with bone uptake to establish a degree of confidence

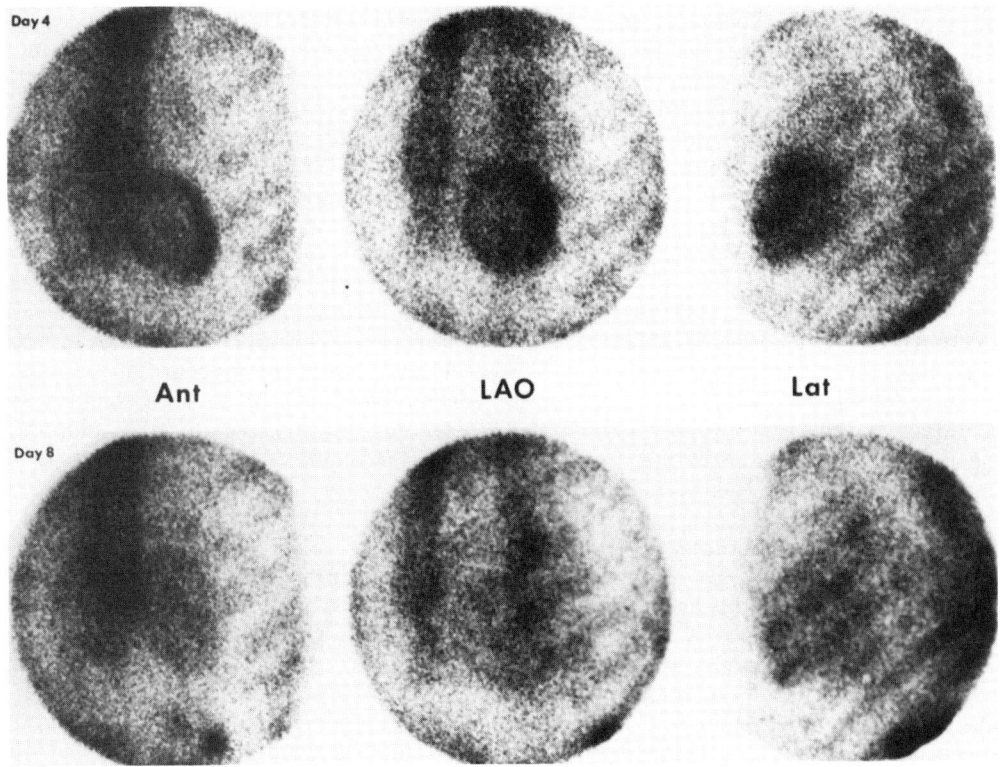

Figure 9-4. Infarct avid: studies obtained 4 and 8 days after extensive acute LV infarction. Images are obtained 2 hours after IV injection of 15 mCi of Tc-99m PPi.

in interpreting the study (Fig. 9-4). A good scheme of grading has been the following:

Uptake Intensity	Score	Interpretation
No uptake	0	Negative
Barely visible	1+	Negative
Diffuse*	2+	Equivocal
Focal, less than sternum	2+	Positive
Equal to sternum	3+	Positive
Greater than sternum	4+	Positive

With this grading scheme, the more positive the study, the greater the confidence that an infarction has occurred. Some allowance should be made for the extent or type of infarction, e.g., transmural versus

*May be prolonged blood pool phase. Some correlation with unstable angina.

subendocardial, because the amount of infarcted tissue will affect the quantity of Tc-99m PPi concentrated in the area. Very extensive acute infarctions may appear early as ring or doughnut uptake patterns because of the slow revascularization of the central area of necrosis, with uptake appearing in the center several days later as revascularization proceeds. Persistent uptake beyond a week may also indicate recurrent infarction. Right ventricular infarctions are often first discovered with Tc-99m PPi imaging.

Myocardial perfusion imaging with Tl-201 is nonspecific in regard to what is causing the myocardial perfusion imbalance (ischemia, old or new infarct) unless one includes consideration of the clinical setting in the process of interpretation. A defect in Tl-201 myocardial concentration in a resting patient who is being evaluated for acute chest pain usually means that the patient does have some form of coronary heart disease and will likely be admitted to or remain in the coronary care unit for evaluation, whereas a similar case, but with normal myocardial perfusion, is likely to have a noncardiac cause for the pain and have his workup proceed on an outpatient basis.

MYOCARDIAL PERFUSION IMAGING

Rationale

One of the chief clinical problems presenting in medical practice is chest pain. Even though the various causes can generally be deciphered from the character or circumstances of the pain, quite frequently there remains some doubt, and tests are ordered for confirmation of clinical suspicions. In the past the treadmill exercise tolerance test was used with ECG monitoring with the expectation that if the patient had ischemic heart disease characteristic changes would be seen in the ST-T wave segments of the ECG during the stress testing. If the exercise tolerance testing were abnormal, the next step might be an invasive one, namely, cardiac catheterization to visualize the coronary artery lesions. Cardiac catheterization is attendant with significant mortality and morbity and therefore nearly always preceded by noninvasive testing. The treadmill exercise tolerance test has a low risk to the patient if guidelines are followed, but it has a sensitivity of only 60 to 70 percent and a significant incidence of false-positive results. The rationale for myocardial perfusion imaging (MPI) is found in the improvement in diagnostic efficiency gained by combining it with the exercise tolerance test. A myocardial perfusion defect together with an ECG ST-T wave segment abnormality induced by exercise is very convincing evidence of ischemic heart disease.

Procedure

The procedure is as follows: An exercise tolerance test is performed by a fasting patient using a standard exercise testing protocol such as the Bruce protocol with 12-lead ECG, blood pressure, heart rate, and visual–verbal monitoring by trained personnel and physicians. When an end point is reached (certain ECG ST-T segment changes, chest pain, or 85 percent of the predicted maximum heart rate), the tracer material, 2.0 mCi of Tl-201 thallous chloride is injected IV and the exercise con-

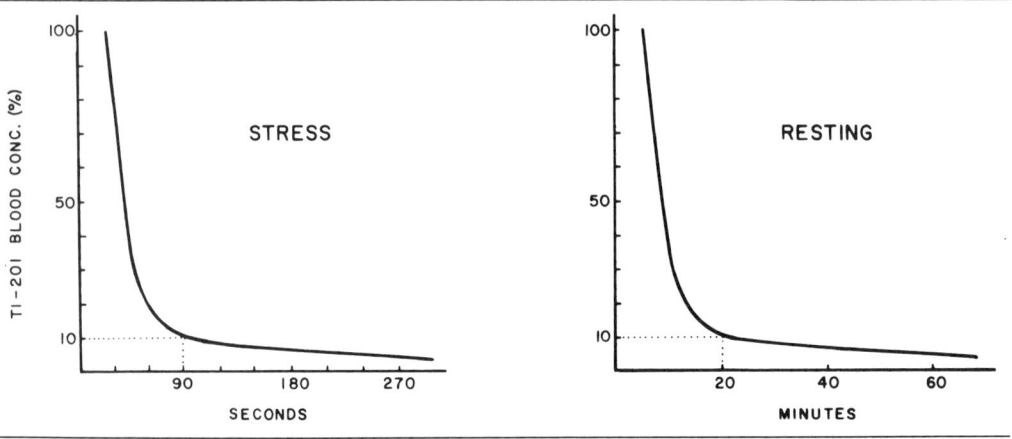

Figure 9-5. Blood disappearance of Tl-201. Note the difference in the time axes.

tinued for 90 seconds at the same level if possible. Most of the Tl-201 is removed from the blood by exercising muscle tissues in that 90 seconds, and it is important that the myocardial perfusion imbalance be maintained throughout that time (Fig. 9–5). Initial imaging should be started immediately and completed within 30 minutes if possible. Images obtained at 45 minutes will begin to show the effects of Tl-201 redistribution out of normal and into recovering ischemic myocardium (Fig. 9–6). Redistribution images are usually obtained from 2 to 4 hours after injection. Stress and redistribution images obtained for a certain number of counts will show the relative or regional myocardial perfusion. If quantitative information, e.g., from washout–washin rate studies, is desired, the stress and redistribution images must be obtained for a fixed period of time. Emission computed tomography aids considerably in the identification and sizing of myocardial perfusion defects (Fig. 9–7).

The procedure for resting studies is somewhat different. At rest blood flow is diminished to muscle and increased to the splanchnic area. It is therefore preferable to have patients fasting for 4 hours and to have them walk around without exertion and then stand while the injection is made. Blood clearance is slower at rest, and 20 minutes should pass before imaging (Fig. 9–5).

Pharmaceuticals

A myocardial perfusion agent should be distributed in direct proportion to flow and remain in place long enough for imaging to be completed. Redistribution and metabolic properties allow additional information to be obtained. Tl-201 is a potassium analogue, i.e., it is distributed to and taken up by muscle cells similarly to potassium. Other myocardial perfusion agents differ from Tl-201 most importantly in the redistribution phase. This is due to biologic property differences and will affect interpretation accordingly. Labeled fatty acids, e.g., decanoic acid derivatives, appear to be metabolized by the myocardium.

Affinity for myocardium, nonaffinity for nearby structures, a major photon yield between 100 to 200 keV, and a high photon flux are highly desirable properties for a myocardium-imaging agent. Tl-201 is dis-

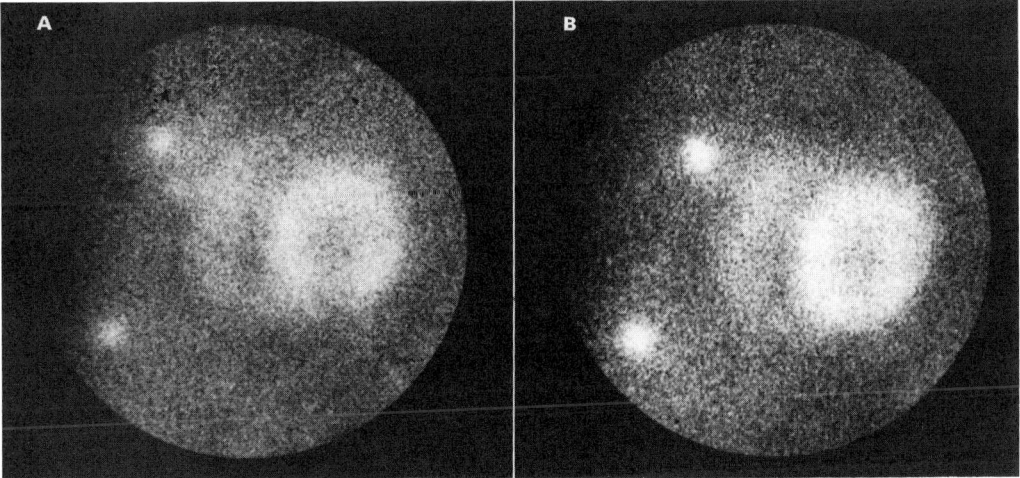

Figure 9-6. Myocardial ischemia; 40-degree left anterior oblique (LAO) exercise (A) and 4-hour redistribution (B) cardiac planar images after IV injection of 2 mCi of Tl-201 thallous chloride that demonstrate an ischemic defect inferiorly with delayed image fill-in.

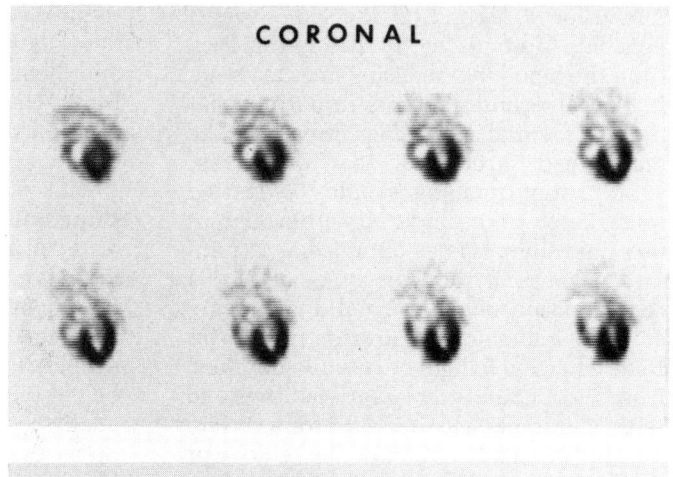
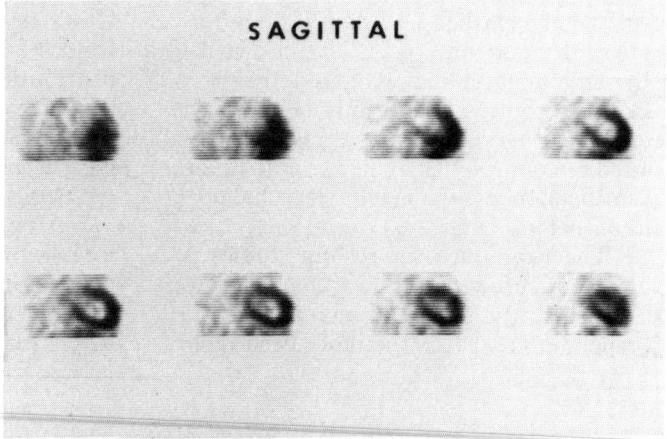
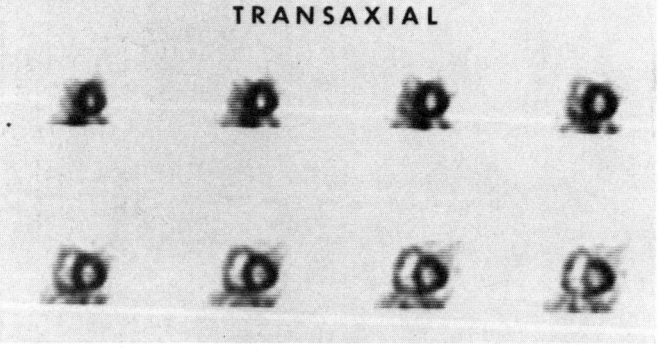

Figure 9-7. Oblique single-photon emission computed tomography (SPECT) reconstructed arrays of the resting myocardium obtained beginning 20 minutes after the injection of 2 mCi of Tl-201 thallous chloride. Perfusion defects are more apparent with this technique than with planar imaging.

tributed in proportion to flow and has some affinity for the myocardium but lacks the other properties; however, Tl-201 is the major myocardial perfusion agent in use today and has achieved that status because it can be imaged with the ordinary gamma camera and because it has wide commercial availability. These two features helped Tl-201 to become a first-hand experience for the practicing community cardiologist.

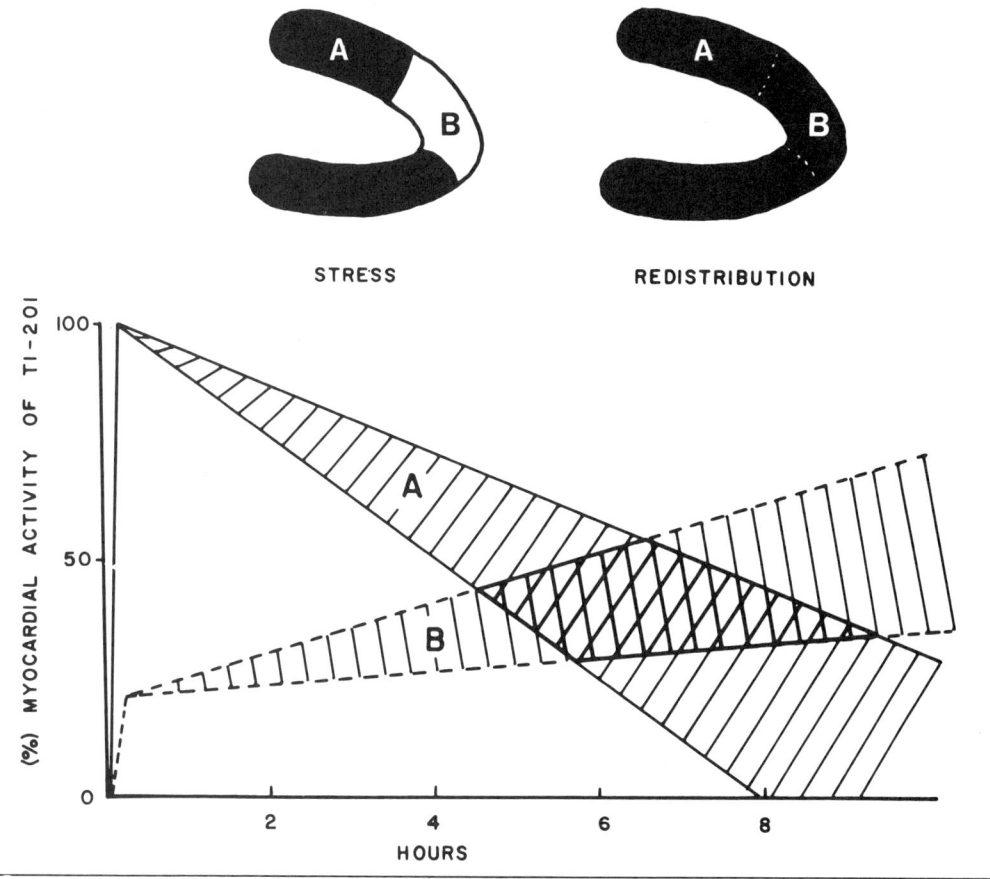

Figure 9-8. Time course of Tl-201 activity in normal myocardium (A) and ischemic myocardium (B).

Interpretation

A Tl-201 myocardial image demonstrates viable myocardium where the tracer is seen. The absence of tracer indicates the absence of live muscle cells or ischemia, depending upon conditions at the time of injection (Fig. 9-8). A single Tl-201 image cannot be used to determine the age of an infarct. A persistent defect seen on a 4-hour redistribution image is most likely going to be due to a previous infarction; however, there is a slight chance it may be prolonged ischemia. Resolution of the latter dilemma may require a resting Tl-201 study 1 week later to ensure that prolonged poststress ischemia was not the problem.

Quantitative Tl-201 imaging, i.e., acquisition for a fixed time (e.g., 10 minutes) into a computer, is done to measure more closely the biologic or effective half-life of Tl-201 in the myocardium. Myocardial punch biopsy findings in dogs indicate that the biologic $T^{1/2}$ of Tl-201 is between 4 and 7 hours (Fig. 9-8).[31] Clinical experience in exercised normal humans indicates that we can expect at least a 33 percent washout of the Tl-201 on planar images from normally perfused myocardium at 4 hours poststress and that ischemic zones show a lesser net washout rate or occasionally even accumulation if the ischemic zone is large enough. It has been claimed that triple-vessel coronary disease with nearly uniform degrees of stenosis can be detected by this method, whereas such a condition would be missed on preset count limited images because of the even distribution of the Tl-201.

RADIONUCLIDE VENTRICULOGRAPHY

Rationale

Radionuclide ventriculography initially achieved widespread usage as a cardiac chamber-imaging procedure primarily because it was a noninvasive technique that could be performed easily on outpatients. Additionally, it involved lower radiation doses than cardiac catheterization, had virtually no risk of iodinated contrast reaction, and had greater accuracy for determining the fraction of blood ejected from the ventricular chambers.

The radionuclide method for determining the ejection fraction is independent of the geometric constraints of the cardiac catheterization and echographic techniques and is now considered the "gold standard" for the ejection fraction of either the left or right ventricular chamber. It is the only really practical method for determination of the right ventricular ejection fraction because of the right ventricle configuration.

$$\text{Ejection fraction} = \frac{\text{End diastolic counts} - \text{End systolic counts}}{\text{End diastolic counts} - \text{Background}}$$

Radionuclide ventriculographic techniques are competitive with myocardial perfusion imaging in the investigation of ischemic heart disease as the cause of chest pain. Physiologically, the order of events after the induction of imbalanced or inadequate coronary artery perfusion is as follows:

1. Ischemia
2. Ventricular wall motion abnormality
3. ST-T wave ECG changes
4. Chest pain

The immediate result of ischemia is the development of a ventricular wall motion abnormality, and if the latter is large enough, there will be an adverse effect on the ejection fraction, volumes, etc. Many clinicians feel they are getting much more functionally significant information from this study than from the myocardial perfusion Tl-201 images.

A more detailed list of indications for radionuclide ventriculography includes the investigation for ischemic heart disease as the cause of chest pain, the further workup of suspected false-positive treadmill-ECG exercise tolerance tests, prognostic grouping of postmyocardial infarction patients, investigation of the functional significance of coronary artery lesions seen at catheterization, the follow-up of coronary artery bypass graft patients with chest pain, and the elucidation of apparent right ventricular dysfunction after an acute myocardial infarction. Other commonplace indications include the classification and baseline function of cardiomyopathies, the investigation of congestive heart failure, the response to pharmacologic therapy of heart failure and arrhythmias, the observation of the wave of contraction (onset of mechanical systole) spreading through the atria and ventricles in patients with conduction system abnormalities and ectopic arrhythmias, the measurement of the cardiotoxic effects of the anthracycline group of drugs (e.g., doxorubicin), and observation of the effect of pulmonary function on right ventricular function. The radionuclide ventriculogram has a significant role to play in patients with valve disease, particularly in the use of the regurgitant fraction index for confirmation of significant valvular insufficiency and in the assessment of ventricular reserve in aortic and mitral valve regurgitant lesions by the measurement of ejection fraction and volume changes with exercise.

Procedure

There are two essentially different techniques involved in the radionuclide ventriculogram, namely, the single or first-pass radionuclide angiogram, which may or may not be ECG gated, and the equilibrium ECG gated cardiac blood pool acquisition. The latter also goes by the names multigated acquisition, gate synchronous acquisition, synchronous multigated acquisition, etc. Either technique has been used separately for most of the indications listed; however, because each technique has strong and weak points, it has been desirable to have the ability to do both techniques whenever indicated. The first-pass technique is particularly useful when it is desirable to acquire the data in the shortest possible period of time. The equilibrium technique yields a higher resolution image and a more representative beat cycle because of greater data integration.

First-Pass Technique. The first-pass technique involves the rapid injection of a small volume of high-concentration tracer material into a vein near the heart, e.g., the right external jugular, for rest studies. For stress first-pass studies, the median basilic arm vein is chosen because the circulation time is much shorter during exercise and it is necessary to slow the bolus down somewhat by using an injection site at an intermediate distance from the heart. Before injection, the tracer volume is loaded into plastic tubing proximal to the needle or catheter, with tiny bubbles separating the tracer from the normal saline bolus chaser to avoid dilution. Injection is accomplished at the appropriate time, and the transit of the bolus through the central circulation observed. As the bolus of tracer enters the cardiac chamber of interest, the patient is instructed to suspend respiration temporarily to minimize heart motion resulting from breathing. The first-pass technique is generally accomplished with the gamma camera in a 30-degree right anterior oblique (RAO) or anterior position (Fig. 9–9).

Equilibrium Technique. The equilibrium technique technique involves labeled blood elements, usually RBCs, and gating of the acquisition with the R wave of the patient's ECG. Gating is necessary because the computer program requires a starting point for the framing of each heart beat. The rising portion of the normal R wave coincides with end–diastole exactly. At least one of the equilibrium views must be angled individually by trial and error to afford the best separation of the left ventricle from the right ventricle and left atrium for the determination of the left ventricular ejection fraction. This is called the modified left anterior oblique view. Modified means the camera usually has 5 to 15 degrees of craniocaudal tilt.

Pharmaceuticals

When both techniques are to be used, the patient is given stannous ion IV as stannous pyrophosphate 5 to 30 minutes before the injection of Tc-99m pertechnetate. Injection of the Tc-99m tracer serves the purpose of the first-pass angiogram and labels the red cells for the equilibrium study. If two first-pass studies are needed, e.g., rest and stress, then the first one should be accomplished with an agent cleared from the blood pool rapidly, e.g., Tc-99m DTPA or Tc-99m pertechnetate 1 hour before giving the stannous ion and proceeding with the second first-pass and equilibrium studies. A reasonable alternative is to administer the stannous ion, then do the first-pass study under the conditions most likely to show an abnormality, i.e., maximal exercise, and if the abnormality is not seen, then the baseline function is assumed to be normal, and the second first-pass study at rest is not done. If the abnormality does occur and is seen involving the inferior wall of the left ventricle under stress, the patient must have a resting first-pass study on a subsequent day to evaluate the inferior wall. Short-lived, high–photon flux, gamma-emitting nuclides such as tantalum-193 or gold-195m offer the opportunity to do multiple first-pass studies without the difficulties just detailed; however, each has its own drawbacks, not the least of which is the radiation dosimetry to the nuclear medicine staff.

Most laboratories use the in vivo method for preparing Tc-99m–labeled

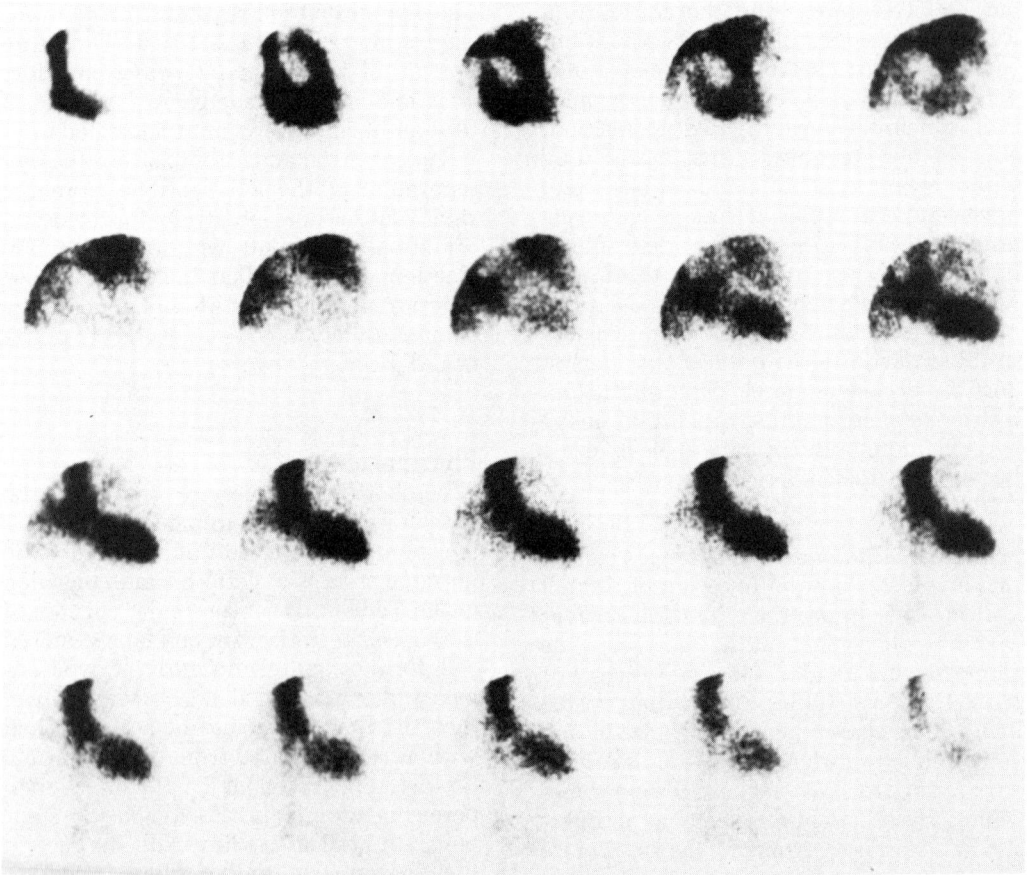

Figure 9-9. Angiogram. One-second frames in a 30-degree RAO view of the heart blood pool after a bolus IV injection of 20 mCi of Tc-99m sodium pertechnetate. The third row shows the left ventricular phase.

RBCs for equilibrium imaging because of its convenience. The Brookhaven kit for stannous ion gives a significantly higher binding efficiency and an improved target-to-background ratio but requires more preparation handling time (30 minutes) and has too large a volume for a compact first-pass bolus. Tc-99m-tin-labeled red cell study patients may be imaged for up to 6 hours without the administration of additional tracer material, allowing serial studies, whereas Tc-99m-labeled albumin study patients usually cannot be imaged beyond 1 hour because of seepage of the albumin out of the intravascular space.

Interpretation

Radionuclide ventriculographic studies yield two basic categories of information: focal and global. Focal information refers to localized wall motion abnormalities seen at rest or occurring under stressful conditions. This type of information is usually obtained from looking at movies of the beating heart acquired under resting or stressful conditions. Some information is also obtained from a variety of functional images designed to represent three-dimensional changes in a planar image. These functional images are derived, for instance, by subtracting end-systole from end-diastole to show the distribution of the blood volume that was ejected from the ventricle during systole.

Global refers to the quantifiable information derived from these studies, e.g., ejection fraction, end-diastolic volume, left ventricular output, and dV/dt, etc. Together, focal and global information from cardiac chamber imaging provides insight into the functional status of the heart. It cannot provide the anatomic detail of a coronary artery lesion needed by the surgeon before bypass grafting, nor can it provide a direct measure of pressures within the heart or visualization of the heart valves. These are the province of contrast angiographic and echographic techniques.

REFERENCES

1. Hillis LD, Braunwald E: Myocardial ischemia. N Engl J Med 296:971, 1977
2. Willerson JT, Parkey RN, Bonte FJ, et al: Pathophysiologic considerations and clinicopathological correlates of technetium-99m stannous pyrophosphate myocardial scintigraphy. Semin Nucl Med 10:54, 1980
3. Chervu LR: Radiopharmaceuticals in cardiovascular nuclear medicine. Semin Nucl Med 9:241, 1979
4. Lebowitz E, Green MW, Fairchild R, et al: Thallium-201 for medical use I. J Nucl Med 16:151, 1974
5. Atkins HL, Budinger TF, Lebowitz E, et al: Thallium-201 for medical use. Part 3: Human distribution and physical imaging properties. J Nucl Med 18:133, 1977
6. Ritchie JL, Hamilton GW: Biologic properties of thallium. In Ritchie JL, Hamilton GW, Wackers FJ Th (eds): Thallium-201 Myocardial Imaging. New York, Raven Press, 1978, pp 9–28
7. Britton J, Blank M: Thallium activation of Na-K-ATPase of rabbit kidney. Biochim Biophys Acta 159:160, 1968
8. Holman BL, Lesch M, Zweimann FG, et al: Detection and sizing of acute myocardial infarcts with Tc-99m (Sn) tetracycline. N Engl J Med 291:159, 1974
9. Nelson MF, Melton RE, Van Wazer JR: Sodium trimetaphosphate as a bone-imaging agent. 1. Animal Studies. J Nucl Med 16:1043, 1975
10. Subramanian G, McAfee JG, Blair RJ, et al: Technetium 99m methylene diphosphonate—A superior agent for skeletal imaging: Comparison with other technetium complexes. J Nucl Med 16:744, 1975
11. Dewanjee MK, Anderson GS, Wahner HW: Pharmacodynamics of stannous-chelates administered with technetium-99m chelates for radionuclide imaging. In Sodd VS, Hoogland DR, Allen DR, Ice RD (eds). Radiopharmaceuticals II. New York Society of Nuclear Medicine, 1979, pp 421–434
12. Buja LM, Tofe AJ, Kulkarni PV, et al: Sites and mechanisms of localization of technetium 99m phosphorous radiopharmaceuticals in acute myocardial infarcts and other tissues. J Clin Invest 60:724, 1977
13. Rhodes BA: Considerations in the radiolabeling of albumin. Semin Nucl Med 4:281, 1974
14. Nusynowitz MI, Straw JD, Benedetto AR, et al: Blood clearance rates of technetium-99 albumin preparations: Concise Communication. J Nucl Med 19:1142, 1978
15. Smith TD, Richards P: A simple kit for the preparation of Tc-99m red blood cells. J Nucl Med 17:126, 1976
16. Srivastava SC, Chervu LR: Radionuclide labeled red blood cells. Current status and future prospects. Semin Nucl Med 14:68, 1982
17. Chandler WM, Shuck LD: Effect of tin on pertechnetate distribution. J Nucl Med 16:690, 1975
18. Pavel DG, Zimmer AM, Patterson VN: In vivo labeling of red blood cells with Tc-99m: A new approach to blood pool visualization. J Nucl Med 18:305, 1977
19. Zimmer AM, Pavel DG: Technical parameters involved in the in vivo red cell labeling technique. J Nucl Med 18:637, 1977
20. Hamilton RG, Alderson PO: A comparative evaluation of techniques for rapid and efficient in vivo labeling of red cells with Tc-99 pertechnetate. J Nucl Med 18:1008, 1977
21. Callahan RJ, Froelich JW, McKusick KA, et al: A modified method for the in vivo labeling of red blood cells with Tc-99m: Concise communication. J Nucl Med 23:315, 1982
22. Srivastava SC, Babich JB, Richards P: A new kit method for the selective labeling of erythrocytes in whole blood with technetium-99m. J Nucl Med 24:P128, 1983
23. Dewanjee MK: Binding of Tc-99m ion to

hemoglobin. J Nucl Med 15:703, 1974
24. Straub RF, Srivastava SC, Meinken GE, et al: Transport, binding and uptake kinetics of tin and technetium in the in-vitro Tc-99m labeling of red blood cells. J Nucl Med 26:P130, 1985
25. Larson SM, Hamilton GW, Richards P, et al: Kit-labeled technetium 99m red blood cells (Tc-99m-RBC's) for clinical cardiac chamber imaging. Eur J Nucl Med 3:227, 1978
26. Stevenson JS, Eckelman WC, Sobocinski PZ, et al: The toxicity of Sn-pyrophosphate: Clinical manifestations prior to acute LD50. J Nucl Med 15:252, 1974
27. Coffey JL: Oak Ridge Associated Universities, Oak Ridge, Tenn. Personal communication.
28. Hladik WB III, Nigg KK, Rhodes BA: Drug-induced changes in the biologic distribution of radiopharmaceuticals. Semin Nucl Med 12:184, 1982
29. Hegge FN, Hamilton GW, Larson SM, et al: Cardiac chamber imaging: A comparison of red blood cells labeled with Tc-99m in vitro and in vivo. J Nucl Med 19:129, 1978
30. Leitl GP, Drew HM, Kelly ME, et al: Interference with Tc-99m labeling of red blood cells (RBCs) by RBC antibodies. J Nucl Med 21:P44, 1980
31. Bellar GA, Watson DD, Ackell P, et al: Time course of thallium-201 redistribution after transient myocardial ischemia. Circulation 61:791, 1980

CHAPTER 10

Lung

Lung-imaging radiopharmaceuticals may be divided into two main categories: (1) lung perfusion agents and (2) lung ventilation agents. Typically the perfusion agents are radiolabeled particles that are temporarily trapped in the pulmonary arterioles and capillaries and provide diagnostic information regarding regional blood flow. Ventilation agents are either radioactive gases or radioaerosols used to demonstrate the patency of the lung airways and parenchyma.

PHYSIOLOGIC ANATOMY OF THE LUNG

The lung may be divided into three functional zones: the conducting zone, the respiratory zone, and the intermediate or transitory zone.[1] The conducting zone is comprised of the bronchi and bronchioles, which distribute inspired gas to and collect expired gas from the terminal airway units. In addition, the pulmonary arteries and veins distribute and remove, respectively, blood to the capillary bed. In the respiratory zone, which is comprised of a complex of alveoli and capillaries, air and blood come into closest contact, thus facilitating gas exchange. This zone is sometimes termed the gas exchange apparatus (Figs. 10–1 and 10–2). The intermediate zone links together the conducting and respiratory zones.

Figure 10–1 illustrates the branching pattern of the airways from the trachea to the alveolar sacs.[2] The bronchi and bronchioles function only to conduct air to the more peripheral zones. After inspiration fresh air moves into the lungs by bulk flow up to the respiratory bronchioles, i.e., to where the transition zone begins, but from there the movement of oxygen into the alveolar ducts and alveoli occurs by diffusion. Higher tidal volumes of air penetrate deeper by bulk flow, but never reach the end of the alveolar system.[3]

Under normal conditions air freely moves into and out of the airways and respiratory zone, and airway resistance is minimal. In the presence of disease, however, airway resistance may increase both at inspiration and expiration. In less severe cases of asthma or emphysema, for example, air may enter the bronchioles and alveoli readily because chest expansion and the inflow of air inflates these structures. Expiration,

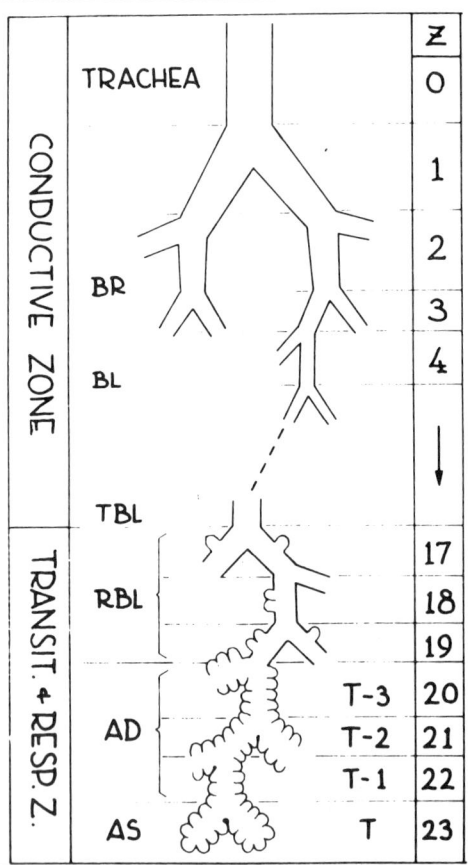

Figure 10-1. Branching pattern of the airways from the trachea to the alveolar sacs. BR, bronchi; BL, bronchioles; TBL, terminal bronchioles; RBL, respiratory bronchioles; AD, alveolar duct; AS, alveolar sac. *(From Weibel ER: Morphometry of the Human Lung. New York, Academic Press, 1963, with permission.)*

however, is more difficult because the weakened, diseased bronchioles collapse from the pressure of the thoracic cage against the lungs, which leads to air trapping in the alveoli. In advanced disease air intake also may be obstructed because of inflamed bronchi and bronchioles and the presence of mucous plugs, which occur often in bronchial asthma.

The pulmonary artery has 22 to 26 branches. At about the 24th branch, a short connector artery of 125-μm diameter divides at right angles to form two distribution arteries (Fig. 10-3). The smallest diameter distribution arteries range between 60 and 100 μm, and from these vessels short precapillary arterioles of 25-μm diameter arise at right angles. These vessels then break up into alveolar capillary beds. The basic elements of the alveolar capillary bed are the capillary segments, which have the shape of short cylindrical tubes. The segments are modified at their ends in the form of wedges to allow each segment to join at either end with two adjacent segments. The average internal diameter of the capillary segment is 8 μm (range 6 to 10 μm).[2]

It is clear from the structure of the alveolar capillary network that blood entering each precapillary arteriole has many alternative routes to reach the postcapillary venule. This fact is important in that pulmonary hemodynamics will not be appreciably affected by a routine lung-scanning dose of radiolabeled particles unless advanced lung disease and pulmonary hypertension are present.

Normal blood flow in the lung is influenced by hydrostatic pressure. In the upright position the mean pulmonary arterial pressure is 3 mm Hg at the top of the lung, 13 mm Hg in the midzone, and 21 mm Hg at the bottom of the lung. This pressure difference alters blood distribution between the upper and lower parts of the lung. Studies whereby xenon-133 dissolved in saline is injected and counted over the lung have shown that in normal subjects a change from the upright to the supine position results in a doubling of blood perfusion to the upper lung zones at the cost of the lower zones, the midzones recording no change.[4] For this reason lung-scanning agents are usually injected while the patient is supine.

Blood flow to the lung is affected by various pathologic conditions. The presence of a pulmonary embolus not only mechanically blocks blood flow to the lung area distal to the blockade but also may cause local vasospasm, which further decreases blood flow to the region.[5] In the case of air-

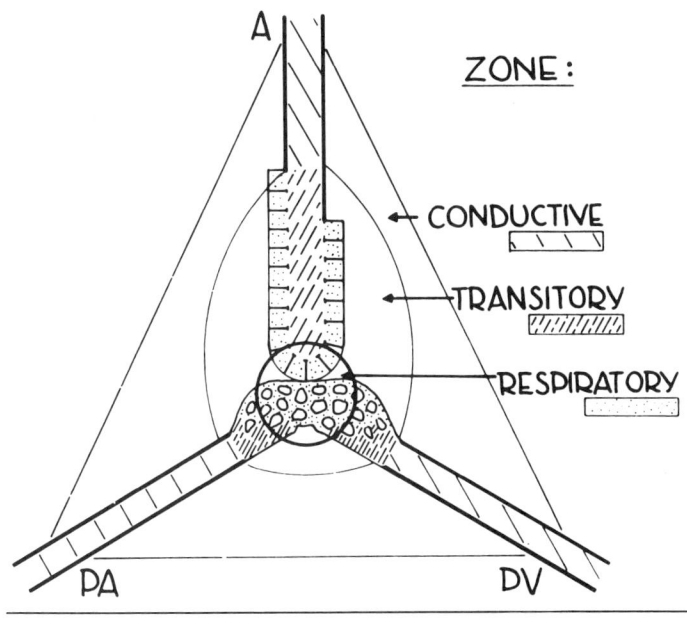

Figure 10-2. The three functional zones of the lung: conductive, transitory, and respiratory (gas exchange apparatus). *(From Weibel ER: Morphometry of the Human Lung. New York, Academic Press, 1963, with permission.)*

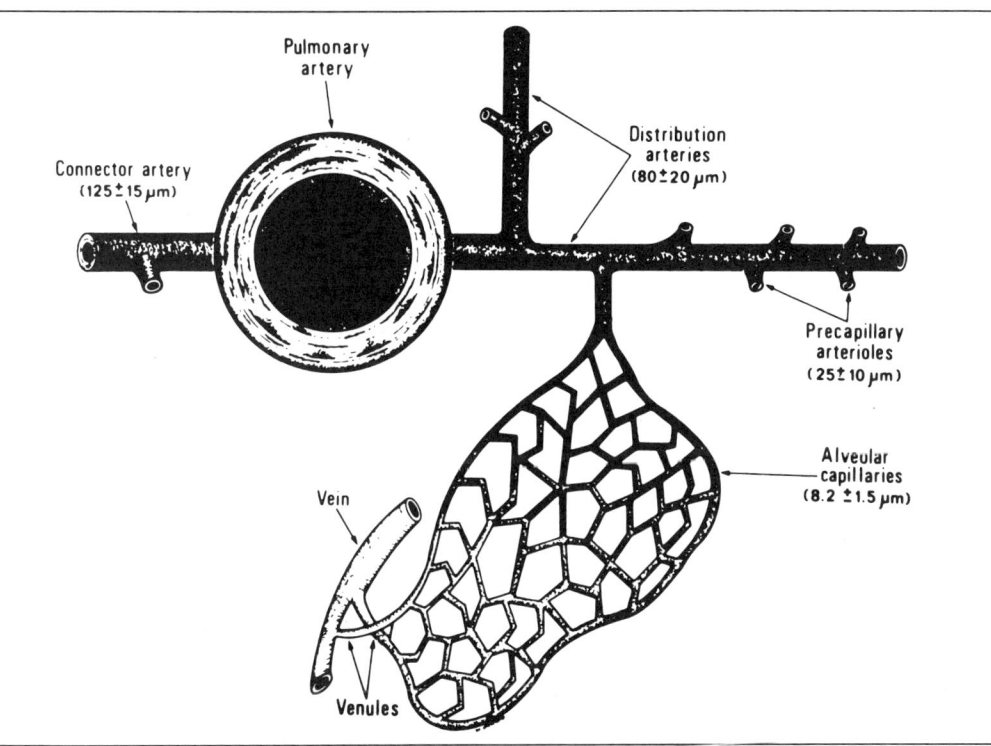

Figure 10-3. Schematic representation of the pulmonary vasculature with an emphasis on the alveolar capillary network demonstrating the totally anastomotic nature of the capillary bed. *(From Davis MA, 1975, p 267, with permission.[15])*

237

way disease such as emphysema, destruction of many alveolar walls also causes destruction of their capillaries. This results in increased vascular resistance to blood flow. Additionally, a physiologic decrease in local blood perfusion occurs in emphysema because emphysematous alveoli have poor exchange of air with the atmosphere. The resulting alveolar hypoxia causes vasoconstriction of blood vessels, which shunts blood to other areas of the lung that are better aerated.[5] Ventilatory disease may thus cause blood perfusion defects to be visualized in the lung scan.

LUNG PERFUSION IMAGING AGENTS

Site-specific localization of radioactivity in the lungs began with Au-198 labeled to 50-μm-sized carbon particles to irradiate tumor tissue.[6]

The diagnostic value of radioactive particles entrapped within the lung was investigated in dogs in 1963.[7-9] Taplin et al prepared I-131 human serum albumin (HSA) macroaggregates (I-131 MAA) and demonstrated their ability to be trapped and eventually cleared from the lungs. They performed the first toxicity studies to demonstrate the safety of injecting large numbers of particles intravenously. After these studies, from 1965 to 1970, I-131 MAA became accepted for routine clinical use in humans as the agent of choice for lung imaging of suspected emboli.

The search for an agent with more favorable imaging properties than I-131 led to the development of particles labeled with shorter half-lived radionuclides. These included In-113m ferric hydroxide[10] and Tc-99m ferrous hydroxide macroaggregates; however, toxic reactions associated with the use of these preparations led to their disuse.[11]

In 1969, Tc-99m human albumin microspheres (HAM) were developed by Zolle et al and Rhodes et al.[12,13] The HAM could be microsieved to control particle size and were biodegradable in vivo. A kit form using sodium thiosulfate as the tagging agent became available from the 3M Company.[13] Labeling efficiency was only 60 to 70 percent, however, and insonation was necessary to break up aggregation of microspheres.

Subramanian et al[14] developed Tc-99m MAA as an "instant kit" using stannous chloride as the tagging agent. Labeling yields were quantitative and required no separation of unbound pertechnetate. The Tc-99m MAA kit became commercially available in the mid 1970s, soon to be joined by a Tc-Sn HAM kit. These two radiopharmaceuticals are currently the agents of choice for lung perfusion imaging.

The Tc-Sn-MAA Kit

Kits for the routine preparation of Tc-99m MAA are available from several commercial sources. Kits may be prepared extemporaneously if the need arises by the following method.

Solution A	Sodium acetate anhydrous	1.0 g
	Human serum albumin injection (25%)	0.1 g
	Sterile water for injection	qs 10.0 ml
Solution B	Stannous chloride dihydrate	0.025 g
	HCl, 12 M	0.4 ml
	Sterile water for injection	qs 5.0 ml

All solutions are prepared under a nitrogen atmosphere. To prepare the reaction mixture, 5 ml of solution A followed by 1 ml of solution B are added through a 0.22-μm sterile membrane filter to 19 ml of sterile water for injection contained in a 30-ml serum vial with a Teflon stirbar. This pH 5 mixture is heated with stirring in an 80 to 85°C water bath for 2 to 3 minutes. The soft aggregate formed is removed into a 50-ml syringe and then forced into a new 30-ml vial through a 27-gauge needle. The shearing force breaks the soft aggregate into 1- to 5-μm-sized particles. Subsequently, the suspension is heated with stirring for 15 minutes at 73 ± 1°C to form firm 20- to 50-μm-sized aggregates. One milliliter of suspension, containing approximately 5 million particles, is aliquotted into sterile 10-ml vials that are frozen in dry ice and then kept for 1 to 2 months in a freezer before use.

The suspension must be checked before final packaging to assure the absence of large clumps (by visual inspection) and to determine particle size and number (by microscopic inspection). Sterility and pyrogen tests must be performed and the product radiolabeled with Tc-99m pertechnetate to check radiochemical purity. Biologic distribution studies in animals must be performed to confirm appropriate organ distribution.

Commercial kits are usually lyophilized and vary widely in the number of particles per kit (Table 10–1). Kits may contain added substances to facilitate particle dispersion during reconstitution with pertechnetate.

The Tc-Sn HAM Kit

The production of albumin microspheres is quite an involved process. The general procedure requires rapid mixing of a small volume of aqueous albumin solution in a large volume of vegetable oil to produce an emulsion of minute spheres dispersed in oil. Sphere size depends on mixing speed and the ratio of albumin to oil. Subsequently, the oil is heated to evaporate water from the spheres to solidify them. Ether is added to the mixture, and the spheres are separated by filtration followed by ether washings to remove residual oil. Dried spheres are then sieved to obtain the appropriate size for lung studies (15 to 30 μm). The selected spheres are then treated with a stannous chloride solution to incorporate stannous ion into the spheres. Finally, the spheres are packaged into serum vials and lyophilized.

The vial contains Pluronic F-68, which aids in dispersing the spheres during reconstitution with Tc-99m pertechnetate. Quality control testing for microspheres is similar to MAA.

Preparation and Dispensing Tc-99m MAA or Tc-99m HAM for Lung Imaging

Daily preparation of these kits simply requires the addition of Tc-99m pertechnetate. Generally, the particles of MAA or HAM disperse readily after a sharp snap of the wrist while holding the vial between the thumb and forefinger. Insonation of the HAM kit is suggested to assure dispersion of any aggregated spheres. Individual spheres will not be broken down further by this process. The MAA kits, however, should *not* be insonated to disperse particles because this process may break the soft aggregates into smaller-sized particles that will pass through the lung capillaries.

The appropriate amount of activity of Tc-99m pertechnetate should be added to the kit to assure that each patient dose contains a sufficient number of particles for the lung scan. A typical adult dose is 3 mCi injected intravenously and contains between 100,000 and 600,000 particles as recommended by the various manufacturers. If a Sn-MAA kit contains 5 million particles, adding 100 mCi of Tc-99m pertechnetate will thus provide 150,000 particles per 3-mCi dose. Remember that the particle number per dose will increase with time because of Tc-99m decay so that, for example, 6 hours later the same 3-mCi dose will contain 300,000 particles.

Tc-MAA or -HAM particles will settle out of solution quite rapidly; therefore, before obtaining a dose the vial should be shaken gently to redisperse the particles. The same problem exists for doses in syringes that sit for some time before injection. The syringe should be mixed just before injection, otherwise solution may be injected without a sufficient number of particles. During injection blood should not be drawn into the syringe and mixed with particles because clumping of particles may occur, which leads to "hot spots" on the lung scan. In some instances the number of par-

TABLE 10-1. Tc-99m KITS FOR LUNG PERFUSION IMAGING

Manufacturer	Composition	Quantity	No. of Particles per Kit	Particle Size—Range (μm)
A	Human albumin aggr	2.0 mg	$8 \pm 4 \times 10^6$	10-90
	Human albumin	0.5 mg		
	$SnCl_2 \cdot 2\, H_2O$	120 μg		
	Lactose	80.0 mg		
	Succinic acid	24.0 mg		
	Sodium acetate	1.4 mg		
B	Human albumin aggr	0.34 mg	$2.0 \times 10^6 \pm 25\%$	15-90 (90%)
	Stannous tartrate	0.27 mg		
	Isotonic saline	0.6 ml		
C	Human albumin aggr	1.0 mg	$3.6-6.5 \times 10^6$	10-90 (90%)
	Human albumin	10.0 mg		
	Sodium chloride	10.0 mg		
	Stannous chloride (max)	0.07 mg		
D	Human albumin aggr	1.5 mg	$4-5 \times 10^6$ (avg)	10-90 (90%)
	Human albumin	10.0 mg		
	$SnCl_2 \cdot 2\, H_2O$ (min)	0.06 mg	$1.0-8.0 \times 10^6$	Avg size, 20-40
	Stannous and stannic chloride (max)	0.16 mg		
	Sodium chloride	1.8 mg		
E	Human albumin aggr	2.0 mg	$6.8 \pm 0.8 \times 10^6$	10-90 (90%)
	Stannous tin (min)	0.095 mg		
	$SnCl_2 \cdot 2\, H_2O$ (max)	0.21 mg		
	Sodium chloride	17.0 mg		
F	HAM	5.0 mg	$1.0-1.5 \times 10^6$	10-35 (95%)
	Tin (as stannous and stannic chloride pentahydrate)	100-250 μg		
	Pluronic F-68	5.0 mg		

Manufacturers: A, Mallinckrodt; B, Medi-physics; C, Dupont-NEN; D, Squibb; E, Syncor; F, 3M Co.

ticles injected must be limited because of the patient's age (pediatrics) and condition (pulmonary hypertension). These exceptions are discussed in more detail under particle toxicity.

Before dispensing patient doses the suspension should be inspected visually to ensure the absence of any large clumps. Microscopic inspection may also be necessary to confirm proper particle size. Storage of the radiolabeled product in a refrigerator (2 to 8 °C) is encouraged because these products contain protein and no bacterial preservative.

Manufacturer Suggested Average No. of Particles/Study	Lung Half-life		Kit Storage Before Labeling	Kit Storage After Labeling	Expiration Time After Labeling
	Biologic	Effective			
600,000 (200,000–1,200,000)	10.8 hr	3.8 hr	15–30°C	2–8°C	8 hr
350,000 (200,000–700,000)	—	—	2–8°C	2–8°C	6 hr
350,000 (200,000–700,000)	5.6 hr	—	15–30°C	2–8°C	8 hr
350,000	2 to 3 hr	—	2–8°C	2–8°C	6 hr
350,000 (200,000–700,000)	—	—	2–8°C	2–8°C	6 hr
100,000 (90,000–600,000)	3 hr 13 hr (microspheres alone)	2 hr	15–30°C	2–8°C	8 hr

BIODISTRIBUTION AND MECHANISM OF LUNG LOCALIZATION

More than 90 percent of Tc-99m MAA or Tc-99m HAM is extracted by the pulmonary arterioles and capillaries in the first passage through the lungs. The mechanism of localization is by physical entrapment of particles that are larger than the blood vessel lumen. Distribution of particles in the lung is a function of regional blood flow; thus, in a normal lung radiolabeled particles are distributed uniformly throughout the lung tissue, and it appears "hot." Where blood flow is occluded or restricted because of emboli or vessel constriction, particles are prevented from passage beyond these points. This is seen as perfusion defects or "cold spots" distal to the point of obstruction. Large emboli block larger-sized vessels and produce larger-sized perfusion defects.

PROPERTIES OF RADIOLABELED PARTICLES FOR LUNG IMAGING

A number of factors must be considered in the design and use of labeled particles for lung perfusion imaging. The most basic considerations are particle size, particle number, quality or hardness, and chemical composition. These factors influence the biodistribution, metabolic fate, and potential toxicity of lung perfusion agents.

Particle Size

The first criterion for localization in the lung is a particle size large enough to be trapped in the pulmonary arterioles and capillaries. Because the smallest capillaries have an internal diameter of 6 to 10 µm, particles smaller than 10 µm are unsatisfactory because they will readily pass through the lung. On the other hand, particles too large will obstruct larger arterioles, which are fewer in number, potentially producing a serious reduction in blood flow and elevation of pulmonary arterial pressure. Davis[15] has concluded that the ideal vessels to block in the lung are the capillary segments because they are highly anastomotic and blockade of one or even several capillary segments will not substantially alter blood flow or pressure. Davis recommends that the ideal particle size is 13.5 ± 1.5 µm to achieve a high extraction efficiency into the capillary bed, but he concedes that because of technical problems of production 15 ± 5-µm (10- to 20-µm range) particles are more practical. Such a tight size range is very impractical for MAA, however, and additionally the soft-textured 10- to 20-µm MAA particles clear the lung too rapidly ($T_{1/2}$, 30 minutes) to be useful for lung imaging. For this reason most commercial MAA kits contain particles in the 10- to 90-µm range, with the majority in the 20- to 60-µm range. Because of their method of production microspheres can be produced in the 10- to 20-µm range, and because they are harder particles, their slower clearance rate ($T_{1/2}$, 1 to 2 hours) makes them useful for lung imaging. Figure 10–4 illustrates the microscopic appearance of MAA and HAM particles.

Particle Number

In response to reported problems of acute toxicity from administering too many particles, several investigators embarked on the task of determining the ideal number of particles that would produce a satisfactory lung scan. In 1974 Heck and Duley[16] reported the results of their investigation to determine the number of particles of Tc-99m albumin microspheres (15 to 30 µm) required to provide satisfactory lung images. Their analysis demonstrated that increasing the number of counts by increasing the collection time did not improve image uniformity unless an adequate number of particles were present in the lungs. Spurious scan abnormalities (patchy scans) resulted when less than 15,000 particles were administered. When a dose containing 30,000 particles was injected, scan patchiness near the periphery of the lung was observed. This abnormal pattern was noted first in the periphery because this area of the lung has minimal tissue thickness. Further, because the total number of particles viewed by the detector was lowest in this region, the percent variability of particle distribution was greatest near the lung edge. Because of these results and the observation that a syringe may retain particles, particularly with small-volume doses, a minimum of 60,000 microspheres was recommended for an adequate lung image.

In 1977 Dworkin et al[17] reported the results of a similar study that determined the effect of particle number on lung images with 10- to 50-µm-size particles of Tc-99m

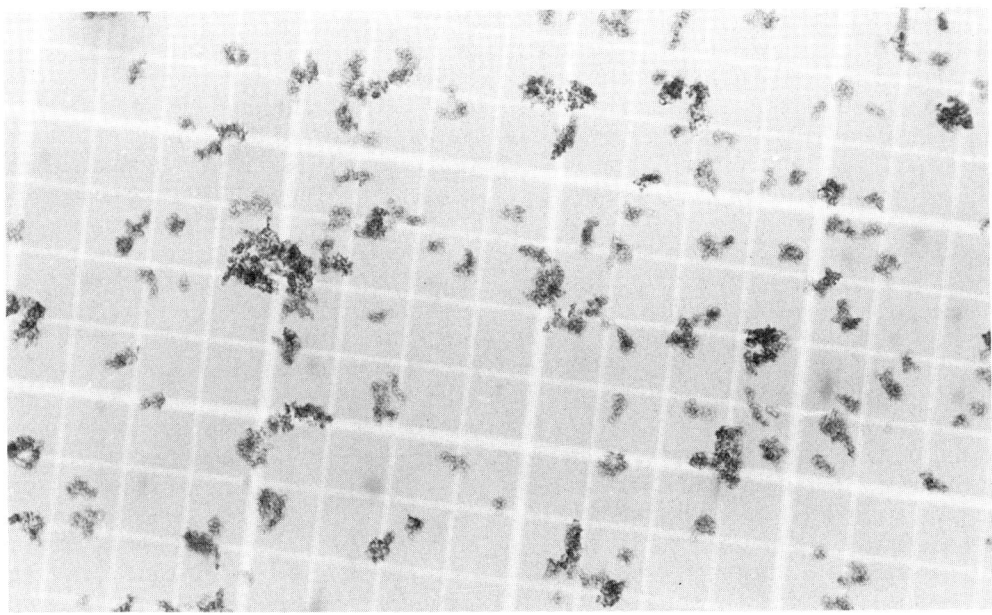

Figure 10-4. A. Photomicrograph of MAA particles used for perfusion lung imaging. The distance between lines equals 50 μm.

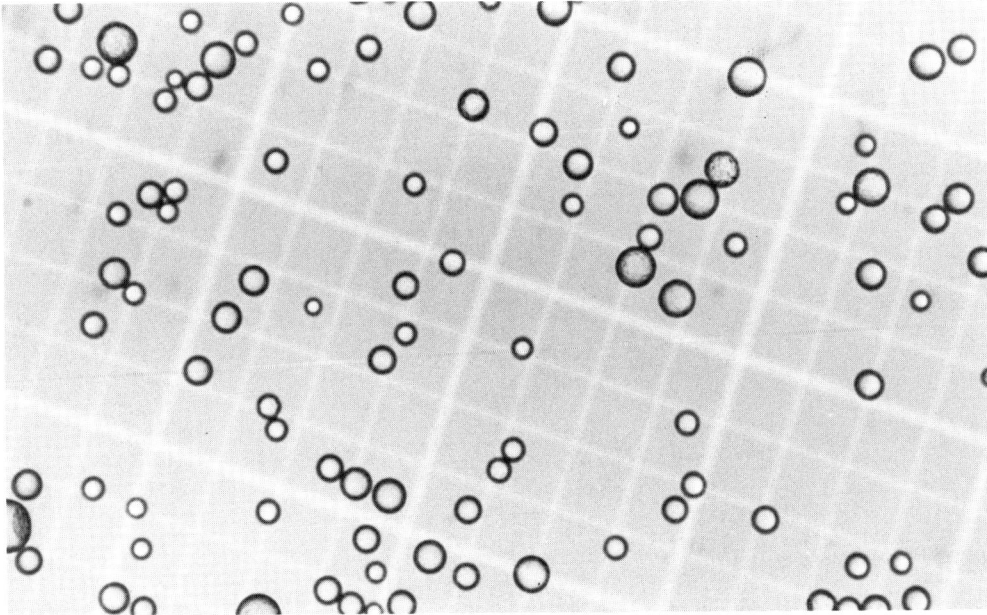

Figure 10-4. B. Photomicrograph of HAM used for perfusion lung imaging. The distance between lines equals 50 μm.

stannous MAA in dogs. The results confirmed the work of Heck and Duley, and they concluded that the minimum number of particles required for a satisfactory lung scan was 60 particles/g of lung or 60,000 particles/study if one assumes that the weight of the lungs in an average human is 1000 g. An upper limit of 250,000 particles for a lung scan was suggested because little is to be gained above this number whereas the chances of toxicity are increased.

Particle Hardness and Chemical Composition

Ideally, particles that lodge in the pulmonary blood vessels should be biodegradable and produce no local tissue reactions. For these reasons, HSA is routinely used because it is a natural body constituent. Additionally, it can be heated to the desired hardness to achieve proper clearance from the lung.

In the early days of lung scanning concern was focused on the potential antigenic effects of the denatured protein particles. After extensive testing, Iio and Wagner[18] demonstrated that there was no evidence to prove that aggregated human albumin was antigenic to humans. This was corroborated by Taplin et al.[8]

Generally, for a given size particle a higher heating temperature will produce a harder particle that will take longer to break up and clear from the lungs. Zolle et al[12] demonstrated that albumin microspheres prepared at 118°C, 146°C, and 165°C had biologic half-times in dog lungs of 2.4, 7.2, and 144 hours, respectively.

Although albumin particles demonstrated no tissue reactions, pathologic changes were reported with the no-longer-used Tc-99m iron hydroxide macroaggregates.[15] Flushing reactions were also reported to occur with the latter, thus sug-

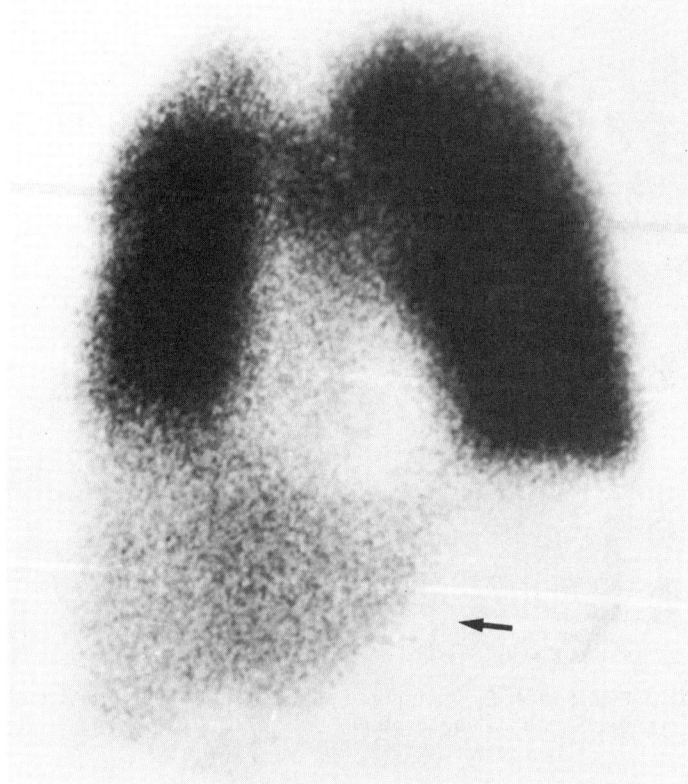

Figure 10-5. Anterior perfusion lung scan with Tc-99m MAA. Liver activity (*arrow*) is evident because particles that are too soft or too small readily pass through the lung capillaries.

gesting that its chemical composition was a factor in causing the reactions.

LUNG CLEARANCE AND METABOLIC FATE OF PARTICLES

The biodegradation of the MAA or HAM particles and their radiolabel must be slow enough to provide ample time for imaging, yet once imaging has been accomplished, the particles should then degrade as rapidly as possible.

It was shown by Taplin and MacDonald,[19] using an in vivo cinemicroscopic technique, that the mechanism of MAA clearance from the lungs is due to particle fragmentation by blood cell bombardment and by continuous forward and backward movement within arterioles until the aggregates are small enough to traverse the capillary lumina. Albumin microspheres do not fragment, as do MAA particles, but undergo dissolution, probably through the enzymatic action of pulmonary phagocytes.[20] Phagocytosis was not observed by Taplin when studying MAA particles.

The rate of particle clearance from the lung is a function of particle size distribution and number, method of preparation (related to particle hardness), and the state of lung health.

Smaller-sized particles are expected to have faster clearances. Taplin and MacDonald[19] demonstrated in dogs that I-131 MAA doses with particle sizes of 5 to 25 μm, 10 to 70 μm, and 10 to 150 μm had biologic half-times of 30 minutes, 4 to 6 hours, and 18 to 24 hours, respectively. Particles that are too soft because of inadequate heating or too small in size readily pass through the lungs and become localized in the liver. This is undesirable because of the close apposition of the right lung and liver, which is demonstrated in Figure 10-5.

The patient's condition may affect lung clearance of particles. Davis[21] determined that the average clearance half-time of Tc-99m iron hydroxide particles from the lung in normal subjects averaged 19 hours but was significantly slower in various degrees of pulmonary embolism (105 hours) and chronic lung disease (222 hours). Busse et al[22] demonstrated that the lung clearance rate of I-131-MAA was slower in asthmatics and in patients receiving steroid and immunosuppressive therapy, with viral pneumonia, and with chronic interstitial lung disease. In such cases, if multiple follow-up lung scans are anticipated, it is probably wise to administer the minimum number of particles necessary for a good-quality scan.

The half-times of several radiolabeled particles used in perfusion lung imaging are listed in Table 10-1. It is important to note that the activity present in the lungs at any particular time is not necessarily proportional to the number of particles present. In other words, the rates of activity clearance and of particle clearance per se may be different because a particle may partially dissolve or break up and release a portion of its activity, but the particle would still be blocking the vessel. In this circumstance we find a decrease in lung activity but no change in the number of particles remaining or vessels occluded. Activity loss half-life may thus be significantly shorter than particle loss half-life. This concept is discussed in detail by Davis.[15]

Once the particles are cleared from the lungs they are engulfed by the reticuloendothelial system (RES), primarily in the liver. Taplin and MacDonald[19] demonstrated that I-131 aggregates of albumin undergo proteolytic digestion in the Kupffer's cells as evidenced by the presence of I-131-labeled tyrosine, peptides, and free radionuclide in the plasma and urine during the first few hours after injection. Their biologic half-time in the liver was 9 to 10 hours. Tc-MAA is also metabolized in the liver, with urinary excretion of 30 to 75 percent of the dose in 24 hours depending on which commercial product is used. Kitani and Taplin[23] noted that excretion can also occur into the gallbladder and intestine with Tc-MAA produced by the iron–ascorbate method. The fate of Tc-MAA produced by the stannous chloride method is not known for certain but probably involves enzymatic digestion of albumin, which releases Tc-labeled amino acids and pertechnetate, which are excreted into the urine. A fraction of the activity also remains in the liver, probably as insoluble Tc-colloid. The biologic fate of dual-labeled Tc-HSA colloid labeled with carbon-14 HSA and Tc-99m support this mechanism.[24] Such an agent used for liver imaging demonstrated a biologic half-life of C-14 activity in the liver of 4 hours and 11 hours for Tc-99m activity.

PARTICLE TOXICITY

Safety and effectiveness considerations with particulate lung-scanning agents have been reviewed.[25] In the early days of lung scanning with I-131 MAA a typical lung-scanning dose (LSD) contained 1×10^6 particles. Studies performed by Taplin and MacDonald[19] in normal dogs demonstrated that a wide margin of safety existed when such doses were administered. These studies showed that the first sign of acute toxicity, observed as a rise in pulmonary arterial pressure (PAP), occurred at a dose of 20 mg/kg body weight, which was greater than 1000 times the average LSD and about 5000 times the minimum lethal dose. This safety factor can be appreciated more fully when one considers that in the normal lung less than 1 percent of the arterioles and capillaries are blocked by such doses.[15]

Despite this wide margin of safety in normal subjects, several deaths[26-29] have been reported to be associated with the administration of MAA for lung scanning. Evaluation of these cases revealed that the patients suffered from severe pulmonary hypertension. Their underlying diseases had caused narrowing and occlusion of the pulmonary blood vessels. In each case, immediately after injection of the MAA dose, clinical deterioration occurred and was manifested by respiratory distress, cyanosis, hypertension, and eventual death. Each of these reports discussed the need in such cases to decrease the number of particles injected and to restrict their size to below 50 µm, preferably in the 10- to 30-µm range.

It has been shown by Davis and Taube[30] and Allen et al[31] that the primary cause of cardiopulmonary toxicity associated with lung-scanning agents is the size and number of particles injected. Large particles, when compared with the same size dose of small particles, were more effective in raising the PAP. This inverse relationship between particle size and number in producing an acute toxic response is derived from the fact that larger particles block larger-sized pulmonary arterioles, which are fewer in number in the lung.

Allen et al[32] demonstrated that the safety factor for an LSD of 1×10^6 particles of Tc-stannous-MAA (30 to 50 µm) was 125 based on the elevation of PAP. That is to say, it would take 125 times the LSD to produce a 10 to 20 percent elevation of the PAP in normal lung. If only 100,000 particles are administered for a lung scan, this safety factor would be ten times larger (1250); this emphasizes why it is desirable to limit the number of particles administered to only that number that will give satisfactory lung scans, i.e., not more than 250,000. Although safety factors for 100,000 particles appear large, it must be emphasized that they are for normal lung and must be considered with caution in patients with severe pulmonary disease. In patients with pulmonary hypertension only the minimum number of particles (60,000) is recommended if a lung scan is performed.

In addition to patients with pulmonary hypertension, the pediatric patient requires special consideration. Heyman[33] makes note that a significant increase in the number of alveoli and pulmonary arteries occurs during the first few years of life and reaches adult levels at about 8 years of age. Further, the increase in alveolar development is 10 to 30 percent of adult values during the first year of life and up to 50 percent the adult number of 3 years. He suggests limiting the number of particles to 50,000 in the newborn infant and 165,000 in children up to 1 year old. Under such circumstances Davis and Taube[34] describe a technique for preparing pediatric doses whereby excess particles from MAA kits are discarded and a number that can be radiolabeled with Tc-99m pertechnetate to achieve the desired concentration for pediatric doses is retained.

In summary, several factors must be considered before a lung-scanning dose of radiolabeled particles is administered to a patient. Most important are particle size and number and the patient's condition or age. It appears that the minimum number of particles required for a satisfactory lung scan is 60,000, with a recommended maximum of about 250,000. Commercially available MAA kits contain most of the particles in the 10- to 90-μm range, but each kit varies considerably in its total number of particles (Table 10–1). A protocol should thus be established in each department for the preparation of LSDs based on the type of kit used and the age and condition of the patient. It is also strongly recommended that separate protocols be established for the preparation of LSDs for normal adults, patients suspected of pulmonary hypertension who should receive only the minimum number of particles, and pediatric patients who should receive the appropriate fraction of the adult dose.

Another concern that was considered when lung scanning was first established was the threat of cerebral microembolization resulting from particles that enter the systemic circulation either after degradation in the lung or through a right-to-left cardiac shunt. In this regard Taplin et al[8] reported that suspensions of albumin particles, which show initial pulmonary retention, are subsequently cleared from the lungs and transposed to the liver and spleen. It thus appeared that if the small particles were able to traverse the pulmonary capillaries they would also do so through cerebral vessels without significant danger of microembolization. In other studies Taplin and MacDonald[19] estimated the margin of safety for particles that were not degraded into smaller sizes in the lungs but entered the systemic circulation directly through a right-to-left cardiac shunt. These studies were performed in monkeys receiving direct carotid arterial injections of MAA. From these results, it was estimated that the margin of safety (based on no evidence of behavioral abnormalities or histologic changes in brain tissue) was greater than 2000 if one injected less than 1 mg of aggregates (10 to 60 μm) for a lung scan. In this size range, 1 mg of aggregates contained approximately 5 million particles. This margin of safety also assumed that there was a 50 percent shunt to the general circulation, including 10 percent to the head and 3 percent to each hemisphere.

LUNG VENTILATION IMAGING AGENTS

The ventilation lung scan became an important diagnostic tool in nuclear medicine because it improved the specificity of the perfusion lung scan in the diagnosis of pulmonary embolism (PE). Taplin and Chopra[35] reviewed the combined perfusion–ventilation lung scan and summarized the important findings. Before the establishment of the ventilation lung scan as a procedure, a diagnosis of PE was based on clinical suspicion and on finding one or more segmental or lobar perfusion defects in the face of a normal chest radiograph. When it was realized that the normal chest radiograph could not exclude all nonembolic causes of perfusion defects, particularly in cases involving chronic obstructive pulmonary disease, the ventilation lung scan (V) gained acceptance as a method for evaluating regional ventilation. It was shown to have diagnostic value in the early detection of obstructive pulmonary disease[35] where chest radiographs were relatively insensitive. More importantly, it added specificity to lung perfusion scanning (P) by demonstrating that perfusion defects of embolic origin (proven angiographically) were nearly always well ventilated, whereas those caused by parenchymal or obstructive airway disease were neither perfused nor ventilated (P/V matching). The finding of poorly perfused but well-ventilated regions (P/V mismatch) in radiographically normal lung was thus considered strong evidence for pulmonary embolism.[35]

METHODS AND MECHANISMS IN PERFUSION-VENTILATION IMAGING

Under ideal circumstances in a patient with suspected pulmonary embolism (PE) the perfusion lung scan is performed first because, if it is normal, there is generally no need for further evaluation. If perfusion defects are found, a subsequent ventilation scan will aid in obtaining a more definitive diagnosis. One very important consideration when the perfusion study is performed initially is that Tc-99m activity will be present in the lung during the ventilation study because the Tc-99m albumin particles will not have cleared from the lungs sufficiently before the ventilation study begins.

To perform a satisfactory ventilation study the ventilation agent used must have a photon energy greater than the 140-keV photon of Tc-99m. This will allow discrimination from the Tc-99m activity during the ventilation study. This is usually accomplished by using radionuclide gases (xenon-127, krypton-81m) of higher gamma energy. As an alternative method, Xe-133 gas (81 keV) or Tc-99m DTPA aerosol ventilation imaging can be performed before the Tc-99m MAA perfusion study. This method is less desirable, however, because subjects who demonstrate a normal perfusion scan will undergo an unnecessary ventilation study. It is the best alternative though if high-energy gases are not available. Further discussion on this matter will appear later in this chapter.

The general procedure followed in ventilation imaging with radioactive gases involves a three-part study: gas washin, equilibrium, and gas washout. The patient is attached to a closed-circuit breathing system supplied with oxygen. The study begins by having the patient breathe in a bolus of xenon gas (washin). Subsequently the patient rebreathes from the system for 5 minutes to equilibrate the gas between the system and the lung. Finally, the patient breathes in room air and exhales the xenon activity (washout). In normal lung, inhaled gas will diffuse readily into all areas of lung parenchyma, and upon exhalation, the radioactive gas will wash out readily from the lung. In lung where air flow and diffusion are impaired by obstructive airway disease, gas washin will be delayed or absent in obstructed areas; however, during the equilibrium phase where the patient rebreathes the radioactive gas, the gas atoms eventually diffuse into partially obstructed areas. Upon washout, normal areas lose activity readily whereas poorly ventilated areas clear gas slowly and therefore appear as hot areas of trapped gas. Examination of the washout phase makes xenon gas studies a more sensitive and quantifiable indicator of obstruction, especially in peripheral airways.[35] When areas of gas trapping coincide with areas of perfusion defects seen on the Tc-MAA scan, the probability for PE is low, and for obstructive airway disease it is high.

An alternative to the Tc-MAA perfusion–xenon ventilation study just described is to perform a xenon perfusion–xenon ventilation study. This technique is useful in patients for whom particle injections would pose a high risk; however, to see more than one lung surface in the perfusion phase, multiple injections must be performed. With this method xenon dissolved in saline is given intravenously during a breath hold at maximum lung capacity. This is maintained for 30 seconds. During this time xenon activity in the lung delimits blood flow to identify perfusion defects. Subsequently, the activity leaves the blood to enter the alveolar air because of the high air-to-blood partition coefficient for xenon. The patient then rebreathes from the breathing system for 5 minutes to establish equilibrium conditions. After this, the washout phase is imaged.

INERT RADIOACTIVE GASES

The most widely used agents for lung ventilation studies are the radioactive noble gases. This primarily grew out of the early work of Knipping et al[36] who developed a technique whereby patients inhaled Xe-133 and the accumulation of radioactivity in various regions of the lung was measured with external counters. In this way they were able to detect regional differences in ventilation caused by local disease.

One requirement for assessing regional ventilation is that the gas must be relatively insoluble in body fluid. The noble gases meet this requirement quite well because they are inert and poorly soluble in water.

Xenon-133

In the mid-1960s Xe-133 was first used for ventilation lung imaging. In the 1970s it gained clinical acceptance and became more widely used because it could be produced inexpensively in large quantities.

Xe-133 is produced commercially in a nuclear reactor as a by-product of uranium fission. It is available in unit-dose vials ready for patient use in 10-mCi and 20-mCi sizes, or it can be purchased in bulk 1-Ci size for in-house packaging. It is also available dissolved in sterile saline for intravenous use. A method of in-house packaging of xenon will be described later in this chapter.

Xe-133 has a 5.3-day half-life so that sufficient quantities can be kept in the nuclear medicine lab ready for use. Generally, new supplies need to be purchased weekly. The primary disadvantage of Xe-133 is poor image quality because of low photon abundance (35 photons/100 disintegrations) and low tissue penetration of the principal 81-keV gamma ray. Additionally, the 81-keV gamma requires the ventilation study to be performed before the perfusion scan with Tc-99m. This means that patients who have normal perfusion scans will receive a ventilation scan unnecessarily, whereas patients with abnormal perfusion scans may not be imaged in the optimal projection during the xenon study. For these reasons isotopes with gamma energies higher than 140 keV are more desirable.

Xenon-135

In 1968 Newhouse et al[37] introduced Xe-135 for ventilation studies. Xe-135 had the advantage of a 250-keV gamma with a 95 percent photon abundance that was ideal for camera imaging after the Tc-99m perfusion scan; however, it was not cost-effective because its short half-life (9 hours) precluded having a ready supply in the hospital except through daily shipments.

Xenon-127

In 1973 Hoffer et al[38] reported that improved quality images could be obtained using Xe-127 compared with Xe-133. This was due to higher photon energies and abundances, the primary gamma being 203 keV at a 68 percent abundance. This allowed ventilation imaging after the Tc-99m perfusion scan. Other benefits from Xe-127 were lower radiation dose because of no beta radiation and a longer shelf life because of the 36.4-day half-life. Several other reports[39-42] document the advantages of Xe-127, thus making it the agent of choice for ventilation imaging. Two precautions with the use of Xe-127 are the requirement for heavier lead shielding because of high-energy gammas (375 keV) and the contamination hazard of the long physical half-life.

Xe-127 is produced in a particle accelerator by the bombardment of a cesium target with protons. The production of large, multicurie quantities can only be accomplished in very large machines capable of accelerating protons up to several hundred MeV. These facilities include the Brookhaven Linac Isotopes Producer (BLIP) at the Brookhaven National Laboratory, the Los Alamos Meson Production Facility (LAMPF) at Los Alamos National Laboratory, and the cyclotron at the Tri University Meson Facility (TRIUMF) in Vancouver, British Columbia.

For several years the principal supplier has been Brookhaven, where Xe-127 is produced by bombarding cesium with 80- to

200-MeV protons according to the following reaction: ^{133}Cs(p,2p5n)^{127}Xe. After irradiation the cesium chloride target is held for 21 days before processing to allow shorter-lived xenon impurities (Xe-129m, 8 days; Xe-131m, 12 days) to decay to acceptable levels. At this time it is heated to melt the salt while sweeping off the Xe-127 and contaminants with helium gas. The contaminants, mostly radioiodine, are removed, and the Xe-127 is stored at liquid nitrogen temperature in a stainless steel ampule. Xe-127 is transferred from the storage ampule to glass shipping ampules by cryogenic pumping. At the hospital the Xe-127 activity is transferred from the bulk ampule into unit-dose vials for patient use. Five and 10-mCi unit-dose vials are available commercially.

Krypton-81m

In the mid-1970s Kr-81m gas became available as the daughter product of rubidium-81 decay in a generator system (^{81}Rb $\xrightarrow{4.5\ hr}$ ^{81m}Kr). The advantage of Kr-81m is a 190-keV gamma of 66 percent abundance that allows post perfusion imaging. When a perfusion defect is seen during the Tc-99m study, Kr-81m is immediately inhaled by the patient. This allows viewing of the patient in the best projection so that perfusion–ventilation match–mismatch combinations can be visualized. Because of its 13-second half-life, however, only gas washin images can be obtained. No equilibrium or washout gas–trapping images are possible. One advantage of the short half-life is insignificant radiation contamination problems. The primary disadvantage of this system is the 4.5-hour Rb-81 parent, which requires close proximity to the accelerator production facility for daily shipments. For this reason Kr-81m is not widely used.

Table 10–2 compares the properties of radioactive gases used for ventilation imaging.

BIOLOGIC DISTRIBUTION OF XENON

The amount of xenon that enters the body during a ventilation study is directly related to the lung air concentration, the duration of exposure, and xenon's solubility in tissue fluid. The poor solubility of xenon in water (12 percent at 25 °C) is the reason for its slow absorption into the body. It requires about 30 hours of rebreathing for xenon to reach an equilibrium concentration in other tissues.[43] Within the short time of 10 minutes required for a ventilation study, only about one third of the administered activity of xenon enters the body, assuming a lung volume of 2.5 L and a ventilation system volume of 10 L. About two thirds of this

TABLE 10–2. RADIOACTIVE GASES FOR LUNG VENTILATION IMAGING

Gas	Production and Decay	$T_{1/2}$	Gamma E (keV)	Photon Abundance (%)
Xe-133	^{235}U(n,f)^{133}Xe $\xrightarrow{\beta^-}$ ^{133}Cs	5.3 d	81	36
Xe-135	^{235}U(n,f)^{135}Xe $\xrightarrow{\beta^-}$ ^{135}Cs	9.1 hr	250	95
Xe-127	^{133}Cs(p,2p5n)^{127}Xe $\xrightarrow{EC}$ ^{127}I	36.4 d	145	4
			172	25
			203	68
			375	18
Kr-81m	^{81}Rb $\xrightarrow{4.5\ hr}$ ^{81m}Kr $\xrightarrow{IT}$ ^{81}Kr	13 sec	191	66

TABLE 10-3. BIOLOGIC DISTRIBUTION OF XENON

Body Compartment	% Distribution in the Body	Biologic $T_{1/2}$
Lung–air	68	22 sec
RBC–hemoglobin	9	3 min
Muscle	11	0.4 hr
Nonadipose fat	8	2.7 hr
Adipose tissue	4	7.6–17 hr

(Data from Susskind H, et al, 1977, p 462.[43])

amount is in the lung and the remainder in other tissues as shown in Table 10-3.

The amount of xenon distributed to various tissues and their subsequent rate of clearance is related to blood flow, tissue mass, and the tissue-to-blood partition coefficient. For example, the fat-to-blood coefficient is 7.9 whereas the skeletal muscle-to-blood coefficient is only 0.7[44]; therefore, all things being equal, fat tissue will concentrate far more xenon than muscle, and its rate of clearance will be slower. A greater fraction of the administered dose is distributed in muscle, however, because of its larger mass and greater blood flow.

The clearance rate of xenon from the tissues varies considerably, being fastest from the lungs ($T_{1/2}$, 22 seconds) and slowest from fat ($T_{1/2}$, 8 to 17 hours). Obese people will therefore retain xenon for longer periods of time than lean people.

RADIATION DOSE FROM RADIOXENONS

The radiation dose from a given amount of xenon activity depends on (1) the relative volumes of the breathing system and the patient's lung, (2) the length of xenon breathing time before washout, and (3) the rate of gas washout from the lung. For an average lung air volume of 2.5 l, a breathing system of 10 l, and a 5-minute rebreathing time before a 2-minute washout, the radiation-absorbed dose to the lung for Xe-127 is 4.4 mrad/mCi administered.[45] This assumes that the Xe-127 dose contains 0.1 mCi each of Xe-129m and Xe-131m as impurities, which is a conservative estimate.

A typical 5-mCi dose of Xe-127 will give a lung dose of 22 mrad. As a comparison, the lung dose for Xe-133 is 6.5 mrad/mCi or 65 mrad for a typical 10-mCi dose. The radiation dose from a Xe-127 lung study is thus about one third that of a Xe-133 lung study. Because these isotopes have identical biologic properties, the primary reason for the disparity in radiation dose is the mode of decay, Xe-133 by beta emission and Xe-127 by electron capture. The radiation dose to the airway mucosa has been shown to be greater than the lung dose.[41] Based upon a spirometer xenon concentration of 0.1 µCi/ml during a 3-minute rebreathing and a 3-minute washout, the mucosal dose is estimated to be about 15 mrad/mCi of Xe-127 and 116 mrad/mCi of Xe-133.

CONSIDERATIONS IN HANDLING RADIOXENON

The use of Xe-133 and Xe-127 in nuclear medicine presents two primary concerns to the user: how to package and store it in a convenient form ready for use and how to handle the used gas without environmental contamination. Licensing agencies usually address radioxenon use separately from all other medical radionuclides because of its unique properties. We shall therefore discuss these properties and handling methods.

Packaging and Storage of Xenon

Little precaution is necessary for xenon purchased in unit-dose vials. These vials are sealed tightly with a synthetic rubber closure that retards loss by permeation to less than 1 percent per day.[46]

Large institutions that perform numerous lung scans each week or perform research investigations with xenon often purchase Xe-133 or Xe-127 in a bulk ampule. The transfer of activity from this highly concentrated form to smaller-size vials requires careful manipulation. A primary concern when packaging or storing xenon is to keep it out of contact with oils, greases, or other lipophilic material. Because of its fat solubility xenon will be concentrated in these materials over time and be unavailable for use.

Several commercial devices are available for handling xenon gas in a bulk ampule; however, a very simple, effective, and inexpensive device can be made by the user for transferring the concentrated activity in the bulk ampule into unit-dose vials for patient use. The accuracy and reproducibility of this method has been previously described.[47] Figure 10–6 illustrates a U-tube device containing water under equilibrium conditions. The volume of air space in the right arm of the U-tube is predetermined by the user and will be the space into which the xenon activity is transferred. The concentration of xenon activity in mCi/ml can be determined from this volume and the total activity transferred. Once the xenon is confined to this space, it does not readily diffuse out because of its poor solubility in water. Additionally, the concentration remains constant during vial filling because the water level rises in proportion to the volume of gas removed.

Transfer of Xenon from an Ampule to the U-Tube Device

1. Raise the water level to the top of the right arm in the U-tube with alternating stopcock and syringe manipulation (Fig. 10–6, A and B). Record the volume. The stopcock should be set as in S-1 at the end.
2. Attach the transfer needle (18 g, 3.5 inches) to the stopcock and leave the syringe attached with the plunger fully depressed.
3. Assay the xenon ampule in the dose calibrator and record the activity.
4. Attach the air vent (20 g, 1 inch) to the ampule through its rubber closure. Next, thrust the transfer needle through the rubber closure to break the inner glass seal. Extend the needle to the end of the ampule. Air will enter the ampule through the air vent to relieve negative pressure (Fig. 10–6, C).
5. Position the stopcock as in S-2. Allow the water in the right arm to fall to the equilibrium level to draw xenon activity into the U-tube (Fig. 10–6, D).
6. Reposition the stopcock as in S-1. Remove the ampule and reassay. Record the residual activity and calculate the activity transferred to the U-tube. Calculate the activity concentration in mCi/ml in the U-tube.
7. Remove the transfer needle and attach a 27-g, 0.5-inch needle.

Filling Unit-Dose Vials

1. Calculate the volume of gas needed for the desired xenon activity. Remove the volume of air from a unit-dose vial using a separate syringe and needle. Do not remove more air than required for the dose. Typically 2-ml-sized serum vials are used, stoppered with butyl or Viton rubber stoppers.
2. Position the stopcock as in S-3. Draw the required volume of xenon gas into the syringe. The water level will rise proportionately in the right arm of the U-tube (Fig. 10–6, E).
3. Reposition the stopcock as in S-1. Attach a previously evacuated unit-dose vial to the stopcock and expel the xenon dose into the vial (Fig. 10–6, F).
4. Reposition the stopcock as in S-3. Remove the filled vial from the assembly and assay.
5. Repeat steps 1 to 4 for subsequent vials until all the xenon is packaged.

When preparing unit-dose vials, five vials each of 5, 8, 10, and 12 mCi (to allow for decay before use) provide sufficient Xe-127 for 20 patients during a 4- to 5-week period, each patient receiving about 5 mCi per dose. If Xe-133 is packaged, vials should

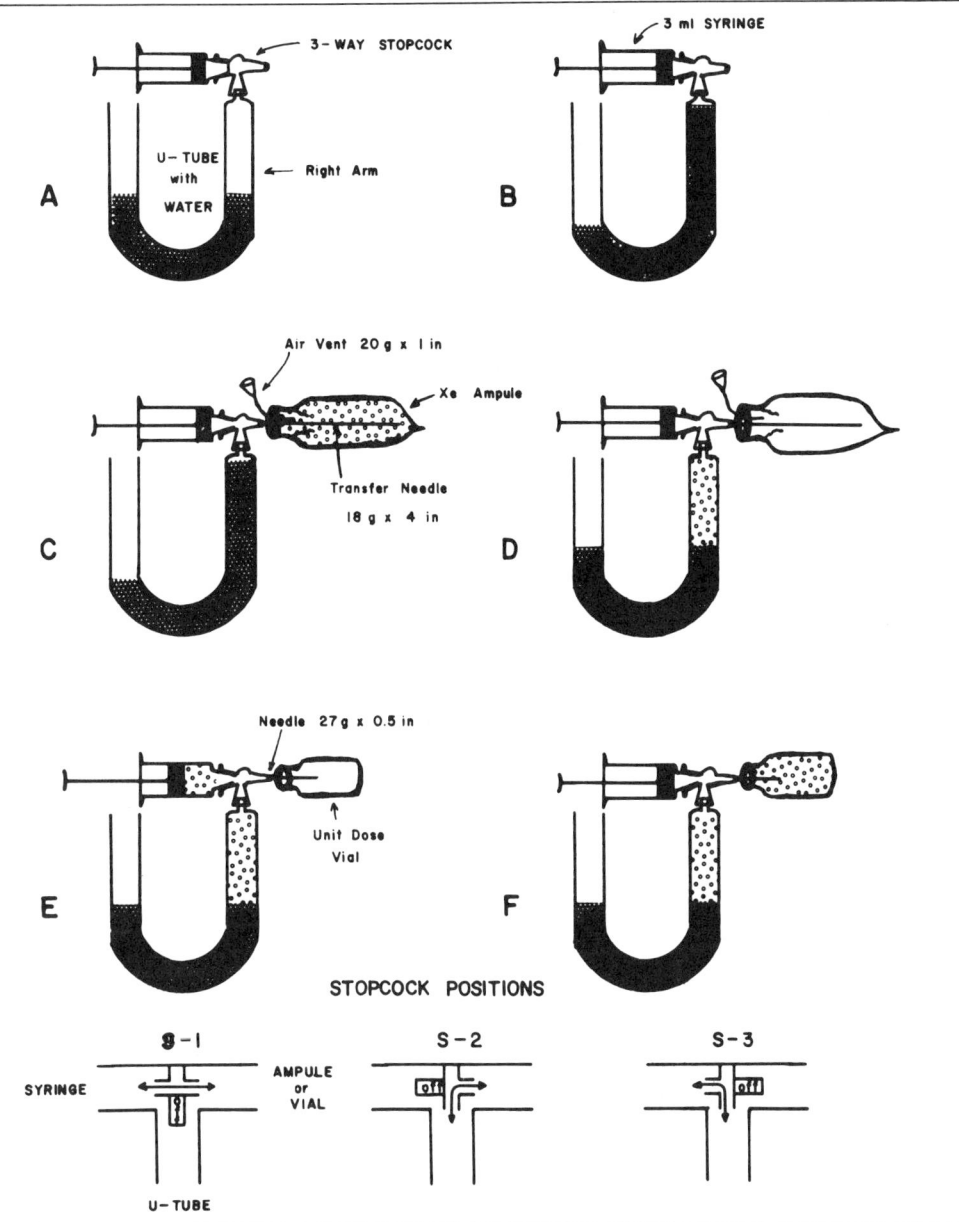

Figure 10-6. A device to transfer radioxenon from a large activity ampule to unit-dose vials containing sufficient activity for patient use. See the text for an explanation of its operation.

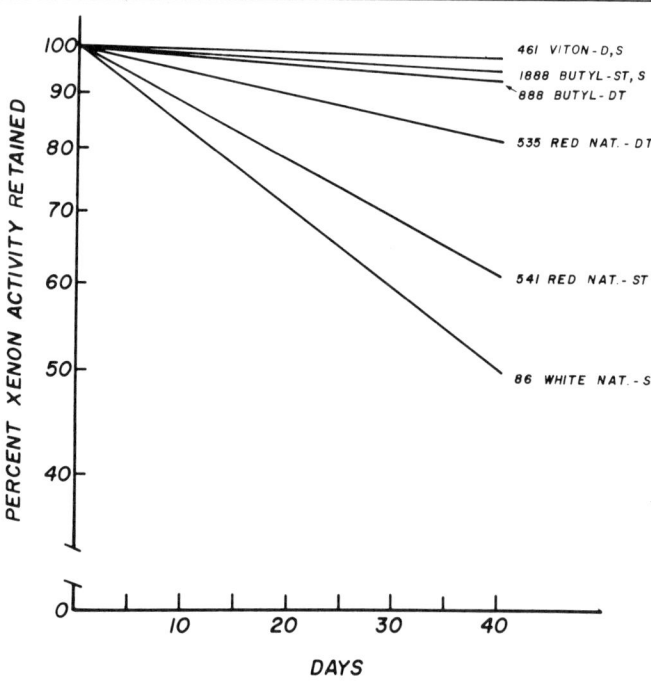

Figure 10-7. Xenon retention in unit-dose vials stoppered with various elastomeric closure materials: Viton, butyl, red natural, and white natural rubbers. D, disk; S, stopper; ST, Teflon-faced stopper; DT, Teflon-faced disk. (From Kowalsky RJ, 1979, p 222, with permission.[46])

contain two to three times more activity because patient doses are larger and its half-life is much shorter.

Retention by and removal from vials of xenon activity depends on the type of rubber closure used and the storage temperature.[46] Synthetic rubber closures of Viton or butyl rubber retard the loss of xenon better than natural rubber (Fig. 10–7). Vials should be stored in a cool area, preferably in an exhaust hood.

XENON PATIENT ADMINISTRATION SYSTEMS

A ventilation study with Xe-133 or Xe-127 is performed with the patient attached to a closed breathing system. Many systems are available commercially. The essential components include a leak-resistant circuit (most problems with leaks occur around the patient's face mask), a CO_2 absorber, a moisture absorber (essential for efficient charcoal trap operation), an expansion device (spirometer or breathing bag), bacterial filter (to protect the system), appropriate valves to control air flow and to admit oxygen when needed, and a means to exhaust the used xenon once the study is complete. Figure 10–8 shows a simple xenon breathing circuit.

Once the patient is acclimated to the breathing system, the xenon gas is flushed into the system close to the patient's mouth during an inspired breath (the washin phase). The xenon is flushed from the vial into the system with a special gun device. A double needle punctures the vial stopper; air is pumped into the vial through one needle, and xenon activity exits through the other needle (Fig. 10–9).

The study continues through a rebreathing phase (5 to 10 minutes) and finally the washout phase. At this time the xenon is either exhausted into a large bag that is eventually released to outside air through a special exhaust system, or the xenon is detained by adsorption on activated charcoal. This is typically referred to

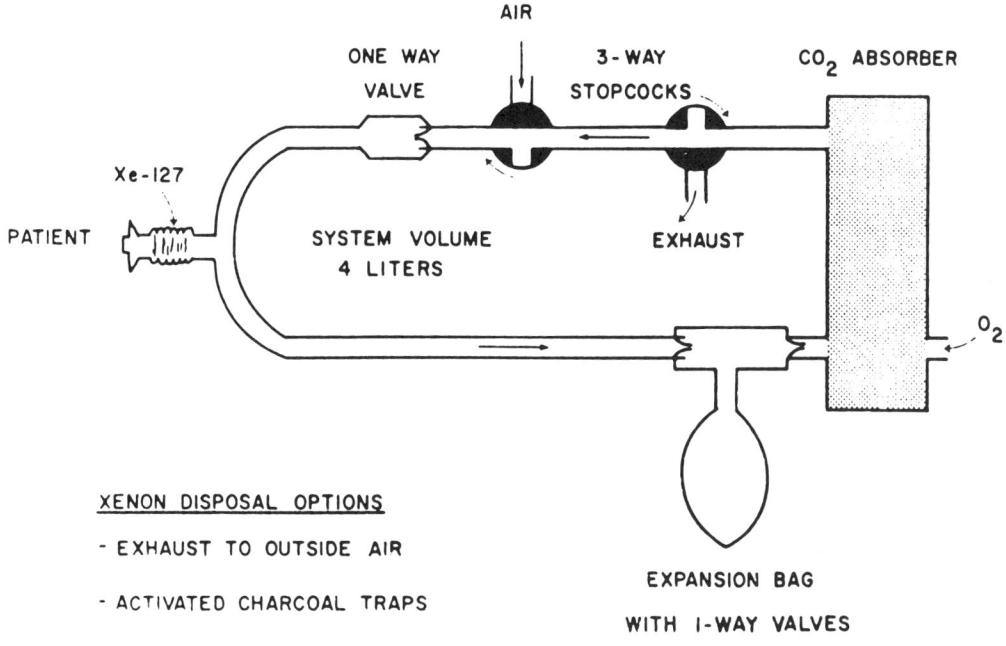

Figure 10-8. Diagram of a simplified closed breathing circuit for administering radioxenon gas during lung ventilation studies. The charcoal trap, moisture absorber, bacterial filters, and motorized blowers are omitted for simplicity.

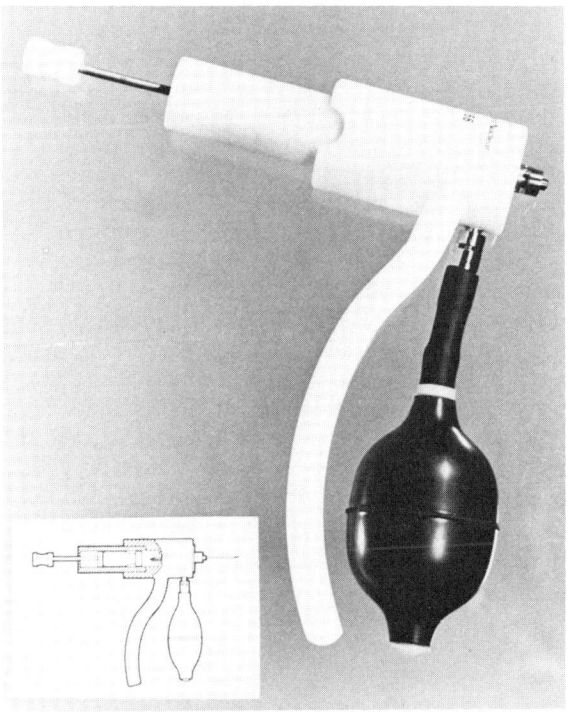

Figure 10-9. Hand-held device for administration of xenon gas. The device uses forced air to transfer xenon gas from the unit-dose vial to the patient breathing circuit. *(From DuPont Company, NEN Medical Products Division, with permission.)*

as charcoal trapping, but in reality the charcoal only slows transit of xenon atoms long enough to allow decay before exiting from the trap.

The use of xenon for patients using ventilators has caused concern over potential contamination of the ventilator by xenon combining with lubricants. The possibility of this occurring should be fairly easy to check with a radiation survey instrument, and the contaminated ventilators can be cleaned.

Factors in Charcoal Trapping

There are several factors to consider for the proper operation of a charcoal trap. These factors include airflow velocity, moisture content of the air, size of the trap, and temperature.

A charcoal trap is simply a series of cylindrical canisters containing activated charcoal. The charcoal is activated by chemical treatment and high heat to produce a large adsorptive surface area where xenon atoms can bind. The adsorption of xenon atoms is more effective when airflow through the trap is slow and if other gaseous molecules do not occupy the binding sites. Water vapor is a primary "poison" for charcoal traps, and for this reason a moisture trap must be included in the breathing circuit ahead of the charcoal. The flow rate of expired air from the patient is normally too fast to allow efficient adsorption to occur, and therefore breathing systems usually use an expansion interface (a large balloon reservoir) to store the exhausted xenon temporarily. The xenon is then pumped at a controlled rate from the reservoir into the charcoal trap.

Because traps accumulate xenon activity with use, they must be heavily shielded with lead, especially for Xe-127. Additionally, the use of Xe-127 requires a longer trap, usually twice that for Xe-133 because of Xe-127's longer half-life. All traps eventually become saturated with contaminating gases and moisture and must be replaced, otherwise the xenon activity will break through and contaminate the work environment.

Temperature greatly affects the effectiveness of charcoal adsorption of xenon. Lower-temperature traps greatly enhance binding efficiency. A refrigerated xenon trap is commercially available* and increases the trapping efficiency. At $-20\,°C$ the xenon adsorptive capacity of activated charcoal is about five times greater than at $20\,°C$.

PERMISSIBLE CONCENTRATIONS OF XENON IN AIR

Federal and state regulations have been established to limit the concentration of radioactive material that can be expelled into water and air. These limits are designated the maximum permissible concentrations or MPCs. The limits are established to protect radiation workers and the general public from injurious exposure to radiation. The MPC of a particular radionuclide is that concentration in $\mu Ci/ml$ to which an individual may be continuously exposed for a given length of time and not exceed the maximum permissible radiation dose (MPD) allowed for the whole body or a specified critical organ. For example, the MPD for whole-body exposure to a radiation worker is 5 rem/yr. The MPC for Xe-133 is $1 \times 10^{-5}\ \mu Ci/ml$ in air for a 40-hour workweek. This means that a radiation worker who is continuously exposed to a Xe-133 atmospheric concentration of $1 \times 10^{-5}\ \mu Ci/ml$ for 40 hr/wk for 50 wk/yr, would receive a 5-rem total-body radiation dose. This assumes also that exposure to no other kind of radiation source occurred during that time. MPC values calculated for a restricted area are based on exposure 40 hr/wk for 50 wk/yr and a MPD of 5 rem/yr. A restricted area is an area exposed only to radiation workers. MPC values calculated for an unrestricted area are based on continuous exposure 168 hr/wk for 52 wk/yr and a MPD of 0.5

Victoreen/Nuclear Associates, Carle Place, NY.

TABLE 10-4. MPCs OF RADIOXENON IN AIR

Radionuclide	MPC (μCi/ml)	
	40 hr/wk (Restricted Area)	168 hr/wk (Unrestricted Area)
Xe-133	1×10^{-5}	3×10^{-7}
Xe-127	9×10^{-6}	2×10^{-7}

(Data from George DL, 1978, p 105.[48])

rem/yr. An unrestricted area is an area exposed to the general public. The general public is allowed to receive only one tenth the exposure of the radiation worker. The MPC values for Xe-133 and Xe-127 are listed in Table 10–4.

Calculations for Safe Emission of Radioxenon into Restricted and Unrestricted Areas

Two basic questions can be posed regarding the use of radioxenon: (1) what is the quantity that can be released into the nuclear medicine room without exceeding the MPC for a restricted area and (2) what quantity can be released to the outside air without exceeding the MPC for an unrestricted area. To answer each question the following assumptions will be made in an illustrative example: (1) the imaging room size where xenon studies will be performed is 3000 cubic feet (8.5×10^7 ml), (2) air is exhausted to outside atmosphere at 600 cubic feet per minute, (3) the maximum activity used per week is 30 mCi of Xe-127, and (4) 25 percent of the activity escapes into the room from leakage and inadvertent release.

Exhaust to the Imaging Room (Restricted Area)

1. Air volume exhausted

   600 ft³/min × 28,320 ml/ft³ ×
   60 min/hr × 40 hr/wk =
   4.08×10^{10} ml/wk

2. Xe-127 concentration released into the room

$$\frac{(3 \times 10^4 \, \mu\text{Ci/wk}) \times 0.25}{4.08 \times 10^{10} \text{ ml/wk}}$$
$$= 1.84 \times 10^{-7} \, \mu\text{Ci/ml}$$

3. Percentage of MPC

$$\frac{1.84 \times 10^{-7} \, \mu\text{Ci/ml} \, (100)}{9 \times 10^{-6} \, \mu\text{Ci/ml}} = 2\%$$

Emergency Considerations in the Imaging Room. The imaging room has a total volume of 3000 cubic feet (8.5×10^7 ml); with the exhaust airflow at 600 ft³/min the room air turnover time is

3000 ft³/600 ft³/min = 5 min/change.

To consider an emergency situation, assume that a full 5-mCi dose of Xe-127 gas is accidentally released instantaneously. The concentration in the room, evenly distributed, would be

$5 \times 10^3 \, \mu\text{Ci}/8.5 \times 10^7$ ml =
$5.9 \times 10^{-5} \, \mu\text{Ci/ml}$

Half the airborne activity is considered to be removed with each room air change. The time required to reduce the Xe-127 concentration to below $9 \times 10^{-6} \, \mu\text{Ci/ml}$ (MPC) is calculated from the equation $A = A_0 e^{-\lambda t}$. Thus:

$9 \times 10^{-6} \, \mu\text{Ci/ml} = 5.9 \times 10^{-5} \, \mu\text{Ci/ml} \times e^{-0.693/5 \text{ min/chg} \, (x \text{ min})}$

$$\frac{\ln 9 \times 10^{-6}}{5.9 \times 10^{-5}} = -0.139x$$

$$x = 13.5 \text{ min}$$

Therefore 13.5 minutes is the estimated time required to reduce the Xe-127 concentration to the MPC value.

Exhaust to Outside Air (Unrestricted Area)

1. Air volume exhausted

   600 ft^3/min × 28,320 ml/ft^3 × 60 min/hr × 168 hr/wk = 1.71 × 10^{11} ml/wk

2. Xe-127 concentration released to the outside air

   $$\frac{(3 \times 10^4 \text{ μCi/wk}) \times 0.25}{1.71 \times 10^{11} \text{ ml/wk}} = 4.38 \times 10^{-8} \text{ μCi/ml}$$

3. Percentage of MPC

   $$\frac{4.38 \times 10^{-8} \text{ μCi/ml (100)}}{2 \times 10^{-7} \text{ μCi/ml}} = 22\%$$

The released Xe-127 concentration in this example is thus about one fifth the established MPC. The user should be aware that the room exhaust should be a separate unit and not enter the air return to the hospital. It should exhaust directly to outside air, and the terminal exhaust duct shuld be located at least 30 feet from the nearest air intake.

RADIOAEROSOL VENTILATION IMAGING

Radioaerosol lung imaging actually predates the use of xenons for ventilation because the radioaerosol image was essentially static and could be imaged with a rectilinear scanner, whereas the washin and washout phases of xenon imaging required the speed of Anger-type gamma cameras. Radioaerosol imaging was only slowly accepted, however, and one of the reasons was the inability to produce aerosol droplets small enough to achieve adequate diffusion into the lung periphery. Droplets larger than 3 to 5 μm in diameter cause hyperdeposition of aerosol in the trachea and major airways in subjects without airway obstruction, which leads to false-positive scans. A droplet size smaller than 2 μm is necessary for good distribution and minimal large airway deposition.

A significant development has revitalized the use of radioaerosol ventilation imaging.[49] With this technique a settling bag is placed between the nebulizer and the patient's mouthpiece. The bag removes most of the droplets larger than 2 μm in size by sedimentation, impaction, and turbulence.

Further research efforts have led to the development of nebulization systems that efficiently produce aerosol droplet particles 1 μm or less, thus obviating the need for a settling bag. Commercially produced disposable systems are now available for routine use in nuclear medicine for radioaerosol inhalation studies. Figure 10–10 illustrates one of these systems. The usual operating procedure requires placing 30 to 50 mCi of Tc-99m DTPA in a 2- to 3-ml volume into the nebulizer. Aerosol droplets are generated by forcing air or oxygen through the nebulizer at 8 to 10 l/min at 25 to 50 psi. The patient inhales the radioaerosol during normal breathing through the mouth with the nose clamped shut. Radioaerosol that is not used by the patient or is exhaled during breathing is trapped in a particle retentive filter. The amount of radioactivity that deposits in the patient's lungs depends on the initial nebulizer concentration, the length of breathing time and the patient's condition. Generally, with a normal subject and an initial Tc-99m DTPA concentration of 30 mCi/3 ml, the lung deposition of activity is approximately 0.1 mCi per minute of breathing time. A typical study requires between 5 and 10 minutes of breathing time to acquire sufficient activity (0.5 to 1.0 mCi) to perform inhalation imaging. The efficiency of delivering activity from the nebulizer to the lungs is only about 2 to 5 percent, which is why such a large amount of activity is placed into the nebulizer initially. After inhalation of radioaerosol, the unit is removed, and the patient is transported to the gamma camera for imaging.

Radioaerosol ventilation studies have also been used after perfusion lung imaging in lieu of radioxenon studies. Although the washout phase of the xenon study is the most sensitive method for detecting localized obstructive airway disease,[35] radioaero-

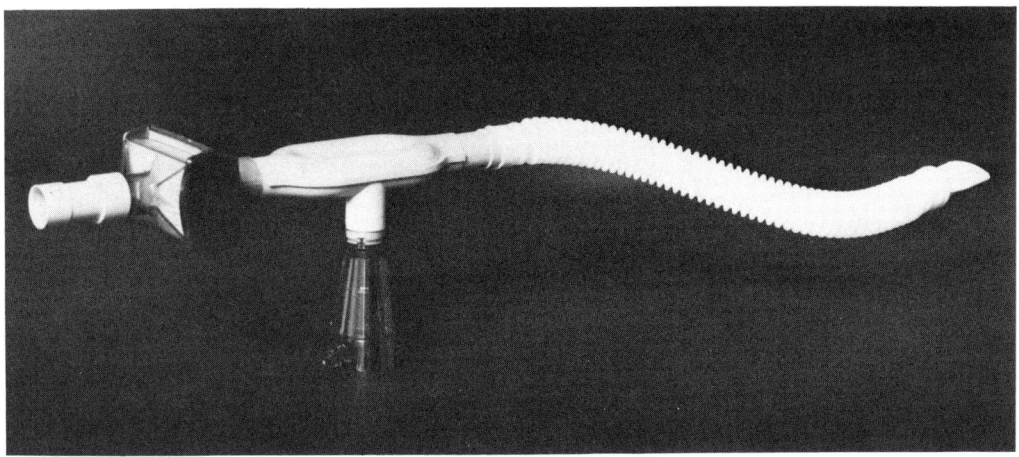

Figure 10-10. The UltraVent aerosol delivery system for production and administration of Tc-99m DTPA radioaerosol for lung inhalation studies. *(From Mallinckrodt, Inc, with permission.)*

sol studies provide an alternative method of evaluation when xenon is not available. Ideally, a radioaerosol with a gamma energy higher than 140 keV should be used. Because it is more convenient to use a Tc-99m aerosol, however, the perfusion, aerosol ventilation technique must be modified to achieve a satisfactory study. The technique developed[35,50] requires that the Tc-99m particle perfusion scan be done with only 0.5 to 1 mCi (instead of 3 mCi) and the aerosol study with 3 to 5 mCi deposited in the lung. The rationale for this method is that embolic perfusion defects will fill in on the aerosol study. Complete filling in, however, requires that the activity of Tc-aerosol present in the lung exceed that of the MAA injected by four or five times.[35]

The technetium agent of choice for radioaerosol imaging is Tc-99m DTPA. Its rate of lung clearance into the blood is somewhat slower than Tc-99m pertechnetate[51] because of DTPA's large molecular weight ($K = 1.5$ percent/min for DTPA; $K = 5.1$ percent/min for TcO_4^-), and DTPA has a faster and more complete elimination from the body by urinary excretion.

Clinical Evaluation of the Lung with Radiopharmaceuticals

RATIONALE

Indications for perfusion and ventilation lung imaging include suspected pulmonary thromboembolism, preoperative evaluation of patients with chronic obstructive pulmonary disease, inhalation injury in burn patients, foreign body aspiration, and right-to-left shunt quantitation.

By far the most common indication for perfusion lung imaging is the clinician's suspicion that pulmonary thromboembolism has occurred. The clues that initiate this suspicion usually are a sudden outset of breathlessness or pleuritic chest pain, especially in a patient in a high-risk category, e.g., one who is bedridden, is on oral contraceptives, or has cancer or deep venous disease of the lower extremities. Laboratory tests, e.g., arterial blood gas measurements and electrocardiographic abnormalities, seem to be of significantly less value in arriving at the diagnosis than the clinician's original suspicion followed by perfusion–ventilation imaging and possibly pulmonary angiography. Doppler ultrasound and impedance electroplethysmography are useful in establishing the diagnosis of deep venous thrombosis in the lower extremities but do not confirm the diagnosis of PE in patients with breathlessness.

Statistics on PE put the incidence at about half that of acute myocardial infarction and three times as common as strokes. Of the patients who survive the first hour after embolization, approximately 70 percent are not diagnosed or treated properly. Treatment does improve survival significantly. It is for these reasons that clinicians have been encouraged to request a lung scan at the time of the first clinical suspicion of pulmonary embolization.

The value of perfusion lung imaging lies in its ready availability, noninvasiveness, and safety. More meaningful information is obtained from this one test than from all the other tests commonly obtained other than pulmonary angiography. The latter is invasive and does entail a certain, albeit low, morbidity from the procedure. It is generally felt that lung scanning is more sensitive but less specific than pulmonary angiography except in certain interpretive categories.

A normal perfusion lung scan virtually eliminates the possibility of pulmonary embolism (Fig 10–11A). In the setting of multiple perfusion defects, if the largest defect is at least segmental, in a clear zone on the chest radiograph, and shows normal ventilation, then these findings warrant interpretation as a very high probability for acute pulmonary embolization, and there is no need for angiographic confirmation unless the patient is at extreme risk of hemorrhaging while receiving anticoagulant therapy. When pulmonary angiography must be done to confirm a diagnosis, the lung scan serves as a useful guide to the angiographer by shortening the procedure and lowering the risk to the patient. A useful alternative to angiography is serial lung scanning. Most patients with acute pulmonary embolization show detectable improvement in perfusion within 1 to 2 weeks.

PROCEDURE

The procedure for the performance of a lung scan should begin with evaluation of a current chest x-ray. After it is concluded that a lung scan may be helpful and that the patient does not have severe pulmonary hypertension, a perfusion lung scan may be initiated.

Under normal circumstances, the patient is injected intravenously with Tc-99m MAA particles while in a supine position. This results in a predominant distribution of particles to the dependent-most portions of the lung because of normal perfusion dynamics. Some centers inject half the dose with the patient supine and half with the patient prone so as to improve the distribution of particles. It is necessary to use this fractional injection technique in patients who are to have a preoperative evaluation before lung resection. Injection is best accomplished at an unused venipuncture site. Injecting through intravenous tubing often results in the labeling of intravenous line clots, with resultant microembolization and hot spots in the lung images. Within 5 minutes after injection of the particles, the lungs are imaged with the patient in a seated position whenever possible to achieve full expansion of the lungs. Images should be obtained in the four standard views plus four obliques or with a single-photon emission computed tomography system in a rotational mode of acquisition. It is important

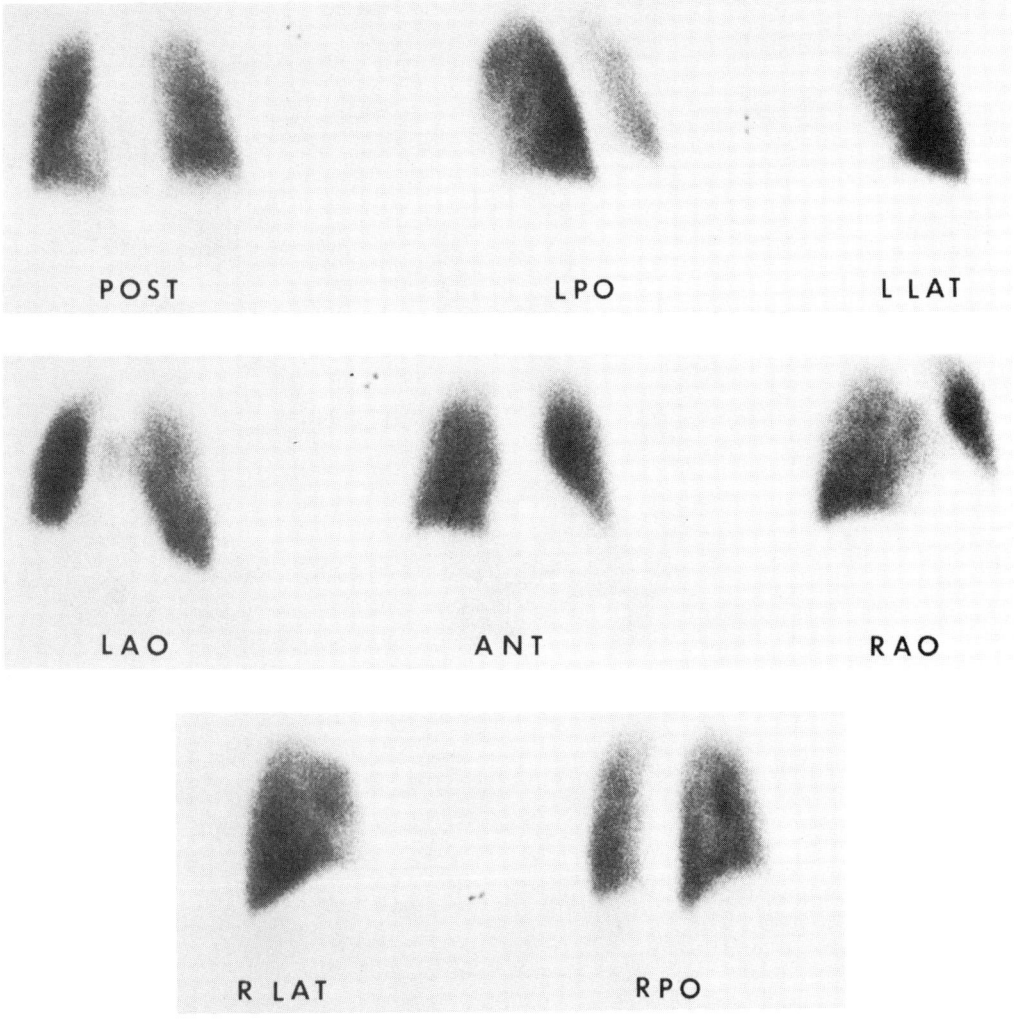

Figure 10-11. A. Normal perfusion lung scan in a patient after an intravenous injection of 3 mCi of Tc-99m MAA. Illustrated are the eight standard views: posterior (POST), left posterior oblique (LPO), left lateral (L LAT), left anterior oblique (LAO), anterior (ANT), right anterior oblique (RAO), right lateral (R LAT), and right posterior oblique (RPO).

to see all surfaces of the lungs from at least two angles to determine the size and character of any perfusion abnormalities.

Pulmonary hypertension necessitates the use of fewer than the normal number of particles. In this disease the normal number of pulmonary arterioles and capillaries has been markedly decreased because of a process called pruning. The total number of particles given to patients with pulmonary hypertension should be reduced to 50,000 to 60,000 to avoid plugging an excessive percentage of pulmonary endarterioles and capillaries, with potentially disastrous consequences.

Ventilation studies may be performed

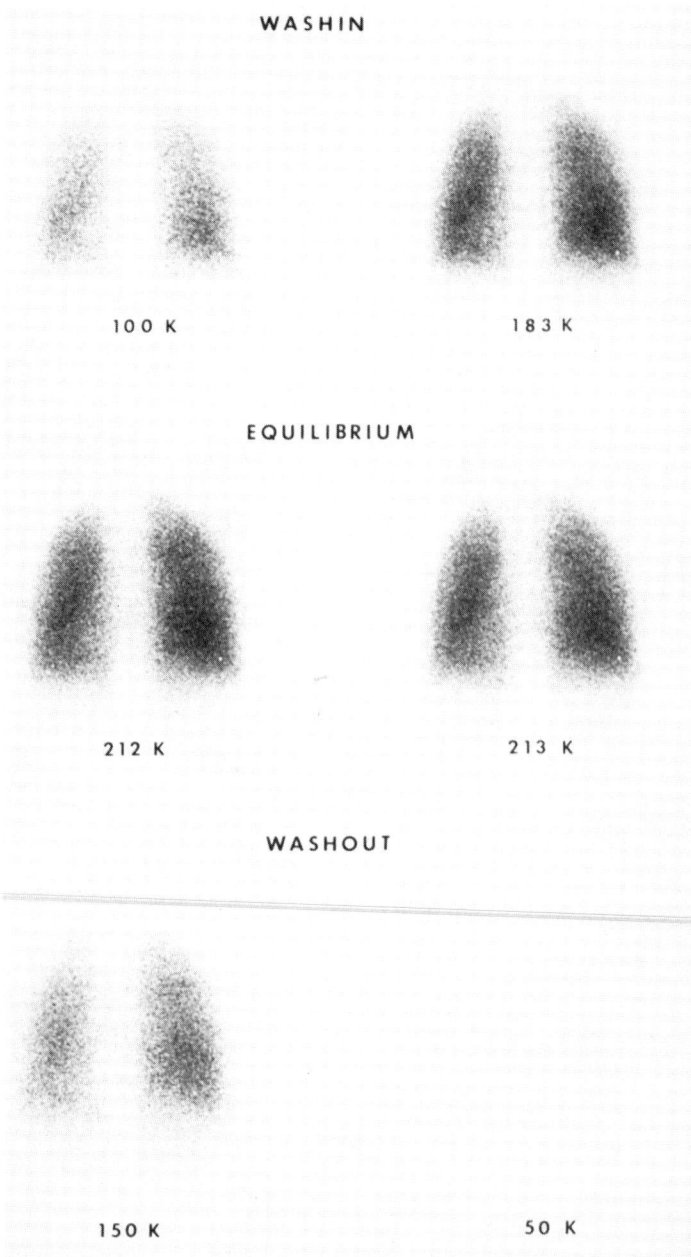

Figure 10-11. B. Normal ventilation lung scan in the same patient after inhalation of 10 mCi of Xe-133 gas from a closed-circuit breathing system. Illustrated are the three standard phases of the ventilation study: washin, equilibrium, and washout. In this case the ventilation study was performed before the perfusion study with Tc-99m MAA because of Xe-133's lower gamma energy (81 keV) compared with Tc-99m (140 keV).

with one of the noble gases or with radioaerosols. The former are preferred by the majority of centers. The choice of gas will affect the technique for ventilation. Kr-81m ventilation is limited essentially to the washin phase. Xe-133 will demonstrate all three phases of ventilation, namely, washin, equilibrium, and washout, but must be used before the perfusion study to demonstrate all of these (Fig. 10–11B). Xe-127 is the ideal choice for ventilation because the optimal viewing position can be selected after evaluating the perfusion study and repeated ventilation studies may be performed to evaluate multiple perfusion defects.

Ventilation with the gases is best accomplished with the patient sitting up to optimize lung expansion. A closed rebreathing system with CO_2 and xenon gas exhaust traps is used. Some centers emphasize that the initial inhalation be a single, deep breath that is held for 30 to 60 seconds to show the initial ventilatory distribution. The equilibration phase should last for 5 minutes to ensure the distribution of gas into poorly ventilated areas, which then are visualized as gas trapping in the washout phase.

Radioaerosol ventilation requires careful attention to aerosol particle size. This has been controlled somewhat better with the addition of a settling bag between the aerosolizer and the patient or by use of the newer aerosol systems now commercially available. Under optimal conditions radioaerosol ventilation yields information similar to the single-breath gas washin. There may be some deposition in the airways. Distribution will be abnormally affected by bronchial disease.

In the quantitation of right-to-left shunts, whole-body computer images are used to calculate the percentage of particles shunted to the systemic circulation according to the following equation:

$$\% \text{ R-to-L shunt} = \frac{\text{Total-body counts} - \text{Total-lung counts}}{\text{Total-body counts}} \times 100 - 4$$

PHARMACEUTICALS

Perfusion lung imaging is most commonly done with Tc-99m–labeled MAA. Usually 250,000 to 500,000 particles are used with 2 to 4 mCi of Tc-99m. The particle size distribution usually runs from 10 to 90 μm, with the majority within a 10- to 40-μm range. When stricter particle size control is desired, HAM particles are used because they have been sieved to a 15- to 30-μm size.

HAM preparations have shown a slightly higher incidence of adverse reactions in the past.* HAM preparations have been the choice for right-to-left shunt quantitation because the obligatory amount of radioactivity bypassing the lungs is only 4 percent in the first 15 minutes after injection.

Ventilation imaging is best done with one of the xenons. Kr-81m has a higher energy emission than Tc-99m and therefore may be used after the perfusion study, but its very short half-life precludes evaluation of equilibrium or washout phases. Xe-133 can show the three phases of ventilation, but because of its lower energy emission than Tc-99m, the ventilation must precede the perfusion study without knowing the optimal viewing position. Xe-127 has sufficient half-life and emission energy such that all three phases of ventilation may be seen after optimum positioning based on the perfusion study findings. Other advantages of Xe-127 are its longer half-life and lower radiation dosimetry. It must be noted, however, that a medium-energy collimator should be used and perfusion abnormalities should be ventilated in silhouette so that there is no normal lung behind the perfusion defect from which Xe-127 photons could emerge and appear to fill in the defect.

INTERPRETATION

For the most common indication, pulmonary embolization, the classic findings are multiple perfusion defects, with the largest being an anatomic segment, lobe, or lung, and normal ventilation of one of the latter (Figs. 10–12A and 10–12B). Occasionally there may be a mild washin ventilatory abnormality in the area of a pulmonary embolus perfusion defect because of the bronchoconstrictor–vasoconstrictor effects of serotonin, bronchoalveolar hypocapnia, or reduction of surfactant. Gas

---

* *SNM Adverse RXN's Registry, 1967–1975; HAM, 11; MAA, 1.*

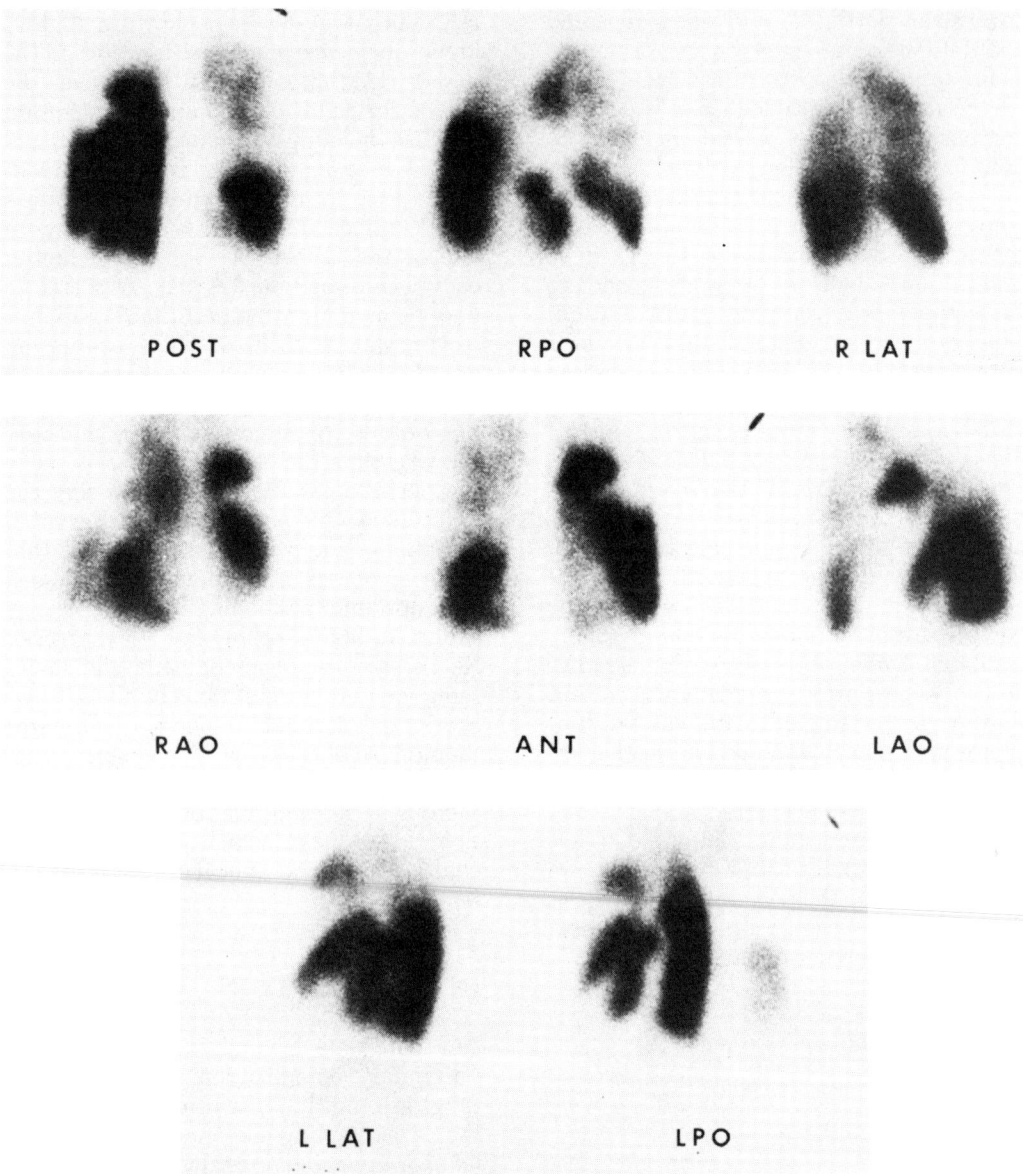

Figure 10-12. A. Pulmonary embolism. Abnormal perfusion lung scan in a patient following an intravenous injection of 3 mCi of Tc-99m MAA that illustrates multiple perfusion defects, several of which correspond to anatomic lung segments.

trapping in the area of a perfusion defect is, however, indicative of obstructive pulmonary disease, asthma, or a ball valve type of airway obstruction resulting from inspissated mucus or a foreign body (Figs. 10–13A and 10–13B). With the latter mechanisms, a perfusion abnormality occurs in response to hypoxia. Emphysema generally causes both washin and washout ventilatory abnormalities.

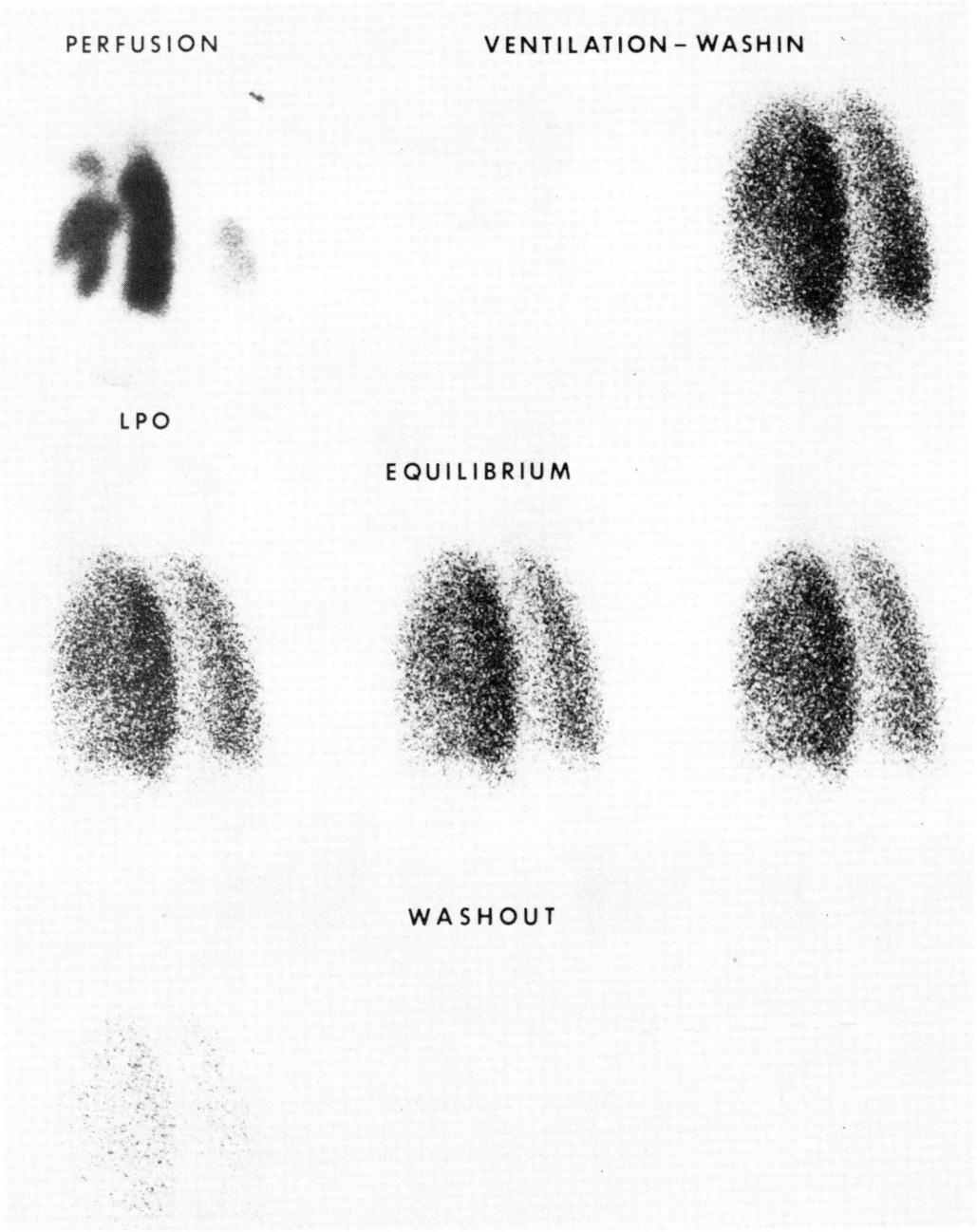

Figure 10-12. B. Normal postperfusion ventilation lung scan in the same patient in the LPO view with 4 mCi of Xe-127 gas. The normal distribution of gas during washin and washout phases demonstrates a dramatic mismatch between the prior abnormal perfusion scan and the ventilation scan and represents a high probability for PE in this patient.

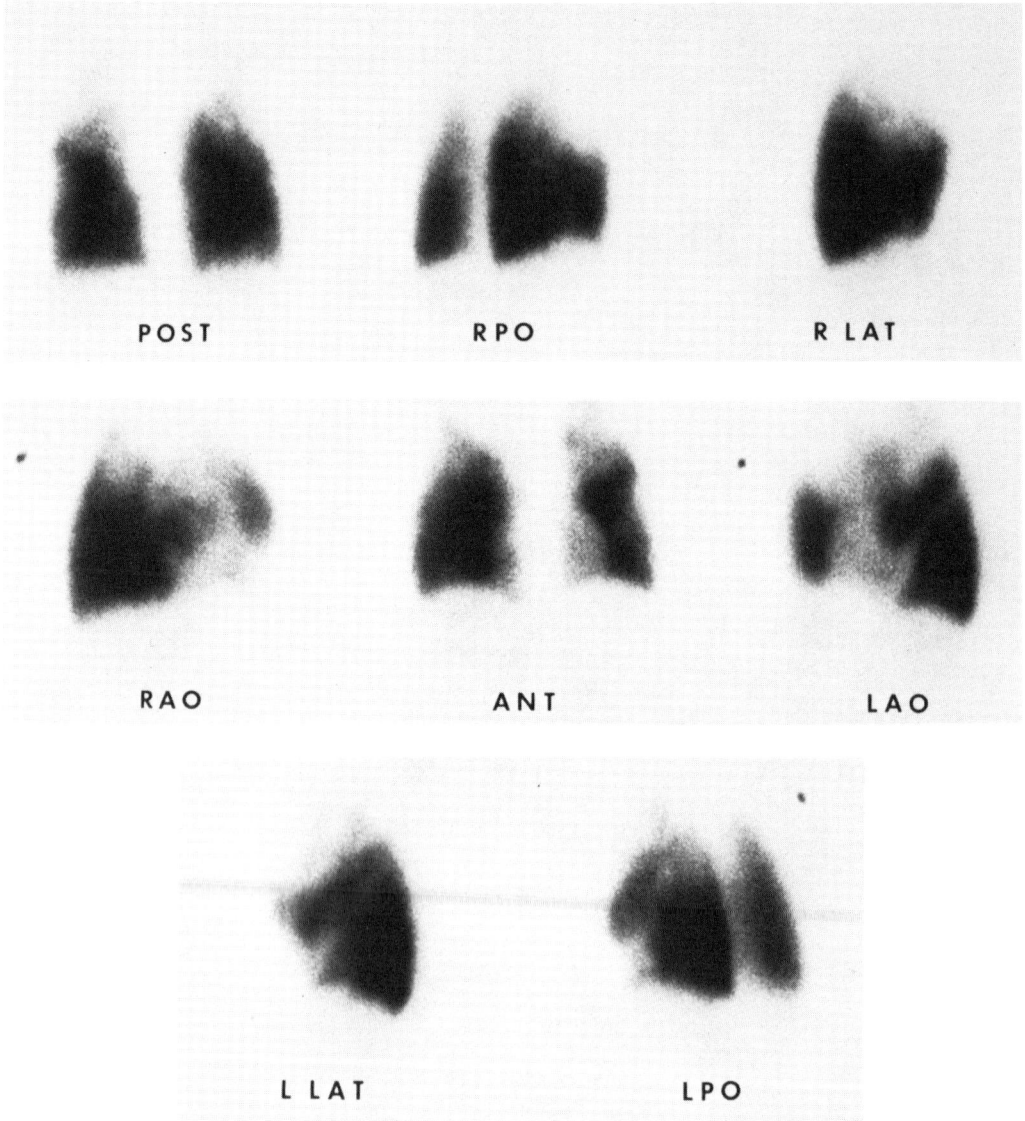

Figure 10-13. A. Obstructive pulmonary disease. Abnormal perfusion lung scan in a patient with 3 mCi of Tc-99m MAA that demonstrates extensive perfusion defects in the lung apices. Perfusion to the lung bases is essentially normal, but note the "fissure sign" along the left lung major fissure.

In the preoperative evaluation of patients for viability after lung resection for tumor, the perfusion study is used to quantitate the remaining postoperative function and to predict survival. Digitally stored anterior and posterior lung perfusion images are used to calculate the 1-second forced expiratory volume (FEV_1) remaining after the proposed surgery. A predicted postoperative contralateral FEV_1 greater than 800 ml translates to an 85 percent postoperative survival rate, which is considered acceptable for surgery of that magnitude.

The incidence of inhalation injury in

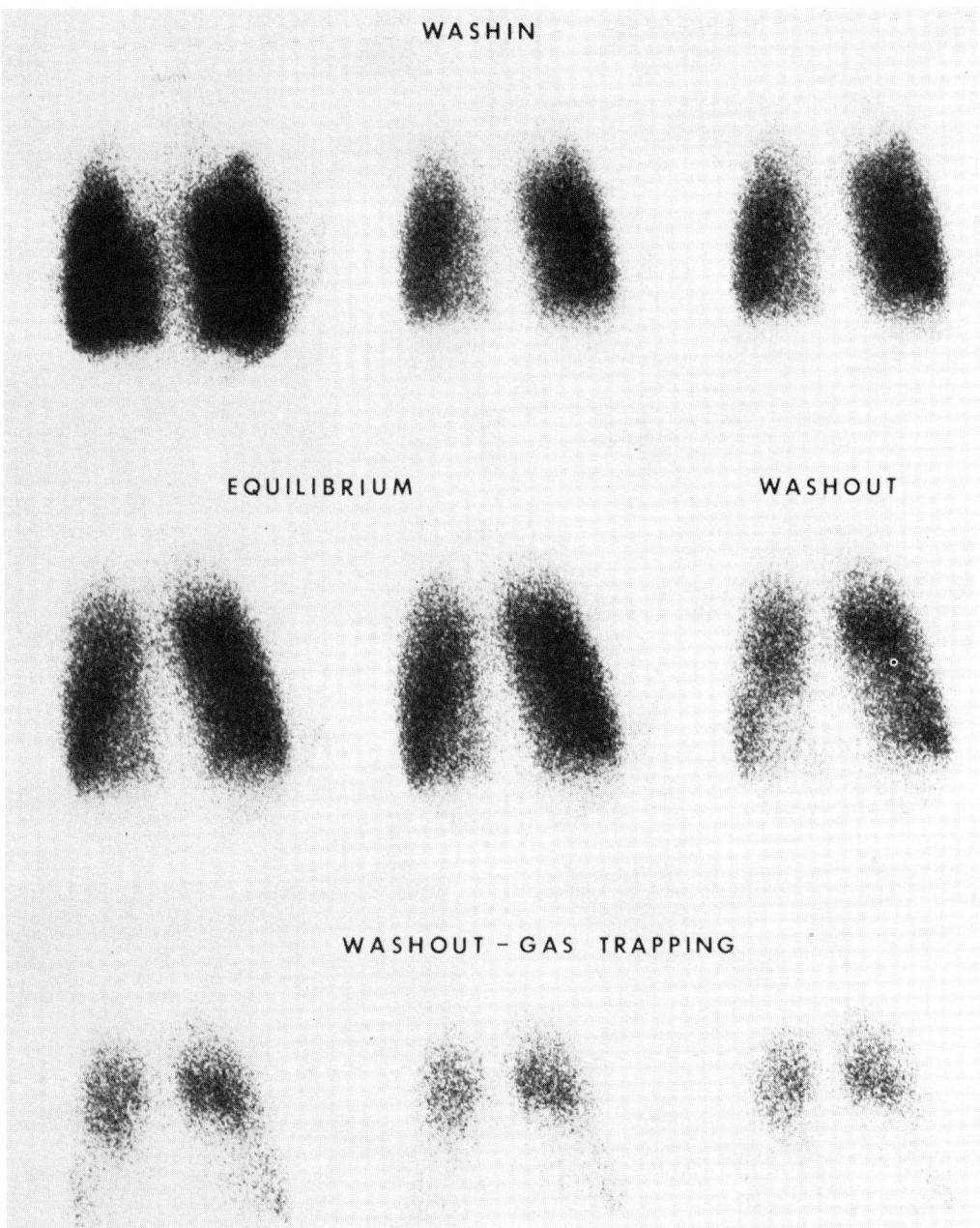

Figure 10-13. B. Abnormal postperfusion ventilation scan in the same patient with 5 mCi of Xe-127 gas that demonstrates gas trapping in the lung apices during the washout phase corresponding to defects seen on the perfusion scan. Ventilation of the lung bases is normal. These findings of matching perfusion–ventilation defects indicate obstructive pulmonary disease in both upper lung fields.

burn patients has been estimated at 35 percent. There are two phases to thermal inhalation injury, namely, an early, asymptomatic, and radiographically normal phase and a later symptomatic phase that is difficult to treat. Tracheobronchial mucosal edema, severe inflammatory reaction, and generation of fluid and mucus leading to alveolar air trapping occur in the early phase. A ventilation study in this phase will demonstrate abnormalities with an overall accuracy of 90 percent, which allows the institution of corrective measures before the symptomatic phase.

With aspiration of foreign bodies, both ventilation and perfusion studies have been of benefit. Their usefulness has been in localizing the approximate site of the obstructed airway before bronchoscopy when the foreign body is not visible on a chest x-ray. In an emergency situation, the ventilation study will be most useful in showing the airway obstruction if the patient can cooperate. If the patient cannot cooperate for ventilation or the foreign body is very small and likely to be lodged more peripherally, then a perfusion study will be more efficacious. Under these circumstances the perfusion abnormalities result from hypoxia and shunting of blood away from the hypoxic zone. The perfusion study is more likely to show a small defect than a ventilation study.

Right-to-left shunt quantitation requires careful attention to particle size. HAM particle whole-body distribution is evaluated from data collected digitally within 15 minutes of injection. Greater than 4 percent right-to-left shunting under these conditions is considered abnormal and has been used in the evaluation of various cardiac abnormalities and adult respiratory distress syndrome (ARDS). The margin of safety with this technique is sufficient to warrant its use.

REFERENCES

1. Weibel ER: Morphological basis of alveolar-capillary gas exchange. Physiol Rev 53:419, 1973
2. Weibel ER: Morphometry of the human lung. New York, Academic Press, 1963
3. Weibel ER: Morphological basis for V/Q distribution. In Hutas I, Debreczeni LA (eds): Advances in Physiological Sciences Vol 10—Respiration, Budapest, Pergamon Press, 1980, pp 179–189.
4. Bryan AC, Bentivoglio LG, Beerel F, et al: Determination of regional variations in ventilation and perfusion in normal subjects using xenon 133. J Appl Physiol 19:395, 1964
5. Guyton AC: Textbook of Medical Physiology. Philadelphia, Saunders, 1976
6. Muller JH, Rossier PH: A new method for the treatment of cancer of the lungs by means of artificial radioactivity. Acta Radiol 35:449, 1951
7. Haynie TP, Calhoon JD, Nasjleti CE, et al: Visualization of pulmonary artery occlusion of photoscanning. JAMA 185:306, 1963
8. Taplin GV, Johnson DE, Dore EK, et al: Suspensions of radioalbumin aggregates for photoscanning the liver, spleen, lung an other organs. J Nucl Med 5:259, 1964
9. Lindeman JF, Quinn III JL: The recent history of clinical procedures in nuclear medicine. In Gottschalk A, and Potchen EJ (eds): Diagnostic Nuclear Medicine. Baltimore, Williams & Wilkins, 1976, pp 8–13
10. Stern HS, Goodwin DA, Wagner HN, et al: In-113m—A short-lived isotope for lung scanning. Nucleonics 24:57, 1966
11. Robinowitz M, Mathew J, Eckelman W, et al: Fatal reactions following Tc-99m ferrous hydroxide lung scans. J Nucl Med 14:445, 1973
12. Zolle, I, Rhodes BA, Wagner HN Jr: Preparation of metabolizable radioactive human serum albumin microspheres for studies of the circulation. Int J Appl Radiat Isot 21:155, 1970
13. Rhodes BA, Stern HS, Buchannan JA, et al: Lung scanning with Tc-99m microspheres. Radiology 99:613, 1971
14. Subramanian G, Arnold RW, Thomas FD, et al: Evaluation of an instant Tc-99m labeled lung scanning agent. J Nucl Med 13:790, 1972
15. Davis MA: Particulate radiopharmaceuticals for pulmonary studies. In Subramanian G, Rhodes BA, Cooper JF, Sodd VJ (eds): Radiopharmaceuticals. New York, Society of Nuclear Medicine, 1975, pp 267–281
16. Heck LL, Duley JW: Statistical considerations in lung imaging with Tc-99m albumin particles. Radiology 113:675, 1974

17. Dworkin HJ, Gutkowski RF, Porter W, et al: Effect of particle number on lung perfusion images. J Nucl Med 18:260, 1977
18. Iio M, Wagner HN Jr.: Studies of reticuloendothelial system (RES) I. Measurement of the phagocytic capacity of the RES in man and dog. J Clin Invest 42:417, 1963
19. Taplin GV, MacDonald NS: Radiochemistry of macroaggregated albumin and newer lung scanning agents. Semin Nucl Med 1:132, 1971
20. Burdine JA, Sonnemaker RE, Ryder LA, et al: Perfusion studies with technetium-99m human albumin microspheres (HAM). Radiology 95:101, 1970
21. Davis MA: Long-term retention and biologic fate of Tc-99m iron hydroxide aggregates. In Radiopharmaceuticals and Labeled Compounds. Vienna, IAEA, 1973, Vol 2, pp 43–63
22. Busse W, Reed C, Tyson I, et al: Prolonged retention of radioactivity following perfusion lung scan in asthmatic patients. J Nucl Med 14:837, 1973
23. Kitani K, Taplin GV: Biliary excretion of Tc-99m albumin microaggregate degradation products (a method for measuring Kupffer cell digestive function) J Nucl Med 13:260, 1971
24. Gallagher BM: Personal communication. New England Nuclear Corp, N Billeria, Mass
25. Kowalsky RJ: Safety and effectiveness considerations with particulate lung scanning agents. J Nucl Med Tech 10:223, 1982
26. Dworkin HJ, Smith JR, Bull FE: A reaction following administration of macroaggregated albumin (MAA) for a lung scan. Am J Roentgen 98:427, 1966
27. Vincent WR, Goldberg SJ, Desilets D: Fatality immediately following rapid infusion of macroaggregates of Tc-99m albumin (MAA) for lung scan. Radiology 91:1181, 1968
28. Williams JO: Death following injection of lung scanning agent in a case of pulmonary hypertension. Br J Radiol 47:61, 1974
29. Child JS, Wolfe JD, Tashkin D, et al: Fatal lung scan in a case of pulmonary hypertension due to obliterative pulmonary vascular disease. Chest 67:308, 1975
30. Davis MA, Taube RA: Pulmonary perfusion imaging: Acute toxicity and safety factors as a function of particle size. J Nucl Med 19:1209, 1978
31. Allen DR, Ferens JM, Cheney FW, et al: Critical evaluation of acute cardiopulmonary toxicity of microspheres, J Nucl Med 19:1204, 1978
32. Allen DR, Nelp WB, Hartnett DE, et al: Critical assessment of changes in the pulmonary circulation following injection of lung scanning agent (MAA). In Radiopharmaceuticals and Labeled Compounds. Vienna, IAEA, Vol 2, 1973, pp 37–42
33. Heyman S: Toxicity and safety factors associated with lung perfusion studies with radiolabeled particles. Leter to the editor. J Nucl Med 20:1098, 1979
34. Davis MA, Taube RA: Reply. Letter to the editor. J Nucl Med 20:1099, 1979
35. Taplin GV, Chopra SK: Lung perfusion–ventilation scintigraphy in obstructive airway disease and pulmonary embolism. Radiol Clin North Am 16:491, 1978
36. Knipping HW, Bolt W, Venrath H, et al: Eine neue Methode zur Prüfung der Herz- und Lungen-Funktion, die regionale Funktionsanalyse in der Lungen- und Herzklinik mit Hilfe des radioactiven Edlegases Xenon-133. Deutsch Med Wschr 80:1146, 1955
37. Newhouse MT, Wright FJ, Ingham GK, et al: Use of scintillation camera and xenon-135 for study of topographic pulmonary function. Respir Physiol 4:141, 1968
38. Hoffer PB, Harper PV, Beck RN, et al: Improved xenon images with Xe-127. J Nucl Med 14:172, 1973
39. Atkins HL, Susskind H, Klopper JF, et al: A clinical comparison of Xe-127 and Xe-133 for ventilation studies. J Nucl Med 18:653, 1977
40. Chilton HM, Cooper JF, Friedman BI: Xe-127 ventilation imaging immediately following Tc-99m perfusion studies. Clin Nucl Med 2:152, 1977
41. Goddard BA, Ackery DM: Xenon-133, Xe-127 and Xe-125 for lung function investigations. A dosimetric comparison. J Nucl Med 16:780, 1975
42. McCartney WH, Perry JR, Staab EV, et al: Comparison of Xe-127 and Xe-133 in ventilation–perfusion imaging in diagnosis of pulmonary embolus. J Nucl Med 19:675, 1978
43. Susskind H, Atkins HL, Cohn SH, et al: Whole-body retention of radioxenon. J Nucl Med 18:462, 1977
44. Ponto RA, Loken MK: Radioactive gases: Production, properties, handling and uses. In Subramanian G, Rhodes BA, Cooper JF, Sodd VJ (eds): Radiopharmaceuticals. New

York, Society of Nuclear Medicine, 1975, pp 296–304
45. Atkins HL, Robertson JS, Croft BY, et al: Estimates of radiation absorbed doses from radioxenons in lung imaging. J Nucl Med 21:459, 1980
46. Kowalsky RJ: Stability of xenon-127 in unit dose vials. J Nucl Med Tech 7:222, 1979
47. Kowalsky RJ, Dalton DR, Saylor WL: A simple device for efficient transfer and unit dose packaging of Xe-127. J Nucl Med 19:414, 1978
48. George DL: Permissible concentration in air of xenon-127: Concise communication. J Nucl Med 19:105, 1978
49. Hayes M, Taplin GV, Chopra SK, et al: Improved radioaerosol adminstration system for routine inhalation lung imaging. Radiology 131:256, 1979
50. Hayes M, Taplin GV: Lung imaging with radioaerosols for the assessment of airway disease. Semin Nucl Med 10:243, 1980
51. Rinderknecht J, Shapiro L, Krouthhammer M, et al: Accelerated clearance of small solutes from the lungs in interstitial lung disease. Am Rev Respir Dis 121:105, 1980

CHAPTER 11

Liver, Gallbladder, Spleen, and Bone Marrow

The liver, spleen, and bone marrow form a major part of the reticuloendothelial system (RES) in humans. The venous sinuses of these organs are lined with reticular cells that function to remove from the blood foreign particles or degraded endogenous substances such as effete red blood cells, bacteria, endotoxins, and denatured proteins. The liver, in addition to removing particles, can also excrete certain substances into the bile. A knowledge of the normal function of these organs is essential in understanding the design and use of radioactive drugs for liver, gallbladder, spleen, and bone marrow evaluation.

LIVER

There are two main classes of radiopharmaceutical agents used to study the liver: (1) particulate agents, or radiocolloids, that become entrapped in the liver for a prolonged period of time, permitting the evaluation of liver morphology; and (2) nonparticulate hepatobiliary agents that are actively cleared from the blood by the hepatocytes and excreted into the bile, permitting an evaluation of hepatobiliary function.

PHYSIOLOGIC ANATOMY OF THE LIVER

The gross anatomic relationship of the liver and hepatobiliary system is shown in Figure 11-1. The two main types of cells in the liver are the hepatocytes of the liver parenchyma and the littoral cells of the liver sinusoids. Hepatocytes, sometimes called polygonal cells because of their shape, make up 85 percent of the cell population in the liver and are responsible for the major metabolic functions. The littoral cells constitute 15 percent of all liver cells and serve a phagocytic or blood-cleansing function.

The functional unit of the liver is the lobule, of which there are between 50,000 and 100,000 in the liver. Each lobule consists of a segment of a central vein surrounded by a number of sinusoids in an arrangement similar to the spokes around the hub of a wheel. The sinusoids are vessels that transport blood from the portal vein to the central vein, which eventually delivers blood to the hepatic vein. Two primary

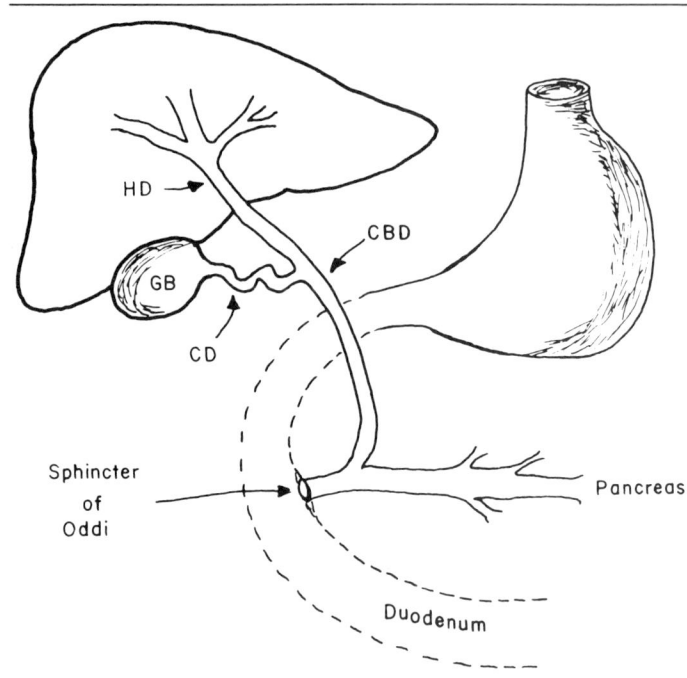

Figure 11-1. Liver and hepatobiliary system: hepatic duct (HD), gallbladder (GB), cystic duct (CD), common bile duct (CBD).

types of cells make up the sinusoids; *endothelial cells* and *Kupffer's cells*. Endothelial cells form the main structure or sinusoidal lining and act as blood filters, whereas Kupffer's cells, which are dispersed along the sinusoid, serve as macrophages. These sinusoidal cells are responsible for the processes whereby various materials are removed from the blood. Surrounding the sinusoids are the hepatocytes. Between the sinusoid and the hepatocytes is the space of Disse. This space ranges in depth from 0.25 to 2.0 µm and contains a reinforcing network of collagen fibers. These features of liver microanatomy are depicted in Figures 11-2 and 11-3 and are described in detail by Elias and Sherrick[1].

Sinusoidal Cells

Morphologically, *endothelial cells* are flat irregularly shaped cells characterized by numerous fenestrae, or pores, that appear throughout their cytoplasm. These pores are approximately 0.1 µm in diameter. Through these pores molecular substances and small particles may leave the sinusoidal blood, enter the space of Disse and have access to the underlying hepatocytes. Larger particles may enter the space also through 0.02- to 1.0-µm slits between the endothelial cells. In addition to this "sieve-like" function, endothelial cells contain pinocytotic vesicles that can sequester into the cell's cytoplasm particles less than 0.1 µm in size. This process has been observed with antimony sulfide particles.

Kupffer's cells have a variable shape but are basically stellate. They lie on or are embedded in the endothelial lining and may also lie at least partly in the space of Disse where their microvilli intermingle with the microvilli of the hepatocytes, which suggests anchorage of these cells. They also tend to accumulate near the branches of the portal veins. This variability in shape and position suggests that Kupffer's cells are mobile. Kupffer's cells have a bulky cytoplasm that is rich in lysosomes, which indicates their ability to digest material. Their membrane is covered with a 70-nm-thick fuzzy coat of

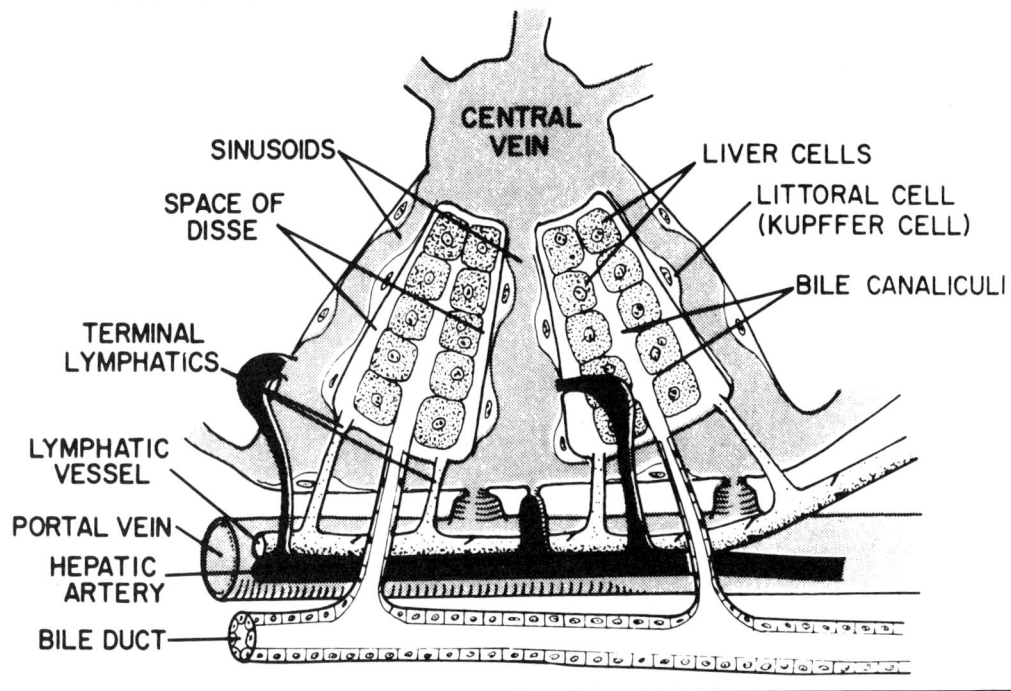

Figure 11-2. Basic structure of a liver lobule showing the hepatic cellular plates, the blood vessels, the bile-collecting system, and the lymph flow system, which comprises the spaces of Disse and the interlobular lymphatics. *(From Guyton AC, et al: Circulatory Physiology II: Dynamics and Control of the Body Fluids. Philadelphia, Saunders, 1975, p 220, with permission.)*

protein-like material that contains pinocytotic structures capable of trapping particles less 0.1 μm such as colloidal gold. Additionally, Kupffer's cells are capable of phagocytosis by pseudopodia, and, in general, particles larger than 0.1 μm are specifically engulfed by them.

Some general properties may be noted regarding Kupffer's cell phagocytosis of particles from the blood. Microscopic studies have shown in several instances, although not with all types of substances, that intravenously injected particles become coated with a serum protein material (opsonin). This coating is believed to be fibrin-like because heparin prevents the reaction. This coating frequently causes the particles to adhere to each other and to the walls of the liver sinusoids. In vivo, particle size may thus be much larger than the preinjection size because of aggregation. A coated particle that adheres to the fuzzy coat of a Kupffer's cell induces the phagocytic process. Once inside the cell lysosomes digest metabolizable particles and dispose of them by reutilization or excretion. Indigestable particles may be stored in the lysosomes or distributed over daughter cells or to other organs by the migration of loaded Kupffer's cells. A complete description of sinusoidal cell function is given by Wisse.[2,3]

Hepatocytes

The hepatocyte is polygonal in shape, about 30μm in diameter, and has eight or more surfaces. These cells are arranged in the form of plates one cell in thickness forming

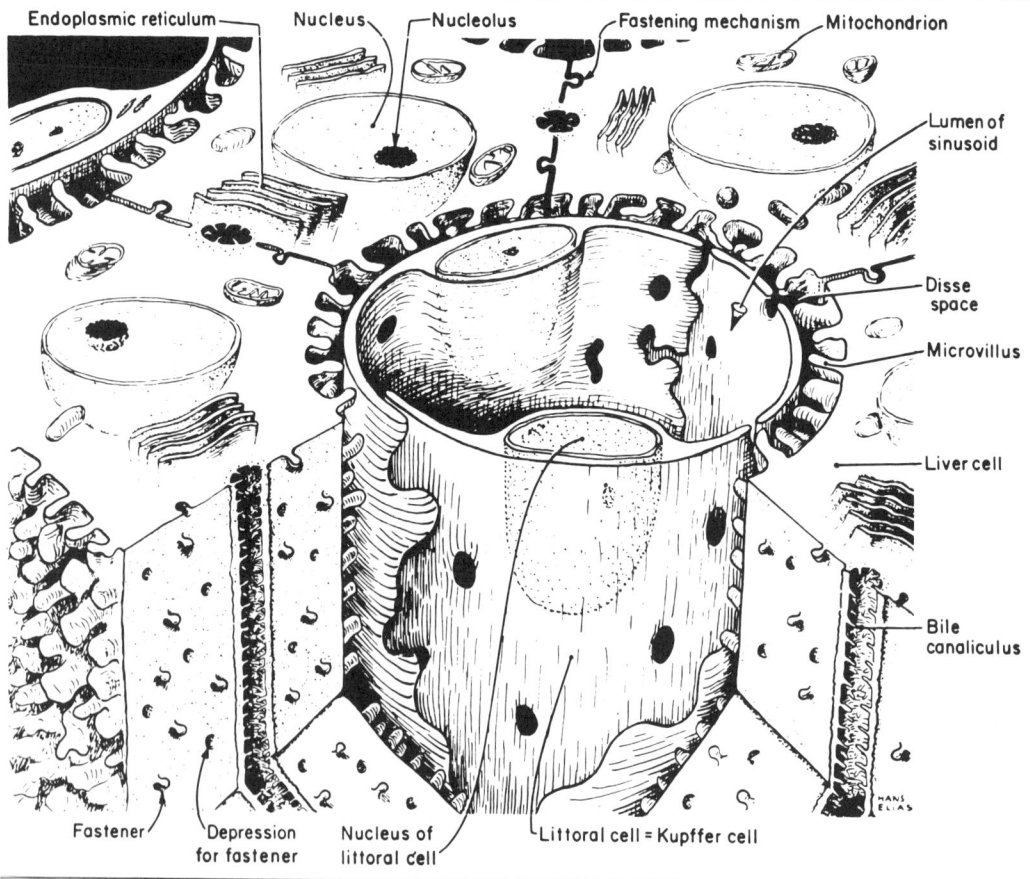

Figure 11-3. Ultrastructure of the mammalian liver. *(From Elias H, Pauly JE: Human Microanatomy. Chicago, DaVinci, 1960, p 135, with permission.)*

an irregular wallwork surrounding the space containing the sinusoids. The hepatocyte has three physiologic surfaces: one that contacts neighboring hepatocytes, a grooved surface that delimits bile canaliculi, and a sinusoidal surface that projects numerous microvilli into the space of Disse.[4]

Soluble substances that leave the sinusoidal blood and enter the space of Disse may reenter the blood back through the sinusoidal pores, or they may interact with specific receptor sites on the hepatocyte membrane. This membrane is capable of four independent carrier-mediated transport pathways that can accommodate either organic anions, organic cations, neutral compounds, or conjugated bile salts (Fig. 11-4).[5] Within the hepatocyte are various protein storage sites and metabolizing organelles that can process substances before transport at the biliary canaliculus into the bile. Any substance that is actively transported at these membrane sites will exhibit a transport maximum and may be inhibited competitively by other substances with similar chemical properties. Bilirubin is excreted by the anionic pathway, and hyperbilirubinemia, therefore, may effectively slow the rate of radiopharmaceutical excretion by this pathway.

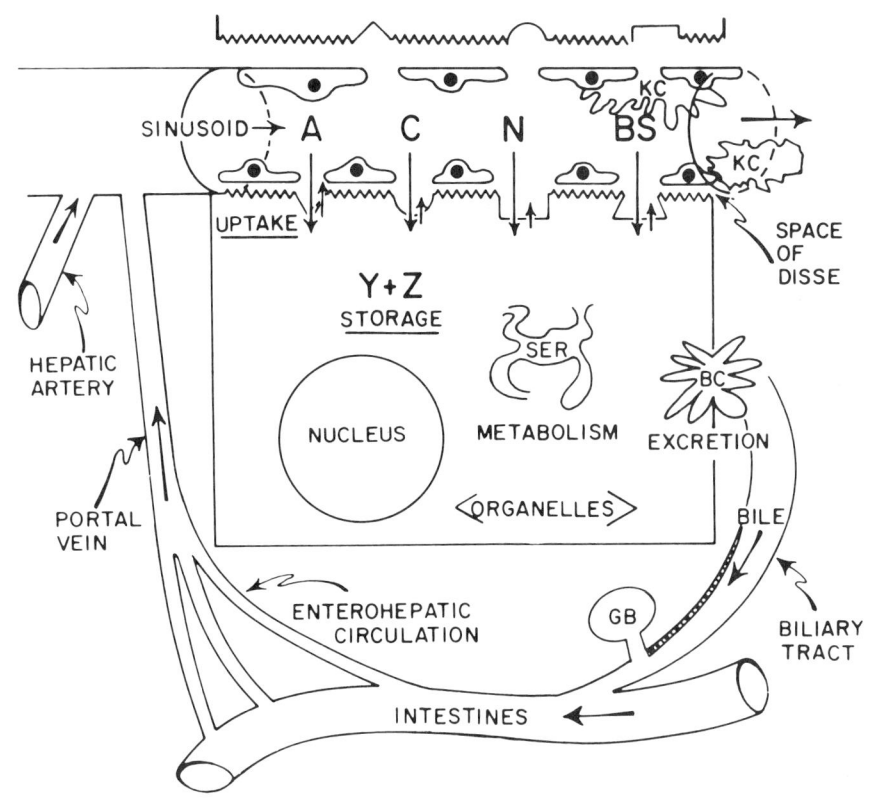

Figure 11-4. Schematic representation of a hepatocyte. Substrates in the blood diffuse through pores in the endothelial lining of the sinusoids and bind to the hepatocyte at one of four membrane-bound carriers: anionic (A), cationic (C), nonionic (N), and bile salt (BS). Inside the hepatocyte the substrate may be stored at specific binging sites such as Y and Z proteins, and it also may undergo metabolic conversion at other sites including the smooth endoplasmic reticulum (SER). Biliary excretion occurs at a biliary canaliculus (BC). Subsequently the substrate in the bile may be stored and concentrated in the gallbladder (GB) or excreted into the intestines. Some biliary components are reabsorbed from the intestines into the portal vein and reextracted by the hepatocyte (enterohepatic circulation). The sinusoids are lined by Kupffer's cells (KC), which are a part of the RES. (From Loberg MD, et al, 1979, p 522, with permission.[5])

DEVELOPMENT OF RADIOCOLLOIDS

Several radioactive agents have been used to study the liver. Early investigations used the radiocolloid P-32 chromic phosphate to study liver blood flow[6] and I-131 human serum albumin (HSA)[7] and colloidal Au-198[8] to make the first liver scans with the newly developed rectilinear scanner. An interesting approach to liver scanning was the administration of Mo-99 as the molybdate anion that localized in hepatocytes by incorporation into xanthine oxidase.[9] Scans were obtained in 24 hours by detection of accumulated Te-99m activity in the liver.

In 1956 Benacerraf et al developed colloidal particles of I-131-HSA to study liver phagocytosis,[10] but this agent was rapidly metabolized and cleared from the liver, thus making it unsatisfactory for use with slow-moving rectilinear scanners.

In 1963 Tc-99m sulfur colloid (Tc-SC) was developed by Richards.[11] The tagging of Tc-99m to sulfur particles was accomplished by air oxidation of hydrogen sulfide gas bubbling through an acidified solution of sodium pertechnetate and gelatin. The preparation was sterilized before use by filtration through a 0.22-μm membrane. The particle size was estimated to be 0.05 to 0.15 μm.[12] Soon afterward the preparation of sulfur colloid was greatly simplified by use of a kit that contained sodium thiosulfate as the source of sulfur.[13]

Several other radiocolloids were developed for diagnostic studies, but none have supplanted the clinical utility of sulfur colloid. Tc-99m antimony sulfide colloid prepared from preformed particles (8 to 12 nm) became more useful for studying the lymphatic system.[14] Indium-113m hydroxide colloid was useful as an alternative for those laboratories with tin-113/In-113m generators.[15] The development of Tc-99m phytate (inositol hexaphosphate), which formed an insoluble calcium chelate in the blood, was sought as a means of altering biologic localization among liver, spleen, and bone marrow.[16]

The impetus for developing Tc-99m stannous albumin colloid was the theoretic reduction of the radiation dose to the liver because of hepatic metabolism. This has not been realized from clinical investigations, however, and the kit offers only instant labeling as an advantage.

Tc-SC appears to remain the drug of choice for RES imaging because of ready availability, ease of preparation, and a long history of use that has developed a clinical familiarity with its pattern of biodistribution and scan interpretation. Table 11-1 summarizes the properties of several radiocolloids.

TABLE 11-1. PROPERTIES OF RADIOCOLLOIDS FOR LIVER IMAGING

Agent	Particle Size (nm)	Half-life Physical	Half-life Biologic	Decay Mode	Gamma Energy (keV)	Activity Administered (mCi)	Radiation Dose to Liver (rad/mCi)
Au-198 colloid	5–50	2.8 d	Very long	β^-	411	0.3	40
Tc-99m sulfur colloid	100–1000	6 hr	Very long	IT	140	5.0	0.34
I-131 albumin colloid	10–20	8 d	60 min	β^-	364	0.2	0.8
In-113m hydroxide colloid	10–20	1.7 hr	30 d	IT	393	2.0	0.5
Tc-99m albumin colloid (Microlite-NEN)	200–1000 (80%) <200 (15%)	6 hr	11 hr (Tc-99m) 4 hr (HSA)	IT	140	5.0	0.34

TABLE 11-2. Tc-99m SULFUR COLLOID KIT

Kit Component	Quantity	Function
Reaction mixture vial		
Sodium thiosulfate ($Na_2S_2O_3$)	12 mg	Source of sulfur
Gelatin	9 mg	Protective colloid
Potassium phosphate (K_2HPO_4)	24.5 mg	pH adjustment > 7.0
Disodium edetate (Na_2EDTA)	2.79 mg	Chelates aluminum ion
Acid syringe		
Hydrochloric acid (HCl)	18 mg	Lowers pH at reaction time
		Hydrolysis of thiosulfate
Buffer syringe		
Sodium hydroxide (NaOH)	20 mg	Neutralizes excess HCl
Sodium phosphate (NaH_2PO_4)	70 mg	and buffers final product to pH 5-6

PRODUCTION OF Tc-99m SULFUR COLLOID

Tc-SC is prepared daily using the kit method developed in the early 1960s. Although kit formulations vary between manufacturers, the basic principle of production is the same. One of the commercial Tc-SC kits will be used to illustrate the important aspects of colloid production. Listed in Table 11-2 are the kit components and ingredient function. Table 11-3 compares several colloid kits for liver imaging.

To prepare Tc-SC, Tc-99m pertechnetate is added to the reaction vial followed by hydrochloric acid. The mixture is immediately placed into a boiling water bath for 10 minutes. During this time the Tc-SC is formed. The vial is then removed from the water bath and allowed to cool, and the buffer solution is added to adjust the solution pH before patient administration. Chromatography is done to measure the radiolabeling efficiency. The US Pharmacopeia (USP) states that not less than 92 percent of the activity must be in the form of Tc-SC.

During the reaction the initially clear solution turns cloudy because of the release of elemental sulfur according to the following reaction:

$$S_2O_3^{2-} + 2H^+ \longrightarrow S + SO_2 + H_2O$$

The acid hydrolysis of thiosulfate goes through the formation of thiosulfuric acid, $H_2S_2O_3$, which rapidly decomposes to form primarily sulfur, sulfur dioxide, and water but is also known to form hydrogen sulfide, H_2S. The Tc-99m is probably converted to the heptasulfide Tc_2S_7 because it has been demonstrated that carrier pertechnetate (Tc-99) in an acid solution will precipitate Tc_2S_7 on the addition of H_2S.[17] As the sulfur atoms are produced, they aggregate to form the colloidal particles of sulfur that contain the Tc_2S_7 by coprecipitation. It is interesting to note that in this chemical form technetium is not reduced but maintains the 7+ valence state, which is an exception to the usual requirement of pertechnetate reduction before radiolabeling.

The gelatin is present to control particle size formation during the reaction and to stablize the colloid. Gelatin is a macromolecular protein whose molecules serve as seed nuclei for the aggregation of sulfur atoms into colloidal sized particles. Gelatin coats the particles as they form; this controls particle size and gives the final product stability against precipitation. If the preparation is made without gelatin, the particles grow large in size and will precipitate onto the glass surface, making it very difficult to redisperse the particles.

Disodium edetate (Na_2EDTA) is present in the product to chelate any aluminum ion that may be present in the pertechnetate solution. If edetate is not present, free

TABLE 11-3. Tc-99m COLLOID KITS FOR LIVER-SPLEEN IMAGING

	Reaction Vial		Syringe A		Syringe B	
Colloid	Component	Quantity	Component	Quantity	Component	Quantity
Sulfur colloid (Mallinckrodt)	Phosphoric Acid (H_3PO_4)	100 mg in 2 ml	Gelatin $Na_2S_2O_3$ NaCl qs ad	13.2 mg 6.6 mg 0.99 mg 1.65 ml	Gelatin $NaC_2H_3O_2$ Na_2EDTA NaCl qs ad	21.6 mg 0.544 mg 4.0 mg 5.4 mg 1.6 ml

Preparation:

1. Add 0.1 to 5.0 ml Tc-99m pertechnetate (400 mCi max) to reaction vial.
2. Add contents of syringe A to the reaction vial.
3. Place the vial into a shielded boiling water bath for 8 min.
4. Add contents of syringe B to the reaction vial.
5. Place the vial into a boiling water bath for 2 min.
6. Cool the vial 15 min before use.
7. Store the labeled product at 15 to 30°C, and use within 6 hr of preparation.

Sulfur colloid (Syncor)	$Na_2S_2O_3$ Na_2EDTA Gelatin (lyophilized)	2.0 mg 2.3 mg 18.1 mg	HCl (0.148 M)	1.5 ml	NaH_2PO_4 NaOH qs ad	38.8 mg 11.1 mg 1.5 ml

Preparation:

1. Add 1 to 3 ml Tc-99m pertechnetate (500 mCi/ml max) to the reaction vial.
2. Add contents of syringe A to the reaction vial.
3. Place the vial into a shielded boiling water bath for 3 to 10 min.
4. Cool the vial for 3 min.
5. Add contents of syringe B to the vial
6. Store the labeled product at 15 to 30°C, and use within 6 hr of preparation.

Sulfur colloid (Squibb)	$Na_2S_2O_3$ Gelatin K_2HPO_4 Na_2EDTA qs ad	12.0 mg 9.0 mg 25.5 mg 2.79 mg 3.0 ml	HCl (0.25 M)	2 ml	NaH_2PO_4 NaOH qs ad	80 mg 20 mg 2 ml

Preparation:

1. Add 0.1 to 5.0 ml Tc-99m pertechnetate to the reaction vial.
2. Add contents of syringe A to the reaction vial.
3. Place the vial into a shielded boiling water bath for 10 ± 2 min.
4. Allow the vial to cool for 5 min.
5. Add contents of syringe B to the reaction vial.
6. Store the labeled product at 15 to 30°C, and use within 6 hr of preparation.

(continued)

TABLE 11-3. (Continued)

Colloid	Reaction Vial		Syringe A		Syringe B	
	Component	*Quantity*	*Component*	*Quantity*	*Component*	*Quantity*
Sulfur colloid (Medi-Physics)	HCl (1.0 M)	0.5 ml	$Na_2S_2O_3$ qs ad	1.9 mg 1.1 ml	Gelatin $NaC_2H_3O_2$ qs ad	5.3 mg 177.0 mg 2.1 ml

Preparation:

1. Add 0.1 to 5.0 ml Tc-99m pertechnetate (400 mCi max) to the reaction vial.
2. Add contents of syringe A to the reaction vial.
3. Place the vial into a shielded boiling water bath for 5 ± 0.5 min.
4. Add contents of syringe B to the reaction vial.
5. Cool the vial to room temperature before use.
6. Store the labeled product at 15 to 30°C, and use within 6 hr of preparation.

Colloid	Component	Quantity
Albumin colloid (Dupont/NEN)[a]	Albumin colloid	1.00 mg
	Normal HSA	10.0 mg
	$SnCl_2 \cdot 2H_2O$ (min)	0.006 mg
	$SnCl_2 \cdot 2H_2O$ (max)	0.17 mg
	Poloxamer 188	1.1 mg
	Medronate disodium	0.12 mg
	Sodium phosphate anhydrous	10.0 mg

Preparation:

1. Add 2 to 8 ml Tc-99m pertechnetate (75 mCi max) to the reaction vial.
2. Swirl for 1 min; let stand for 1 to 2 min before use.
3. Store labeled product at 2 to 8°C, and use within 6 hr of preparation.

[a]Store the kit at 15 to 30°C before labeling with Tc-99m.

---

aluminum ion will react with the phosphate buffers to form insoluble aluminum phosphate, which precipitates from solution and carries with it the Tc-SC. Intravenous injection of such a product will produce uptake of activity in the lungs because of the large particle size. Figures 11-5 through 11-9 illustrate some results of changing formulation parameters in the production of Tc-SC.

PHYSICAL AND CHEMICAL STABILITY OF Tc-99m SULFUR COLLOID

In general the preparation of Tc-SC from commercial kits does not present any significant problems if manufacturers' directions are followed closely. Once formed, the technetium–sulfur bond is quite stable. A few considerations during preparation, how-

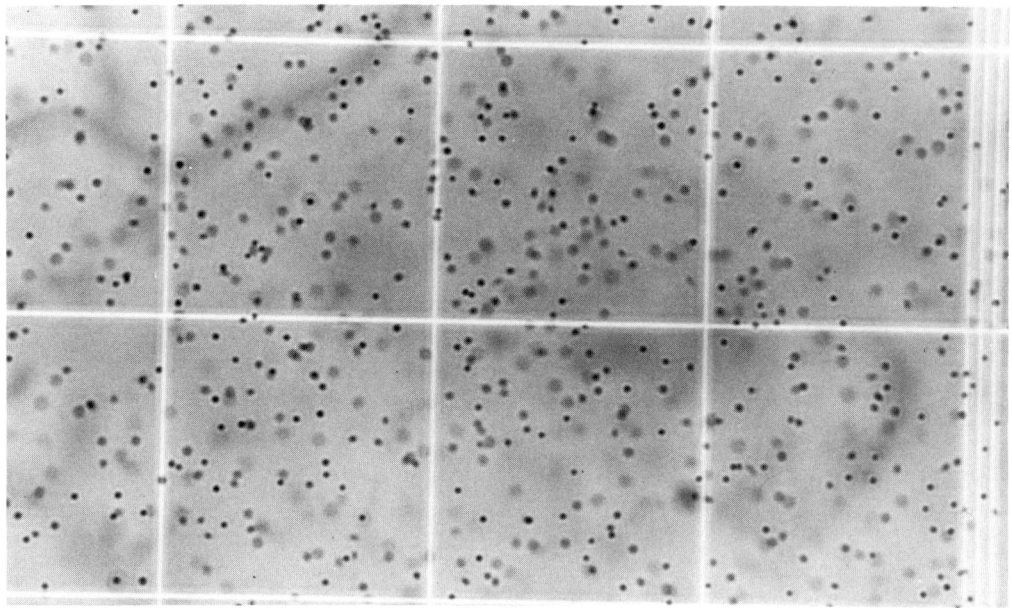

Figure 11-5. A. Microscopic appearance of sulfur colloid prepared with gelatin. Magnification, 450 ×; distance between lines, 50 μm.

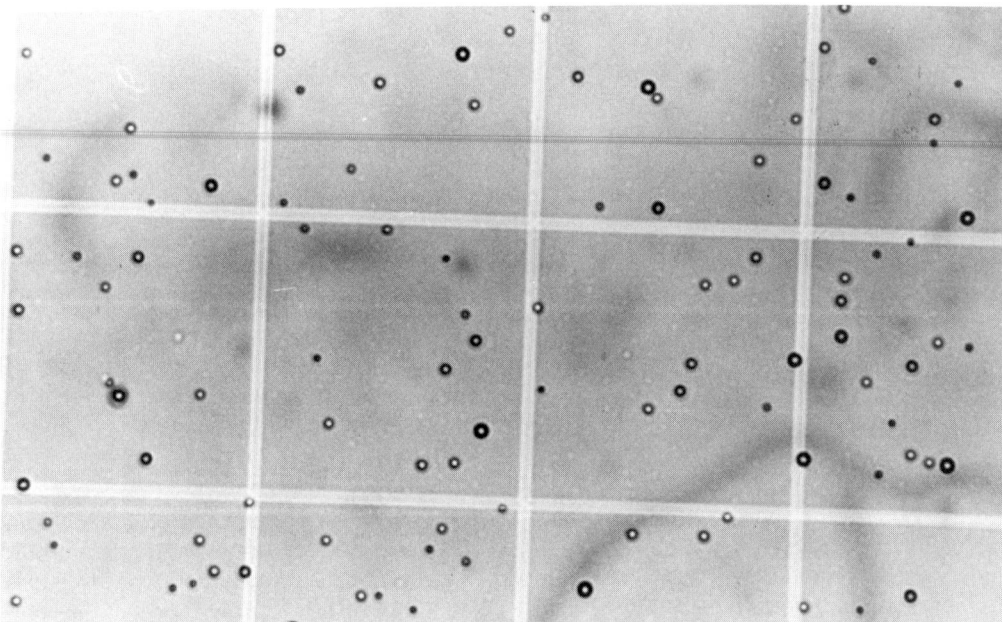

Figure 11-5. B. Microscopic appearance of sulfur colloid prepared without gelatin. Note that the particle size is larger than that in Figure 11-5A. Magnification, 450 ×; distance between lines, 50 μm.

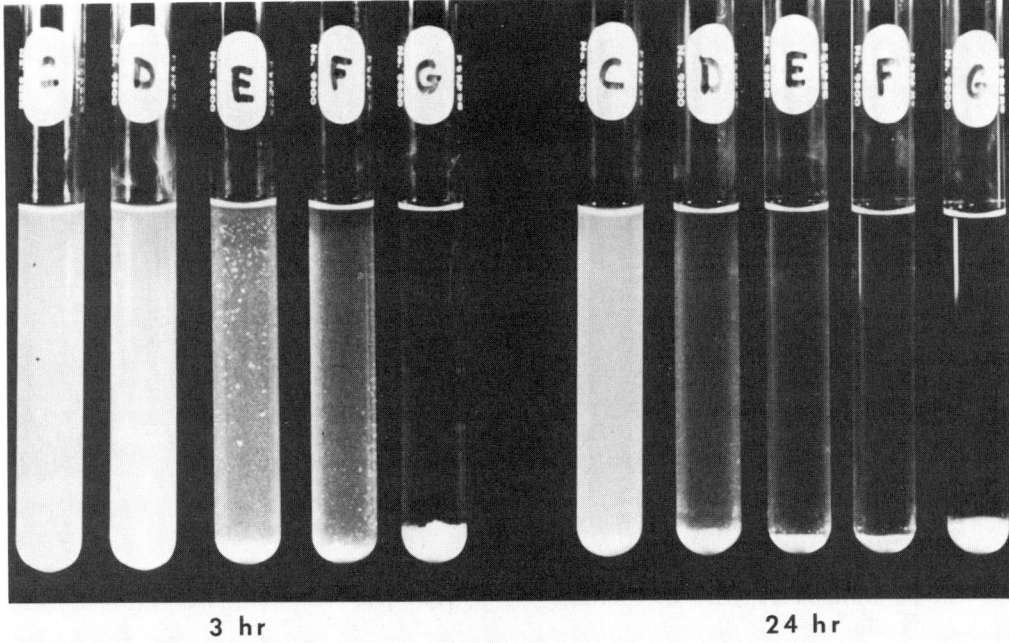

Figure 11-6. Flocculation of sulfur colloid with time by aluminum ion. The product does not contain EDTA. Aluminum ion concentration (µg/ml): C, 1; D, 3; E, 5; F, 30; G, 50.

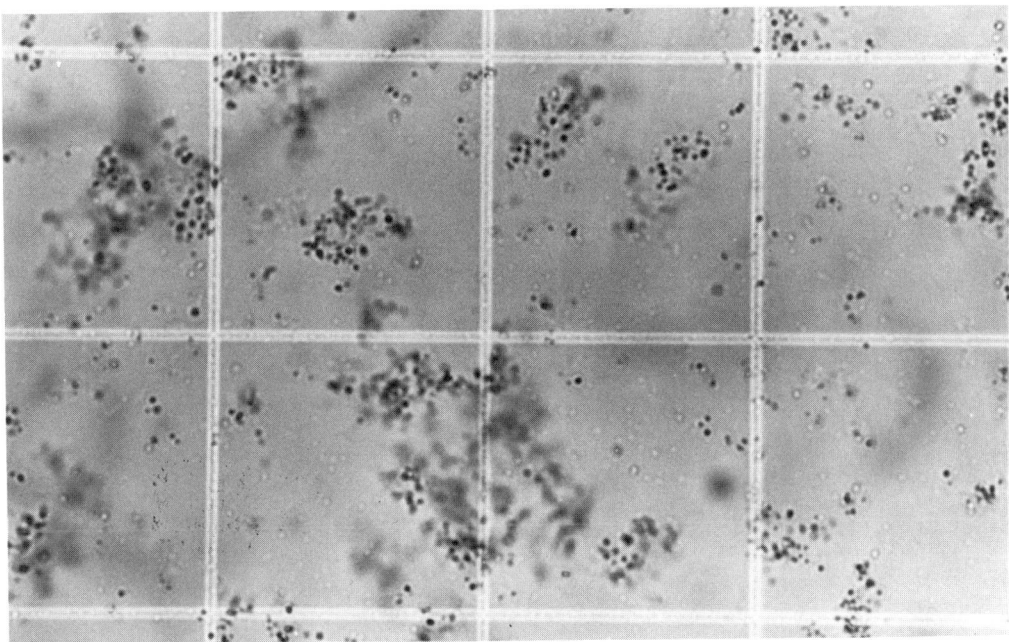

Figure 11-7. Flocculated particles of aluminum phosphate containing sulfur colloid particles. Magnification, 450 ×; distance between lines, 50 µm.

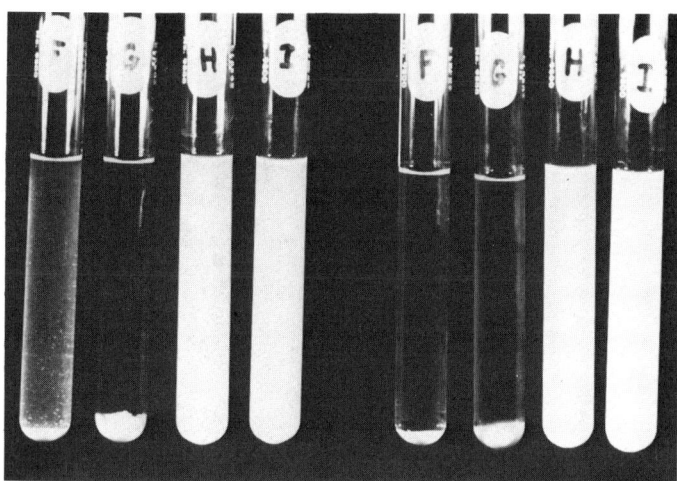

Figure 11-8. Influence of a buffer system on sulfur colloid stability. Tubes F and G, phosphate buffer; tubes H and I, acetate buffer; tubes F and H, 120 μg Al ion; tubes G and I, 360 μg Al ion. The product does not contain EDTA.

ever, are noteworthy.[18] Kits containing thiosulfate and EDTA together in the reaction vial to which pertechnetate has been added should not be allowed to stand for any length of time before heating because the thiosulfate can reduce the pertechnetate to a lower-valence state. The reduced technetium will then complex with EDTA to produce a radiochemical impurity in Tc-SC. In actual practice this may amount to only a few percent of the total activity, but Tc-EDTA formaton can be minimized if

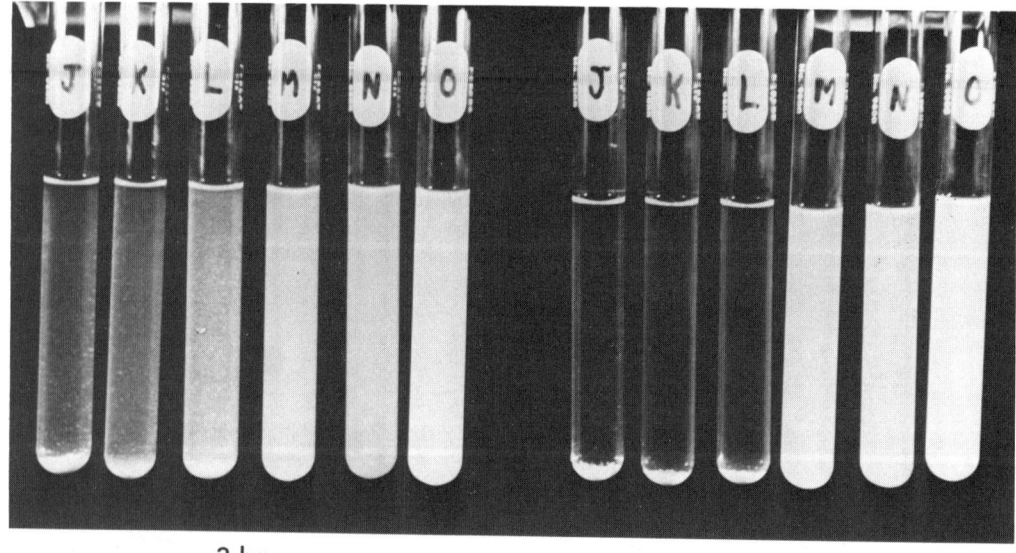

Figure 11-9. Stabilizing effect of EDTA against aluminum phosphate flocculation in sulfur colloid. EDTA:Al ion molar ratio: J, 0.125; K, 0.25; L, 0.5; M, 1.0; N, 2.0; O, 4.0.

the reaction vial is heated immediately after the addition of pertechnetate and acid. The ideal kit would require acidification of pertechnetate first, followed by the addition of thiosulfate, and then heating. Heating should be for the entire length of time stipulated for each kit at a rolling boil (95 to 100°C) to assure complete reaction. Finally, the completed preparation of Tc-SC should be buffered to pH 6. An alkaline pH decomposes the sulfide to release free pertechnetate.

BIODISTRIBUTION OF Tc-99m SULFUR COLLOID

After intravenous administration in humans Tc-SC leaves the vascular space rapidly with a clearance half-time of 2 to 3 minutes[12] and localizes in the liver, spleen, and bone marrow. Within 10 to 15 minutes (about five half-times), about 97 percent of the dose is remove from the blood, and liver imaging may begin. The start of imaging may be delayed in patients with severely diseased livers because of slow blood clearance. By 92 hours 4 percent of the injected activity is excreted in the urine and 3 percent in the feces.[12] The remaining activity is retained in the body with an effective half-life of 6 hours.

Several factors have been shown to influence the blood clearance and distribution of intravenously injected colloids in general including Tc-SC.[19] Some of the more important factors include organ blood flow, disease state, particle size, particle dose, and serum factors.

Blood Flow

Extraction of trace doses of radiocolloids by the liver is directly related to the volume of blood flow through the organ. In a healthy individual about 85 percent of a Tc-SC dose will localize in the liver, with 4 to 8 percent in the spleen and the remainder in the bone marrow.[20] This disproportionate localization is due, primarily, to the fact that the liver receives about 30 percent of the cardiac output compared with only about 5 percent for the spleen.[21]

Disease States

In liver disease a significant number of cells will be injured or destroyed, and this factor can decrease the absolute concentration of colloid deposited in the liver. Severe cirrhosis produces a backpressure in portal blood flow, which also influences radiocolloid distribution. In cirrhosis a decreased liver uptake of radiocolloid with a concomitant shunting of excess particles to the spleen and bone marrow is frequently observed.

The presence of certain infectious diseases that produce high levels of sytemic endotoxin may stimulate overall RES activity in the body. Using metabolizable microaggregates of radioiodinated albumin, Wagner and Iio[22] demonstrated that bacterial infections caused an increased RES functional capacity in humans. This suggests that organs with normally diminished RES activity may localize radiocolloids in disease; indeed, experimental studies in animals have demonstrated increased lung uptake of Tc-SC in endotoxin-treated animals compared with nontreated controls.[23] This phenomenon may be responsible for the occasional increased lung uptake of Tc-SC seen in patients during a liver scan.

Particle Size

Tc-SC produced by the original H_2S method provides an essentially monodisperse colloidal preparation, with 90 percent of the particles having a size of 0.09 ± 0.01 μm.[17] The thiosulfate method gives a more nonuniform size distribution as prepared from commercial kits. Using Nuclepore filtration, Davis et al[24] determined the size distribution of thiosulfate-generated particles to be as follows: less than 0.1 μm (15%), less than 0.4 μm (70%), 0.1 to 1.0 μm (80%), and greater than 1.0 μm (5%).

In general, larger particles are cleared faster from the blood and have greater deposition in the liver and spleen and less in the bone marrow. Atkins et al[25] compared small-sized particles of Tc-SC produced by the H₂S method with particles of Tc-SC ten times larger produced by the thiosulfate method. As the dose of smaller-sized particles increased, the percent uptake in the liver decreased whereas uptake in bone marrow increased; spleen uptake was unaffected. For the larger particles there was always more in the liver and spleen and less in bone marrow than with the smaller-sized particles. The reasons for this are not clear but may relate to the processes involved with particle localization. It may be that larger particles are not only subject to phagocytosis from the blood but may also be physically trapped within the liver's space of Disse whereas smaller particles readily move into and out of this space. If smaller particles are less likely to be trapped in the space of Disse, their systemic circulation time will be increased, and the probability of bone marrow phagocytosis is therefore increased.

Blood Clearance and Serum Opsonins

When colloidal particles (Au-198) are administered to rats in small numbers (less than 1×10^{13} particles/kg body weight) the rate of blood clearance is constant, having a half-time of 2.5 minutes.[26] Similar clearance half-times are reported for Tc-SC.[12] This is similar to the situation of administering trace doses of radiocolloids to humans for liver scans. In these situations the rate of liver uptake is related to its blood flow rather than its RES capacity. When the dose administered to rats is greater than 1×10^{13} particles/kg, the rate of blood disappearance decreases with increasing dose. This indicates a condition of RES depression, and this phenomenon has also been observed in humans. It has been suggested that this depression is due to saturation of the RE cell capacity, but several experimental observations reveal that it may also be due to depletion of the specific serum opsonin pool for that particular colloid.[19] Support for the role of opsonins is given by the fact that RES depression in animals and humans appears to be particle specific in that the injection of one type of colloid will induce a state of RES depression relative to the subsequent blood clearance of that particular colloid, whereas the clearance of a dissimilar colloid is less affected. Figure 11–10 illustrates this point.

It may be inferred, then, that the localization of particles by phagocytosis may be controlled by both antibody-like opsonins in the blood and specific macrophages that recognize a specific opsonin–particle complex. Recognition may be influenced by particle change or other chemical properties of the particle surface.

MECHANISM OF LOCALIZATION AND METABOLIC FATE OF RADIOCOLLOIDS

A common belief is that colloidal particles are localized in the liver by Kupffer's cell phagocytosis. Although this is true to some extent, it may not completely explain the process, and a few reports indicate that other mechanisms of localization may be involved. Chaudhuri et al[27] using autoradiography, demonstrated in mice that although colloidal Au-198 was primarily engulfed by Kupffer's cells Tc-SC maintained a generalized distribution throughout the liver with no apparent concentration in Kupffer's cells. This may be due to differences in the particle size of these two colloids or to their chemical properties. Brucer[28] states that phagocytosis of small colloids (<0.1 μm) is a primary function of Kupffer's cells, whereas larger particles, (0.1 to 1.0 μm) which leave the sinusoidal blood through the slits between endothelial cells, may become trapped in the network of hepatocellular microvilli and collagen fibrils in the space of Disse. In other experiments,[29] analysis of isolated rat liver sinusoidal cells after intravenous administration of radiocolloids demonstrated that a size distribution of sinusoidal cells exists. In this regard there was preferential localization of small col-

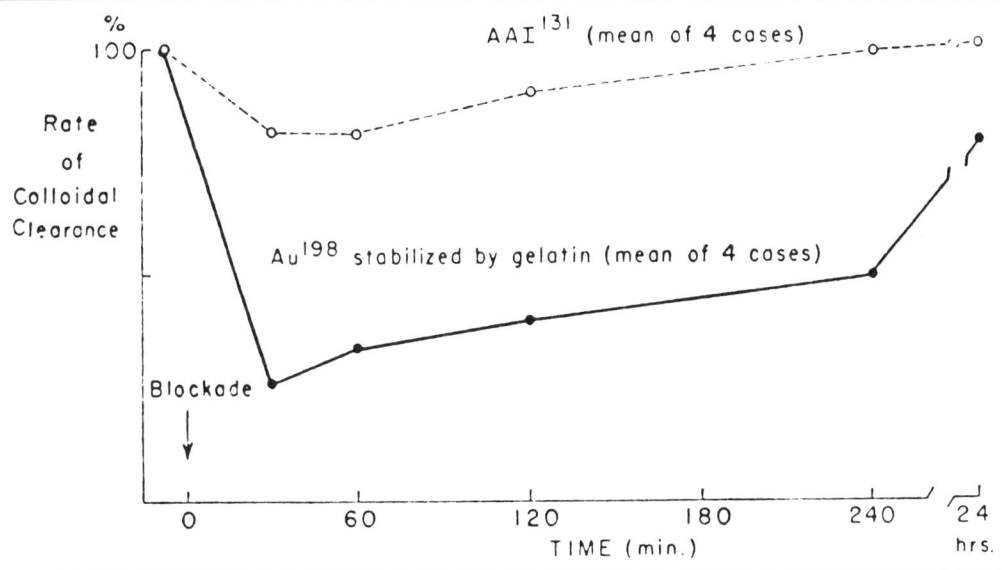

Figure 11-10. Effect of RES blockade with gelatin (50 mg/kg) on aggregated albumin iodine-131 and Au-198 colloid stabilized by gelatin in humans. *(From Wagner HN, et al, 1964, p 1525, copyright of the American Society for Clinical Investigation, with permission.[22])*

loids (0.005 to 0.05 μm) such as colloidal Au-198 in the smaller cells, which were in the majority, whereas larger colloids (0.8 to 1.5 μm) such as Tc-SC localized primarily in the larger sinusoidal cells, which included only 15 to 25 percent of all cells. It thus appears that larger colloidal particles may only be phagocytosed by a discrete and limited number of cells in the liver and that the high degree of liver extraction of colloids is due, primarily, to physical entrapment in the space of Disse.

Regarding particle fate in the liver, Brucer[28] states that particles trapped in the space of Disse are presumed to drain into portal and hepatic lymph nodes, a process requiring weeks to months. Although no evidence could be found to support this contention, it seems reasonable because colloids have been used to study the lymphatic system and are readily transported in the lymph.

Similarly, no firm evidence is available to demonstrate the fate of particles engulfed by phagocytes. Unless specific enzyme systems are present to transform these inert sulfur particles into chemically excretable forms (e.g., SO_4^{2-}), these particles are probably stored in the cytoplasm of Kupffer's cells. Because these cells are eventually replaced by new cells, the particles may simply be transferred from cell to cell with each succeeding generation. One study, however, suggests a mode of excretion from the body. Easton[30] reported that, in mice, macrophages loaded with thorium dioxide colloid eventually pass from the liver into the circulation and migrate to the lungs. Upon passing into the airway mucosa they ascend the respiratory passages and are either swallowed and excreted in the feces or are eliminated in the saliva. A considerable fraction (one third to half) of the administered dose, however, was retained for up to 1 year. A small amount was excreted in bile through parenchymal liver cells and a small amount into the urine, but only during the first 10 days.

ADVERSE REACTIONS AND TOXICITY FROM RADIOCOLLOIDS AND RADIATION DOSE

When a substance is retained for an indefinite period of time in the body, toxicity becomes a concern. Fortunately for diagnostic radiocolloids, chronic and acute toxicity is of small concern because these agents are usually administered only once or twice to the same patient and in extremely small amounts. Additionally, when the RES is challenged with high doses of colloids, recovery from RES depression is rapid and complete because of the regenerative capacity of the RES.[22] One exception to this has been noted. Colloidal indium hydroxide has been shown to produce hepatocyte toxicity in mice, but this is of minor significance because the dose used was 10,000 times the usual diagnostic doses of In-113m or In-111 in humans.[31]

One exceptional situation where adverse effects may be serious is with potential misadministration during therapeutic use of radiocolloids. This situation refers to the administration of the wrong salt form of the radionuclide P-32. For instance, if 10 to 15 mCi of P-32 as soluble sodium phosphate instead of insoluble colloidal chromic phosphate is administered intracavitarily for therapy for effusions, severe bone marrow depression may result.[32] This occurs because the soluble sodium salt is readily absorbed into the blood from the peritoneal cavity or any other extracellular fluid space and is translocated to the bone marrow.

With Tc-SC no toxic reactions have been observed in mice given intravenous doses 1000 times the usual adult dose.[33] Pyrogenic or allergic reactions have, however, been reported with the use of Tc-SC that were attributed to stabilizers used in the formulations.[32]

Radiation dose estimates for Tc-SC under various conditons of liver health are listed in Table 11-4. Note that the radiation dose to organs other than the liver increases as liver disease becomes more advanced because of altered distribution of radiocolloid.

HEPATOBILIARY AGENTS

In 1955 an interest in hepatic reticuloendothelial function led George Taplin to investigate the excretion of rose bengal dye into the biliary system. It was presumed, at that time, that excretion of the dye was through Kupffer's cells. Further studies with radioiodinated I-131 rose bengal, however, led to the discovery that the dye was excreted, instead, by the hepatocytes and that it was not absorbed by the bowel. This information eventually led Taplin et al to introduce I-131 rose bengal as the radiopharmaceutical for studying hepatobiliary excretion,[35] and it remained in use for nearly 20 years.

TABLE 11-4. RADIATION DOSE FROM Tc-99m SULFUR COLLOID (rad/5mCi Administered)

Organ	Normal Liver	Diffuse Parenchymal Disease	
		Early-Intermediate	Intermediate-Advanced
Liver	1.7	1.1	0.8
Spleen	1.1	1.4	2.1
Bone marrow	0.14	0.23	0.4
Testes	0.0055	0.0105	0.016
Ovaries	0.028	0.0405	0.06
Total body	0.095	0.095	0.09

(From MIRD Report No. 3, 1975, p 108, with permission.[34])

During this time other agents were investigated to replace I-131. Short-lived radionuclides with more favorable physical properties were sought so that more activity could be administered with less radiation dose to the patient. Only the I-123 analogue of rose bengal offered a significant clinical advantage. It substantially reduced the radiation dose and improved image quality, but because of its relative unavailability and the need for in-house preparation and testing, I-123 rose bengal was not widely used.

A large number of Tc-99m agents were developed for hepatobiliary scintigraphy to replace I-131 rose bengal. The most successful agents used were Tc-99m–labeled pyridoxylidene glutamate (Tc-PYG) and derivatives of N-substituted iminodiacetic acid, the first being Tc-99m N-2, 6-dimethylacetanilido iminodiacetic acid (Tc-HIDA).[5] The primary disadvantage of Tc-PYG was that the extent and speed of its hepatobiliary clearance was less than that of I-131 rose bengal. Tc-HIDA, however, was found to clear the blood more rapidly than rose bengal and to possess a nearly identical hepatobiliary clearance.[5]

Several derivatives of the original Tc-HIDA compound have been prepared and investigated. Many of these agents have demonstrated superior hepatobiliary clearance properties and are now considered the drugs of choice for studying hepatobiliary function in humans.

Tc-99m-Labeled N-Substituted Iminodiacetic Acid Analogues

Development of Tc-99m–labeled N-substituted iminodiacetic acids (Tc-IDA analogues) began with the idea of producing a bifunctional radiopharmaceutical agent, that is, one having a strong chelating portion (iminodiacetic acid) that could chelate radionuclide metals, and a biochemical or drug portion (N-substituted group) that could be modified chemically and that would govern biologic distribution. The structure of iminodiacetic acid is shown in Figure 11-11. The N-substituted group is designated by the letter R. The generic names and acronyms respectively are as follows: lidofenin (HIDA), etilfenin (DIDA), iprofenin (PIPIDA), butilfenin (BIDA), and disofenin (DISIDA).

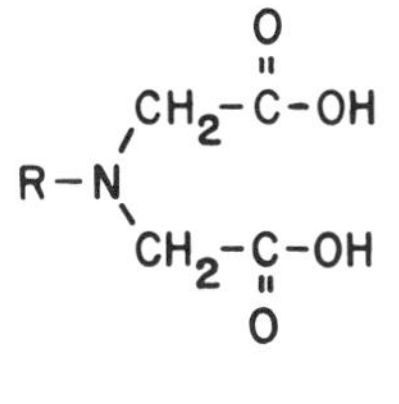

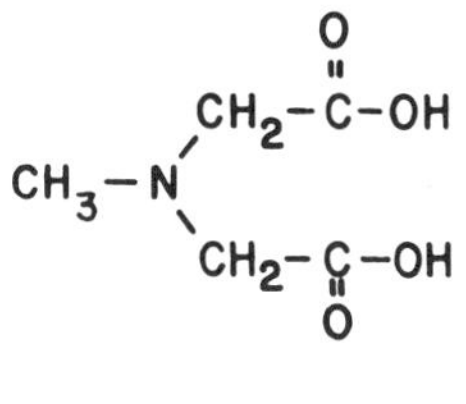

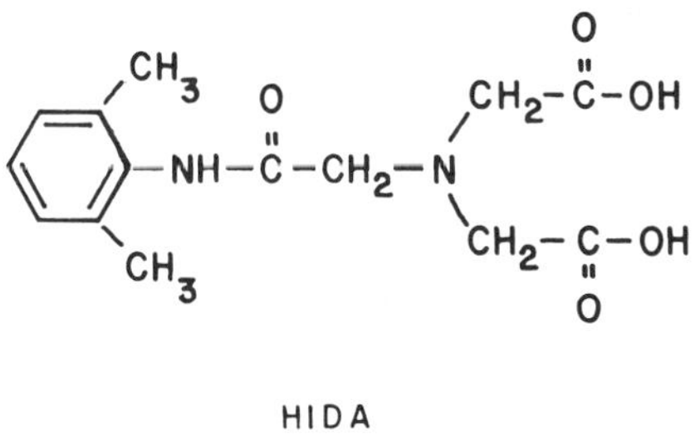

Figure 11-11. Chemical structure of N-substituted IDA and the first-used analogues, methyl-substituted (MIDA) and 2,6-dimethylacetanilido-substituted (HIDA).

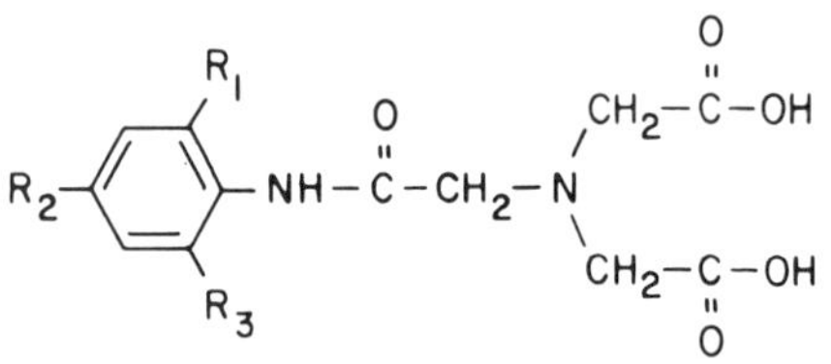

ANALOGUE	ACRONYM	R-1	R-2	R-3
2,6-dimethylacetanilido-IDA	HIDA	CH_3	H	CH_3
2,6-diethylacetanilido-IDA	DIDA	C_2H_5	H	C_2H_5
paraisopropylacetanilido-IDA	PIPIDA	H	$CH(CH_3)_2$	H
parabutylacetanilido-IDA	BIDA	H	C_4H_9	H
2,6-diisopropylacetanilido-IDA	DISIDA	$CH(CH_3)_2$	H	$CH(CH_3)_2$

Figure 11-12. Names and structures of N-substituted IDA analogues used as hepatobiliary imaging agents when labeled with Tc-99m.

The first two agents studied were stannous Tc-99m-labeled methyliminodiacetic acid (Tc-MIDA) and Tc-HIDA. Biodistribution studies in animals demonstrated that Tc-MIDA had rapid excretion into the urine whereas Tc-HIDA was excreted primarily by the liver into the bile.[36] This excretory pattern was not completely unpredictable because MIDA is quite hydrophilic and such compounds favor urinary excretion. The HIDA compound had lipophilic properties because of the substituted ring system, which favored liver excretion. It is interesting to note that the initial intent for synthesizing Tc-IDA compounds was to develop a technetium-labeled agent for heart imaging based on the structural similarities between the HIDA and lidocaine molecules. The high liver extraction of one of the first compounds tested, however, prompted the acronym HIDA, for hepatobiliary-IDA, and changed the course of direction toward development of a hepatobiliary imaging agent. The ability to add chemical substituents to the aromatic ring in the HIDA molecule stimulated much interest in the development of other Tc-IDA analogues. Figure 11-12 depicts several of these analogues that have been labeled with Tc-99m for clinical use.

Production of Tc-IDA Analogues

These agents are available as radiopharmaceutical kits that contain the particular IDA analogues and stannous chloride in lyophilized form. The Tc-99m complex is formed by the simple addition of pertechnetate to the vial. Thin-layer chromatography is performed to check for radiochemical impurities. The final product is stable for at least 6 hours after reconstitution with pertechnetate.

Chemical Structure and Properties of Tc-IDA Analogues

The Tc-IDA analogues have been studied more rigorously than most Tc-99m agents. One very interesting finding from the original work with Tc-HIDA is that the final complex formed with Tc-99m is believed to exist as a dimer, with two molecules of the chelating agent (HIDA) reacting with one atom of Tc-99m as shown in Figure 11–13.[5] The dimeric configuration, with Tc serving as a bridging atom between two ligand molecules, is a key factor that determines hepatobiliary excretion. This fact was determined from experiments that compared the hepatobiliary clearance of Tc-99m HIDA with that of carbon-14 HIDA and Sn-113 HIDA in dogs.[37] The results demonstrated that, 90 minutes after intravenous injection of these agents, 71 percent of the Tc-HIDA dose was excreted in the bile whereas only 0.15 percent and 0.02 percent of C-14 HIDA and Sn-113 HIDA, respectively, were excreted in bile. The technetium atom present in the complex thus exerts a strong influence on the biologic distribution of these agents. This contrasts with other Tc-99m agents whose biologic distribution is primarily determined by the properties of the particular ligand that binds technetium.

The dimeric structure also confers stability to the technetium complex. This fact has been substantiated by in vitro and in vivo experiments.[38] Ligand exchange reactions between Tc-HIDA and EDTA, also known to form very strong chelates with Tc, have demonstrated that Tc-EDTA does form in such incubation mixtures, but the rate of Tc release from HIDA is pH dependent and is extremely slow at physiologic pH. Although Tc-HIDA is not as thermodynamically stable as Tc-EDTA, it is thus kinetically inert and is expected to be very stable in vivo. This fact has been borne out in dogs injected with Tc-HIDA where the contents of the urinary bladder and gallbladder were obtained and reinjected.[36] The results showed an excretory pattern similar to the original compound. This suggests that Tc-HIDA is excreted in its original radiochemical form, having been minimally dissociated or metabolized.[36] Although similar studies have not been reported with other Tc-IDA derivatives, they are expected to behave similarly. In vivo stability of these agents is an important factor regarding their clinical use because metabolic degradation could produce metabolites with altered excretory patterns that might confuse the diagnostic interpretation. This could be especially important when delayed images are obtained 18 to 24 hours postinjection where potential pertechnetate impurity, localized in the gastrointestinal (GI) tract, could be misleading.

The hepatobiliary excretion of a substance has been shown to be related to several physicochemical properties[39,40] that include the requirements of (1) a molecular weight between 300 and 1000; (2) the presence of a strong polar group, usually

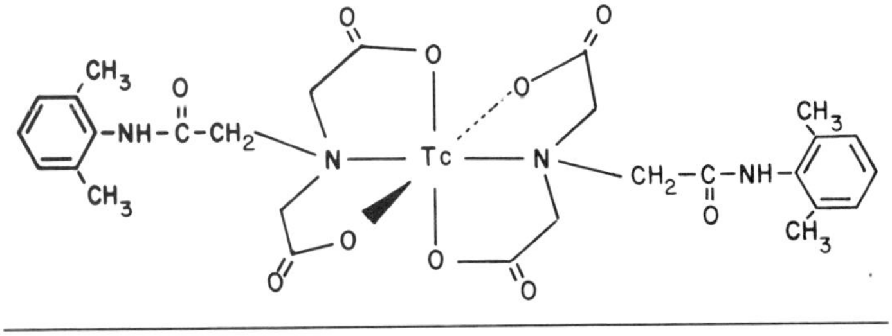

Figure 11-13. Dimeric structure of Tc $(HIDA)_2$.

ionized at plasma pH and typically anionic; (3) the presence of nonpolar groups, usually as aromatic rings; (4) a lipophilic character enhanced by ring substitution; and (5) binding to plasma albumin, which may promote transfer into the hepatocyte and limit urinary excretion.

In Tc-HIDA, the Tc atom is in the 3 + valence state and complexed by ionic and coordinate covalent bonds. It therefore satisfies three of the four negatively charged carboxylate oxygens and leaves a net charge of minus 1 on the complex. It has a molecular weight of 782, is lipophilic, and has both polar and nonpolar groups within its structure. All of these properties promote hepatobiliary excretion.

An ideal hepatobiliary agent should have the following characteristics: (1) rapid extraction from the plasma by the hepatocytes, (2) effective competition with bilirubin excretion, (3) rapid transit through the hepatocyte, (4) high biliary concentration, (5) minimal renal excretion, and (6) ready availability in kit form with high Tc-99m-labeling yields. Several of the Tc-IDA analogues have these characteristics with a more rapid rate and greater extent of biliary excretion than I-131-Rose Bengal (Table 11–5).

Mechanism of Localization and Excretion of Tc-IDA Analogues

The normal intrahepatic handling of Tc-HIDA and other derivatives is characterized by active transport at the anionic site of the hepatocyte membrane. This follows with transport through the hepatocyte cytoplasm and the biliary canaliculus into the bile ducts, with accumulation in the gall bladder and excretion into the intestine, usually visualized 10 to 20 minutes after injection.[37]

Confirmation of the anionic site of hepatocyte excretion has been made through competition experiments that demonstrate that sulfobromophthalein (BSP), known to be excreted at this site, effectively competes with the excretion of Tc-IDA compounds.[42] This has clinical importance in jaundiced patients. In studying the jaundiced patient, a radiopharmaceutical should be chosen with a low rate of renal excretion because this would afford the liver's saturated anionic clearance mechanism a better opportunity to concentrate and secrete the radiopharmaceutical. In a comparison of Tc-IDA derivatives Wistow et al[43] concluded that the parabutyl derivative BIDA may be preferred in the jaundiced patient because of its slower rate of renal clearance. Although the most desirable property of the IDA agents is high liver extraction, some degree of renal clearance appears to be essential, however, because it is the main mechanism for reducing blood background and allowing scintigraphic visualization of intestinal radioactivity.

Some comparison has been made between the various Tc-IDA derivatives regarding their rates of hepatobiliary clearance in the presence of elevated serum bilirubin levels. All agents will exhibit in-

TABLE 11–5. COMPARATIVE BILIARY EXCRETION OF TC-LABELED IDA ANALOGUES AND ROSE BENGAL I-131

Agent	Cumulative Percent Dose in Bile		
	30 min	60 min	90 min
DISIDA	43.7	76.2	86.8
DIDA	38.5	65.0	88.9
PIPIDA	34.6	64.3	73.8
BIDA	28.3	58.1	70.0
Rose bengal	13.0	40.1	57.9

(Data from Wistow NW, et al, 1978, p 793.[41])

creased renal excretion in various degrees of jaundice. In normal subjects the urinary excretion of Tc-HIDA is virtually complete by 24 hours and represents 14 percent of the injected dose, whereas in jaundiced patients, 22 percent is present in the urine at 90 minutes, increasing to 53 percent by 18 to 24 hours.[37] In the same subjects, the first and second half-lives of blood clearance increased, respectively, from 4.6 minutes and 31.5 minutes in normals to 5.3 minutes and 118 minutes in jaundiced subjects. Experience with Tc-HIDA has shown that, for serum bilirubin levels of 5 mg/dl or lower, serial imaging can distinguish between medical and surgical jaundice, but that at higher levels the degree of liver uptake is severely diminished and results are of qualified value.[44] In such instances, Ryan et al[37] suggest doubling the administered activity to provide sufficient activity for evaluating delayed images.

The newer Tc-IDA derivatives appear to be more effective than Tc-HIDA at elevated bilirubin levels. Tc-PIPIDA was shown to have four to five times greater uptake into isolated hepatocytes than Tc-HIDA at similar bilirubin levels.[5] In other comparisons Tc-DIDA was shown to have a hepatic extraction efficiency 2.15 times higher than Tc-PIPIDA and a blood-to-intestine transit time 12 minutes faster.[45] Tc-DISIDA has been shown to be similar to Tc-DIDA but to have a hepatic extraction efficiency 1.16 times higher than Tc-DIDA, with better delineation of liver parenchyma and hepatic ducts and less renal activity in patients with decreased hepatocyte function.[46] An additional report[47] indicates that Tc-DISIDA (now commercially available as disofenin) is the superior agent in detecting acute and chronic cholecystitis and in distinguishing medical from surgical jaundice in patients with elevated bilirubin levels from 1.1 to 24.5 mg/dl. Despite the superior claims of one agent over another, it is important to remember that all agents will suffer decreased hepatic extraction in jaundice, which may hinder diagnosis. Thus, Pauwels et al[48] have shown with Tc-DIDA that in the detection of obstructive jaundice the true positive identification rate declined as bilirubin levels rose, being, respectively, 93 percent (less than 10 mg/dl), 83 percent (10 to 20 mg/dl), and 25 percent (greater than 20 mg/dl).

In summary, it appears that good delineation of the liver and biliary system with Tc-IDA analogues requires a high rate of liver extraction from the blood and a low rate of renal excretion. With all of these agents, however, as the serum bilirubin levels increase, the liver extraction rate decreases and renal excretion increases. The best agent would thus be one that exhibits a smaller decrease in liver extraction with only a slight increase in renal excretion in the presence of decreased hepatocyte function. Tc-DISIDA appears to fit these requirements better than all the other agents and, at present, is considered to be the radiopharmaceutical of choice for hepatobiliary imaging.[46]

RADIATION DOSE

The radiation absorbed doses of Tc-IDA analogues have been calculated for normal subjects.[49] The critical organ is the gallbladder with an absorbed dose range of 690 to 780 mrad/mCi. The radiation dose depends on the degree of gallbladder stimulation, being lowest when a whole meal is used as the method of stimulation and highest in fasting subjects with no gallbladder stimulation. Cholecystokinin stimulation produces an intermediate radiation absorbed dose. A summary of biokinetic parameters and radiation absorbed doses for several Tc-IDA analogues is listed in Table 11-6. The absorbed dose ranges in mrad/mCi for these analogues in other organs were as follows: upper large intestine (320 to 370), lower large intestine (210 to 240), and small intestine (170 to 200). The gallbladder and intestinal doses are 10 to 15 percent higher for Tc-DISIDA than with the other agents, and the absorbed dose to the liver is lower because of more rapid liver excretion. Tc-BIDA produces the highest

TABLE 11-6. BIOKINETIC PARAMETERS AND RADIATION DOSE FOR TC-IDA ANALOGUES IN NORMAL SUBJECTS

Agent	Liver Clearance $T_{1/2}$ Biologic (min)	Renal Clearance Percent Dose in 24 hr Urine	Liver	Urinary Bladder	Radiation Dose (mrad/mCi)		
					Whole Meal	Gallbladder Cholecystokinin	Fasting
DISIDA	18.8	11.1	65	30	780	1030	2090
DIDA	37.3	17.1	73	36	690	1010	1860
HIDA	42.3	15.5	78	33	700	1010	1880
PIPIDA	59.3	14.3	90	33	690	990	1830
BIDA	107.6	5.6	130	23	690	990	1810

(Data from Brown PH, et al, 1982, p 1025.[49])

liver dose because of the longest excretion half-time from the liver. Tc-BIDA has the lowest urinary bladder dose and Tc-DIDA the highest in accordance with their urinary excretions.

SPLEEN

PHYSIOLOGIC ANATOMY

The spleen consists of two main compartments: the white pulp consisting of small lymphocytes and plasma cells and the red pulp, a swampy mass of vascular spaces whose supporting structure contains phagocytic cells of the RES. The spleen has two main functions in concert with its composition: antibody production in the white pulp and particle filtration in the red pulp. There is no significant storage of red or white cells in the human spleen as there is in certain animal species; however, about 30 percent of the body's platelets are sequestered by slow transit in the spleen and can be immediately released into the circulation when needed.[50]

Blood entering the spleen through the splenic arterioles empties first into the white pulp where plasma skimming occurs to remove soluble antigens. Passing through the white pulp, blood enters the red pulp through an open meshwork of large oval cells at the junction of the white and red pulp, termed the marginal zone. This cellular maze appears to serve as an initial filter that removes abnormal cells and allows normal cells to proceed unhindered. Upon entering the red pulp proper, blood cells may enter either of its alternate structures: the sinuses or the cords. Blood that enters the sinuses directly passes out easily from the spleen through the efferent veins. Blood cells that enter the cords, however, must pass through a fenestrated, screen-like basement membrane separating the cords from the sinus before gaining access to the venous drainage system. They are thus delayed to varying degrees in their transit. Because these fenestrae are only 3 µm in diameter, the blood cells must squeeze through, being deformed in their passage. It is at this point that abnormal, misshapen, and chemically altered cells are detained or destroyed. The macrophages that line the cord side of the sinus basement membrane can then phagocytose the cellular debris. The schematic organization of splenic microanatomy is shown in Figure 11-14, and a detailed description of physiologic anatomy is given by Williams et al.[51]

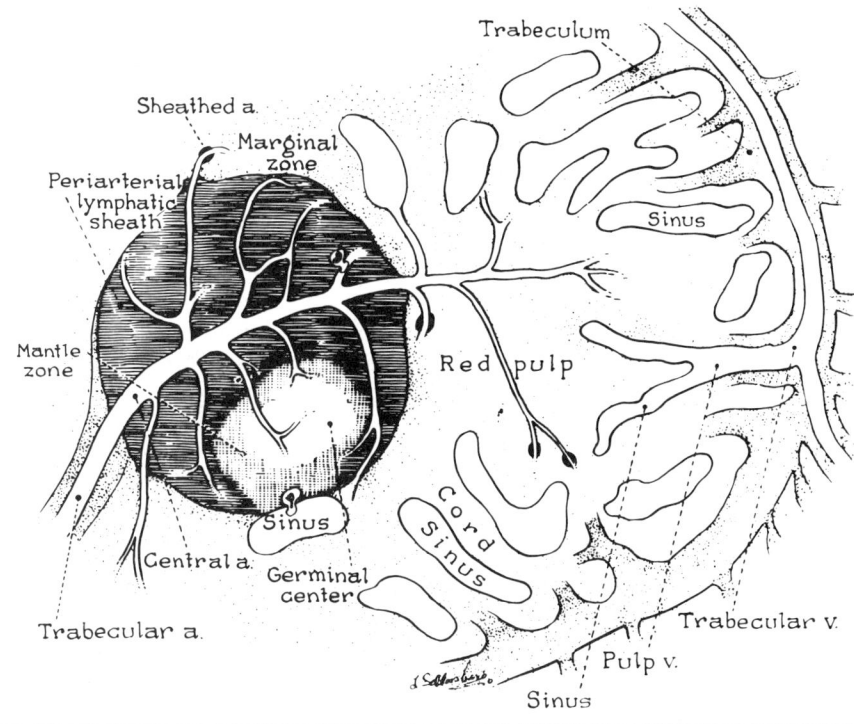

Figure 11-14. Schematic view of the organization of the human spleen. The white pulp has two components: a periarterial lymphatic sheath and a lymphatic follicle. The latter is made up of a germinal center and a surrounding mantle zone. The white pulp is surrounded by a marginal zone. The remainder of the tissue depicted is the red pulp, which consists primarily of splenic sinuses separated by splenic cords. *(From Greep RO, Weiss L: Histology, 3rd ed. New York, McGraw-Hill, 1973, p 397, with permission.)*

SPLEEN-IMAGING AGENTS

Two basic types of radioactive agents have been used to visualize the spleen: (1) radiocolloids, which are localized by splenic phagocytes; and (2) radiolabeled red blood cells, denatured by either chemical or heat damage.

Tc-99m sulfur colloid is frequently used because of convenience and simplicity. Its disadvantage is the lack of specificity because the liver localizes the majority of radioactivity. This incurs an unnecessary radiation dose to the patient and presents difficulty, at times, in obtaining lateral views of the spleen and in separating the left liver margin from the medial edge of the spleen.[51]

Damaged radiolabeled red blood cells offer the advantage of splenic specificity, but this is not without some inconvenience because cells must first be obtained by venipuncture from the patient, radiolabeled, denatured, and then reinjected. In spite of this inconvenience, radiolabeled red cells are the agents of choice for spleen-specific localization.

Radiolabeled Red Blood Cells

The first spleen-imaging agent was heat-damaged chromium-51-labeled red cells. Although adequate splenic localization could be achieved, the low photon yield (9 percent) of the 320-keV gamma emission was quite unsatisfactory for imaging.

In 1964 Wagner et al[52] developed a technique of incubating whole blood with mercury-197-bromomercurihydroxy propane (Hg-197 BMHP), which chemically denatured and radiolabeled the cells simultaneously. With this agent the organic radiomercurial ion (R-Hg$^+$) binds to the sulfhydryl groups within the red cell while causing cell damage. After injection, the labeled cells localize primarily in the spleen, but ultimately the radiomercury is released and translocated to the kidney. This produced a high radiation dose to the kidney, which ultimately led to its discontinued use.

Tc-99m-Labeled Denatured Red Blood Cells

Several different methods have been used to achieve Tc-99m binding to red cells (Tc-RBC); however, the principal efforts were made by the radiochemistry and medical research group at Brookhaven National Laboratory. Although the pertechnetate anion will readily penetrate the red cell membrane, it does not remain bound to the cell unless it is reduced to a lower valence. While developing a labeling method using stannous chloride, Eckelman et al[53] discovered that higher concentrations of stannous chloride produced a damaged red cell that localized in the spleen. Further efforts to improve splenic localization,[54] however, demonstrated that only 10 to 20 percent of the administered dose actually localized in the spleen.

In 1975 Smith and Richards[55] developed a simple kit for the in vitro preparation of Tc-RBCs that could be used for spleen imaging. With this technique red cells are "tinned" by incubation of 3 to 6 ml of whole blood with stannous citrate for 4 minutes. After centrifugation and separation, the packed RBCs are added to Tc-99m pertechnetate to achieve greater than 97 percent labeling yields. Subsequently, the Tc-99m-labeled cells are heated for 15 minutes at 49.5°C to produce heat-damaged red cells that localize in the spleen. A desirable feature of this kit is that if the heating step is omitted, the labeled cells can be used as a blood pool-imaging agent (see Chapter 9) because the low levels of the stannous ion (2 μg) minimize chemical denaturation of the cells, thus giving them a long plasma half-life. The unique feature of this method is that the stannous ion is incubated with the cells before pertechnetate is added. This allows excess tin, not associated with the cells, to be removed before pertechnetate addition, thus minimizing competing reactions with plasma protein and maximizing cell labeling.

It was discovered from this work that carrier Tc-99 levels in some generator eluates may be high enough to interfere with the labeling yields of Tc-99m because of the very low stannous ion concentration in the kit. This potential problem is easily avoided if the number of technetium atoms (Tc-99 and Tc-99m) in the generator eluate added to the kit does not exceed the total number of atoms generated by the decay of 20 mCi of Mo-99. Thus, if 100 mCi of Mo-99 decayed between the previous and present elutions, not more than one fifth of the present eluate should be used in the kit.

The Tc-99m heat-damaged red blood cells prepared using the in vitro kit have been evaluated for splenic sequestration in human subjects.[56] The blood clearance of these cells is rapid ($T_{1/2}$ = 6.3 minutes), and splenic uptake reaches a plateau by 30 minutes. Uptake varies among patients, with the lowest value at 42 percent of the administered activity and the mean at 72 percent. Two hours after dosing, 5 percent of administered activity was excreted in the urine.

The reliability of splenic uptake with the in vitro kit method is apparently due to two factors: (1) the small volume of cells (4 ml) used provides more uniform heating so that adequate cell preparation is achieved in a short time, and (2) the small volume of cells administered presents a lesser possibility of overloading the spleen's sequestering ability than does a larger volume of heated cells.[56]

Mechanism of Localization of Heat-Damaged Tc-99m Red Blood Cells

Localization of damaged red cells in the spleen depends on the degree of cell injury rather than on the type of injury.[57] Heat and chemical denaturation both produce spherocytes, characterized by a loss of red cell membrane and intracellular electrolytes, but heat additionally produces knobby projections from the cell membrane.[57] These changes apparently create a fragile membrane which is more easily subject to lysis. Splenic removal of red cells is a more selective process than removal by the liver and other RES tissue. Insufficient heating of cells produces incomplete denaturation and decreased sequestration by the spleen, whereas overheating creates localization in the liver. Heating must thus be controlled very carefully to produce a spleen-specific agent.

BONE MARROW

PHYSIOLOGIC ANATOMY

In normal adults active bone marrow is found in the vertebrae, ribs, sternum, pelvis, scapulae, skull, and extreme portions of the humeri and femora.[5] The marrow consists of two primary tissues: (1) the hematopoietic marrow, which produces blood cells; and (2) the reticuloendothelial marrow, which provides a phagocytic function. Figure 11-15 shows a cross section of bone illustrating the main constituents of the bone marrow.

Blood supplied to the marrow is through the nutrient arteries that run longitudinally in the central portion of the marrow cavity and send out lateral branches that terminate in capillary beds within bone or at the periphery of the marrow space.[58] The arteriolar capillary blood is drained by postcapillary venules that re-enter the marrow cavity and coalesce to form large, venous sinuses in which the blood flow is back toward the center of the cavity to the central vein.[58]

The hematopoietic marrow is in the form of cords that lie between the venous sinuses. The wall of the venous sinus is primarily composed of a unicellular layer, but in its fullest development it is trilaminar, consisting of a lining cell, basement membrane, and adventitial cell.[59] The wall is fenestrated, which requires the blood cellular elements to squeeze through pores to enter the venous circulation. The adventitial cells provide a phagocytic function by removing foreign particles from the blood as it passes into the sinuses. It is at this point that radioactive colloids are

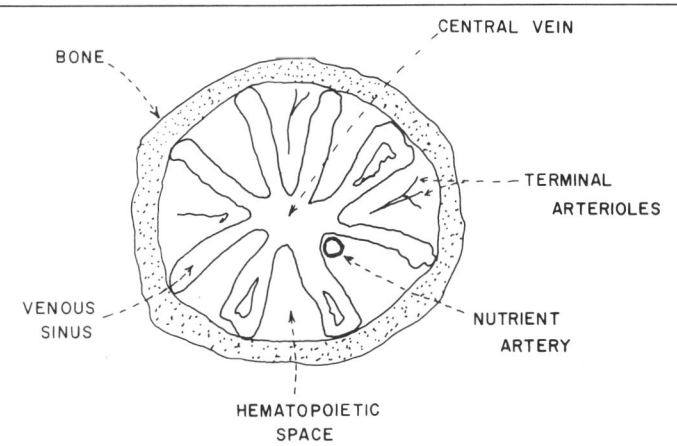

Figure 11-15. Schematic diagram of bone marrow microanatomy.

trapped, thus providing a means to visualize the bone marrow scintigraphically.

RADIOPHARMACEUTICALS FOR BONE MARROW IMAGING

There are two main classes of agents available to evaluate the bone marrow: (1) radioisotopes of iron have been used to quantitate the activity of the hematopoietic marrow because they are incorporated into hemoglobin during RBC formation, and (2) radiocolloids may be used because they are localized in bone marrow phagocytes.

No agent has been developed that has high specificity for bone marrow localization. Although a first choice would be a radioisotope of iron, none of those available has satisfactory imaging properties. The use of iron-52 is limited because it must be made in a cyclotron and used promptly because of its 8-hour half-life. In addition, it requires equipment to detect positron annihilation radiation. Iron-59 is also unsatisfactory because of its high gamma energies of 1.1 and 1.3 MeV.[60]

Radionuclides of indium have chemical properties similar to iron. Ionic indium as In-111 chloride labels plasma transferrin after intravenous injection similar to iron, but beyond this similarity its biologic properties differ significantly from iron. Comparisons have demonstrated striking differences in the metabolic behavior of indium and iron transferrin in the hematopoietic system. In humans the plasma clearance half-time of indium transferrin (6.1 hours) is much slower compared with Fe-59 transferrin (1 to 2 hours), and the liver uptake of indium is greater.[61] Animal studies also demonstrate much less uptake of radioindium into erythrocytes compared with radioiron.[61]

Because of these limitations, radiocolloids have been the agents most widely used for bone marrow evaluation; however, none of the radiocolloids have a high specificity for marrow localization. Subramanian et al[16] reported that about 30 percent of an injected dose of Tc-99m stannous phytate localized in the bone marrow of experimental rats if the phytate-to-stannous ion ratio was high enough, but the distribution in human marrow is not as high. Atkins et al achieved a greater localization of Tc-SC in the bone marrow if smaller-sized (0.1 μm) particles were used and if large doses were administered.[25] Apparently, smaller particles are less likely to be trapped in the liver than larger particles, and the larger doses decrease the efficiency of the liver and spleen to remove particles, the extra particles being left for bone marrow phagocytosis.

Tc-SC is the agent most widely used because of convenience. The dose is usually 10 to 12 mCi, which is two to three times larger than typical liver-scanning doses, to provide an excess of activity to visualize the marrow. The primary limitation in the use of all radiocolloids is the high concentration in the liver and spleen that interferes with marrow activity in the trunk region.[60]

DISTRIBUTION OF COLLOIDS IN BONE MARROW

In normal subjects the distribution of reticuloendothelial marrow is equal to that of active hematopoietic marrow, and therefore the ratio of phagocytic cells to hematopoietic cells is relatively constant, hence the rationale for using radiocolloids to study active bone marrow.[60] Normal distribution of radiocolloids is limited to the active marrow as determined by co-administration of radioiron; however, it must be noted that in the presence of disease the extent of active marrow, estimated by means of radiocolloids, does not always parallel the distribution of functional hematopoietic cells.[60]

Another factor one must recognize is that marrow localization of radiocolloid depends on what fraction of the injected particles does not localize in the liver and spleen. Severe liver disease thus markedly increases the marrow uptake of colloids. This fact is independent of the relationship between marrow reticuloendothelial tissue activity and hematopoietic activity. One should thus establish the status of liver and spleen function at the time of marrow evaluation with colloids. It is evident, then, that care must be taken to interpret bone marrow scans in light of the clinical picture.

Clinical Evaluation of the Liver, Gallbladder, Spleen, and Bone Marrow with Radiopharmaceuticals

LIVER

RATIONALE

The majority of liver–spleen scans are requested as part of a workup for metastatic disease in patients with known tumors. The next most common indications are abnormal liver chemistry results, e.g., increased alkaline phosphatase or transaminases, and a palpable epigastric or right upper quadrant mass. For the former, the question is really whether there is a mass causing compression of a portion of the liver, which in turn is resulting in the elevated enzyme levels. For the latter, the question is whether the palpable mass is a normally functioning but enlarged liver or spleen tissue. Other indications include suspected subphrenic abscess, trauma, and alcoholic liver disease. The liver–spleen scan is quickly and easily performed with little or no discomfort to the patient, and though in the main is regarded as a screening procedure, it often provides some highly specific information about liver and spleen function.

PROCEDURE

The routine liver–spleen scan is performed by injecting 5 mCi of Tc-99m sulfur colloid intravenously with the patient under a large-field-of-view gamma camera. Images are obtained at 5-second intervals to examine the perfusion from the hepatic artery or portal vein of any large defects seen on the 15-minute delayed static views and to observe for gross vascular abnormalities of the aorta in the abdomen (Fig. 11–16A). Many laboratories do not perform the perfusion study. Four standard views (anterior, right lateral, posterior, and left lateral) and a right anterior oblique view are obtained (Fig. 11–16B). A space-occupying lesion must be 2 to 3 cm in size and near the periphery of the liver to be seen well. If there is suspicion of a defect that is not convincingly seen, then end-expiratory gated or upright images should be obtained to try to eliminate the breathing motion blur of the defect. Deep-seated lesions will be seen best with the use of emission-computed tomographic imaging systems (Fig. 1–17). Sometimes differences in the sulfur colloid preparation procedure result in an imbalance in the distribution to the liver and spleen because of a change in the particle size. The best clue should be to see the same effect in other liver–spleen scans done from the same batch of sulfur colloid that day.

PHARMACEUTICALS

Although there has been some interest in a Tc-99m microalbumin preparation, it seems that Tc-99m sulfur colloid will re-

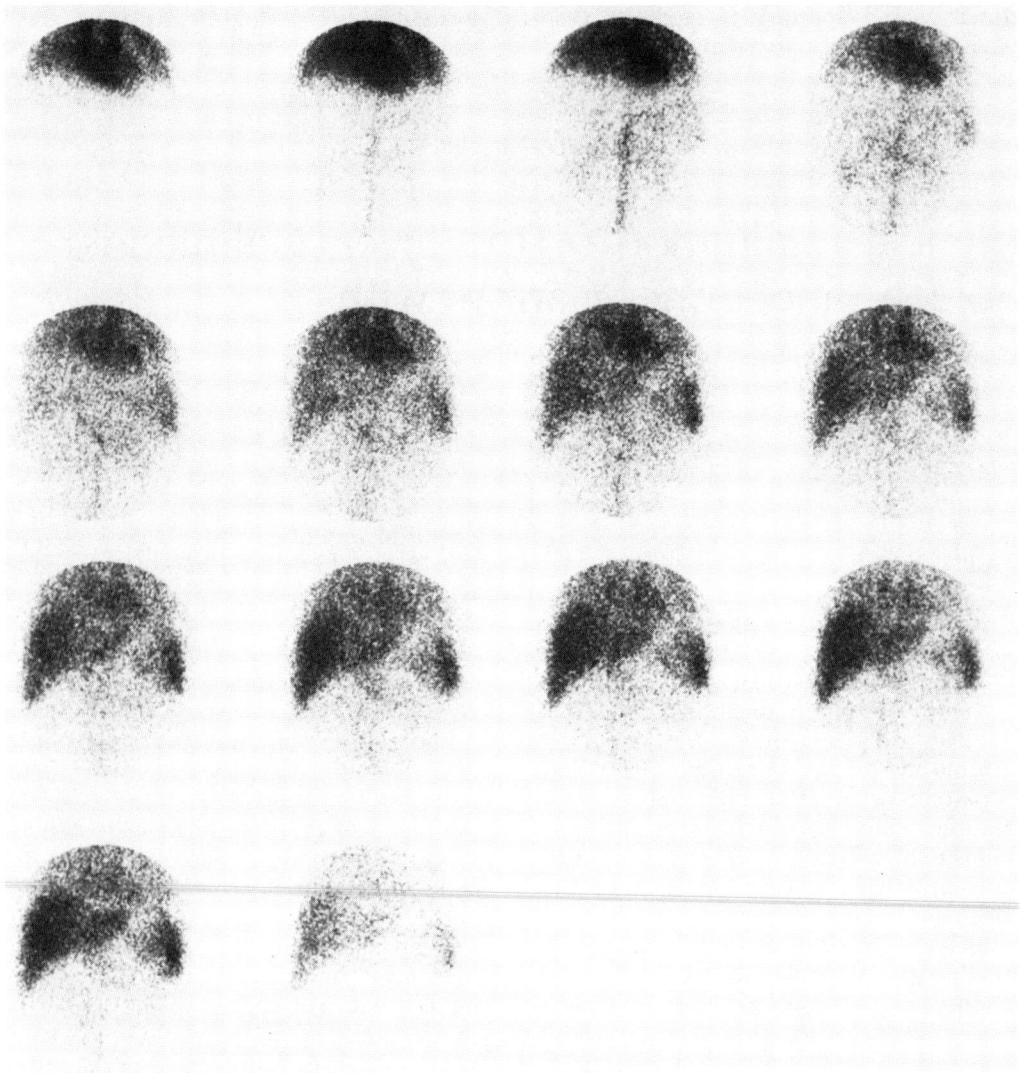

Figure 11-16. A. Normal anterior liver blood flow study in a patient after intravenous injection of 5 mCi of Tc-99m sulfur colloid. Sequential images taken at 5-second intervals demonstrate the normal distribution of activity in the heart, abdominal aorta, liver, and spleen.

main the mainstay of liver–spleen imaging. The property that these liver–spleen scanning preparations have in common is the general particle size. It is the RES that is taking up the microparticles. Roughly 90 to 95 percent of the RES is contained within the liver and spleen of normal individuals. It is nearly impossible to saturate the reticuloendothelial system with sulfur colloid.

INTERPRETATION

Normally, sulfur colloid appears uniformly distributed in the liver with an equal concentration in the spleen. Areas of lesser

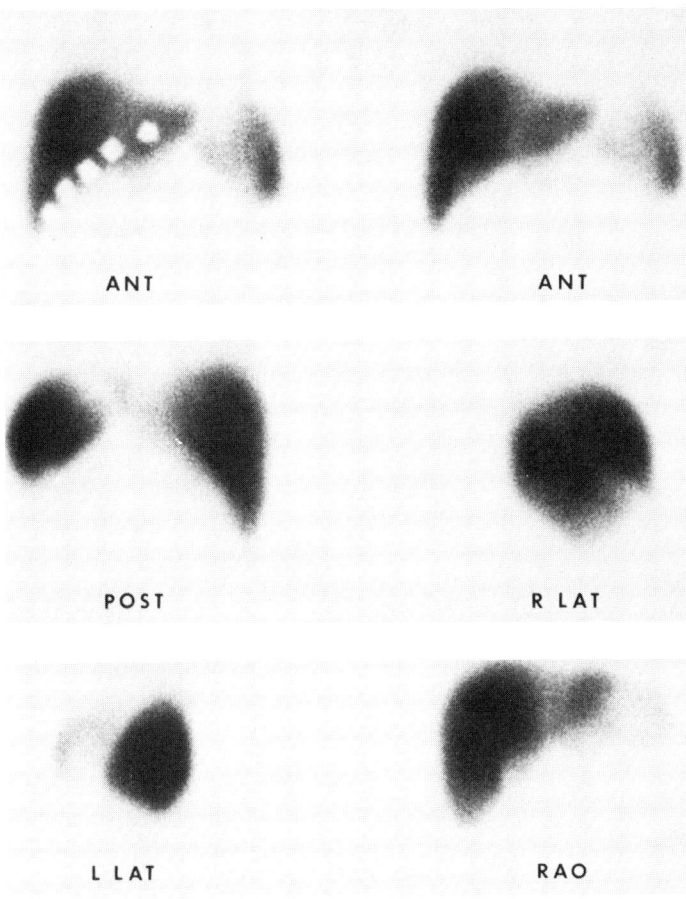

Figure 11-16. B. Normal static liver-spleen scan in the same patient obtained 15 minutes after the liver flow study. Four standard views (anterior, right lateral, posterior, and left lateral) and a right anterior oblique view are shown.

concentration may normally be seen in the gallbladder fossa, the confluence of hepatic veins, the bed of the falciform ligament, the fissure between the right and left lobes anteriorly, and the left lobe in the region of the porta hepatis (Fig. 11-16B). Other defects in the distribution of sulfur colloid in the liver or spleen bear explanation. The clinical history and liver chemistries may make the likelihood of metastatic disease high without further studies.

Examination of the perfusion-phase study may aid in differentiating tumors from cysts. One third of the hepatic blood supply is arterial and accounts for the first phase of perfusion. The other two thirds is delayed and represents portal vein perfusion. Cysts are not expected to show any perfusion. Metastatic tumors and hepatomas will show arterial-phase perfusion and the absence of portal vein perfusion (Fig. 11-18A and B and 11-19A and B). Regenerative liver nodules will most likely show both arterial and portal venous phases of perfusion and may or may not be seen as a defect on the static images at 15 minutes plus. In some instances scanning with another radiopharmaceutical may greatly improve specificity, e.g., hepatoma uptake of gallium-67 citrate.

An increased distribution of colloidal particles to the spleen and marrow documents the existence of hepatocellular disease (Fig. 11-20A and B), and if dis-

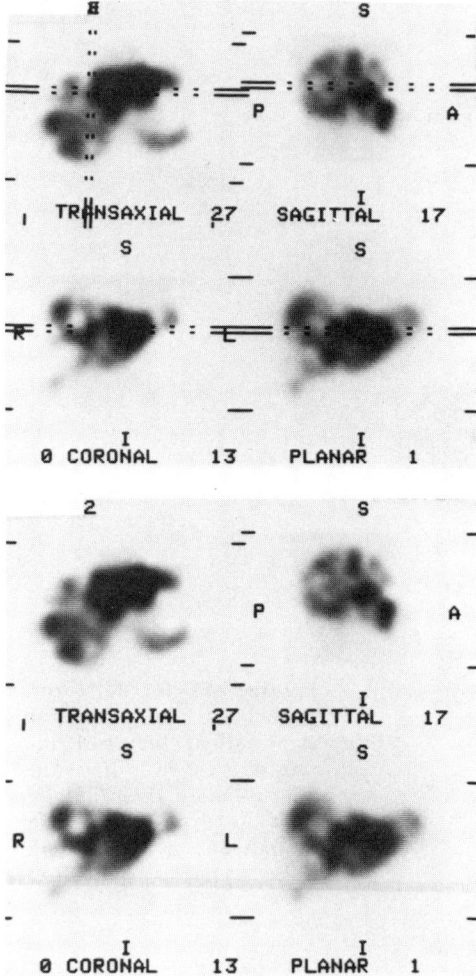

Figure 11-17. Liver single-photon emission computed tomography (SPECT) orthogonal views obtained using 5 mCi of Tc-99m SC demonstrating multiple peripheral and deep-seated defects in a metastatic carcinoma patient being followed for effectiveness of therapy.

tribution includes the lungs, it may portend an increased mortality rate. Maldistribution of colloid to the lungs is seen most commonly in patients with severe hepatocellular disease, septicemia, and carcinomatosis.

Specific questions about the spleen, e.g., the presence of accessory spleen tissue after splenectomy or splenic sequestration of red cells, will be best answered by using a spleen-specific or spleen function agent.

HEPATOBILIARY SYSTEM

RATIONALE

Hepatobiliary imaging is used primarily for demonstrating the functional status of the hepatocytes and biliary tree. Indications include stones, infection, tumor, atresia, and hepatocellular dysfunction. Hepatobiliary imaging is most commonly requested to observe for (non)patency of the common bile duct and common hepatic duct in patients with right upper quadrant pain thought to be due to gallstone obstruction, i.e., acute or chronic cholecystitis. Empyema of the gallbladder will preclude its visualization. The point of obstruction may be seen in patients with painless jaundice resulting from external compression or tumor invasion of the lower portions of the biliary system. Biliary atresia can usually be differentiated from neonatal hepatitis with this technique, and by way of comparison, the hepatobiliary imaging agents are more sensitive to liver (hepatocyte) dysfunction than is sulfur colloid (RES) imaging and can serve to confirm liver disease.

PROCEDURE

For most of the aforementioned indications, the technique involves sequential imaging during the first hour after the injection of 5 mCi of a Tc-99m-labeled IDA agent while making certain to obtain right lateral and posterior views after the early anterior views of the liver (Fig. 11-21). Very often it is not clear on anterior views alone whether the gallbladder has actually been visualized because it may directly overlie activity ex-

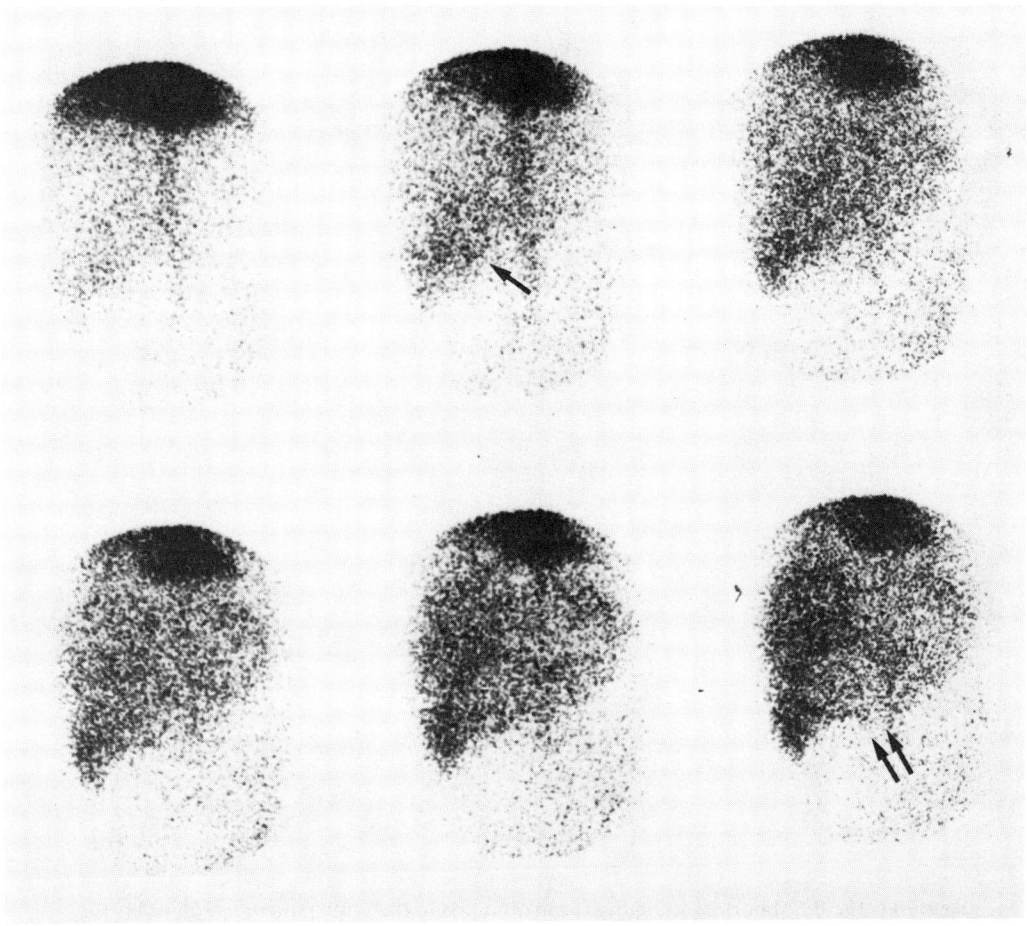

Figure 11-18. A. Abnormal anterior liver flow study typical of a tumor in the liver. The arterial phase shows perfusion of the tumor (single arrow) whereas the venous phase shows a relative lack of perfusion (double arrow) because of decreased RES function.

creted into the duodenum. Right lateral views obtained as activity appears below the liver serve to differentiate the gallbladder from the duodenum. Sometimes it is necessary, because of unusual location or configuration of the gallbladder, to mark the presumed location of the gallbladder on overlying skin and take the patient for ultrasound confirmation. Posterior views help to clarify renal excretion of tracer material from a poorly filling gallbladder in patients with markedly impaired hepatocyte–biliary canalicular cell function. If both gallbladder and intestinal activity are not seen by 1 hour, imaging should proceed at more widely spaced intervals for the next 3 hours or until both structures have been convincingly visualized. Infants under investigation for biliary atresia will usually have been prepared for the study by the administration of phenobarbital for the previous 5 days. When the purpose for hepatobiliary

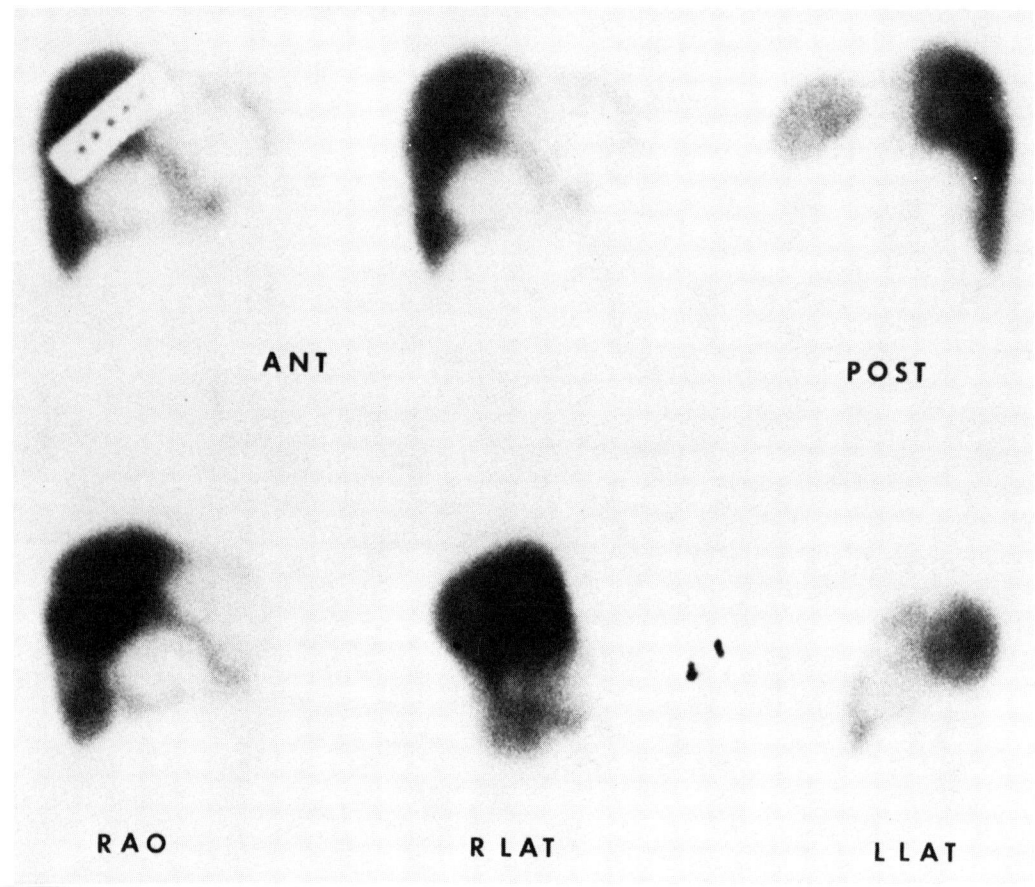

Figure 11-18. B. Abnormal static liver scan obtained in the same patient as Figure 11-18A demonstrating large focal defects 10 minutes after the flow study with 5 mCi of Tc-99m sulfur colloid.

imaging is to delineate a suspected lesion in the liver parenchyma, the images must be obtained in the first few minutes after injection, before most of the tracer is transported into the biliary system.

PHARMACEUTICALS

Years ago hepatocyte and canalicular cell functions were investigated with I-131 rose bengal. Anatomic detail was poor, however, because of the limited amount of activity that could be administered and decreased gamma camera efficiency with I-131. The development of Tc-99m-labeled IDA compounds was met with great interest because of the much improved visualization of the biliary system these radiopharmaceuticals showed and because of the high incidence of diseases of the biliary system. At one time there were 27 IDA compounds available for investigation. Desirable properties that served to narrow the choices were the compound's propensity for the hepatic rather than the renal

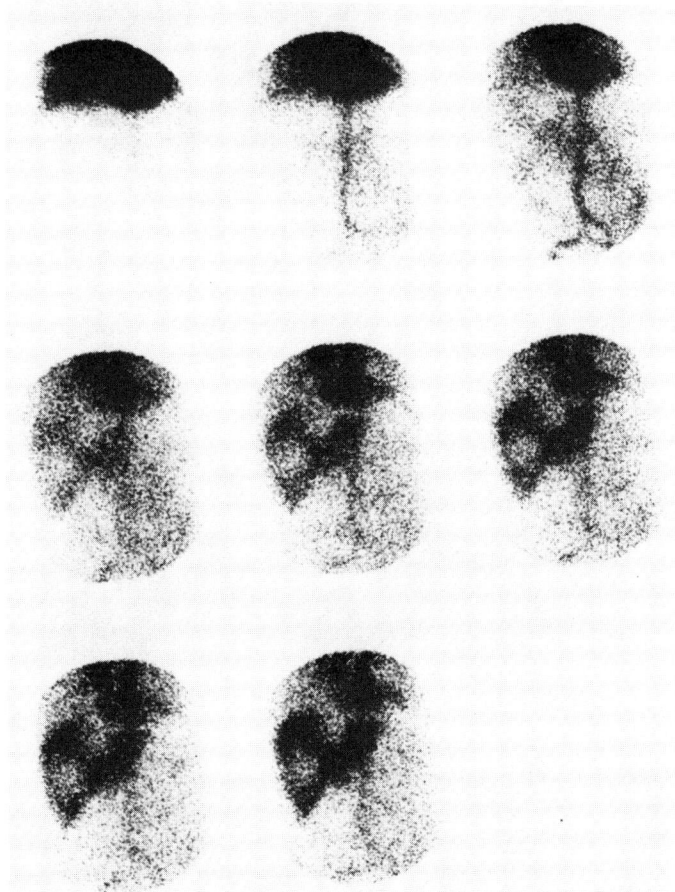

Figure 11-19. A. Liver flow study typical of a cyst or tumor with a necrotic center demonstrating the lack of perfusion during the arterial and venous phases.

excretory route and biliary system visualization at serum bilirubin levels in the twenties. Unless more of these compounds are developed, the best choice would appear to be DISIDA (disofenin).

INTERPRETATION

The primary usefulness of the hepatobiliary imaging agents is to demonstrate the patency of the common bile duct and patency of the biliary system to the intestine. Timing is important because nonvisualization of the gallbladder during the first hour of imaging generally means acute cholecystitis (Figs. 11-22 and 11-23), whereas visualization of the gallbladder between 1 and 4 hours usually means chronic cholecystitis. These agents are a sensitive indicator of impaired liver function, which will be observed as a slow clearance from the nearby cardiac blood pool or delayed excretion into the intestine. Nonvisualization of intestinal activity on delayed images indicates obstruction (Fig. 11-24A, B, and C). An infant with jaundice resulting from neonatal hepatitis should show some (albeit little) excretion into the intestine after 5 days of preparation with phenobarbital (to improve

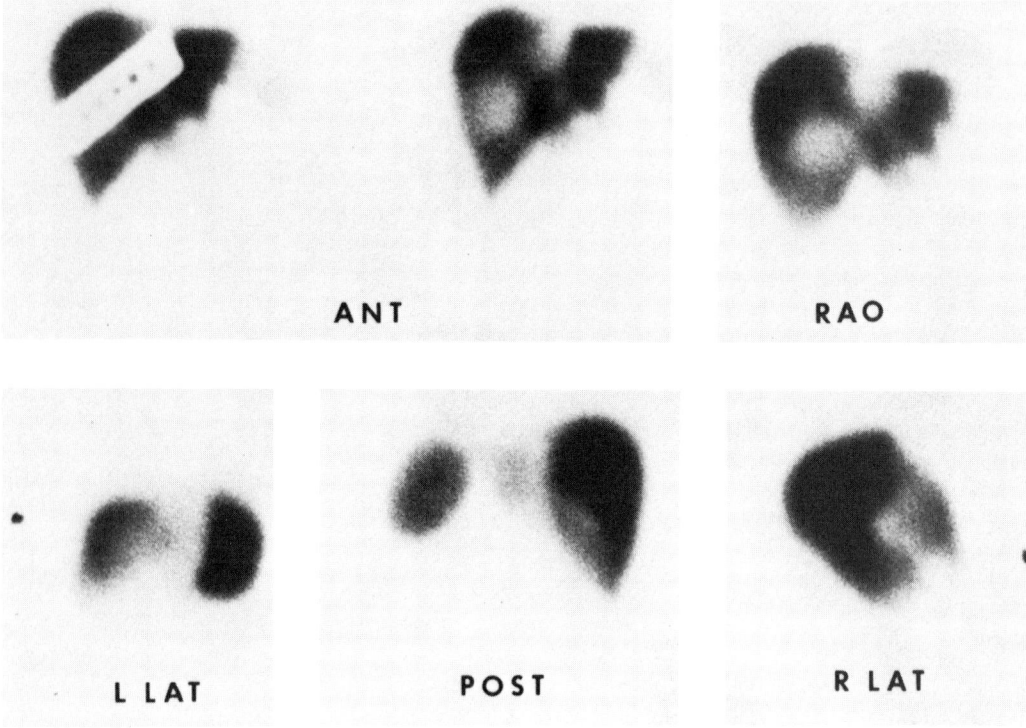

Figure 11-19. B. Static Tc-99m sulfur colloid images of the patient in Figure 11-19A demonstrating focal defects.

conjugation of bilirubin and subsequent excretion), whereas the infant with biliary atresia will fail to show patency to the intestine. Liver parenchymal defects seen on sulfur colloid images should show evidence of function if they are regenerative nodules instead of hepatoma or metastatic tumor.

There is a difference between anatomic and functional imaging with regard to clinical importance. Anatomic imaging techniques, e.g., ultrasound or cholecystography may demonstrate the presence of gallbladder stones in a patient with right upper quadrant pain and suggest the diagnosis of cholecystitis, but a nonvisualized gallbladder abnormality demonstrated with the hepatobiliary imaging agent greatly increases the likelihood of the diagnosis because it shows that abnormal function is present.

SPLEEN (SPECIFIC)

RATIONALE

Spleen-specific imaging, that is, as a separate organ from the liver, is usually done for one of the following reasons: (1) to delineate the spleen from nearby structures and determine its true size and contour; (2) to determine the presence and location of accessory spleens in patients who

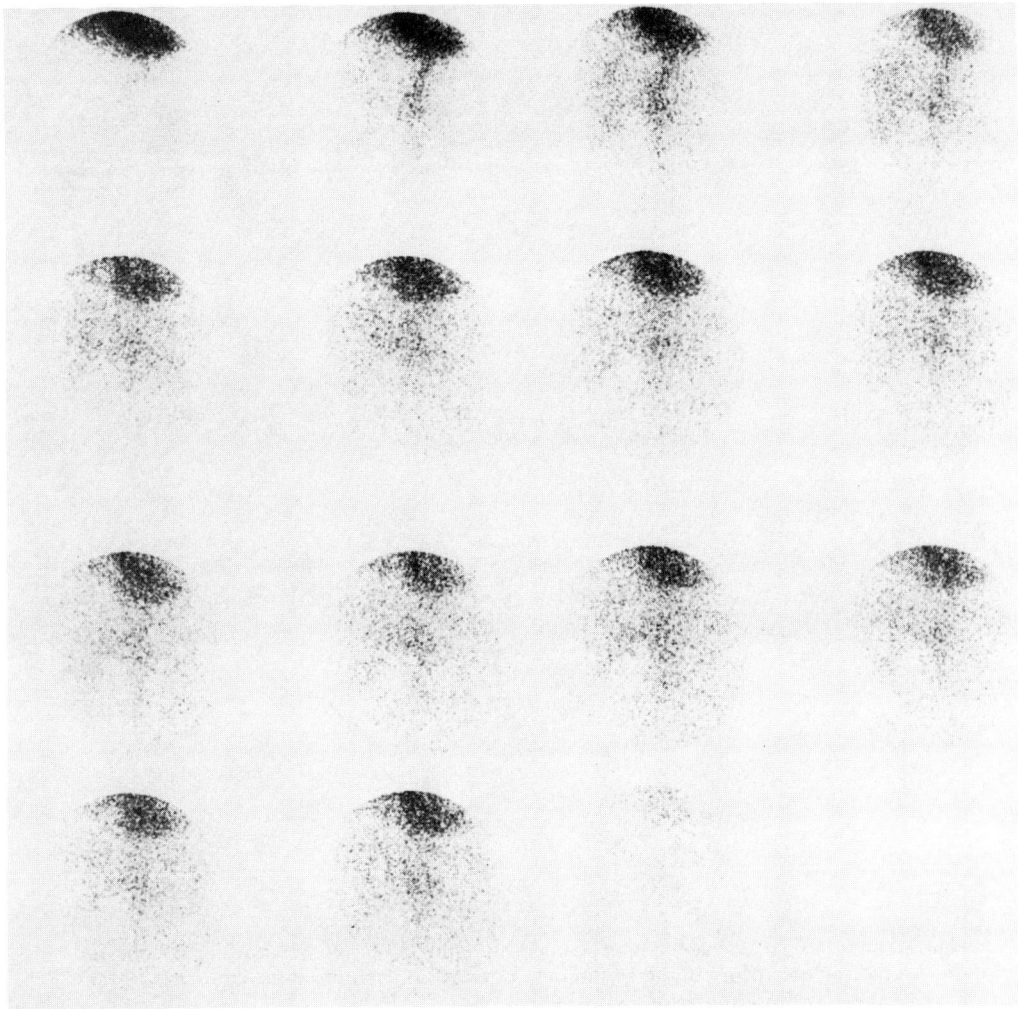

Figure 11-20. A. Anterior liver flow study in a patient with hepatocellular dysfunction secondary to alcoholic cirrhosis that demonstrates poor liver perfusion and a decreased rate of clearance of tracer activity from the heart blood pool.

have had a splenectomy; or (3) to delineate trauma, infarction, or tumor in the spleen. An unexplained mass in the left upper quadrant will frequently require spleen-specific imaging in conjunction with computed tomographic (CT) or ultrasound (US) imaging. Spleen-specific imaging is a sine qua non in the search for accessory spleen tissue that may be causing a patient with idiopathic thrombocytopenic purpura to have a very low platelet count and resulting bleeding diathesis (Fig. 11-25).

PROCEDURE

One millicurie of heat-damaged Tc-99m RBCs is administered, and images are ob-

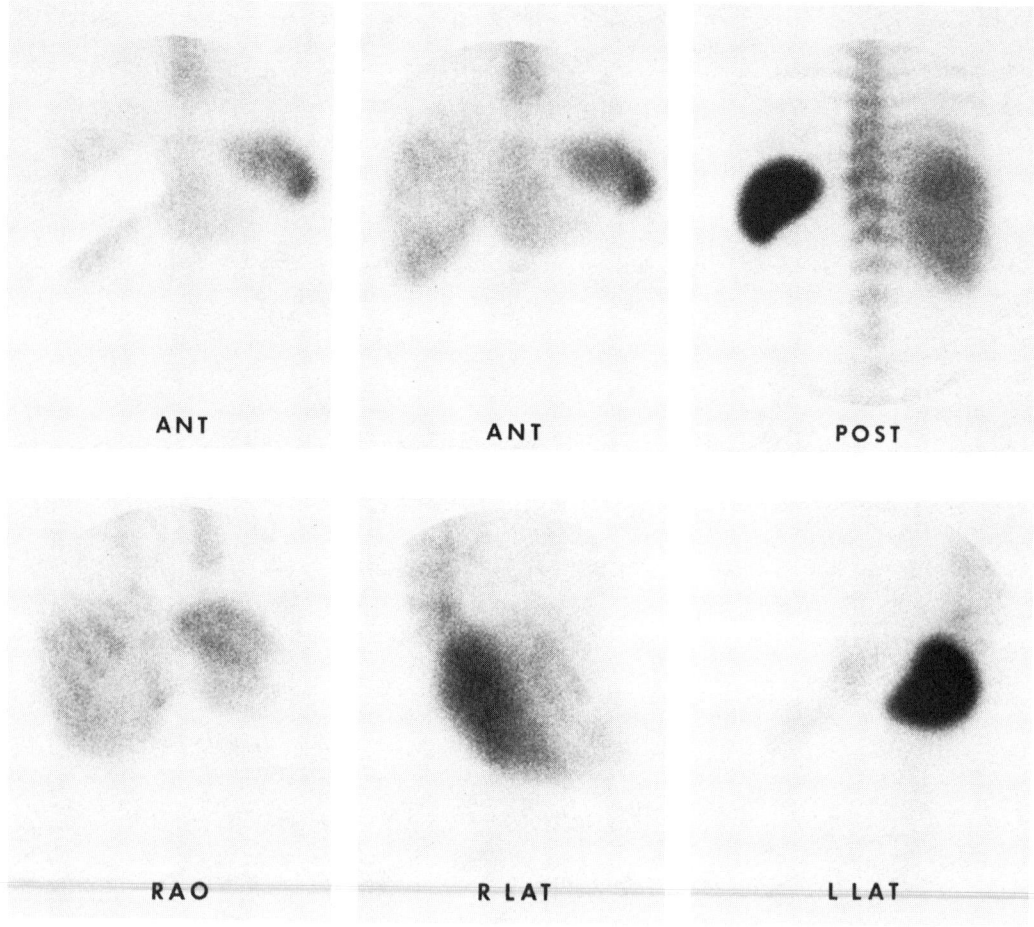

Figure 11-20. B. Static liver–spleen scan in the same patient demonstrating a decreased uptake of Tc-99m sulfur colloid in the liver but with a compensatory increased uptake in the spleen and bone marrow.

tained beginning at 30 minutes. Damaged RBCs are removed from the blood by splenic tissue; therefore, focal accumulations should be spleen specific. Sufficient time must have elapsed for the sequestration to occur. The blood clearance time will be determined by the amount of heat damage, the volume of sequestering tissue, and the volume of administered cells. Clinically, the most reliable way of assessing the clearance of damaged, tagged red cells from the blood is with sequential imaging that includes a blood pool area, e.g., the heart. The entire abdomen and pelvis should be imaged when searching for accessory spleens.

PHARMACEUTICALS

Various radiopharmaceuticals have been used in the past; however, the agent of choice is now heat-damaged Tc-99m tinned RBC.

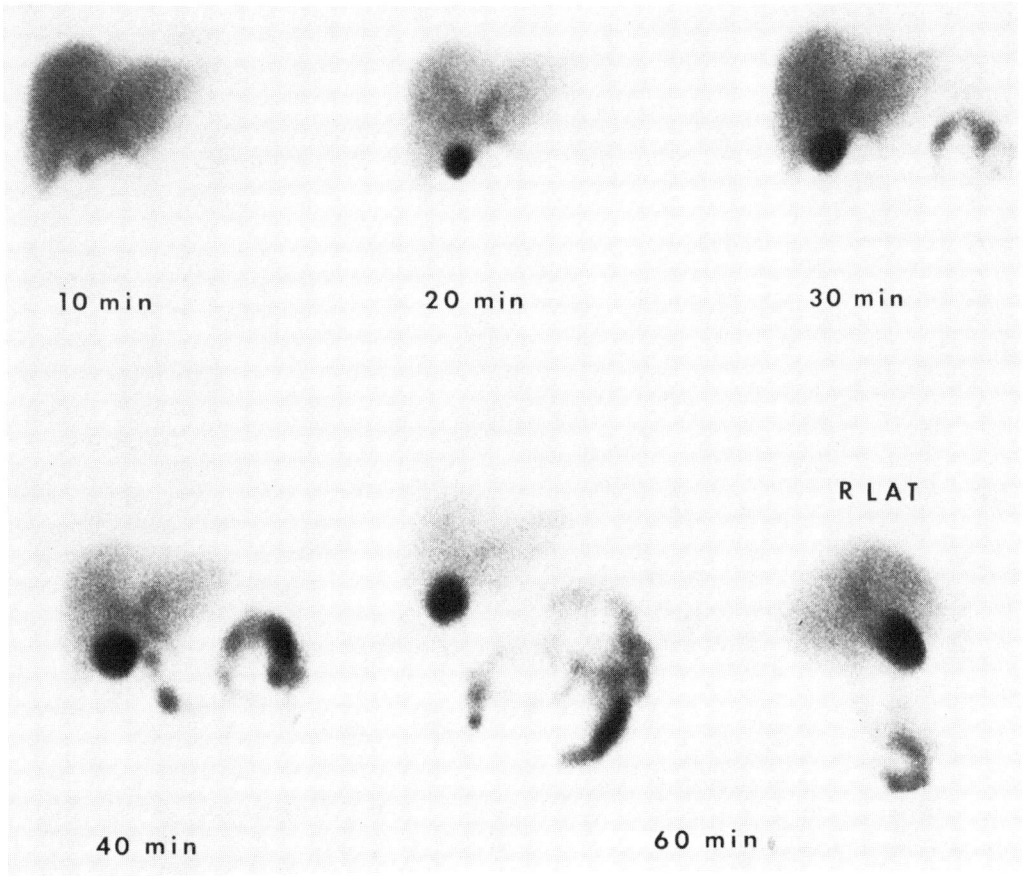

Figure 11-21. Normal hepatobiliary study. After intravenous injection of 5 mCi of Tc-99m disofenin there is a prompt clearance of tracer material by the hepatobiliary system. At 10 minutes there is evidence of activity in the gallbladder and small intestine that becomes more prominent at later times.

INTERPRETATION

Correlation of anatomic (CT or US) and functional spleen-specific images will be necessary in most cases to determine the nature of a left upper quadrant mass. Though accessory spleens may have been seeded anywhere in the abdomen, most of them are located in the left upper quadrant. The spleen-specific technique is particularly useful in these instances when compared with the sulfur colloid scan because the latter may obscure splenic tissue in close proximity to the liver.

The morphologic character of a spleen image abnormality is helpful in determining the cause; for instance, wedge-shaped defects are usually due to fracture hematomas or infarcts, whereas round defects are more likely to be due to tumor involvement or granulomata. Rarely the spleen may fail to be visualized; this occurs in a process called functional asplenia.

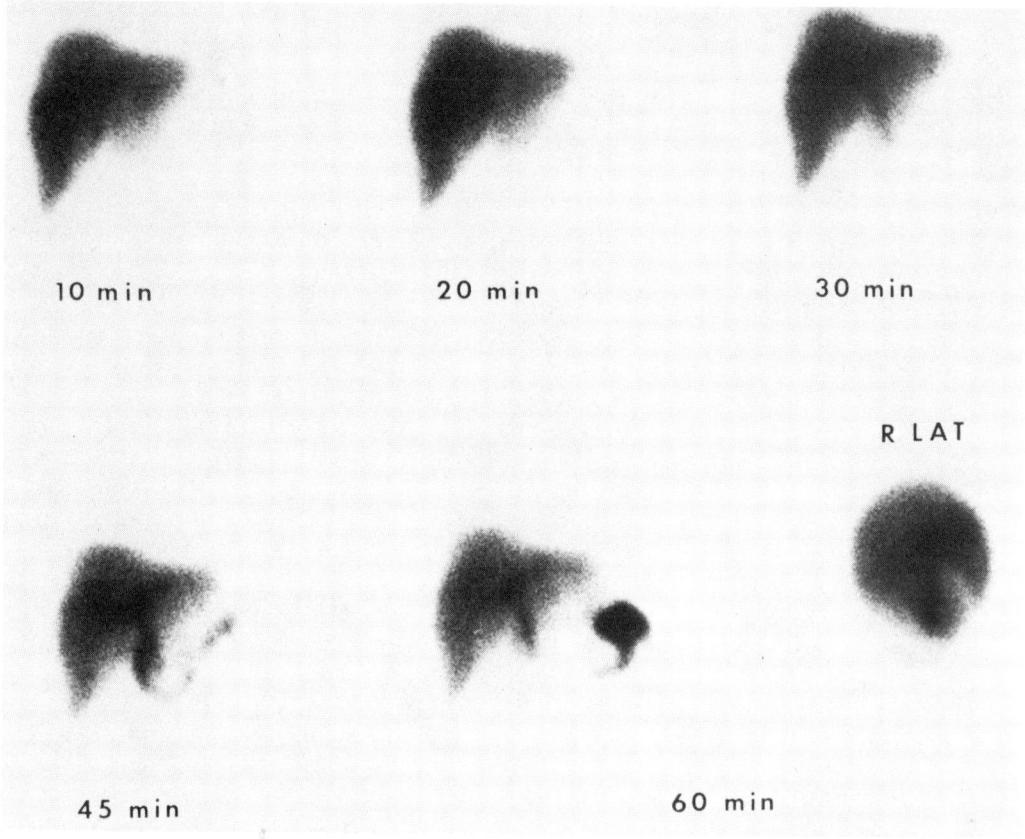

Figure 11-22. Acute cholecystitis. After intravenous injection of 5 mCi of Tc-99m iprofenin there is visualization of tracer material in the common bile duct and proximal bowel at 45 minutes. Nonvisualization of the gallbladder by 60 minutes and 3 hours (image not shown) is consistent with cystic duct obstruction and acute cholecystitis.

BONE MARROW

RATIONALE

Two cell lines in the bone marrow, the erythrogenic or red marrow and the RES or white marrow, may be imaged with radiotracer techniques. The red marrow is imaged to look for active sites in the body, whereas the white marrow is generally imaged to look for inactivity, though the latter also may be used to look for activity on the assumption that both cell lines usually will be present if one is. Erythrogenic activity centers are sought in various forms of anemia to locate marrow biopsy sites or to find sites for studying hematopoiesis with iron kinetic studies. Lack of RES activity in the femoral head is sought to confirm the suspicion of avascular necrosis.

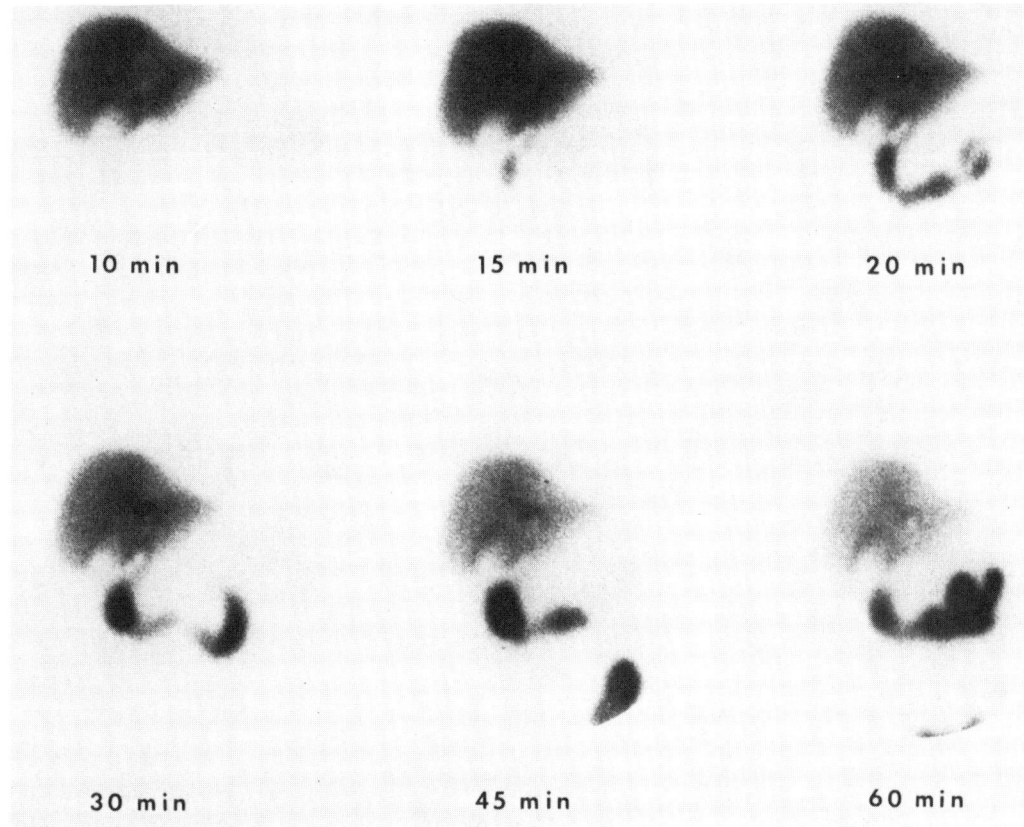

Figure 11-23. Acute gangrenous cholecystitis. After an intravenous dose of 5 mCi of Tc-99m disofenin, activity is promptly excreted into the bowel and demonstrates a patent common bile duct. Activity is not seen in the gallbladder, but note the rim of increased parenchymal activity adjacent to the gallbladder fossa, which is most prominent on the 60-minute image. This characteristic pattern is frequently seen in acute gangrenous cholecystitis.

PROCEDURE

The erythrogenic marrow is best imaged 24 to 48 hours after the injection of 1 to 2 mCi of In-111 chloride by using both photon peaks and a medium-energy collimator on a large-field-of-view gamma camera. Imaging of the RES marrow requires much less time and preparation for the procedure because it may be readily accomplished with 5 to 10 mCi of Tc-99m sulfur colloid. When making separate views of the hips, care must be taken that the images are taken for the same amount of time for right–left comparison purposes and that the information density is adequate to see anatomic detail.

PHARMACEUTICALS

For erythrogenic marrow imaging the only practical choice in radiotracers is In-111

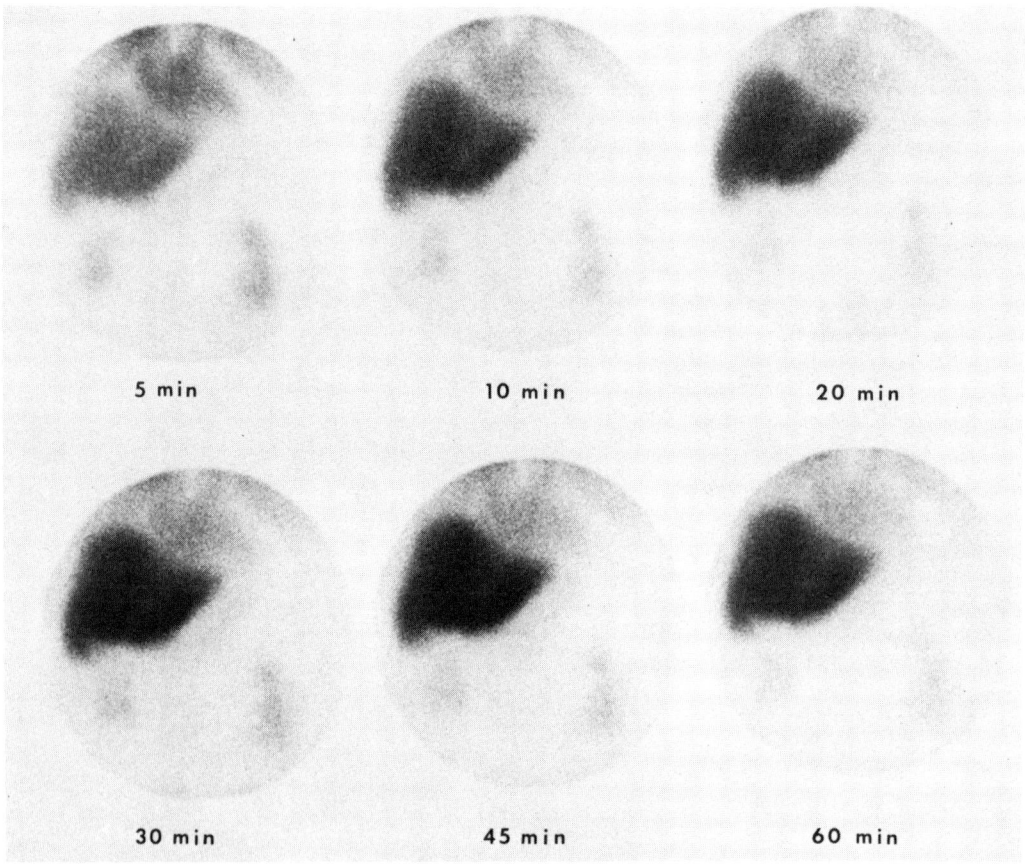

Figure 11-24. Obstruction. **A.** After intravenous injection of 5 mCi of Tc-99m iprofenin, tracer material is seen to clear slowly from the blood. Liver activity is evident.

chloride with its 67-hour half-life and photon peaks at 173 keV (90 percent) and 247 keV (94 percent). Indium must be at or below pH 3 at injection for the subsequent attachment to plasma transferrin to occur. For marrow RES imaging the primary qualification of the radiopharmaceutical is a particle size of about 0.1 μm. Sulfur colloid is most commonly used; however, microaggregated albumin is an alternative choice.

INTERPRETATION

The information obtained from marrow-imaging studies is basically the demonstration of the presence or absence of marrow activity, the meaning of which is inherent to the disease process under study. One should be careful to observe that the presence of activity in one of the cell lines does not necessarily guarantee that the other cell line is present and active in that same area.

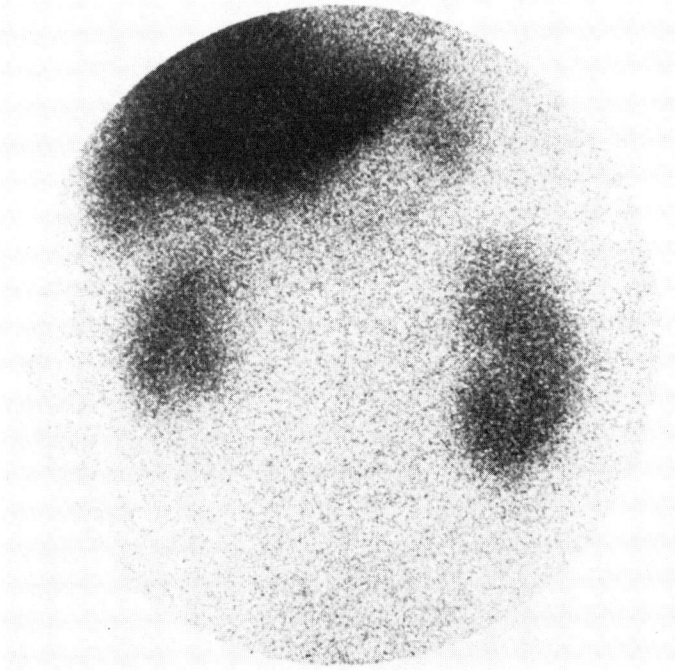

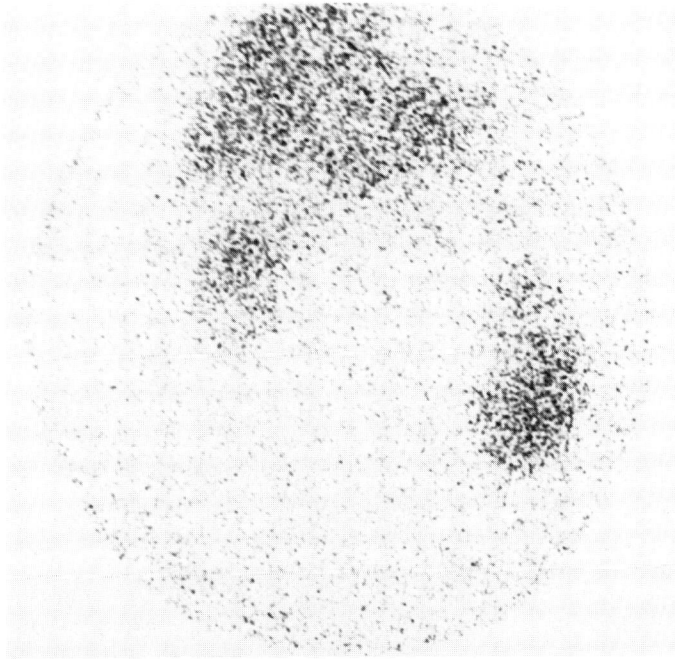

Figure 11-24. B, C. The lack of bowel activity on delayed images at 5 hours (**B**) and 24 hours (**C**) and the presence of kidney excretion is consistent with complete obstruction. A transhepatic cholangiogram demonstrated a stone obstructing the common bile duct distally and two stones in the gallbladder.

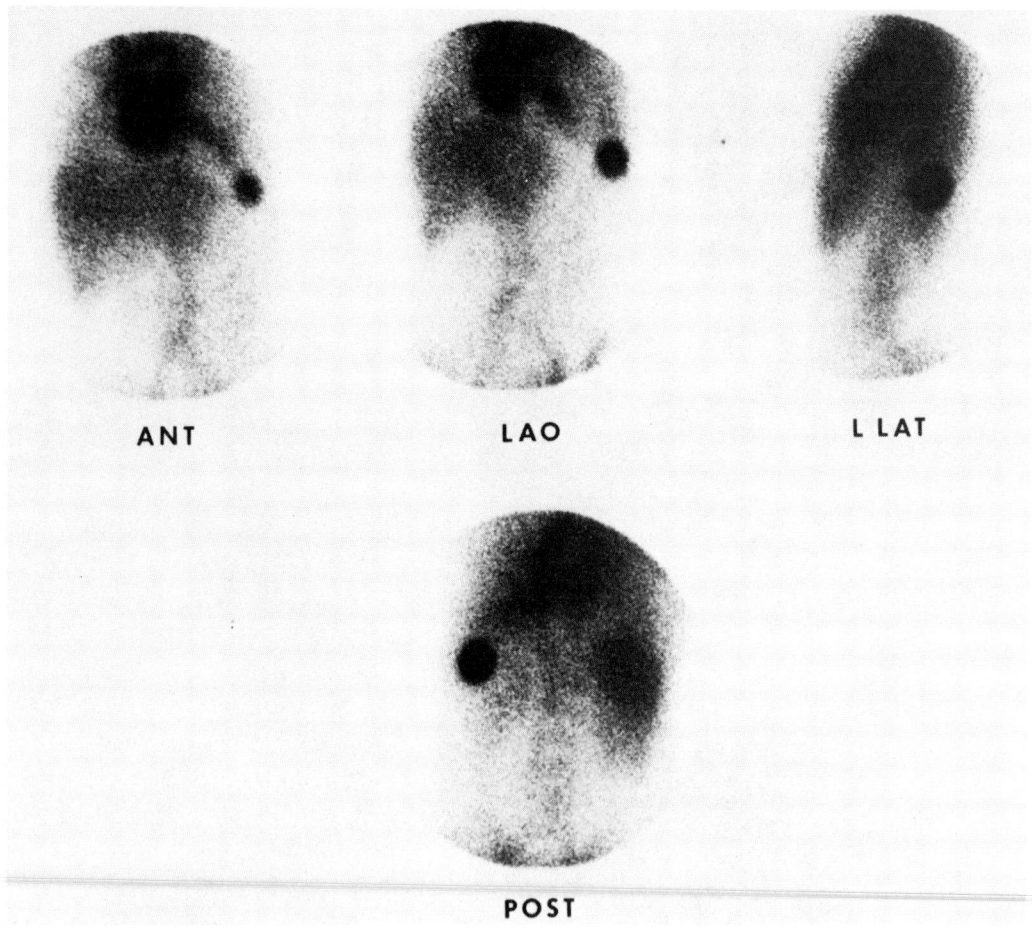

Figure 11-25. Accessory spleen localized in the left upper quadrant of the abdomen in a patient who underwent a splenectomy for thrombocytopenia 10 years earlier. The spleen image was obtained 20 minutes after injection of 1.7 mCi of heat-damaged Tc-99m-labeled autologous RBC prepared by the Brookhaven kit method.

REFERENCES

1. Elias H, Sherrick JC: Morphology of the Liver. New York, Academic Press, 1969
2. Wisse E: Ultrastructure and function of Kupffer cells and other sinusoidal cells. In Wisse E, Knook DL (eds): Kupffer Cells and Other Liver Sinusoidal Cells. Amsterdam, Elsevier North Holland, 1977, pp 33–60
3. Wisse E, DeZanger RB: On the Morphology and other aspects of Kupffer cell function—Observations and speculations concerning pinocytosis and phagocytosis. In Liehr H, Grun M (eds): The Reticuloendothelial System and the Pathogenesis of Liver Disease. Amsterdam, Elsevier North Holland 1979, pp 3–9
4. Rouiller CH: The Liver—Morphology, Biochemistry, Physiology. New York, Academic Press, 1963, Vol 1
5. Loberg MD, Porter DW, Ryan JW: Review and current status of hepatobiliary imaging agents. In Sorenson JA (ed): Radiopharmaceuticals II: Proceedings of the 2nd International Symposium on Radiopharmaceuticals. New York, Society of Nuclear Medicine, 1979, 519–543

6. Dobson EL, Jones HB: The behavior of intravenously injected particulate material: Its rate of disappearance from the blood stream as a measure of liver blood flow. Acta Med Scand 144 (Suppl 273):1–71, 1952
7. Stirrett LA, Yuhl ET, Libby RL: The hepatic radioactivity survey. Radiology 61:930, 1953
8. Stirrett LA, Yuhl ET, Cassen B: Clinical applications of hepatic radioactivity surveys. Am J Gastroenterol 21:310, 1954
9. Sorensen LB, Archambault M: Visualization of the liver by scanning with Mo-99 (molybdate) as tracer. J Lab Clin Med 62:330, 1963
10. Benacerraf B, Biozzi G, Halpern B, et al: A study of phagocytic activity of the reticuloendothelial system toward heat denatured human serum albumin tagged with I-131. Res Bull 2:19, 1956
11. Richards P: A survey of the production at Brookhaven National Laboratory of radioisotopes for medical research. In V. Congresso Nucleare, Rome, 1960. Rome, Comitato Nazionale Ricerche Nucleari, 1960, Vol 2, pp 223–244
12. Harper PV, Lathrop KA, Richards P: Tc-99m as a radiocolloid. J Nucl Med 5:382, 1964
13. Stern HS, McAfee JG, Subramanian G: Preparation, distribution and utilization of technetium 99m sulfur colloid. J Nucl Med 7:655, 1966
14. Ege GN, Warbick A: Lymphoscintigraphy: A comparison of Tc-99m antimony sulfide colloid and Tc-99m stannous phytate. Br J Radiol 52:124, 1979
15. Goodwin DA, Stern HS, Wagner HN, et al: In 113m colloid: A new radiopharmaceutical for liver scanning. Nucleonics 24:65, 1966
16. Subramanian G, McAfee JG, Mehta A, et al: Tc-99m stannous phytate: A new in-vivo colloid for imaging the reticuloendothelial system. J Nucl Med 14:459, 1973
17. Srivastava SC, Richards P: Technetium-labeled compounds. In Rayudu GUS (ed): Radiotracers for Medical Applications. Boca Raton, Fla, CRC Press, 1981, pp 90–92
18. Fortman DL, Sodd VJ: Tc-99m sulfur colloid-evaluation of preparation parameters for kits from four commercial manufacturers. In Sorenson JA (ed): Radiopharmaceuticals II, Proceedings of the 2nd International Symposium on Radiopharmaceuticals. New York, Society of Nuclear Medicine, 1979, pp 15–24
19. Saba TM: Physiology and physiopathology of the reticuloendothelial system. Arch Intern Med 126:1031, 1970
20. Nelp WB: An Evaluation of Colloids for RES Function Studies. In Subramanian G, Rhodes B, Cooper JF, Sodd VJ (eds): New York, Society of Nuclear Medicine, 1975, pp 349–356
21. Guyton AC: Textbook of Medical Physiology, 6th ed. Philadelphia, Saunders, 1981
22. Wagner HN, Iio M: Studies of the reticuloendothelial system (RES) III. Blockade of the RES in man. J Clin Invest 43:1525, 1964
23. Quinones JD: Localization of technetium–sulfur colloid after RES stimulation. J Nucl Med 14:443, 1973
24. Davis MA, Jones AG, Trindade H: A rapid and accurate method for sizing radiocolloids. J Nucl Med 15:923, 1974
25. Atkins HL, Hauser W, Richards P: Factors affecting distribution of Tc-99m sulfur colloid. J Nucl Med 10:319, 1969
26. Cohen Y, Ingrand J, Caro RA: Kinetics of the disappearance of gelatin protected radiogold colloids from the blood stream. Int J Appl Radiat Isot 19:703, 1968
27. Chaudhuri TK, Evans TC, Chaudhuri TK: Autoradiographic studies of distribution in the liver of Au-198 and Tc-99m sulfur colloids. Radiology 109:633, 1973
28. Brucer M: Liver Scans, Clearances, and Perfusions. New York, Krieger, 1977
29. Bissell DM, Hammaker L, Schmid R: Liver sinusoidal cells—Identification of a subpopulation for erythrocyte catabolism. J Cell Biol 54:107, 1972
30. Easton TW: The role of macrophage movements in the transport and elimination of intravenous thorium dioxide in mice. Am J Anat 90:1, 1952
31. Castronovo FP, Wagner HN: Comparative toxicity and pharmacodynamics of ionic indium chloride and hydrated indium oxide. J Nucl Med 14:677, 1973
32. Atkins HL: Adverse reactions. In Rhodes BA (ed): Quality Control in Nuclear Medicine. St Louis, C.V. Mosby, 1977, pp 263–267
33. Haney TA, Ascanio I, Gigliotti JA, et al: Physical and biological properties of a Tc-99m sulfur colloid preparation containing disodium edetate. J Nucl Med 12:64, 1970
34. MIRD Report No. 3: Summary of current

radiation dose estimates to humans with various liver conditions from Tc-99m sulfur colloid. J Nucl Med 16:108A, 1975
35. Taplin GV, Meredith OM, Kade H: The radioactive (I-131 tagged) rose bengal uptake: Excretion test for liver function using external gamma-ray scintillation counting techniques. J Lab Clin Med 45:665, 1955
36. Loberg MD, Cooper M, Harvey E, et al: Development of new radiopharmaceuticals based on N-substitution of iminodiacetic acid. J Nucl Med 17:633, 1976
37. Ryan J, Cooper M, Loberg M, et al: Technetium 99m labeled N-(2,6-dimethylphenyl carbamoylmethyl) iminodiacetic acid (Tc-99m HIDA): A new radiopharmaceutical for hepatobiliary imaging studies. J Nucl Med 18:995, 1977
38. Loberg MD, Fields AT: Stability of Tc-99m labeled N-substituted iminodiacetic acids: Ligand exchange reaction between Tc-99m HIDA and EDTA. Int J Appl Radiat Isot 28:687, 1977
39. Firnau G: Why do Tc-99m chelates work for cholescintigraphy? Eur J Nucl Med 1:137, 1976
40. Hirom PC: The physicochemical factors required for the biliary excretion of organic cations and anions. Biochem Soc Trans 2:327, 1974
41. Wistow NW, Subramanian G, Gagne GM, et al: Experimental and clinical trials of new Tc-99m labeled hepatobiliary agents. Radiology 128:703, 1978
42. Fritzberg AR, Whitney WP, Klingensmith WC: Hepatobiliary Transport Mechanism of Tc-99m-Diethyl IDA. In Sorenson JA (ed): Radiopharmaceuticals II. New York, Society of Nuclear Medicine, 1979, pp 577–586
43. Wistow BW, Subramanian G, Van Heertum RL, et al: An evaluation of Tc-99m labeled hepatobiliary agents. J Nucl Med 18:455, 1977
44. Rosenthall L: Clinical experience with the newer hepatobiliary radiopharmaceuticals. Can J Surg 21:297, 1978
45. Klingensmith WC, Fritzberg DR, Spitzer VM, et al: Clinical comparison of Tc-99m diethyl-IDA and Tc-99m PIPIDA for evaluation of the hepatobiliary system. Radiology 134:195, 1980
46. Klingensmith WC, Fritzberg AR, Spitzer VM, et al: Clinical comparison of diisopropyl-IDA Tc-99m and diethyl-IDA Tc-99m for evaluation of the hepatobiliary system. Radiology 140:791, 1981
47. Weissman HS, Badia JD, Hall T, et al: Tc-99m diisopropyl iminodiacetic acid (DISIDA): The best overall cholescintigraphic radionuclide for the evaluation of hepatobiliary disorders. J Nucl Med 21:P18, 1980
48. Pauwels S, Piret L, Schautens A, et al: Tc-99m diethyl-IDA imaging: Clinical evaluation in jaundiced patients. J Nucl Med 21:1022, 1980
49. Brown PH, Krishnamurthy GT, Bobba VR, et al: Radiation-dose calculation for five Tc-99m IDA hepatobiliary agents. J Nucl Med 23:1025, 1982
50. Erslev AJ, Gabuzda TG: Pathophysiology of Blood, 2nd ed. Philadelphia, Saunders, 1979, pp 15–18
51. Williams WJ, Beutler E, Erslev AJ, Rundles RW: Hematology. New York, McGraw-Hill, 1972, pp 513–514
52. Wagner HN Jr, Weiner IM, McAfee JG, et al: 1-Mercuri-2-hydroxypropane (MHP). A new pharmaceutical for visualization of the spleen by radioisotope scanning. Arch Intern Med 113:696, 1964
53. Eckelman W, Richards P, Hauser W, et al: Technetium labeled red blood cells. J Nucl Med 12:22, 1970
54. Atkins HL, Eckelman WC, Hauser W, et al: Splenic sequestration of Tc-99m labeled red blood cells. J Nucl Med 13:811, 1971
55. Smith TD, Richards P: A simple kit for the preparation of Tc-99m labeled red blood cells. J Nucl Med 17:126, 1975
56. Atkins HL, Goldman AG, Fairchild RG, et al: Splenic sequestration of Tc-99m labeled, heat treated red blood cells. Radiology 136:501, 1980
57. Wagner HN, Jr, Razzak MA, Gaertner RA, et al: Removal of erythrocytes from the circulation. Arch Intern Med 110:90, 1962
58. Weiss L, Chen LT: The organization of hematopoietic cords and vascular sinuses in bone marrow. Blood Cells 1:617, 1975
59. Weiss L: The structure of bone marrow. J Morphol 117:467, 1965
60. Van Dyke D, Shkurkin C, Price D, et al: Differences in distribution of erythropoietic and reticuloendothelial marrow in hematologic disease. Blood 30:364, 1967
61. McIntyre PA: Agents for bone marrow imaging: An evaluation. In Subramanian G, Rhodes B, Cooper JF, Sodd VJ (eds): Radiopharmaceuticals. New York, Society of Nuclear Medicine, 1975, pp 343–348

CHAPTER 12

Kidney and Genitourinary Systems

The kidney is the primary organ responsible for the elimination of metabolic waste products from the body. Drug substances administered to humans for diagnostic or therapeutic purposes are also eliminated through the kidney either as metabolites or as unchanged drug. Renal elimination of several radiopharmaceuticals provides a means to measure kidney function. In addition, some of these agents are bound within the kidney cells for a prolonged period of time, thus providing a means to visualize the organ for morphologic information as well.

PHYSIOLOGIC ANATOMY

The functional unit of the kidney is the nephron illustrated in Figure 12–1. It consists of the glomerulus, proximal convoluted tubule, loop of Henle, distal convoluted tubule, and collecting duct that leads to the renal pelvis. Tubular urine flows through the nephron in this order. There are approximately 1.5 million nephrons in each kidney. About 85 percent of the nephrons reside in the kidney cortex with their glomeruli in the outer two thirds of the cortex; about 15 percent of the nephrons are juxtamedullary with glomeruli in the corticomedullary junction; no glomeruli are found in the kidney medulla. In cortical nephrons, the loops of Henle are short, penetrate only a short distance into the medulla, and have thin descending and thick ascending limbs; in juxtamedullary nephrons, the loops of Henle are long, penetrate the medulla, and return to the cortex; those that penetrate deeply have thin descending and thin ascending limbs that lead into thick ascending limbs.

Blood enters the nephron through the afferent arteriole that branches off the interlobular artery. It subsequently flows through the glomerular capillaries, exists from the glomerulus through the efferent arteriole, and enters peritubular capillaries that bathe the tubules. Blood then leaves the nephron through the cortical venule, which flows into the interlobular vein. About 85 percent of renal blood perfuses the cortex and bypasses the medulla; 10 percent perfuses the corticomedullary junction; 2 percent perfuses the medulla, and 3 percent flows through arteriovenous shunts that bypass the cortical glomerular and peritubular capillary systems and, hence, does not con-

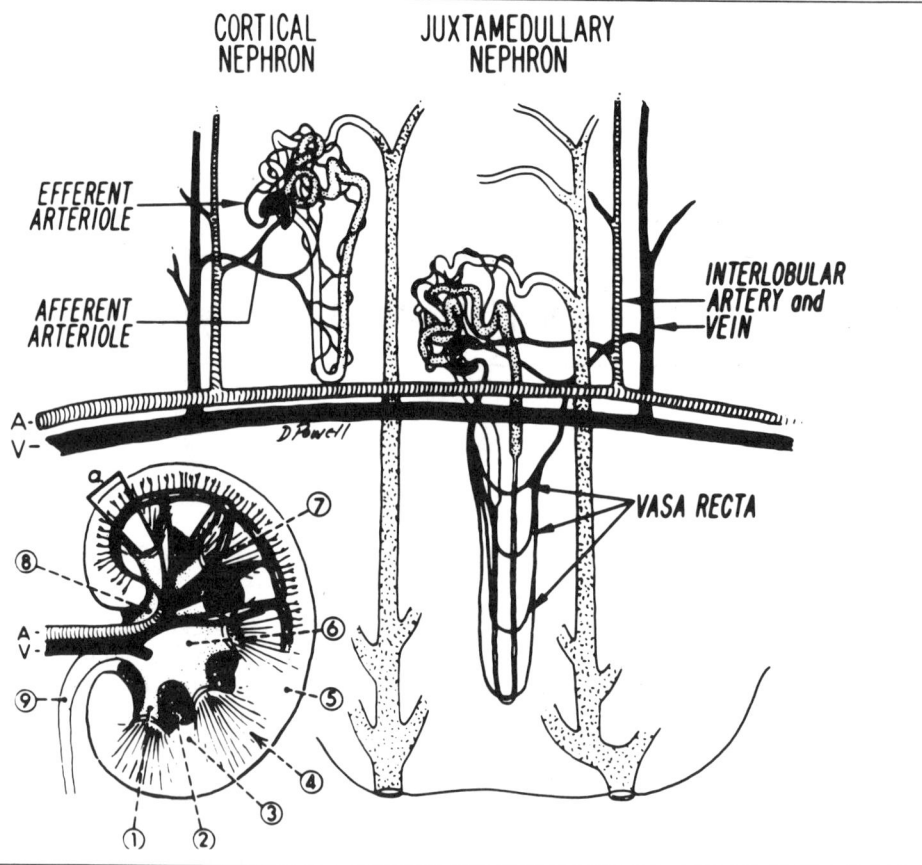

Figure 12-1. The sagittal surface of a bisected kidney is illustrated diagrammatically (lower left). Numbers 1 through 9 indicate the following: 1, minor calix; 2, fat in sinus; 3, renal column of Bertin; 4, medullary ray; 5, cortex; 6, pelvis; 7, interlobar artery; 8, major calix; and 9, ureter. The letter A indicates the renal artery, and the letter V indicates the renal vein. Insert (a) from the upper pole is enlarged to illustrate the relationships between the juxtamedullary and the cortical nephrons and the renal vasculature. (From Brenner BM, Rector Jr FC: The Kidney. Philadelphia, Saunders, 1976, Vol 1, p 5, with permission.)

tribute to glomerular filtration or tubular secretion–reabsorption processes. Drug substances in the blood will follow these pathways through the kidney.

KIDNEY EXCRETION MECHANISMS

The net renal excretion of drugs and other substances from the blood results from the combination of glomerular filtration and tubular secretion and reabsorption. Excretion can take place by passive or by active processes and is influenced by the physicochemical properties of the substance being excreted.

Passive transport is a process whereby a compound diffuses across a biologic membrane from a compartment of higher concentration of the compound to one of lower concentration. With drugs in general, only the non-protein-bound un-ionized, lipid-soluble species in body fluids can be transported by passive diffusion; therefore, the pKa value of the drug, which determines its degree of ionization at a given pH, and its degree of protein binding greatly influence passive transport of the drug. Passive transport is one of the basic operative processes occurring in renal tubular reabsorption. For example, chloride and bicarbonate followed by water are all passively reabsorbed by the tubule because of the electrochemical gradient produced by the active reabsorption of sodium ion.

Active transport is a process characterized by the movement of a compound across a membrane against a concentration gradient, i.e., uphill, from a lower to a higher concentration. Active transport requires energy expenditure and the use of membrane carriers because work is required to move against the concentration gradient. Active transport exhibits saturation of transport so that as drug concentration increases the rate of transport approaches a limiting value of transport maximum, Tm. For example, glucose is actively reabsorbed completely by the tubule in normal individuals, but it spills over into the urine of uncontrolled diabetics because their tubule concentration of glucose exceeds the Tm value. Active transport of a drug can be competitively inhibited by other compounds sharing the same transport system. This aspect was used to advantage in the days when penicillin was scarce. For example, by coadministration of probenecid, which is actively secreted by the same tubular transport system as penicillin, urinary excretion of penicillin was decreased, and plasma levels were prolonged. This allowed the administration of smaller penicillin doses to achieve the desired therapeutic effect.

Active tubular secretion is known to occur by at least two independent pathways: one for organic anions and one for organic cations. Of importance to diagnostic radiology and nuclear medicine is the active tubular secretion of organic anions including the iodinated benzoates, such as diatrizoate, and the hippurates, such as *p*-aminohippuric acid (PAH) and *o*-iodohippuric acid (OIH).

A more in-depth review of renal physiology and excretion mechanisms is given by Gottschalk and Lassiter[1] and Nielsen and Rasmussen.[2]

Important factors influencing the rate and extent of renal excretion of a drug are (1) molecular size and protein binding and their influence on glomerular filtration; (2) active transport through the renal tubules; (3) lipid solubility and the drug's pKa, which influence passive tubular reabsorption; and (4) the volume of distribution of the drug in the body.[2,3]

To enter the glomerular filtrate a substance must satisfy two criteria: be non–protein bound in the plasma and have a small molecular size. The glomerular capillaries are about 100-fold more permeable to water and salt than capillaries in general, but despite this increased permeability, substances with molecular weights greater than 50,000 daltons are almost completely excluded from the glomerular filtrate, whereas non-protein-bound drugs with molecular weights less than 5,000 daltons are filterable.[3] A drug that enters the glomerular filtrate will be excreted in the urine provided it is not reabsorbed across the tubular epithelium back into the blood. Generally, un-ionized, lipid-soluble drugs readily diffuse back into the blood, whereas ionized, water-soluble species remain in the urine unless reabsorbed by an active transport process.[4]

The degree of ionization of a drug depends upon the type of drug, its pKa, and the urinary pH, in accordance with the Henderson–Hasselbalch equation. For drugs that are weak organic acids this equation is as follows:

$$\text{pH} = \text{pKa} + \log \frac{\text{ionized drug}}{\text{un-ionized drug}}$$

Consider, for example, a weakly acidic drug with a pKa of 6. At a urinary pH of 5 it will be 90 percent un-ionized, which favors passive tubular reabsorption, whereas at pH 7 it will be 90 percent ionized and less drug will be reabsorbed.

The removal of a drug from the blood by the kidney can be quantitated by measuring its renal clearance. The renal clearance of a drug may be defined as the minimal volume of plasma required to supply the amount of drug excreted in the urine in a given period of time.[1] The clearance concept is applicable to all substances excreted into the urine and is expressed by the formula:

$$C_x = \frac{U_x \cdot V}{P_x}$$

Where

- U_x = urine concentration of the drug
- P_x = plasma concentration of the drug
- V = urine volume per unit time
- C_x = renal clearance in milliliters per minute

Consider for example, the clearance of Na^+. If $V = 1$ ml/min, $U_{Na} = 280$ mEq/l, and $P_{Na} = 140$ mEq/l, then $C_{Na} = 2$ ml/min. In other words, an amount of sodium equal to that contained in 2 ml of plasma (0.28 mEq) is excreted in the urine each minute. The clearance volume is a virtual volume, however, not a real volume, and one should not infer that all of the Na^+ has been removed from the 2 ml of plasma. On the contrary, only some of the sodium is removed from a much larger volume of blood.

Drug clearance occurs by glomerular filtration, tubular secretion, or a combination of both functions. Reabsorptive processes work against clearance. If a drug is known to be cleared only by a particular function such as glomerular filtration, then the drug may be used to quantitatively measure that function. The normal glomerular filtration rate (GFR) is 125 ml/min in humans and represents about 20 percent of the total renal plasma flow (TRPF). Normal TRPF is 650 ml/min. A small molecular weight substance that is not bound to plasma protein can enter the glomerular filtrate. If it is not metabolized, reabsorbed, or secreted by the tubule, it will remain in the urine with a clearance of 125 ml/min. The polysaccharide inulin best satisfies these requirements and is the standard substance used to measure the GFR.

That is to say, under a steady-state intravenous (IV) infusion of inulin when the GFR is normal, the amount of inulin contained in 125 ml of plasma will appear in the urine each minute by the glomerular filtration process.

Although the clearance of a drug does not delineate the specific mechanism involved with its renal excretion, some idea can be gained regarding the processes involved. For example, if a freely filterable drug has a clearance less than the GFR, then it must undergo tubular reabsorption as well. Glucose is a substance that is readily filtered, but because it is completely reabsorbed by active processes, its clearance in the normal individual is zero. If, on the other hand, a substance has a clearance greater than the GFR, then it must be secreted by the tubules as well.

Renal clearance only provides information regarding the amount of drug removed from the blood that appears in the urine. It is not applicable to substances that are stored, synthesized, or metabolized by the kidney.[5] On the other hand, the extraction ratio (ER) is a measure of both the amount of drug eliminated into the urine and that retained by the kidney. This ratio is defined by Smith[6] as the fraction of substance removed from plasma during one circulation through the kidney. It is expressed by the following equation:

$$ER = \frac{A - V}{A}$$

Where

- A = the renal arterial concentration of a substance
- V = the renal venous concentration of a substance

If a drug has an extraction ratio of 1.0, it will thus be completely removed in a single pass through the kidney. If none of the drug appears in the urine, all of it will be retained by the kidney. A radiopharmaceutical with this property would be the ideal renal imaging agent. On the other hand, if all of the drug appears in the urine, none will be retained in the kidney, and its clearance will be equal to the total renal plasma flow (650 ml/min). Such a drug would be the ideal substance for measuring renal function.

The clearance of PAH (C-PAH) is used to estimate the renal plasma flow, but because its extraction ratio (E-PAH) is only 0.92, its clearance is termed the effective renal plasma flow (ERPF).[6] The ERPF averages about 600 ml/min. TRPF is determined by the following relationship:

$$\text{TRPF} = \frac{\text{C-PAH}}{\text{E-PAH}} = \frac{600 \text{ ml/min}}{0.92} = 650 \text{ ml/min}$$

The total renal blood flow is determined by the relation TRPF/(1-hematocrit).[6] Because only 92 percent of PAH is extracted per pass through the kidney, 8 percent remains in the renal vein. Wesson[7] lists several possible reasons for incomplete extraction: (1) parenchymal bypass in which a small amount of blood that enters the renal vein does not pass through the tubules; (2) red cell transport in which drug that enters red cells does not readily diffuse out during blood transit through the cortical tubules; (3) incomplete cortical extraction, which is due to incomplete drug dissociation from plasma protein and diffusion from plasma to tubule cells; and (4) less extraction of drug from blood that passes through the medulla.

A drug's excretion rate is influenced by its volume of distribution (Vd). This volume is actually an apparent volume rather than a real one because a drug may concentrate in a body compartment of small physical size and give the impression that it is widely distributed in a large volume. In general, the larger the apparent Vd of a drug, the slower will be its rate of excretion. For example, Goldstein et al[4] have shown that theoretically, if a drug is distributed only in plasma water (Vd = 3 l) and is completely cleared per pass through the kidney (ER = 1.0), its plasma elimination half-life would be 3 minutes according to the following equation:

$$T_{1/2} = \frac{0.693 \text{ Vd}}{\text{Clearance}} = \frac{0.693 \ (3000 \text{ ml})}{650 \text{ ml/min}} = 3 \text{ min}$$

If its distribution were extracellular fluid (Vd = 12 l) or the total body water (Vd = 41 l), then its half-life would be 13 and 44 minutes, respectively.

DEVELOPMENT OF RADIOPHARMACEUTICALS FOR KIDNEY STUDIES

A very large number of radiopharmaceuticals have been investigated for renal studies, but only the more widely used agents will be discussed in this chapter. A more extensive review has been provided by Chervu and Blaufox.[8] Figures 12–2 and 12–3 illustrate the chemical structures of some important renal agents.

Radiopharmaceuticals for renal studies can be grouped into two main categories: (1) agents for renal clearance, which may be further subdivided into agents for assessing the GFR and agents for measuring tubular function and renal plasma flow; and (2) agents for renal imaging that bind to the renal cortical cells. The ideal agents for routine kidney studies in nuclear medicine should measure a particular function of the kidney by virtue of their excretion mechanisms. Agents with exclusive routes of excretion are rare, and most radiopharmaceuticals have mixed processes of excretion by the kidney.

The presence of unilateral renal disease cannot be easily recognized by routine kidney function tests because the unaffected kidney soon compensates for the diseased one. This fact prompted Taplin et al to introduce the radioisotope renogram in 1956.[9] The renogram permitted the evaluation of individual kidney function in a noninvasive manner. The original study consisted of a two-channel detection system, each kidney having its own scintillation detector connected to a ratemeter and recorder. After IV administration of a radiopharmaceutical that was cleared primarily by tubular secretion, the activity flowing through each kidney over time could be recorded. The first agent used was iodine-131 iodopyracet (Diodrast). The main problem with iodopyracet was a liver uptake that interfered

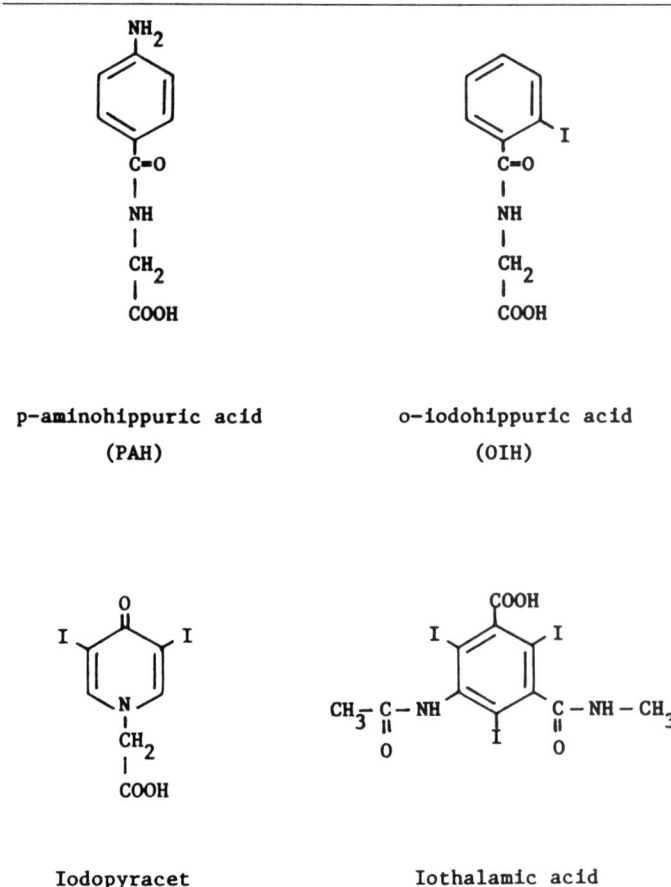

Figure 12-2. The structure of PAH and iodinated compounds that have been used for kidney imaging.

with the activity cleared by the right kidney. This problem stimulated the search for a better agent. PAH was the ideal choice to consider because of its high renal extraction, but it could not be labeled with a gamma-emitting nuclide. Further efforts culminated with the development of I-131 OIH (or Hippuran) in 1960 by Tubis et al.[10] Hippuran was excreted solely by the kidneys. Although Hippuran became the agent of choice for renograms and assessing tubular function, its rapid excretion and lack of kidney retention made it unsatisfactory for performing static kidney scans.

In 1960 Hg-203 chlormerodrin was being used for brain scanning and was known to be concentrated in the kidney. It was a likely choice for renal imaging because 5 to 10 percent of the administered dose was bound in each kidney with an effective half-life of 28 days.[11] This permitted visualization of the size, shape, and position of the kidneys and the presence of space-occupying lesions that appeared as areas of decreased activity. The mercury compound was bound by sulfhydryl-containing proteins in the tubular cells. A disadvantage of Hg-203 was the high radiation dose to the kidney (117 rad/mCi) because of its beta emission and long half-life, which prompted its replacement by Hg-197. Hg-197, which decays by electron capture, produced a significantly lower radiation dose (6 rad/mCi) but had its own disadvantage of low-energy photons (77 keV) that were easily scattered or absorbed in

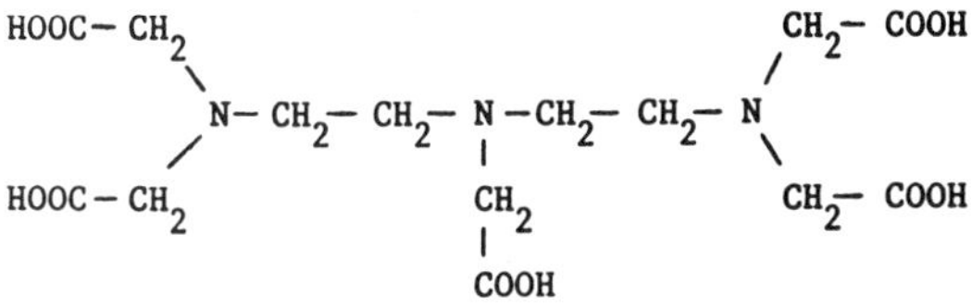

HOOC—CH₂\
           N—CH₂—CH₂—N—CH₂—CH₂—N\
HOOC—CH₂ | CH₂—COOH / CH₂—COOH\
                              CH₂\
                              COOH

DiethyleneTriaminePentaacetic Acid (DTPA)

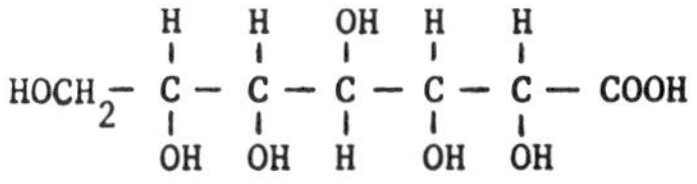

HOCH₂—C(H,OH)—C(H,OH)—C(OH,H)—C(H,OH)—C(H,OH)—COOH

GlucoHeptonic Acid (GHA)

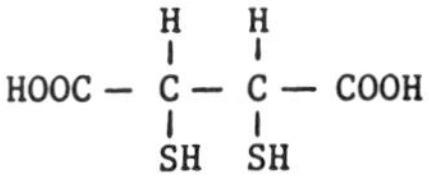

HOOC—C(H,SH)—C(H,SH)—COOH

2,3-DiMercaptoSuccinic Acid (DMSA)

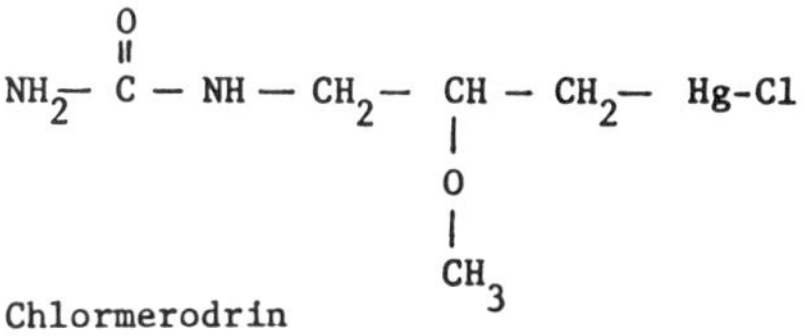

NH₂—C(=O)—NH—CH₂—CH(O—CH₃)—CH₂—Hg-Cl

Chlormerodrin

Figure 12-3. The structure of chlormerodrin and the complexing agents DTPA, GHA, and DMSA for labeling with technetium-99m for kidney imaging.

tissue and did not produce as good a resolution as Hg-203 photons (279 keV). It was clear that a short-lived radionuclide with better imaging properties was needed.

In 1966 Harper et al[12] developed a Tc-99m iron ascorbic acid complex. Approximately 8 percent of the administered activity localized in the distal convoluted tubules and remained in the kidneys for 4 to 20 hours. The significance of a Tc-99m agent was the ability to administer larger activities, which shortened study time and improved counting statistics while producing a low radiation dose.

Subsequently, several different technetium agents were developed for renal studies, most notably chelates of DTPA, DMSA, and glucoheptonate (GH). Figure 12-3 shows the chemical structures of ligands used to complex Tc-99m.

A number of Tc-DTPA preparations were investigated including the ferrous iron-reduced complex, Tc-iron ascorbate DTPA (Renotec) developed by E. R. Squibb, and the stannous tin-reduced product by Eckelman and Richards.[13] The biologic behavior of these three DTPA preparations were compared by Atkins et al[14] with the principal findings that the iron- and tin-reduced products had identical urinary excretion, with negligible binding to the kidney, whereas Renotec was similar to Tc-iron ascorbate. It was concluded that although Renotec contained DTPA the final product did not behave as a true chelate excreted solely by glomerular filtration and, therefore, should not be used to estimate the GFR. Presently, stannous DTPA kits are available commercially, and Tc-DTPA is used primarily to visualize renal perfusion, the collecting system, and to estimate the GFR.

In 1973 Tc-GH was developed at New England Nuclear Corp and Tc-DMSA at Medi-Physics, Inc.[15] Tc-DMSA reaches high concentrations in the renal cortex, which makes it a good choice for imaging the renal parenchyma. Its blood clearance and urinary clearance are slow because of high protein binding, which makes it a poor choice for evaluating the collecting system. Tc-GH is not so highly protein bound and has faster blood and urinary clearance than Tc-DMSA, but the fraction bound in the kidney is lower. Early images after an injection of Tc-GH usually demonstrate the collecting system well, similar to Tc-DTPA, whereas later images show parenchyma alone.[16]

Inulin clearance is regarded as the standard for measuring the GFR. Attempts to prepare radioactive inulin have been successful in that hydroxymethyl carbon-14 inulin shows a high degree of correlation to standard inulin for GFR measurements but requires liquid scintillation counting of the C-14 label. Attempts to prepare inulin with a suitable gamma emitter have not been very successful owing to degradation of the product or to dissimilar renal handling.

In 1965 Sigman et al[17] used I-131 iothalamate to measure the GFR and demonstrated its similarity to inulin. Subsequent studies confirmed its renal clearance to be identical to inulin.[18]

Several metal chelates of EDTA and DTPA have been investigated for GFR studies. Most noteworthy are Cr-51 EDTA, In-111 DTPA, and Tc-99m DTPA. The Cr-51 complex is not ideal for imaging studies because of the low photon abundance (9 percent) of the 320-keV gamma. In-111 DTPA and Tc-99m DTPA have similar biologic properties in humans but are not identical.[19] The In-111 complex has a slightly faster total-body clearance. The slightly greater retention of Tc-99m DTPA in body tissues probably represents Tc-99m nonchelated with DTPA. Tc-99m DTPA thus underestimates the GFR by a few percent, but despite this fact, its ready availability, ideal physical properties, and lower cost compared with In-111 DTPA make it a widely used radiopharmaceutical.

Although numerous agents have been used to study the kidney, the current radiopharmaceuticals of choice include I-131 *ortho*-iodohippurate for tubular function and ERPF measurements; I-125 iothalamate and DTPA complexes of In-111 and Tc-99m for GFR determinations; and Tc-99m complexes of DMSA, GH, and DTPA for renal imaging.

Sodium *Ortho*-iodohippurate I-131 (Hippuran I-131)

Production and Physical Properties. Hippuran I-131 is prepared by the isotope exchange reaction between stable Hippuran I-127 and sodium iodide I-131 according to the following reaction:

$$\text{C}_6\text{H}_4\text{-C(O)-NH-CH}_2\text{-C(O)-ONa} + \text{Na}^{131}\text{I}^* \longrightarrow \text{C}_6\text{H}_3\text{I}^*\text{-C(O)-NH-CH}_2\text{-C(O)-ONa} + \text{Na}^{127}\text{I}$$

Several different techniques have been used to effect exchange of I-131 for I-127 in the aromatic ring.[20] One method requires heating the reactants at pH 6 and 100°C for 4 hours. The unbound radionuclide may be separated from the iodinated Hippuran by ion-exchange chromatography or precipitation methods. The final pH is adjusted between 7.0 and 8.5. Radiochemical purity may be determined using ITLC-SG thin-layer chromatography as the solid phase and chloroform: acetic acid (9:1) as the mobile phase. In this system the Hippuran has an Rf of 1.0, and the radioiodide, 0.1. Radioactivity under the Hippuran peak must be not less than 97 percent. Hippuran I-131 degrades with time. Iodide separation or hydrolysis to *ortho*-iodobenzoic acid may occur. This was illustrated in Chapter 6 (Fig. 6–1). Deiodination is the most common route of degradation. It is primarily caused by radiolytic decomposition whereby a reaction occurs between the drug molecule and free radical species produced by the interaction of ionizing radiation with the aqueous solvent.[21] This process is accelerated in the presence of heat and light and with high specific activity solutions. Radiolytic decomposition reactions can be reduced by decreasing the specific activity and by using stabilizers such as sodium citrate, which act as radical scavengers. Reducing the concentration of water through the use of cosolvents such as propylene glycol may also retard radiolysis.

If the free radioiodide level is too high in a Hippuran preparation, the drug's clearance by the kidney will be prolonged because of radioiodide reabsorption by the tubule. *Ortho*-iodobenzoic acid is also excreted at a rate slower than Hippuran because it accumulates in the liver where it is conjugated with glycine to reform Hippuran, which is subsequently excreted.

Biologic Distribution and Mechanism of Renal Excretion. After IV administration, Hippuran rapidly disappears from the blood by diffusion into the extracellular space and by high renal extraction. It is not metabolized in the body and is excreted unchanged in the urine.[22] It is not stored in the renal tubular cells.[6] Hine et al[23] reported that renal excretion rates of Hippuran in normal subjects closely followed blood disappearance rates. Renal excretion could be accounted for by four exponentials with half-times of 2, 10, and 50 minutes, and a long component ranging from 3 to 13 hours, apparently resulting from iodide impurities. The rapid components of renal excretion are due to the release into the bladder of highly concentrated renal activity that initially accumulates in the kidneys, whereas the slower components reflect back diffusion of more dilute activity from the extracellular space and their subsequent excretion into the urine. In the normal hydrated subject, 70 percent of a single dose of Hippuran is collected in the urine 30 minutes after injection.[24]

Renal excretion of Hippuran is primarily by active tubular secretion, although some degree of glomerular filtration occurs. The exact fraction of injected activity excreted by each process is not known. Theoretically, 20 percent should be filtered and 80 percent secreted if the drug was not protein bound and had 100 percent renal extraction. The overall renal extraction efficiency is less than 100 percent and varies roughly between 65 and 85 percent.[5] The wide range of reported values depends on the conditions of measurement and several intrinsic factors such as binding to blood components, the presence of radioiodide or other impurities in the injected dose, and reabsorption by the tubule.

Hippuran exhibits some degree of red cell[6] and plasma protein binding,[25] and these factors will reduce the amount filtered at the glomerulus to less than the theoretic 20 percent. Protein binding has been reported to be as high as 70 percent, but it is labile.[25] Because only free drug can be secreted by the tubular cells, incomplete dissociation of Hippuran from its blood-binding sites at the blood–tubular cell interface may prevent complete secretion during transit through the peritubular capillaries. Ideally, with a continuous infusion of radiochemically pure, labeled Hippuran and normal renal function, the renal extraction efficiency should approach 90 percent, similar to that of PAH. In practice, however, renal extraction is usually lower, and the ERPF is therefore underestimated. By continuous infusion in normal dogs, the extraction efficiency from plasma is 67 percent.[5] After a single injection in normal dogs, the extraction efficiency of highly purified Hippuran during the first hour is 82 percent from plasma and 65 percent from whole blood, but lower values are obtained with commercial Hippuran.[5] This implies that incomplete red cell diffusion and impurities in commercial Hippuran are, in part, responsible for inefficient renal extraction.

If the injected dose contains free radioiodide, this portion of injected activity will be readily filtered, but about 70 percent will be reabsorbed by the tubule,[26] thus prolonging renal extraction. A comparison of OIH-to-PAH clearance ratios demonstrated that the ratio varied inversely with free radioiodide in OIH preparations, ranging from 0.91 with less than 2.0 percent iodide to 0.80 with greater than 5.0 percent iodide.[22] When radioiodide impurity is high, the rate of blood clearance and urinary accumulation of radioactivity decreases substantially and produces renogram curves with flattened peaks of diminished height followed by a slowed excretory segment.[27]

Once in the tubular urine, Hippuran is presumed to be completely excreted, although studies in rats have demonstrated that passive nonionic tubular reabsorption can occur at various urinary pH values. In one study when urine pH was raised from 6.9 to 7.9, the urinary excretion of Hippuran increased 27 percent.[28] Hippuran is a weak organic acid with a pKa of 3.63, and therefore high urinary pH produces a more highly ionized species that is less likely to be reabsorbed by the tubule. Increased excretion can thus occur at high urinary pH values, and decreased excretion, because of increased tubular reabsorption, is possible at a low urinary pH.

Although the renal extraction efficiency of Hippuran substantially underestimates the ERPF, simultaneous measurement of renal clearance and extraction efficiency would allow a determination of the true renal plasma flow as described earlier, but these measurements are complex, fraught with error, and are attendant with high risk. A simpler method based on a single injection of Hippuran and a single blood sample obtained at a specified time provides a means to measure the ERPF, but this method is not yet commonly used.[24] The routine parameter used to assess renal function in nuclear medicine in a noninvasive manner is the renal transit time of Hippuran and the excretory half-time by external counting with a gamma camera and computer.[29] The accumulation and disappearance of renal activity with time after injection of a single dose of Hippuran is displayed by the renogram curve illustrated in Figure 12–4.

The Renogram. Immediately after injection Hippuran is confined to three primary spaces: the blood, the extracellular space, and the kidney. The blood level initially drops precipitously because of a combination of high renal extraction and rapid diffusion into the extracellular space. The blood level falls continuously thereafter, in a multiexponential manner but at a slower rate because backdiffusion of Hippuran from the extracellular space into the blood predominates. The initial spike of the renogram (Fig. 12–4, curve A) occurs during the first 30 to 60 seconds after injection and depends on the site of injection, the mode of injection, i.e., bolus or IV drip, patient cardiac status, etc. It represents the simultaneous detection of radioactivity in the blood, extracellular space, and in the kidney. Renal parenchymal activity (Fig. 12–4, curve B) is shown by a continual rise during the first few minutes after the initial spike and primarily represents extraction of activity from the blood. During this portion of the renogram curve no radioactivity above tissue background level is detectable in the bladder. Peak renal activity is reached just before the initial appearance of bladder activity and takes 3 to 5 minutes in the normal, hydrated subject. This time-to-peak measure reflects both the average linear rate of movement through the renal parenchyma and the patency of the renal pelvis.[29] A relative prolonged time-to-peak

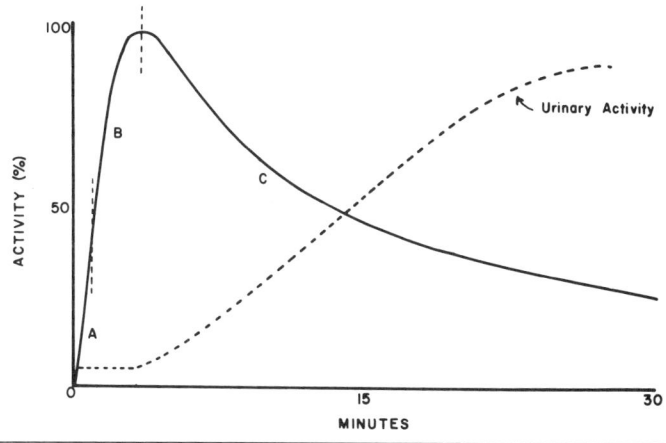

Figure 12-4. A normal renogram curve. See the text for a detailed explanation.

may be seen in low–renal blood flow states (e.g., dehydration or renal arterial stenosis), parenchymal damage (e.g., interstitial nephritis or tubular necrosis), or in urinary tract obstruction. The fall in the renogram curve (Fig. 12-4, curve C) correlates temporally with the abrupt rise in bladder radioactivity. The curve continues to fall because the amount of radioactivity leaving the kidney is greater than that being cleared from the blood by renal extraction.

The time from peak curve amplitude to half this value on the falling segment of the renogram curve in normal subjects is 12 to 15 minutes and can also be used to measure renal function. This time will be prolonged in renal disease and measures the same physiologic events as the time to peak but is less dependent on the injection technique.[29]

The Hippuran renogram is a complex representation of multiple physiologic phenomena, and, as such, is best used as a unique parameter of renal function. Relative funtional differences between kidneys or within comparable segments is more easily evaluated than marginal changes in overall function.

If the physiologic state is comparable, serial studies can be used to evaluate the relative overall renal function while monitoring temporal changes. Figure 12-5 illustrates several renogram curves demonstrating these temporal changes.

Hippuran Use. Hippuran is used to assess renal function. Because most of it is cleared from the renal parenchyma by 30 minutes, abnormal cortical retention of this agent makes it a more sensitive indicator of tubular dysfunction than decreased uptake of the Tc-99m agents. In acute or chronic tubular dysfunction, Hippuran is retained intracellularly in the cortex, and the normal rapid transit into the tubular lumen is delayed. Thus, in uremia, the renal parenchyma may be visualized with Hippuran when the Tc-99m agents fail, particularly in delayed images up to 24 hours, but it is inferior to the Tc-99m agents for delineating focal renal abnormalities.[30]

I-123-labeled Hippuran is now commercially available. Its advantages are a lower radiation dose and improved image quality because of its electron capture mode of decay, 159-keV gamma radiation, and 13-hour half-life. Cost and availability are major disadvantages to its use. Hippuran labeled with I-131 has one major advantage besides lower cost and ready availability. It can be counted independently of Tc-99m by pulse height analysis because of its higher gamma energy. It can thus be used to assess renal tubular function while the mor-

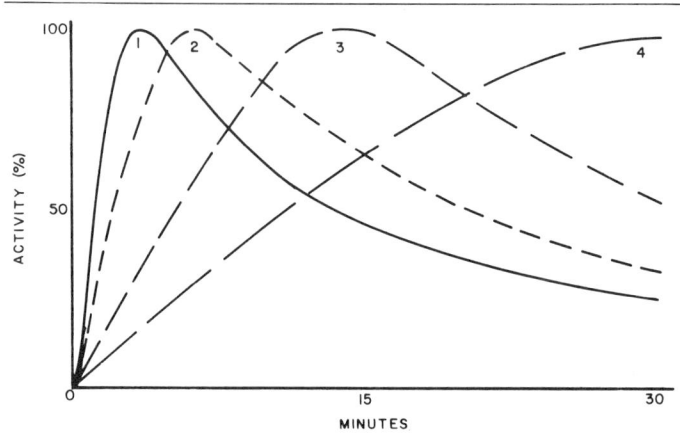

Figure 12-5. Normal renogram curve (1) and curves (2, 3, and 4) depicting progressive kidney deterioration, respectively.

phologic and perfusion abnormalities are examined with a Tc-99m agent.

Radiation Dose. The critical organ after administration of I-131 Hippuran depends on renal function and the radiochemical purity of the product injected. With normal renal function and by using a pure product the bladder wall will be the critical organ because activity rapidly accumulates in the bladder. A pathologic obstruction preventing urinary excretion will decrease the bladder dose but increase the kidney dose commensurate with its ability to extract drug from the blood. When radioiodide impurity is present, the critical organ is the thyroid gland. Its radiation dose will increase significantly in renal disease because of poor urinary excretion of iodide. A patient with normal kidney function and normal thyroid function (assume a 25 percent uptake) who receives 100 µCi of I-131 Hippuran containing the maximum-allowed 3 percent radioiodide will sustain a radiation dose of 9.4 mrad to the kidneys, 4050 mrad to the thyroid gland, and 333 mrad to the bladder wall, assuming a 3-hour void post-injection.[31] In renal failure the thyroid uptake may be 75 percent, thus increasing the gland dose to 12 rad. The radiation dose to the kidney in various stages of renal disease appears in Table 12-1.

TABLE 12-1. RADIATION DOSE TO THE KIDNEYS FROM 100 µCi I-131 HIPPURAN IN VARIOUS DISEASE STATES

		Conditions Assumed	
Disease States	RAD	*Kidney Uptake*	*Transit Time*
Normal	0.01	50%	3.5 min
Dehydration	0.03	50%	10 min
Ischemia	0.03	30%	20 min
Acute tubular necrosis	0.60	50%	4 hr
Glomerulonephritis	6.75	50%	several days
Obstruction			
Recent	40.00	50%	—
1 month	20.00	25%	—
Chronic	4.00	5%	—

(Values from Eliott AT, et al, 1976, pp 293–304[31])

Sodium Iothalamate I-125

Sodium iothalamate labeled with I-125 or I-131 is a radioiodinated derivative of substituted triiodobenzoic acid. Its structure appears in Figure 12-2. The compound is prepared by the isotope-exchange method.

After IV administration iothalamate is excreted by glomerular filtration. It is minimally bound to plasma protein in humans, with reports ranging from 3 percent[17] to 8 to 27 percent.[25] The latter report noted that the renal clearance of iothalamate was greater than inulin clearance if a correction for protein binding was made but that no difference was found without a correction. This suggests that slight tubular secretion may occur in humans. Studies in animals, however, indicate that no tubular secretion or reabsorption occurs and that biliary excretion occurs only in poor or absent renal function.[32] Because of low protein binding, insignificant extrarenal excretion, apparent lack of tubular secretion and reabsorption, and good correlation with inulin clearance,[17] radioiodinated iothalamate is a well-established agent for the estimation of the GFR.

Because of a longer shelf life and greater product stability, the I-125 label is more suitable than I-131, particularly because free radioiodide levels generated through radiolytic decomposition by I-131 will diminish renal clearance values because of tubular reabsorption of iodide.

GFR measurements require the collection of carefully timed blood and urine samples, and some techniques require catheterization. For these reasons GFR measurements are not routinely performed in nuclear medicine. However, I-125 iothalamate remains one of the radiopharmaceuticals of choice for such measurements in humans.

Tc-99m Pentetate (DTPA)

Production and Physical Properties. Tc-99m DTPA is produced routinely in the hospital by simply adding sodium pertechnetate to a sterile kit. The kit contains a lyophilized complex of stannous chloride and 5 to 10 mg of the pentasodium or calcium-trisodium salt of pentetic acid (DTPA). The reason for using a calcium salt is to lessen the chance for depleting calcium ion in plasma, although the routine amounts of DTPA administered are quite small and should not be a cause for concern. The use of a calcium salt was instituted as a precautionary measure when DTPA preparations were being developed for CSF studies. Stannous DTPA kits may be produced by adding stannous chloride to a solution of the DTPA salt and heating under a nitrogen atmosphere.[13] The pH is adjusted to 4, and the product is lyophilized and sealed under nitrogen.

The radiochemical purity of Tc-99m DTPA is tested by the chromatographic method described previously. Hydrolyzed–reduced technetium and pertechnetate are the primary impurities. These are generally not significant, but pertechnetate is more readily generated if the product is exposed to air. Increased levels of pertechnetate may interfere with kidney imaging because of gastric secretion of pertechnetate,[33] but the levels of impurity must be high. The shelf life of Tc-99m DTPA is generally 6 hours after preparation and depends on the amount of activity, presence of oxygen, and the levels of stannous ion. Kits with a higher DTPA-to-Sn(II) molar ratio produce higher yields of the Tc-DTPA complex and lower levels of hydrolyzed technetium impurity.[34]

Biologic Distribution and Mechanism of Renal Excretion. After IV administration of a single dose of Tc-99m-DTPA the plasma disappearance is multiexponential and exhibits half-times of 3.8 minutes, 15.6 minutes, 118 minutes, and 13.6 hours, representing 58, 24, 16, and 2 percent of the injected dose respectively.[19] The early rapid loss from blood represents diffusion into the extracellular space and renal excretion. In the blood of humans Tc-99m DTPA exhibits a slight protein binding of 3 to 5 percent 1 hour after injection[35] and no significant diffusion into red blood cells.[19]

Renal clearance of Tc-99m DTPA is by glomerular filtration, and its rate of clearance approximates that of I-125 iothalamate. It underestimates the latter by about 8 percent, probably because of the small degree of protein binding.[35] It is not secreted by the renal tubules, as shown by no change in renal clearance in dogs treated simultaneously with probenecid,[35] a known competitor for tubular transport of organic anions. Tubular reabsorption of Tc-99m-DTPA also does not appear to occur because the Tc-99m DTPA-to-inulin clearance ratio in dogs remains unchanged when measured at different urine flow rates.[36]

In humans, the peak renal activity is reached by 3 minutes after a single IV dose, at which time 5 percent of the injected activity is present in each kidney.[19] Renal excretion is rapid and relatively complete, with only 4 percent of the dose retained in the body by 24 hours. Sixty-nine percent is eliminated by the kidneys with a biologic half-life of 1.73 hours and the remaining 27 percent with a biologic half-life of 9.23 hours. Insignificant amounts are excreted through the hepatobiliary system into the feces.[19]

Tc-99m DTPA is apparently very stable in vivo, being excreted unchanged into the urine. Atkins et al[14] have shown from gel filtration chromatography of urine samples that 98 percent of the injected activity is still chelated.

Tc-99m DTPA Use. The urinary excretion of Tc-99m DTPA is more rapid than other Tc-99m complexes for renal evaluation (Table 12-2). It is an effective agent for visualizing the pelvicalyceal collecting system and the ureters by simulating the morphologic information of IV urography; thus, it is probably the agent of choice in obstructive uropathy.[30] Because of its negligible cortical retention, however, it may fail to delineate smaller focal parenchymal lesions.[30] Because Tc-99m DTPA is rapidly cleared and not significantly retained in the body, it has usefulness in short-term studies such as cerebral shunt patency evaluation, cerebrospinal fluid (CSF) leak studies, and kidney localization before biopsies or functional studies with Hippuran.

TABLE 12-2. PROPERTIES of Tc-99m RENAL AGENTS

Property	DTPA	GH	DMSA
Blood clearance mean $T_{1/2}$	84 min	27 min	54 min
Plasma protein binding at 1 hr	4%	54%	76%
Percent dose uptake in 2 kidneys			
1 hr	4	9	24
6 hr	2	12	41
Urinary excretion (% of dose)			
2 hr	50	50	16
6 hr	73	64	26
24 hr	96	71	37
Radiation dose (rad/mCi)			
Kidney	0.042	0.17	0.62
Bladder wall	0.55	0.80	0.28
Renal distribution	Collecting system only	Collecting system (early) Parenchyma (late)	Parenchyma only
Renal mechanism	Glomerular filtration	Glomerular filtration Cortical binding Tubular secretion/ reabsorption?	Glomerular filtration Cortical binding Tubular secretion/ reabsorption?

(Data from Arnold RW, et al, 1975, p 357,[16] and McAfee JG, 1982, pp 3-9.[30])

Tc-99m DTPA has been used to measure the GFR.[36] In a comparison of four commercial DTPA preparations with Cr-51 EDTA for GFR measurements, however, it was found that the accuracy of measurements depends on the source of DTPA kits.[37] In this study only the CaNa$_3$ DTPA kits gave accurate results. Several DTPA kit formulations are listed in Table 12–3.

Radiation Dose. The critical organ after administration of Tc-99m DTPA is the bladder wall, which sustains a radiation-absorbed dose of 0.55 rad/mCi, assuming no void of urine,[38] and 0.115 rad/mCi and 0.27 rad/mCi with 2.0-hour and 4.8-hour voiding periods, respectively.[39] For a given blood clearance rate, the radiation dose to the bladder wall will be dependent on the urine content of the bladder at the time of injection, the urine flow rate, and the residence time in the bladder.[31] Adequate hydration and frequent voiding are thus recommended with this and all agents that exhibit major excretion into the urine.

In-111 Pentetate (DTPA)

In vitro the In-111 DTPA complex is considerably more stable than Tc-99m DTPA in that it is not susceptible to oxidation by air. Ionic indium readily hydrolyzes to form the insoluble hydroxide, but when chelated with DTPA, its stability constant is quite high (K = 1 × 10^{28}) so that its rate of dissociation is minimal and no significant hydrolysis occurs.[40]

The biologic distribution and elimination pattern of In-111 DTPA is similar to Tc-99m DTPA, but it is not identical.[19] In normal subjects the plasma clearances of the two chelates are virtually identical 90 minutes after injection. Organ distribution is the same during the first hour, but concentrations of In-111 DTPA become lower by 24 hours. The urinary excretion of In-111 DTPA (50 percent in 1 hour) is somewhat faster than that of Tc-99m DTPA (50 percent in 1.5 hours).[19] With In-111 DTPA 4 to 5 percent of an administered dose is retained in the body, widely distributed in various tissues, and probably represents uncomplexed radionuclide. In-111 DTPA has uses similar to Tc-99m DTPA but is preferred for quantitative GFR measurements along with I-125 iothalamate.[3]

In-111 is a cyclotron-produced radionuclide and is considerably more expensive than Tc-99m. For this reason it is not routinely used for renal imaging but is reserved for studies that take advantage of its physical properties. It is primarily used to evaluate abnormalities in CSF flow. The 2.8-day half-life plus satisfactory photon energy and abundance make it the agent of choice for CSF studies. A more detailed discussion of its production, physical and biologic properties, and use in CSF studies is presented in Chapters 7 and 14.

Tc-99m Succimer (DMSA)

Production and Physical Properties. The chemical structure of DMSA appears in Figure 12–3. It was originally developed and used in China to relieve the symptoms of antimony poisoning resulting from the use of antimony potassium tartrate for the treatment of schistosomiasis. The Tc-99m DMSA complex is routinely prepared for renal imaging by simply adding Tc-99m pertechnetate to a sterile, pyrogen-free kit containing either a reagent solution or a lyophilized powder of stannous-DMSA, waiting 10 minutes, and injecting the patient. The radiolabeled complex is very sensitive to air oxidation and it is recommended to be used within 30 minutes of preparation. The stannous-DMSA reagent solution should not be refrigerated during storage because the complex may precipitate from solution because of low solubility.

Investigative studies have identified the ideal labeling parameters and properties of the Tc-DMSA complex formed. Ikeda et al[41,42] have demonstrated that four Tc-DMSA complexes can form when pertechnetate and Sn(II) DMSA are reacted. A schematic diagram of these complexes is shown in Figure 12–6. Complex II has the highest kidney uptake. The maximum yield of complex II is dependent on the pH of the reaction mixture and the oxygen con-

TABLE 12-3. Tc-99m KITS FOR KIDNEY IMAGING

Manufacturer	Composition Component	Quantity	Maximum Tc-99m Activity	Expiration Time after Labeling	Kit Storage before Labeling	Kit Storage after Labeling
Medi-Physics	DTPA sodium SnCl₂	5.0 mg 0.25 mg	—	1 hr, GFR studies 6 hr, imaging	15–30°C	15–30°C
Squibb	CaNa₃DTPA SnCl₂ · 2 H₂O	10.0 mg 0.5 mg	—	1 hr, GFR studies 6 hr, imaging	15–30°C	15–30°C
Syncor	CaNa₃DTPA SnCl₂ · 2 H₂O	20.6 mg 0.15 mg (min) 0.30 mg (max)	160 mCi	1 hr, GFR studies 6 hr, imaging	15–30°C	15–30°C
Dupont/NEN	Gluceptate sodium SnCl₂ · 2 H₂O	200 mg 0.06 mg (min) 0.07 mg (max)	200 mCi	6 hr	15–30°C	15–30°C
Mallinckrodt	Gluceptate calcium SnCl₂ · 2 H₂O	50 mg 0.7 mg (min) 1.1 mg (max)	300 mCi	6 hr	2–30°C	2–8°C
Medi-Physics	DMSA SnCl₂ H₂O	1.2 mg 0.42 mg 2.2 ml	—	30 min	15–30°C	15–30°C

Preparation note for DMSA: Mix one part by volume of DMSA reagent with one to two parts by volume of pertechnetate; incubate the mixture for 10 minutes before use; protect from light; do not administer more than 2 ml of reagent per patient dose.

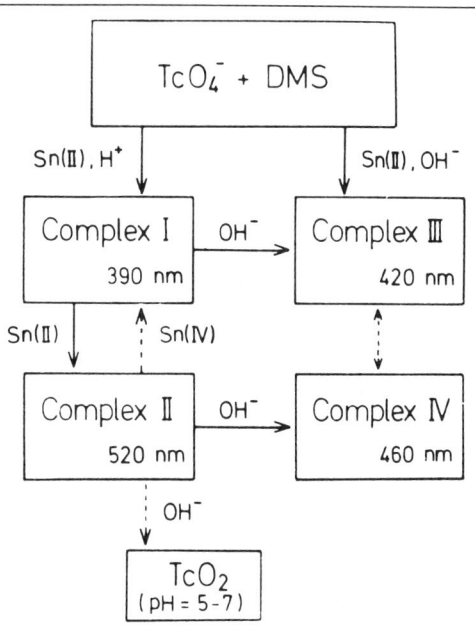

Figure 12-6. Formation of possible Tc-DMSA complexes and their maximum ultraviolet (UV) absorbances. *(From Ikeda I, et al, 1976, p 681, with permission.[41])*

centration in the solution. The highest yield of complex II is achieved at pH 2.5 in the absence of oxygen. At higher pH values urinary excretion of activity occurs with no kidney retention. Kidney localization of complexes prepared at one pH is not appreciably altered if the pH is later changed.[42,43] Complex II formed at pH 2.5 thus reverts to complex IV by raising the pH, but kidney localization diminishes by only 25 percent.[42] Complexes formed at neutral pH do not localize in the kidney if the pH is subsequently lowered to 2.5.

The labeling reaction of Tc-99m DMSA proceeds in two steps: rapid formation of complex I followed by a slower, rate-determining step from complex I to complex II, the latter being greatly affected by oxygen.[42] Once complex II is formed it may revert back to complex I by oxidation. This occurs because Sn(II) is oxidized to Sn(IV), and the reduction potential of the system is decreased. Diminished kidney uptake occurs because complex I is readily excreted. In addition to decreased kidney uptake, increased liver activity has been reported when a Tc-DMSA solution was injected 20 minutes after 1 ml of air was added to the reaction vial.[44]

The following recommendations should be followed when preparing Tc-99m DMSA using Sn(II)-DMSA reagent solution and pertechnetate: (1) the reaction pH should not be greater than 2.5, (2) the volume of pertechnetate should be no greater than twice the volume of Sn(II)-DMSA reagent to diminish the level of dissolved oxidants, (3) admit no air into the reaction vial, and (4) allow 10 minutes for the reaction to occur to provide time for conversion of complex I to complex II.

Analytic studies indicate that the Tc-DMSA complexes do not contain tin as a mixed metal complex of the type Tc-Sn-DMSA.[45] Preliminary structural analysis by nuclear magnetic resonance (NMR)[45] suggests that the chemical structure of the kidney-localizing complex is a dimer consisting of one Tc atom bridging two DMSA molecules as shown in Figure 12-7.

Biologic Distribution and Mechanism of Localization and Excretion. Arnold et al[16] have shown that 75 percent of Tc-99m DMSA is loosely bound to plasma protein initially and during the first 6 hours after IV injection and increases to 90 percent by 24 hours. In vitro dialysis studies also show that Tc-99m DMSA has a high affinity for serum albumin.[40]

The blood disappearance rate is slower than Tc-99m DTPA because of protein binding. The rate of blood clearance can be resolved into three exponential components: 44 percent of the dose has a biologic half-life of 20 minutes; 44 percent, 50 minutes; and 12 percent, 18 hours.[16] Approximately 4 to 5 percent of the Tc-99m DMSA plasma activity is extracted continuously per pass through the kidney in humans.[47] Renal accumulation progresses over a period of hours with a biologic uptake half-time of 1 hour, and no biologic excretion of the

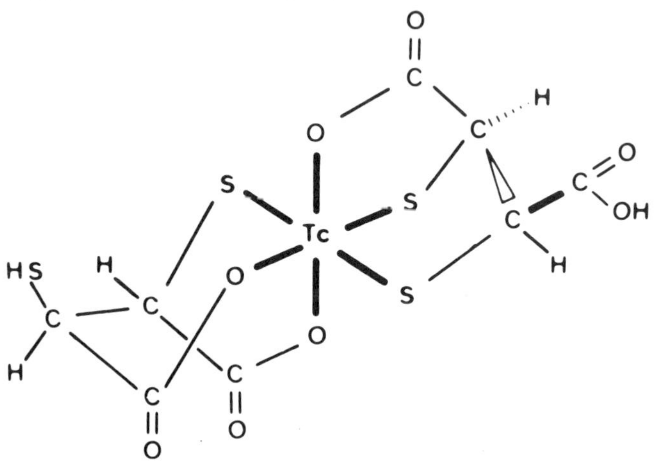

Figure 12-7. A proposed structure for the Tc-DMSA complex. (From Moretti JL, et al, 1982, p 27, with permission.[45])

bound fraction.[16] About 24 percent of the injected dose is bound to both kidneys by 1 hour, increasing to 40 percent by 6 hours.[16] The amount that is not bound by the kidney appears in the urine, with a cumulative urinary excretion by 6 and 24 hours of 26 and 37 percent of the administered dose, respectively. Autoradiographic studies in rats indicate that 96 percent of the renal activity is bound in the cortex and 4 percent in the medulla.[48]

The exact mechanism of renal excretion of Tc-99m DMSA is not known. Because it is highly protein bound, less of the plasma activity will be cleared by glomerular filtration compared with Tc-99m DTPA or Tc-99m GH. This is evident during renal imaging because of poor visualization of the pelvicalyceal collecting system; however, protein binding appears to be important for kidney localization. The Tc-99m DMSA complex formed at a low pH has the highest protein binding and renal concentration.[49] When the complex is formed at higher pH values, progressively lower protein binding and renal concentration occur along with increased liver and bone activity. Renal concentration is not affected by probenecid, a known tubular blocking agent, thus suggesting that DMSA is not secreted, at least not by the same enzyme system as probenecid.[50] Other studies show that ionic mercury (Hg$^+$) effectively decreases the localization of Tc-99m DMSA in the tubular cells.[45] These data suggest that localization of Tc-99m DMSA in the cortical tubular cells occurs either by delivery of the protein-bound complex through the efferent arterial blood to the peritubular fluid where the complex dissociates and binds to the tubular cells or through reabsorption and binding to proximal tubular cells of Tc-99m DMSA filtered at the glomerulus. Subcellular studies indicate that binding occurs to intracellular proteins in the cytosol, microsomes, and mitochondria.[51]

Tc-99m DMSA Use. Tc-99m DMSA mimics the biologic distribution of Hg-197 chlormerodrin by reaching a high concentration in the renal cortex with slow urinary excretion. Imaging at 2 to 4 hours after injection is satisfactory although longer times up to 24 hours allow greater blood clearance and lower background activity.

The cortical morphology of the normal kidney appears in the images as a thin peripheral rim of activity that merges with a central network of activity enclosing four to eight relatively "cold" areas (see illustration on page 345).[47] This pattern probably results from the high activity in the cortical columns of Bertin that extends into the "colder" medulla and separates it into several irregular pyramidal structures. Normal variations of this renal cortical image must be learned to avoid misinterpreting normal structures as renal defects.[47]

DMSA is an excellent agent for detecting focal abnormalities of the renal cortex. Because of its slow urinary excretion, it is a poor agent for demonstrating abnormalities of the collecting system. Because of its high kidney uptake it has been suggested that Tc-99m DMSA may be the best technetium agent for determining relative functional renal mass.

Distribution of Tc-99m DMSA may be altered in severe renal disease or from acid–base imbalance. When renal function is severely impaired, the liver may also accumulate activity as an alternate excretory pathway (Fig. 12–8). These mechanisms are not well understood. Studies conducted in rats with ammonium chloride-induced acidosis producing low urinary pH demonstrated that kidney concentration of DMSA activity was reduced by more than 50 percent and liver activity increased.[50] The reasons for this effect are not known, but the results may bear significance in the quantitative estimation of renal function in patients with acid–base disturbances. Changing kidney-to-liver activity ratios may produce false overestimation of right kidney activity when there is increased hepatic uptake. In particular, this may lead to incorrect analysis in cases of asymmetrical renal disease.[50]

Radiation Dose. The kidney and more specifically the renal cortex is the critical organ for Tc-99m DMSA. Because of high renal uptake the radiation dose diminishes as renal function decreases, but the radiation dose to other organs such as the liver and blood will increase. In the normal kidney with a maximal uptake of 44 percent of the administered activity and no biologic excretion, the radiation dose to the whole

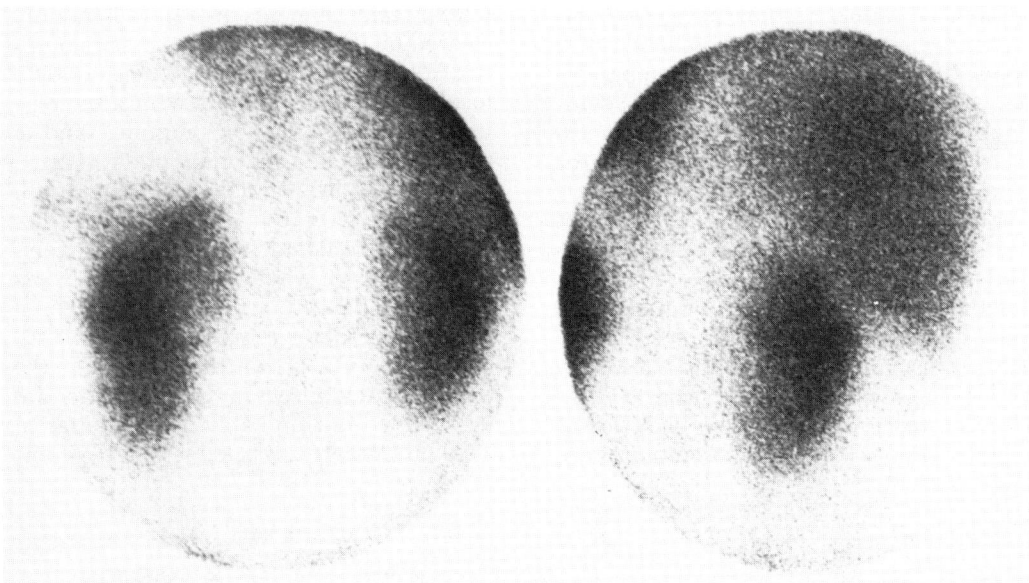

Figure 12-8. Renal scan in a patient with Tc-99m DMSA that demonstrates liver uptake secondary to renal failure.

kidney is 0.62 rad/mCi, and to the renal cortex, 0.76 rad/mCi.[16] For a routine 5-mCi dose, then, each kidney receives an absorbed dose of 3 to 3.5 rad.

Tc-99m Gluceptate (GH)

Production and Physical Properties. Glucoheptonic acid is a seven-carbon carboxylic acid sugar. Its structure appears in Figure 12–3. It is usually available as the sodium or calcium glucoheptonate salts generically named gluceptates. Tc-99m gluceptate (Tc-99m GH) is routinely prepared in the hospital by simply adding Tc-99m pertechnetate to a kit and mixing for 5 minutes to effect dissolution and complexation. The kit contains a sterile, pyrogen-free, lyophilized powder consisting of stannous chloride and either sodium or calcium gluceptate sealed under nitrogen gas. Kits are usually purchased from a commercial source but may be prepared extemporaneously for local use.

Stannous ion is not an absolute requirement to prepare Tc-99m GH because the complex has also been prepared by electrolytic reduction using glassy carbon electrodes[52] or with sodium borohydride. Although commercial kits have a recommended shelf life after radiolabeling of 6 hours, the Tc-99m GH complex is apparently quite stable. A 0.01 M Tc-99 GH solution in saline was shown by spectrophotometric analysis to be chemically stable for more than 200 days at room temperature.[53] The stability of the Tc-99m GH has not been well defined but will be subject to oxidative and radiolytic decomposition. Solutions intended for use beyond the 6-hour expiration time, therefore, should be checked using chromatography before use with the system used for Tc-99m DTPA.

The in vitro and in vivo behavior of Tc-99 GH and Tc-99m GH complexes are identical, indicating that the two isomers give the same complex with glucoheptonate and that there are no chemical differences between the nanomolar (Tc-99m) and the millimolar (Tc-99) concentration ranges.[53] The same study also characterized the chemical structure of Tc-GH as being a biscomplex consisting of one technetium atom bridging two glucoheptonate molecules. The complex has a net anionic charge of -1. The structure of Tc(GH)$_2$ appears in Figure 12–9. The net balanced equation[53] proposed for the production of Tc(GH)$_2$ by stannous ion reduction is as presented below.

Biologic Distribution, Mechanism of Localization, and Excretion. The biologic properties of Tc-99m GH in humans have been described by Arnold et al.[16] In the blood negligible diffusion occurs into red blood cells, but about 50 percent of plasma activity is bound loosely to protein initially after injection; this increases gradually to 75 percent by 6 hours and 90 percent by 24 hours. Tc-99m GH clears rapidly from the blood in a triexponential manner with biologic half-times of 5 minutes (84%), 1 hour (10%), and 24 hours (6%). It is mainly cleared by the kidney, with a maximal uptake of 15 percent of the injected dose localizing in both kidneys with a biologic uptake half-time of 45 minutes and a biologic excretion half-time of 24 hours.[16] Tc-99m GH is eventually eliminated into the urine, with 64 and 71 percent accumulated by 6 and 24 hours, respectively. It is not known whether the complex is excreted unchanged; however, the high in vitro stability suggests that it is.

Uptake and binding mechanisms in the proximal tubular cells in the renal cortex are not defined but probably occur similar to Tc-99m DMSA. It is possible that the com-

---

$$TcO_4^- + 2(C_7H_{13}O_8)^- + Sn^{2+} + H_2O \longrightarrow [TcO(C_7H_{12}O_8)_2]^- + 2H^+ + [SnO_2(OH)_2]^{2-}$$

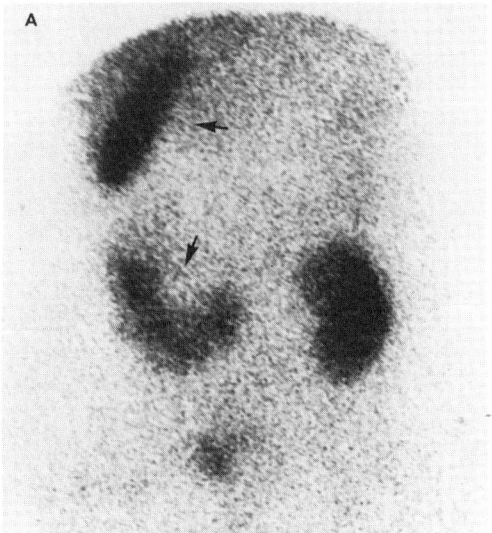

Figure 12-9. The structures of glucoheptonate and Tc (GH). *(From de Kieviet W, 1981, p 708, with permission.*[53]*)*

plex is delivered to the tubular cells by diffusion from the blood and peritubular fluid after dissociation from its plasma protein-binding sites. No data are available to determine whether tubular reabsorption or secretion occurs with Tc-99m GH.

Some fecal excretion of Tc-99m GH amounting to about 4.5 percent of the administered dose in 24 hours, has been reported in dogs.[16] The same authors noted that in clinical studies the gallbladder is occasionally visualized; thus, uptake and excretion by the hepatocytes must also occur to a small extent. Liver activity is expected to be visualized in advanced cases of renal dysfunction (Fig. 12–10).

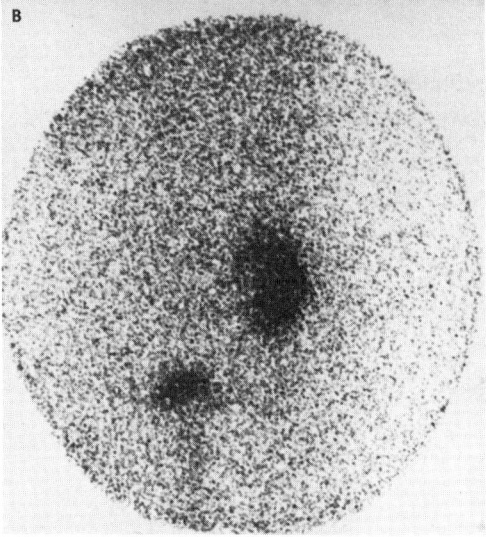

Figure 12-10. A. Demonstration of hepatobiliary excretion (arrows) of Tc-99m GH in a renal transplant patient. **B.** Note the absence of liver excretion on the renogram study with I-131 *ortho*-iodohippurate.

Table 12-2 compares some properties of Tc-99m GH with Tc-99m DMSA and Tc-99m DTPA.

Tc-99m GH Use. Insufficient information is available to determine the precise mechanism of the intrarenal handling of Tc-99m GH. During early imaging times, within 5 minutes after injection, the renal collecting system is well demonstrated with Tc-99m GH, similar to Tc-99m DTPA.[16] It is therefore useful in such conditions as obstructive uropathy and hydronephrosis. The urinary excretion of these two agents during the first 2 to 3 hours is similar, but the excretion of glucoheptonate is less after 3 hours. These data suggest that some glomerular filtration of Tc-99m GH occurs, which can be expected because it is not as highly protein bound as is Tc-99m DMSA. At later times renal parenchymal accumulation occurs, which permits visualization of focal cortical lesions after the activity in the collecting system has cleared into the bladder. Tc-99m GH is a compromise agent between Tc-99m DTPA and Tc-99m DMSA and is probably the Tc-99m agent of choice in the detection of acute tubular necrosis (ATN).[30]

Radiation Dose. The critical organ for Tc-99m GH is the bladder wall because a large portion of the injected dose rapidly accumulates in the urine. The radiation dose is 0.8 rad/mCi, assuming a 4-hour voiding interval.[16] The kidney and cortical dose is less than that of Tc-99m DMSA but more than that of Tc-99m DTPA, being 0.17 rad/mCi for a whole-kidney dose and 0.20 rad/mCi for the renal cortices.[16]

ALTERED BIODISTRIBUTION OF RENAL RADIOPHARMACEUTICALS

The measurement of renal function with Tc-99m DTPA and I-131 Hippuran in patients treated with cyclosporin A, an immunosuppressive agent with known nephrotoxicity, reveals that the renal excretion pattern for these tracers mimics that seen in ATN or rejection.[54] The finding suggests that the differentiation of ischemic ATN and rejection from cyclosporin A nephrotoxicity will be difficult in renal transplant recipients treated with cyclosporin A. Iodinated contrast material has also been shown to significantly decrease ERPF measurements, with I-131 Hippuran requiring 2 weeks for a return to baseline renal function. Drugs that are toxic to the kidney or exert a pharmacologic effect on the kidney can potentially alter renal function and the biodistribution of renal imaging agents. Other drugs that have been implicated in altered renal imaging include phenacetin, a nephrotoxin in large doses, and diuretic agents, notably furosemide. In one study comparing the usefulness of radionuclide renal function studies for evaluation of renal transplant patients, investigators noted instances of acute rejection that were not identified because of interference from the administration of high doses of furosemide.[55,56] Furosemide has been used purposefully as a pharmacologic intervention in Tc-DTPA renal nuclear medicine, primarily in differentiating functional from mechanical hydronephrosis.[57] With conventional radionuclide renography, most dilated upper urinary tract systems demonstrate a progressively increasing concentration of radioactivity to a plateau value followed by prolonged retention. After furosemide administration, however, dilated, nonobstructed systems demonstrate increased urine flow after diuresis that is observed as a decline or washout of activity from the kidney. In significantly obstructed systems, there is a failure of tracer activity to decrease in response to diuresis.

As noted previously, kidney disease or severely decreased kidney function can cause maldistribution of renal radiopharmaceuticals. This may be seen as increased retention of blood pool activity after injection or by evidence of liver excretion.

Clinical Evaluation of the Kidney and Genitourinary Systems

INTRODUCTION

The kidney has long been the object of investigation with radiopharmaceuticals. Mercurials were some of the earliest agents to see widespread use. The earliest renograms were done with probe systems connected to rotating drums with graph paper upon which time–activity curves were transcribed. Special chairs were available to make positioning of the probes easier. Much valuable information was obtained about renal function using these systems; however, because there was no visual means of identifying the renal cortex and collecting system, the time–activity curves of these parts were unavoidably integrated and recorded on the rotating drum graph paper. In time these probe systems were replaced because of the inability to distinguish renal cortical function from the collecting system. They were replaced by image-processing computers that allowed the operator to select the region of interest from which the time–activity curve was to be constructed.

RATIONALE

Renal nuclear medicine studies primarily provide information about kidney perfusion, cortical integrity, and function of the collecting system. When function is expected to be abnormal, the renal nuclear medicine study is particularly useful in showing differences in the function of one side versus the other. In some renal nuclear medicine procedures both functional and anatomic information is obtained. Most of these procedures provide information that is unique in that it either cannot be obtained or is very difficult to obtain by other techniques.

Indications for renal nuclear medicine studies include acute renal failure, agenesis, autonephrectomy, congenital anomalies, decreased function, differential perfusion–function, ectopic kidney, extrinsic mass, hypertension, infarction, infection, mass lesion, obstruction, overall function, postoperative perfusion, renal failure, residual urine, size, thrombosis, toxicity, transplant rejection, trauma, and ureteral reflux. Some of these indications require that only one procedure be done; however, most of them require a multiprocedural approach that is dictated by an understanding of the pathophysiology of the disease process. Probably more than any other nuclear medicine procedure, renal studies are tailored to the clinical indication and patient condition. Not only should a proper sequence of procedures be chosen, but there must also be an appropriate choice of the renal radiopharmaceutical. Sometimes more than one renal radiopharmaceutical must be used to answer the clinical questions.

PROCEDURES

Perfusion studies allow observation of gross and differential blood flow. Perfusion studies usually are composed of a sequence of 5- to 10-second exposure images beginning immediately after IV injection of the tracer material (Fig. 12–11). The series of images is obtained for 1 to 2 minutes depending on the radiopharmaceutical used. Usually the aorta and iliac arteries are well seen during the earlier phases of the study. Oftentimes an inferior vena cava phase can be seen also. It is unusual to see the renal artery itself except in an occasional renal transplant patient where the renal artery is

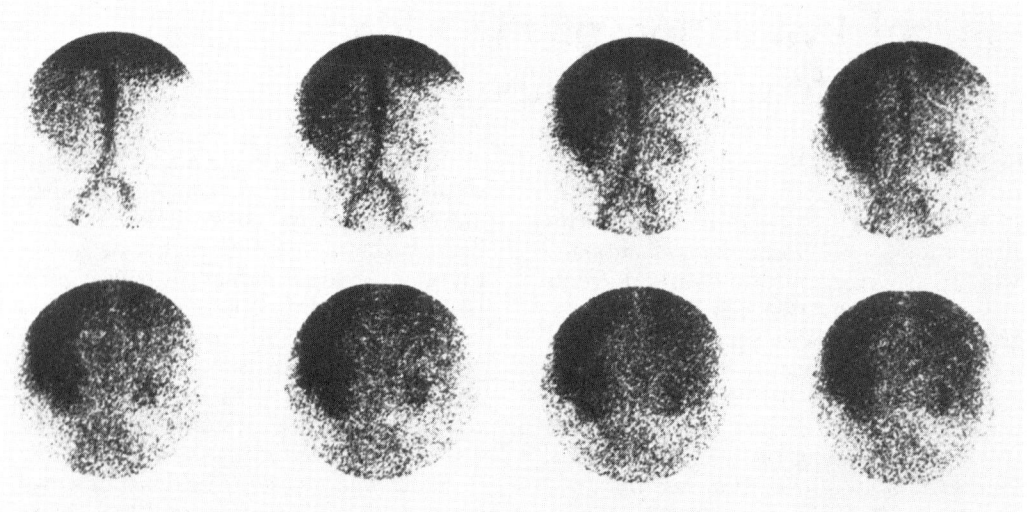

Figure 12-11. Posterior kidney perfusion study recording images at 5-second intervals after IV injection of 10 mCi of Tc-99m DTPA. Early images demonstrate activity in the abdominal aorta and iliac arteries. There is decreased blood flow to a small right kidney because of renal artery stenosis.

close enough to the gamma camera to be resolved. Perfusion studies are indicators of gross blood flow and are not intended to be used for measuring small differences in flow. No patient preparation is necessary for these studies, which is fortunate because many of these studies are done under semiemergency conditions.

Scans are similar to perfusion studies in that they are composed of a series of timed exposures. The difference is that the timed exposures are of longer duration, usually 1 to 5 minutes, and are obtained for a greater period of time, usually for 20 minutes to an hour (Fig. 12-12). Whereas the perfusion study looked at gross blood flow to the kidney, the scan is performed to examine cortical function and function of the collecting system. In this sense a scan is similar to an IV pyelogram, though it lacks the fine anatomic detail of the latter. Scans are best performed with some attention to the hydration status of the patient and sometimes to the position, i.e., upright versus supine or prone, that will best demonstrate the abnormality.

Renograms are functional studies that are acquired into computers. The renogram scan sequence of images is used to define the regions of interest for the generation of time–activity curves (Figs. 12-13 and 12-14). Much flexibility can be used in assignment of the regions of interest to parts or all of the cortex and segments of the collecting system. Body tissue background may be subtracted from the time–activity curves thus generated from the renal cortex to compensate for the diminishing vascular and extravascular activity of the renal radiopharmaceutical and thereby render a more accurate indication of renal cortical function. Renograms require attention to the hydration status of the patient. In most instances it is best to have the patient ingest fluids for an hour and empty the bladder immediately before starting the study. A variation on this procedure is called the *diuretic renogram* (Fig. 12-15) during which a rapidly acting diuretic such as furosemide is given halfway through the study and the effect observed in the time–activity curves and image sequence.

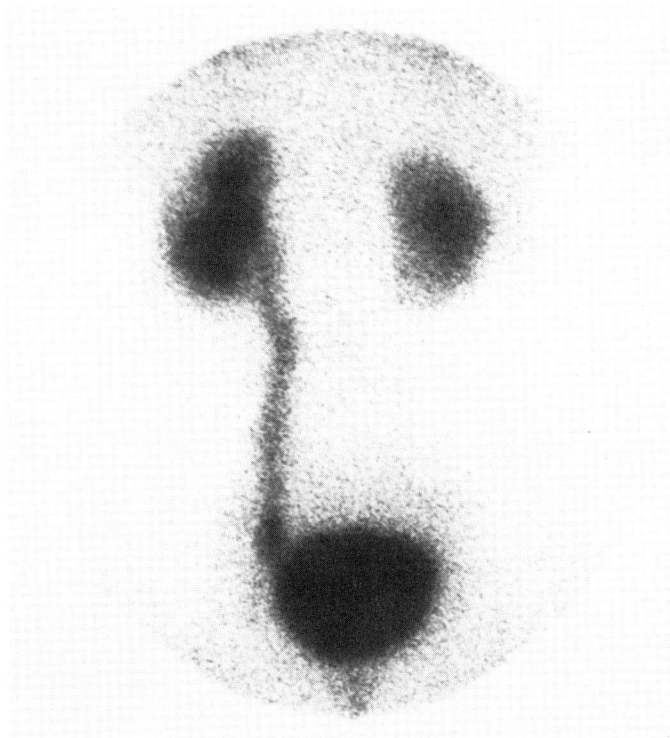

Figure 12-12. Posterior renal scan of the kidneys and urinary bladder 1 hour after the injection of 10 mCi of Tc-99m glucoheptonate. Earlier images at 5, 10, 15, and 20 minutes are not shown. The scan demonstrates left hydronephrosis and hydroureter. The right kidney function is normal. The patient has grade III transitional cell carcinoma of the bladder.

Quantitative renal nuclear medicine studies are performed to measure either differential perfusion–function, effective renal plasma flow, or residual urine. In the *differential perfusion–function* study a renal radiopharmaceutical is chosen that is slowly extracted from the blood stream by the kidney. The images are generally obtained 6 hours after injection to maximize the target-to-background ratio and to avoid interference from collecting system activity. Images are acquired into a computer in order that the counts obtained from each kidney may be used to calculate the percentage of blood flow each kidney receives of total renal perfusion or the percentage of function each kidney provides of total renal function (Fig. 12-16).

Most programs for measurement of *effective renal plasma flow* are highly complicated because they involve multicompartmental analysis. These programs require absolutely punctilious attention to detail in their performance. Careful attention to the radiochemical purity of the pharmaceutical administered, imaging geometry, timing of blood samples, counting geometry, and collection of completely voided urine samples is mandatory for meaningful results. The reader is referred to the documentation accompanying the ERPF program for particulars in regard to the exact procedure to follow because each of these algorithms is different. The reader is recommended to refer to the method published by Dubovsky and Russell.[24]

Residual bladder urine quantitation may be obtained in the latter phases of any procedure involving the use of one of the more rapidly cleared renal radiopharmaceuticals. The correct time for starting this procedure is after most of the tracer material has been cleared by the kidney and is resting in the partially filled bladder. A gamma camera image is acquired into a computer in a prevoiding state and in an

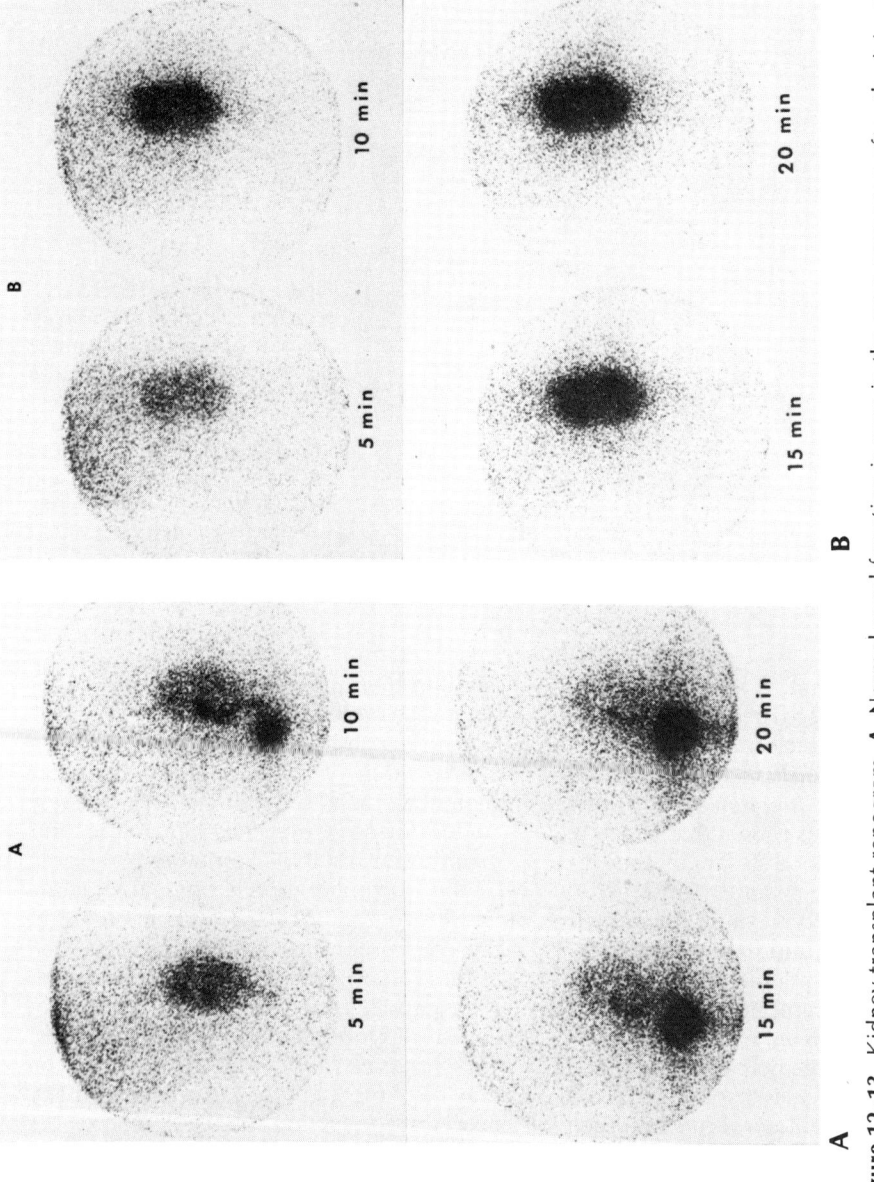

Figure 12-13. Kidney transplant renogram. **A.** Normal renal function is seen in the scan sequence after the injection of 50 μCi of I-131 Hippuran. Cortical activity is seen at 5 minutes, with tracer appearance in the pelvis and bladder by 10 minutes. The renogram curve shown in Figure 12-14A demonstrates a time-to-peak renal activity of 4 minutes with 60 to 65 percent tracer clearance by 20 minutes. **B.** Depressed renal function is found in the same patient 11 days later. No evidence of tracer clearance from the kidney is seen in the images, and the renogram curve (Fig. 12-14B) is consistent with graft rejection or obstruction.

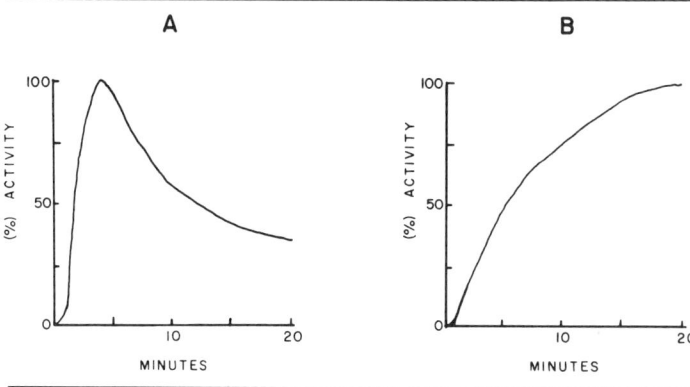

Figure 12-14. **A.** Normal renogram curve. **B.** Renogram curve demonstrating rejection or obstruction.

immediately postvoiding state. The amount of voided urine is measured, and a ratio is made of the product of postvoiding counts and voided volume of urine divided by the previoiding counts of the collecting system minus the postvoiding counts to yield the postvoiding residual urine volume.* It should be pointed out that the latter procedure is noninvasive and thus avoids the possibility of introducing infection, which might occur if the patient were catheterized to obtain the same information.

The *glomerular filtration rate* may be accurately determined with renal radiopharmaceuticals. I-125 iothalamate is the most accurate and probably the most foolproof method for measuring the GFR. It involves multiple plasma and urine samples. Other methods have evolved using chelated radiotracer materials in an effort to estimate the differential GFR. These latter methods assume that plasma clearance can be estimated from the precordial time activity curve and require only one blood sample for plasma concentration. The accuracy of the determination will depend on the source of the DTPA preparation. The reader is referred to the methods described by Piepsz et al[58,59] and Gates.[60]

Reflux may be determined with a procedure very much like the contrast voiding cystourethrogram wherein the patient is catheterized and a small amount (less than 1 mCi) of Tc-99m pertechnetate is instilled into the bladder. This is followed by filling of the bladder with sterile normal saline at a pressure of 30 inches of water. The infused volume is noted concurrently with evidence of ureteral reflux during the bladder instillation phase; however, most commonly, ureteral reflux occurs during micturition when bladder pressures are highest (Fig. 12-17). Though this is primarily a qualitative study, the volume of refluxed urine and the residual urine may be calculated if the patient can cooperate.

PHARMACEUTICALS

It is useful to arrange the four major renal nuclear medicine pharmaceutical agents in order of their overall clearance rate by the kidney after injection. Discussion of their clearance rates and mechanisms is found elsewhere in this chapter. For clinical purposes the order of overall clearance of radiopharmaceuticals by the kidney is as follows (fastest to slowest): OIH, DTPA, GH, and DMSA. This albeit gross means of comparing these greatly different pharmaceutical compounds is useful in the decision-making process for tailoring a clinical study. For instance, renograms are usually performed with OIH or DPTA, whereas

---

* Residual bladder urine volume
$$= \frac{\text{Postvoiding counts} \times \text{voided urine volume}}{\text{Previoiding counts} - \text{postvoiding counts}}$$

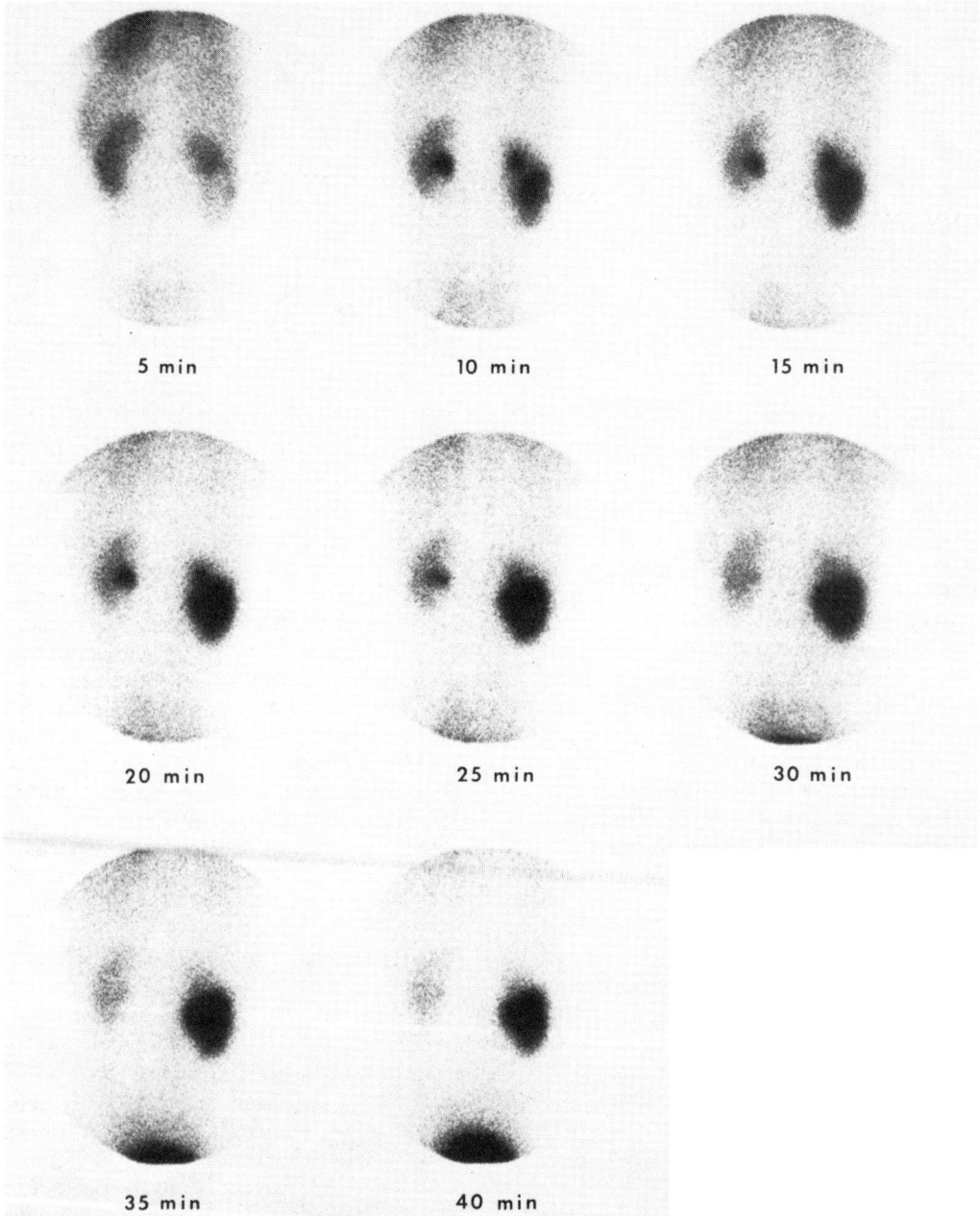

Figure 12-15. A. Diuretic renogram after an IV injection of 3 mCi of Tc-99m DTPA. The sequence of posterior images demonstrates cortical activity on the 5-minute image followed by the presence of activity in the collecting system seen on the 10-minute image. The left kidney shows normal function. The right kidney has a duplicated collecting system with normal function in the upper pole and obstruction in the lower pole evidenced by a lack of tracer washout after 10 mg of IV furosemide given 25 minutes into the study.

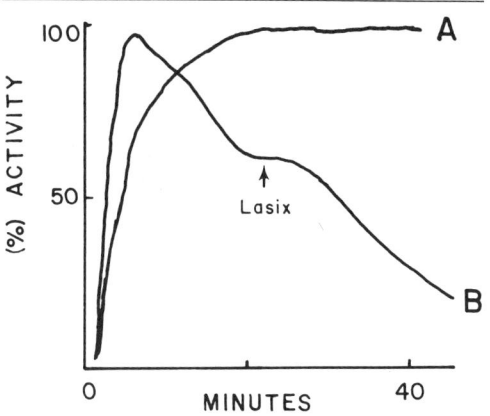

Figure 12-15. B. Renogram plot of kidney activity of Figure 12-15A demonstrating retention of activity in the lower pole of the right kidney (A) and normal time-to-peak and washout of tracer activity in the upper pole of the right kidney (B).

DMSA and GH are more often used for cortical detail or differential function. The collecting system will be evaluated best using DTPA or OIH because of their more rapid clearance. The definitive renogram in effective renal plasma flow studies requires the use of OIH. Of note should be that the last three are Tc-99m-labeled agents and will have a greater photon flux than I-131-labeled OIH. Gross blood perfusion may be best evaluated with DTPA or GH because there is good photon flux from the Tc-99m while minimizing radiation dosimetry.

INTERPRETATION

Perfusion studies give an indication of good gross renal perfusion when the kidneys are visualized simultaneously with the aorta or iliac arteries. This procedure is often needed after abdominal aortic aneurysm repair when there is sudden renal shutdown, after renal transplantation, and after transluminal renal artery angioplastic proce-

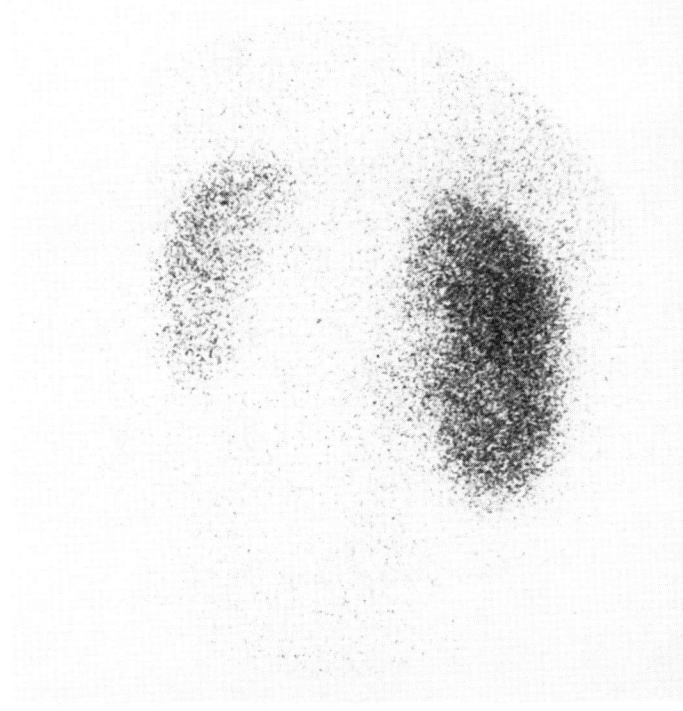

Figure 12-16. Renal scan to evaluate differential kidney function. Images are obtained after an injection of 5 mCi of Tc-99m DMSA. Computer analysis of the images shows a 68 percent uptake in the right kidney and a 32 percent uptake in the left kidney.

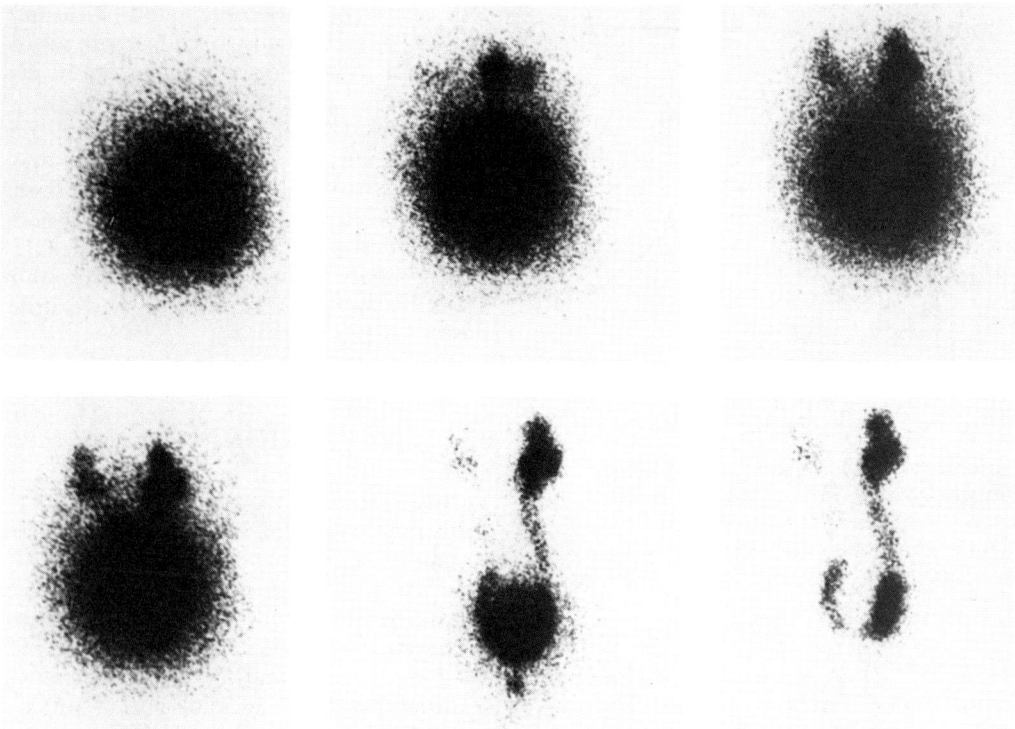

Figure 12-17. Reflux in the ureters and kidney pelves after instillation of 1 mCi of Tc-99m sodium pertechnetate and 25 ml of saline into the bladder. **A.** Bladder filling. **B.** Reflux on right. **C.** Reflux on left. **D.** Catheter removed. **E, F.** Voiding.

dures. One important difference between the two recommended radiopharmaceuticals is that the unwary may be fooled into thinking bilateral renal perfusion is intact when actually the object visualized on the patient's left is the spleen when GH is used. This does not present such a problem with DTPA.

The scan sequence of images gives information about the phases of the kidney cortical and collecting system function. Late imaging obtained with DMSA yields information about cortical anatomic features (Figs. 2–18 and 2–19), renal size, and gross differences in functioning renal mass. Additionally, some information may be obtained about perinephric structures impinging on the renal contour. Ectopic kidney may be positively confirmed using renal scan agents, particularly those with slower clearance rates. Renal failure, e.g., to resolve the question of recoverable or residual renal function versus end-stage renal disease, may be assessed with any of these radiopharmaceuticals; however, the most reliable method uses I-131 OIH with images obtained at 30 minutes, 4 hours, and 24 hours after injection. The complete absence of renal visualization generally indicates end-stage renal disease.

The renogram continues to serve an essential purpose in providing semiquantitative functional and comparative information about cortical function and the status of the collecting system. Water loading or the quicker diuretic renogram may be used to differentiate between functional and mechanical obstruction of the collecting system.

Quantitative studies may be used to

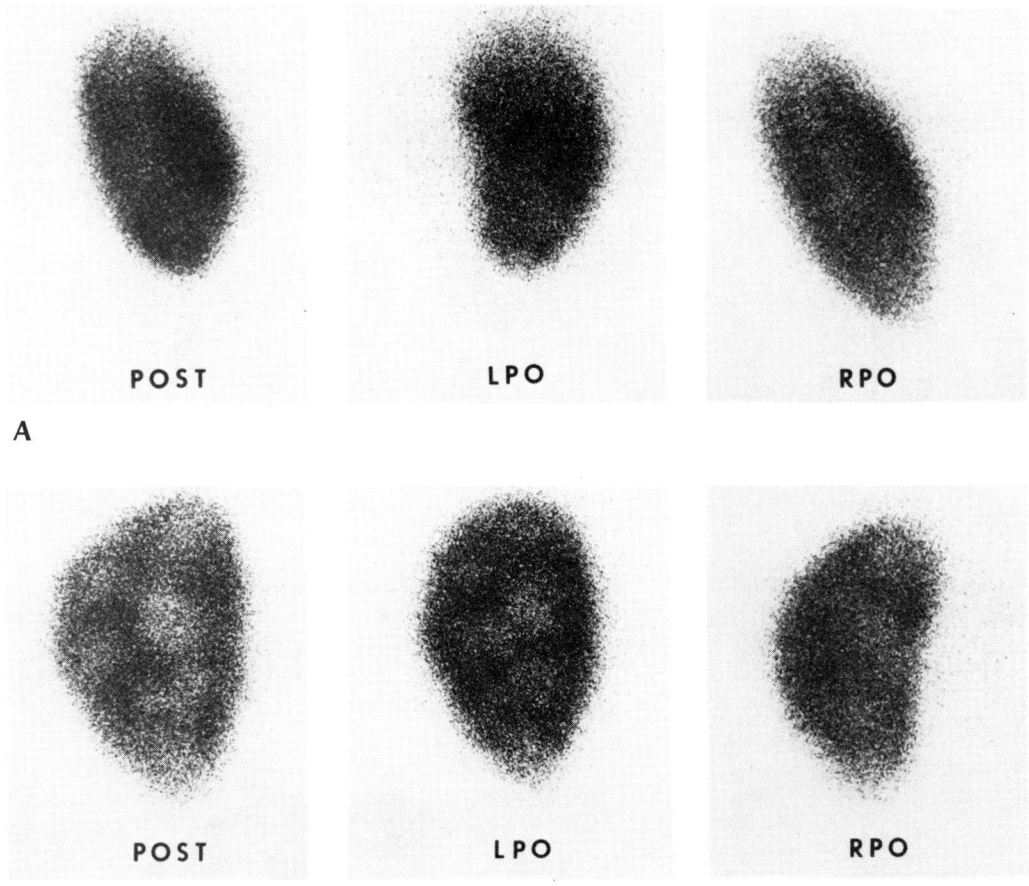

Figure 12-18. Normal renal scan of the right (**A**) and left (**B**) kidneys obtained 7 hours after an IV injection of 5 mCi of Tc-99m DMSA. Note the high concentration in the cortical areas that extend, via the cortical columns of Bertin, into the "colder" medulla (RPO left kidney view).

provide information about differential blood flow and renal function. DMSA is the best agent for this purpose with images obtained in the anterior and posterior projections at 6 hours after injection of the tracer material. Counts from the background-subtracted kidneys are used from the anterior and posterior projections to calculate the geometric mean in order to compensate for differences in renal count attenuation caused by unilateral anatomic displacement of one kidney from the dorsal torso. This method may be used to estimate the differential blood flow to the kidneys if the renal sizes are approximately equal. It does not give a measure of total renal flow or function. To measure the total renal blood flow or function one needs to perform one of the ERPF procedures. Additional information obtained from the latter procedures varies, some including an excretory index and others including total and differential functioning renal mass. The method described for noninvasive quantitation of

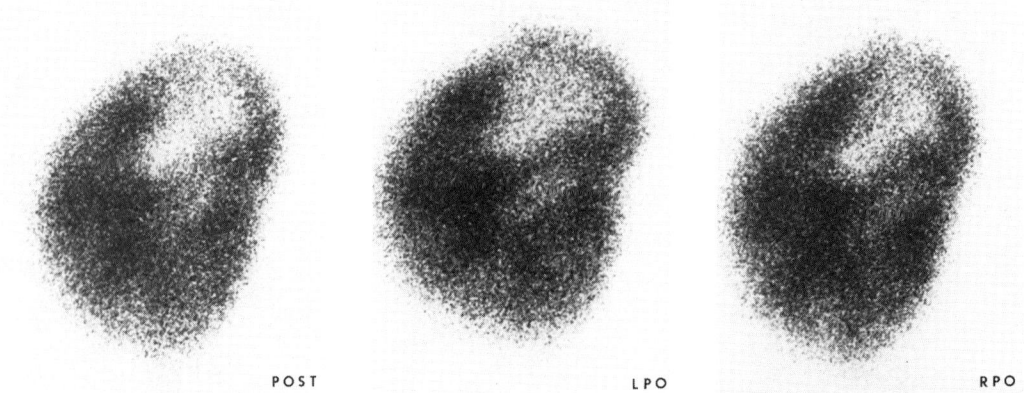

Figure 12-19. Renal scan obtained 4 hours after an injection of 5 mCi of Tc-99m DMSA demonstrating a mass lesion seen as a large photopenic area in the upper pole of the left kidney.

residual urine is vastly underused. The isotopic methods for calculation of the GFR are also underused, especially because the technique using I-125 iothalamate is known to be more accurate than the more commonly used creatinine clearance and the method using DTPA can provide a differential GFR as well.

The urinary reflux procedure has been used primarily in pediatric patients and

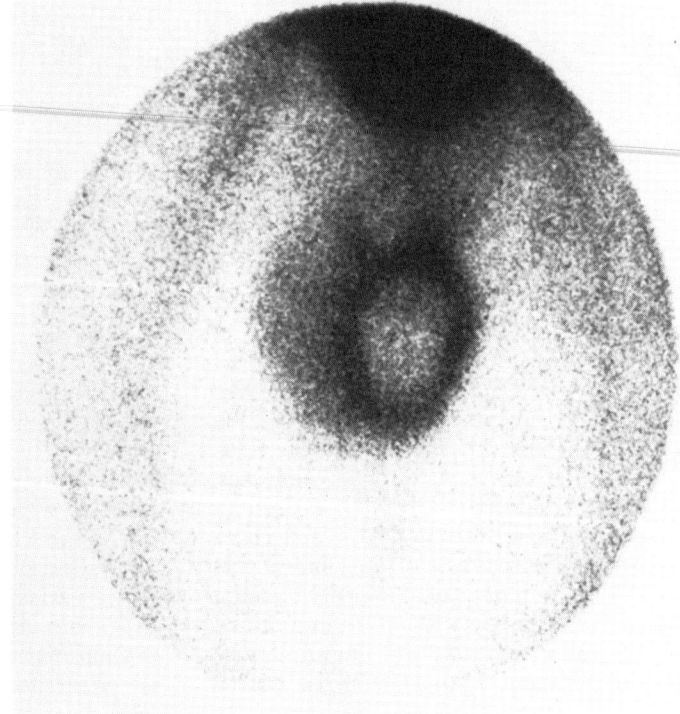

Figure 12-20. Missed torsion (infarct) of the left testicle observed 20 minutes after an IV injection of 10 mCi of Tc-99m sodium pertechnetate. Note the hyperemic halo about the nonperfused left testicle.

young adults to assess the cause of urinary tract infections. The procedure is noted to be at least as sensitive as the x-ray voiding cystourethrogram (VCUG) but with a gonadal radiation burden of only one fiftieth to one hundredth of the x-ray procedure. Even when a decision is made to do the x-ray procedure after the radionuclide reflux study, the radiation dosimetry to the child's gonads should be lower than when the VCUG has been performed first because information has already been obtained from the radionuclide procedure directing the uroradiologist to studying the anatomy on the diseased side. Certainly, interval follow-ups should be done with the radionuclide procedure because it provides both quantitative and qualitative information.

Scrotal imaging after the injection of Tc-99m pertechnetate has been very useful in distinguishing testicular torsion from missed torsion and epididymitis (Fig. 12–20). Perfusion (flow + blood pool) and delayed images are obtained with the scrotum elevated toward the surface of the gamma camera collimator for maximum anatomic resolution. The absence of perfusion suggests impending infarction (torsion) of a testicle. Patterns of increased Tc-99m pertechnetate concentration indicate missed torsion if circumscribing the testicle or epididymitis if assymetrically distributed.

In summary, nuclear medicine procedures are often indicated in the workup of patients with kidney or genitourinary tract problems, especially when functional assessment is required. There is a never-ending need to provide continuing education information to clinicians in regard to what information renal nuclear medicine in particular can provide for their patient problem assessments.

REFERENCES

1. Gottschalk CW, Lassiter WE: Mechanisms of urine formation. In Mountcastle VB (ed): Medical Physiology, 14th ed. St. Louis, C. V. Mosby, 1980, Vol 2, p 1165
2. Nielson P, Rasmussen F: Relationships between molecular structure and excretion of drugs. Life Sciences 17:1495, 1975
3. McAfee JG, Subramanian G: Radioactive agents for imaging. In Freeman LM and Johnson PM (eds): Clinical Scintillation Imaging, 2nd ed. New York, Grune & Stratton, 1975, p 13
4. Goldstein A, Aronow L, Kalman SM: Principles of Drug Action. New York, Harper & Row, Pub, 1969
5. McAfee JG, Grossman ZD, Gagne G, et al: Comparison of renal extraction efficiencies for radioactive agents in the normal dog. J Nucl Med 22:333, 1981
6. Smith HB: The Kidney: Structure and Function in Health and Disease. New York, Oxford University, 1951, p 154
7. Wesson LG: Physiology of the Human Kidney. New York, Grune & Stratton, 1969
8. Chervu RL, Blaufox MD: Renal radiopharmaceuticals—An update. Semin Nucl Med 12:224, 1982
9. Taplin GV, Meredith OM Jr, Kade H, et al: The radioisotope renogram. J Lab Clin Med 48:886, 1956
10. Tubis M, Posnick E, Nordyke RA: Preparation and use of I-131 labeled sodium iodohippurate in kidney function tests. Proc Soc Exp Biol Med 103:497, 1960
11. McAfee JG, Wagner HN Jr: Visualization of renal parenchyma: Scintiscanning with Hg-203 Neohydrin. Radiology 75:820, 1960
12. Harper PV, Lathrop KA, Hinn GM, et al: Technetium-99m Iron Complex. In Radioactive Pharmaceuticals. USAEC Symposium Series 6, April 1966, p 347
13. Eckelman W, Richards, P: Instant Tc-99m DTPA. J Nucl Med 11:761, 1970
14. Atkins HL, Cardinale KG, Eckelman WC, et al: Evaluation of Tc-99m DTPA prepared by three different methods. Radiology 98:674, 1971
15. Lin TH, Khentigen A, Winchell HS: A Tc-99m chelate substitute for organoradiomercurial renal agents. J Nucl Med 15:34, 1973
16. Arnold RW, Subramanian G, McAfee JG, et al: Comparison of Tc-99m complexes for renal imaging. J Nucl Med 16:357, 1975
17. Sigman EM, Elwood CM, Knox F: The measurement of glomerular filtration rate in man with sodium iothalamate I-131 (Conray). J Nucl Med 7:60, 1965
18. Elwood CM, Sigman EM: The measurement of glomerular filtration and effective renal plasma flow in man by iothalamate I-131 and iodopyracet I-131. Circulation 36:441, 1967
19. McAfee JG, Gagne G, Atkins HL, et al: Bi-

ological distribution and excretion of DTPA labeled with Tc-99m and In-111. J Nucl Med 20:1273, 1979
20. Radioisotope Production and Quality Control, Tech Reports Series No. 128. Vienna, IAEA, 1971, pp 861
21. Hotte CE, Ice RD: The in vitro stability of I-131 O-iodohippurate. J Nucl Med 20:441, 1979
22. Burbank MK, Tauxe WN, Maher FT, et al: Evaluation of radioiodinated Hippuran for the estimation of renal plasma flow. Proc Staff Mayo Clinic 36:372, 1961
23. Hine JG, Farmelant MH, Cardarelli JA, et al: Four channel magnetic tape recording and digital analysis of radiohippuran renal function tests in normal subjects. J Nucl Med 4:371, 1963
24. Dubovsky EV, Russell CD: Quantitation of renal function with glomerular and tubular agents. Semin Nucl Med 12:308, 1982
25. Maher FT, Tauxe WN: Renal clearance in man of pharmaceuticals containing radioactive iodine: Influence of plasma binding. JAMA 207:97, 1969
26. Riggs DS: Quantitative aspects of iodine metabolism in man. Pharmacol Rev 4:284, 1952
27. Magnusson G: Influence of varying amounts of I-131 in radiohippuran on the radioactivity measurements. Acta Med Scand (Suppl 378) pp 111–115, 1962
28. Bryan CW, Maher JF: Factors influencing renal excretion of O-iodohippurate. Am J Physiol 225:1220, 1973
29. Farmelant MH, Burrows BA: The renogram: physiologic basis and current clinical use. Semin Nucl Med 4:61, 1974
30. McAfee JG: A review of radiopharmaceuticals in nephrourology. In Joekes AM, Constable AR, Brown NJG, Tauxe WN (eds): Radionuclides in Nephrology. New York, Grune & Stratton, 1982, pp 3–9
31. Eliott AT, Britton KE, Brown NJG, et al: Dosimetry of current radiopharmaceuticals used in renal investigations. In Clutier RJ, Coffey JL, Snyder WS, Watson EE (eds): Radiopharmaceutical Dosimetry Symposium. HEW Publication (FDA) 76–8044, Washington, DC, 1976, pp 293–304
32. Griep RT, Nelp WB: Mechanism of excretion of radioiodinated sodium iothalamate. Radiology 93:807, 1969
33. McKusick KA, Malmud LS, Kirchner PT, et al: An interesting artifact in radionuclide imaging of the kidney. J Nucl Med 14:113, 1973

34. Srivastava SC, Meinken G, Smith TD, et al: Problems associated with stannous Tc-99m radiopharmaceuticals. Int J Appl Radiat Isot 28:83, 1977
35. Klopper JF, Hauser W, Atkins HL, et al: Evaluation of Tc-99m DTPA for the measurement of glomerular filtration rate. J Nucl Med 13:107, 1971
36. Russell CD, Bischoff PG, Kontzen FN, et al: Measurement of glomerular filtration rate: Single injection plasma clearance method without urine collection. J Nucl Med 26:1243, 1985
37. Carlsen JE, Moller ML, Lund JO, et al: Comparison of four commercial Tc-99m (Sn) DTPA preparations used for the measurement of glomerular filtration rate: Concise communication. J Nucl Med 21:126, 1980
38. Hauser W, Atkins HL, Nelson KG, et al: Technetium-99m DTPA: A new radiopharmaceutical for brain and kidney scanning. Radiology 94:679, 1970
39. Package Insert for DTPA Kit, Medi-Physics, Inc, December 1980
40. Welch MJ, Welch TJ: Solution chemistry of carrier-free indium. In Subramanian G, Rhodes BA, Cooper JF, Sodd VJ (eds): Radiopharmaceuticals. New York, Society of Nuclear Medicine, 1975, p 73
41. Ikeda I, Inoue O, Kurata K: Chemical and biological studies on Tc-99m DMS-II: Effect of Sn(II) on the formation of various Tc-DMS complexes. Int J Appl Radiat Isot 27:681, 1976
42. Ikeda I, Inoue O, Kurata K: Preparation of various Tc-99m dimercaptosuccinate complexes and their evaluation as radiotracers. J Nucl Med 18:1222, 1977
43. Kubiatowicz DO, Bolles TF, Nova JC, et al: Localization of low molecular weight Tc-99m labeled dimercaptodicarboxylic acids in kidney tissue. J Pharm Sci 68:621, 1979
44. Taylor A Jr, Lallone RL, Hogan PL: Optimal handling of dimercaptosuccinic acid for quantitative renal scanning. J Nucl Med 21:1190, 1980
45. Moretti JL, Rapin JR, LePoncin M, et al: Dimercaptosuccinic acid complexes: Their structure, biological behaviour and renal localization. In Joekes Am, Constable AR, Brown NJG, Tauxe WN (eds): Radionuclides in Nephrology. New York, Grune & Stratton, 1982, pp 25–31
46. Dewanjee MK: Binding of diagnostic radiopharmaceuticals to human serum albumin

by sequential and equilibrium dialysis. J Nucl Med 23:753, 1982
47. Enlander D, Weber PM, dos Remedios LV: Renal cortical imaging in 35 patients: Superior quality with Tc-99m DMSA. J Nucl Med 15:743, 1974
48. Hosokawa S, Kawamura J, Yoshida O: Basic studies on intrarenal localization of renal scanning agent Tc-99m DMSA. Acta Urol Jap 24:61, 1978
49. Ikeda I, Inoue O, Kurato K: Chemical and biological studies on Tc-99m DMS-I: Formation of complexes by four different methods. Int J Nucl Med Bio 4:56, 1977
50. Yee CA, Lee HB, Blaufox MD: Tc-99m DMSA renal uptake: Influence of biochemical and physiologic factors. J Nucl Med 22:1054, 1981
51. Vanlic-Razumenic N, Petrovic J: Biochemical studies of the renal radiopharmaceutical compound dimercaptosuccinate II. Subcellular localization of Tc-99m DMS complex in the rat kidney in vivo. Eur J Nucl Med 7:304, 1982
52. Steigman J, Chin EV, Solomon NA: Scintiphotos in rabbits made with Tc-99m preparations, reduced by electrolysis and by $SnCl_2$: Concise communication. J Nucl Med 20:766, 1979
53. de Kieviet W: Technetium radiopharmaceuticals: Chemical characterization and tissue distribution of Tc-glucoheptonate using Tc-99m and carrier Tc-99. J Nucl Med 22:703, 1981
54. Klintmalm GBG, Klingensmith WC III, Iwatsuki S, et al: Tc-99m DTPA and I-131 Hippuran findings in cyclosporin A nephrotoxicity in liver transplant recipients. J Nucl Med 22:P37, 1981
55. Clorius JH, Dreikorn K, Zelt J, et al: Renal graft evaluation with pertechnetate and I-131 Hippuran. A comparative clinical study. J Nucl Med 20:1029, 1979
56. Hladik WB III, Nigg KK, Rhodes BA: Drug-induced changes in the biologic distribution of radiopharmaceuticals. Semin Nucl Med 12:181, 1982
57. Thrall JH, Koff SA, Keyes JW Jr: Diuretic radionuclide renography and scintigraphy in the differential diagnosis of hydroureteronephrosis. Semin Nucl Med 11:89, 1981
58. Peipsz A, Dobbeleir A, Erbsman F: Measurement of separate kidney clearance by means of Tc-99m DTPA complex and a scintillation camera. Eur J Nucl Med 2:173, 1977
59. Piepsz A, Denis R, Ham HR, et al: A simple method for measuring separate glomerular filtration rate using a single injection of Tc-99m DTPA and the scintillation camera. J Pediatr 93:769, 1978
60. Gates GF: Glomerular filtration rate: Estimation from fractional renal accumulation of Tc-99m DTPA (stannous). Am J Roentgen 138:565, 1982

CHAPTER 13

Bone

The study of the evolution of humans on Earth from their primordial past to the present has been made possible through radioisotopic analysis of bones and artifacts. The prolonged preservation of human skeletal remains in the earth connotes an inert quality of bone. Living bone, however, is a dynamic and physiologically active organ.

Bone is composed of minute crystals of hydroxyapatite (HA) associated with collagen fibers. The crystals are continually being produced and reabsorbed. Because of the small size of bone crystals, the surface area of bone mineral is quite large. The composition of bone mineral is mainly calcium, phosphate, and hydroxyl ions. The presence of these ions on the large adsorptive surface of bone creates a chemically reactive site for many radionuclidic substances. This provides a means to study bone physiology and to perform diagnostic bone imaging for the detection of radiographically occult lesions.

PHYSIOLOGIC ANATOMY OF BONE

Living bone consists of a variety of tissues as shown in Figure 13–1.[1] The outer layer, which imparts shape and strength, is called cortical bone. Internal to the cortical bone is a spongy cancellous bone. Cancellous bone contains the marrow, which is composed of fat and hematopoietic elements. The articulating surfaces are covered with a layer of cartilage. Tendons, ligaments, and muscle attachments are inserted into cortical bone. Blood vessels penetrate the cortex and permeate the cancellous bone. A fibrous and cellular envelope covers the bone tissue surfaces. This envelope is called the periosteum externally and endosteum internally and contains osteocytes, which are pluripotent in bone remodeling.

Bone Composition

Fresh compact bone is composed of water (9 percent), organic matrix (22 percent), and inorganic salts (69 percent).[1] The organic matrix consists of a noncollagenous or ground substance (10 percent) and collagen fibers (90 percent). The noncollagenous matrix consists of such substances as mucopolysaccharides, glycoproteins, phosphoproteins, phospholipids, etc., and has been assigned the role of mineralization nucleator and inhibitor as well as serving as a glue that occupies the space between collagen fibers. Little is known, however, about the precise distribution and function

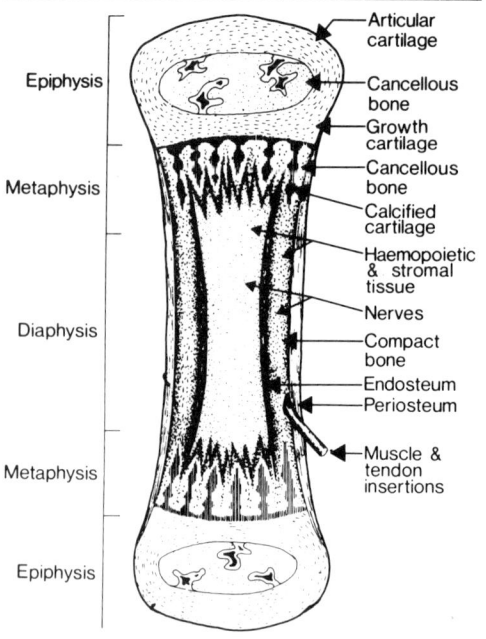

Figure 13-1. Diagrammatic representation of bone as an organ to show the tissues associated with bone tissue. *(From Triffitt JT, 1980, p 46, with permission.[1])*

of noncollagenous matrix in bone. Collagen fibers give bone its powerful tensile strength and provide nucleation centers for the deposition of inorganic salts. These salts are composed essentially of calcium and phosphate and give bone its compressional strength. The principal inorganic salts found in bone are amorphous calcium phosphate (ACP) and HA. ACP is believed to be the precursor to HA, which is the predominant crystalline form found in mature bone. Bone composition is summarized in Table 13–1.

Bone Formation

Osteocytes may function as osteoblasts or osteoclasts. Osteoclasts are instrumental in bone resorption. Osteoblasts are bone-forming cells that lie directly on bone surface. They are responsible for synthesizing the organic matrix, called osteoid, that occupies the space between the osteoblasts and the underlying calcified bone. Soon after the collagen fibers are formed by osteoblasts, ACP precipitates on their surfaces at periodic intervals to form minute nidi that rapidly multiply and grow over a period of days and weeks to form HA crystals. The ACP is not crystalline but is a mixture of hydrated calcium phosphates of varying Ca/P molar ratios consisting mainly of calcium monohydrogen phosphate ($CaHPO_4$, Ca/P = 1.0), octacalcium phosphate ($Ca_4H(PO_4)_3$, Ca/P = 1.33) and tricalcium phosphate ($Ca_3(PO_4)_2$, Ca/P = 1.5).[2] By a process of substitution and addition of atoms, or reabsorption (through osteoclastic activity) and reprecipitation, these ACP salts are converted into the well-crystallized HA ($Ca_{10}(OH)_2(PO_4)_6$, Ca/P = 1.66).

Well crystallized HA is found in mature bone areas such as cortical bone, as needle or rod-like crystallites that measure 200 to 600 Å in length (on the C-axis) and 25 to 75 Å in diameter or as plates 400 Å in length and width and about 50 Å in thickness.[3] The crystals grow most rapidly along the C-axis, and this growth is parallel to the long axes of the collagen fibers. A growing crystal may be likened to a sharpened pencil, with the C-axis represented by the pointed graphite center extending longitudinally.

It is not known precisely what causes calcium salts to deposit in osteoid, but at least two theories are suggested.[4] The first theory is as follows: It is known that osteoblast mitochondria can concentrate large quantities of calcium and phosphate into vesicles. The vesicles can then migrate to the cell wall and extrude minute calcium phosphate crystals onto the osteoid to serve as nucleation centers for HA crystal growth. Another theory is that the osteoblasts secrete a substance into the osteoid to neutralize an inhibitor substance (perhaps pyrophosphate) that normally prevents HA crystallization. Once the inhibitor has been neutralized, then the natural affinity of collagen

TABLE 13-1. BONE COMPOSITION

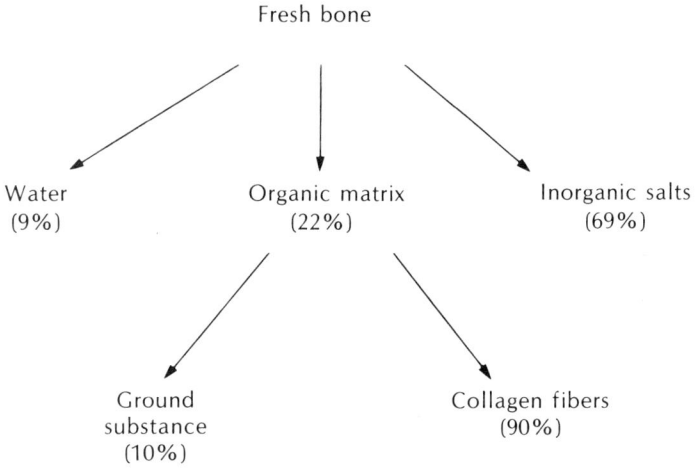

Role: Mineralization nucleator and inhibitor; glue for collagen fibers
 	
Principal substances:
  mucopolysaccharides
  glycoproteins
  phosphoproteins
  phospholipids
	Role: Provides tensile strength of bone and nucleation centers for deposition of inorganic salts of Ca^{2+} and PO_4^{3-}, which provide compressional strength
	
	Principal salts: ACP and HA

fibers for calcium salts supposedly causes the precipitation.

HA crystals are a very stable end product of bone mineralization and do not redissolve readily. Additionally, the crystals formed are microcrystalline in nature, that is, under physiologic conditions HA almost never forms crystals of dimensions greater than a few hundred angstroms in length, breadth, or thickness. Consequently, the HA system has a large surface area (200 m²/g) that provides an enormous opportunity for adsorption and surface exchange of a variety of ions. Indeed, prominent examples include Sr^{2+}, Pb^{2+}, Ra^{2+}, and Mg^{2+} for Ca^{2+}; F^- for OH^-; and CO_3^{2-}, citrate, phosphate esters, diphosphonates, and pyrophosphate for phosphate. It is precisely for this reason that radionuclide species of these substances have been used successfully to study and image the skeleton in humans.

DEVELOPMENT OF BONE-IMAGING AGENTS

The use of self-luminous radium paint on watch dials began in 1908 after an earlier discovery that alpha particles striking a zinc sulfide surface produced luminescence. Radium paint was made by mixing radium chloride and zinc sulfide with a binder. The first hint that radioactive material localized in bone became evident in 1924 when a radium dial painter developed severe osteonecrosis of the mandible and maxilla. Many reports followed this initial discovery of the so-called radium jaw, the cause being traced to isotope localization in bone after chronic inhalation of radon gas and ingestion of radium paint by "tip licking" of the paint brush. It was not uncommon for painters to put a fine point on the brush with their tongues.

Many radionuclides have been used to

study bone, but few of the earlier ones had physical properties desirable for skeletal imaging. The earliest use of bone-seeking radionuclides was for the treatment of bone diseases and metastatic lesions. They included P-32, Ca-45, Ca-47, Sr-89, and Ga-72. In fact, in 1949, Ga-72 was one of the first radionuclides used to detect metastasis to bone, but it was unacceptable because of an extremely high 2.5-MeV gamma.[5] Investigations were switched over to Ga-68 and finally Ga-67 in the early 1950s, but the serendipitous finding by Edwards and Hayes in 1969[6] that carrier-free gallium localized in soft-tissue tumors all but terminated its potential for becoming a bone-imaging agent. Bone localization of radioactive gallium required the coadministration of stable, carrier gallium, which was thought to be potentially toxic. The use of P-32 and Ca-45, being pure beta emitters, was of no value for external detection. Although Ca-47 was a gamma emitter, its 1.31-MeV energy was unwieldy for imaging equipment.

Around 1961, clinical bone scanning had its true beginning when Charkes and Sklaroff at the Einstein Medical Center in Philadelphia began to use Sr-85 bone scans to locate metastasis for rational radiotherapy.[7] Strontium was selected because its metabolism simulated that of calcium and the gamma emission of Sr-85 could be measured by external detection. Additionally, bone metastasis could be detected with Sr-85 before it was evident on x-ray exam. In fact, one report in 1961 found that radiographic changes were demonstrated in only 56 percent of breast cancer patients who had shown abnormal vertebral uptake of Sr-85.[8] Early support for this finding was their quote of a French study in 1948 reporting that a bone lesion must be 30 to 50 percent decalcified to be visible on x-ray. In addition to their clinical work, Sklaroff and Charkes proselytized the idea through numerous publications and lectures that bone scanning was desirable and necessary in the diagnosis and therapy of certain diseases.

Sr-85 was available as nitrate or chloride salts and administered intravenously (IV). The long biologic and physical half-lives of Sr-85 limited the adult dose to 100 µCi, which resulted in prolonged scanning times and poor counting statistics. Although the rate of bone uptake was rapid (90 percent of the maximum in 1 hour), its slow excretion from the body required at least a 2-day delay before scanning to improve the bone-to-background ratio. In 1964 Meckelnburg studied another strontium isotope, Sr-87m citrate, obtained by milking the Y-87/Sr-87m generator.[9] One of the reasons for using Sr-87m was the need to find an agent potentially useful in children and in patients with nonmalignant disease. At the time such uses were hampered because of the high radiation dose of Sr-85 and the AEC restriction of Sr-85 use only in patients with proven malignant bone disease. The Meckelnburg study determined that because of the decay of Sr-87m by isomeric transition and 2.8-hour half-life, the patient radiation dose to bone was 1/160 of an equivalent amount of Sr-85. Although this was an important advance, Sr-87m had several disadvantages of its own, including a short shelf life because of the 80-hour Y-87 parent, the requirement for generator elution and sterilization procedures before use, and the high body background on scans. The 2.8-hour half-life necessitated doing bone scans before adequate blood and tissue clearance was achieved, which increased the potential for both false-positive and false-negative interpretation.

In 1962, Blau et al introduced F-18 as sodium fluoride for bone imaging.[10] Its annihilation radiation was similar in energy to Sr-85 gammas, its radiation bone dose and half-life was similar to Sr-87m, but most important its blood clearance was extremely rapid. These factors, coupled with a high affinity for bone, yielded bone scans with high bone-to-background ratios. Its physical and biologic properties meant that the bone scan could be repeated many times. A significant disadvantage from a logistic point of view was its 1.8-hour half-life requiring the user to be close to a nuclear reactor. In the latter 1960s and early 1970s when F-18 became commercially available, logistics was still a problem, but was solvable with improved transportation schedules from source to user; however, isotope cost was high. As F-18 was finally gaining clinical acceptance, however, the introduction of the new Tc-99m phosphate complexes brought F-18 use to a virtual halt.

The disadvantages posed by strontium and fluorine in bone scanning inspired the search for a better agent. In 1959 Fels et al[11] reported that P-32 polyphosphate localized in the mineral phase of bone to a greater extent than orthophosphate. Influenced by this report, Subramanian and McAfee successfully prepared and investigated in rabbits a complex of Tc-99m ($SnCl_2$ reduced) with sodium tripolyphosphate (STPP) in 1971 and obtained a bone scan.[12] It was one of the key contributions to the field of nuclear medicine because the desirable properties of Tc-99m could be used for studying bone. Their report indicated that Tc-99m STPP achieved a skeletal uptake 65 percent that of Sr-85 only 3 hours after injection. A few months later they reported on an improved agent using synthetic long-chain polyphosphate (46 phosphate moieties).[13] Other investigators also worked with polyphosphates, and a Harvard group had confirmed Subramanian's finding that the average chain length of 40 phosphate units produced the highest bone uptake.[14] The Harvard group only achieved a bone uptake of 25 percent of the injected dose, however, whereas Subramanian reported a 50 percent uptake. Something was awry. About this same time two studies comparing bone uptake as a function of phosphate chain length reported that bone uptake was inversely related to chain length. This was in direct contradiction to previous reports. Additionally, several other reports were published on the use of Tc-99m complexed to pyrophosphate (PPi), a two-unit phosphate chain with high bone uptake. The Harvard group reanalyzed their polyphosphate preparation as well as that of Subramanian to find a changed composition. They found appreciable amounts of ortho- and pyrophosphates present. Further analyses led to the conclusion that the desirable bone-localizing properties of the original long-chain polyphosphates were due to the presence of PPi either as an impurity or as a degradation product.

The introduction of a Tc-99m bone-imaging agent was a significant improvement over other agents. The formal introduction of Tc-99m PPi came in 1972 by Perez and co-workers in Paris, France.[15] PPi had high chemical purity as opposed to the inconsistent chemical purity of polyphosphates. Labeling yields with Tc-99m were higher too (greater than 90 percent), and its blood clearance was more rapid than polyphosphate.

Also in 1972 a different class of Tc-99m-labeled phosphorus compounds were introduced for bone imaging. These were the diphosphonates, organophosphorus compounds characterized by a phosphorus-to-carbon (P-C-P) bond as compared with the phosphorus-to-oxygen (P-O-P) bond of poly- and pyrophosphates. The diphosphonates had previously been found to inhibit dissolution of bone and crystal growth of HA in certain bone diseases. Other studies indicated that the P-C bond was more stable in vivo, not being broken down by phosphatases as were the pyrophosphates.

Three groups almost simultaneously reported on a Tc-99m diphosphonate named ethane-1, hydroxy-1, 1-diphosphonate (EHDP) for bone imaging.[16-18] The advantages claimed for EHDP compared with PPi were a slightly greater bone concentration (50 to 55 percent EHDP versus 45 to 50 percent PPi of the injected dose), an improved in vivo stability (although this was implied), and faster blood clearance, which was its primary advantage. The blood clearance, however, was still not as rapid as F-18, and a number of diphosphonate analogues were studied in an attempt to improve the clearance rate so as to shorten the time between injection and imaging.

In 1975 Subramanian et al introduced Tc-99m methylene diphosphonate (MDP) for skeletal imaging and compared it with EHDP, PPi, and polyphosphate.[19] Their study findings in humans indicated that the diphosphonates were cleared from the blood more rapidly than pyro- or polyphosphates, polyphosphates being the slowest and MDP the fastest. In fact, MDP clearance rates were equivalent to previously reported F-18 clearance data. The slowed blood clearance of poly- and pyrophosphates in part was attributed to their higher plasma protein binding and diffusion into red blood cells. The fraction of the remaining blood activity associated with red blood cells at 24 hours was 22 percent for polyphosphate, 60 percent for PPi, and negligible amounts for EHDP and MDP. Each agent produced excellent bone images, but high-quality images could, as a rule, be obtained 2 hours after IV administration with MDP, whereas 3 to 4 hours were often required for EHDP and 4 hours for pyro- and polyphosphates.

The newer Tc-99m complexes for bone imaging were developed with the goal of producing faster blood clearances to achieve higher bone-to-soft tissue ratios at earlier times after injection. An alternative to faster blood clearance is to increase the affinity of the bone agent for the mineral surface of bone. Investigations during the latter part of the 1970s and early 1980s have demonstrated that affinity for bone surface can be improved by altering the chemical substituents bound to the carbon atom of diphosphonates. In particular, the presence of a hydroxyl group appears to increase the bone uptake of diphosphonates because it provides the opportunity for tridentate binding to calcium on the growing surface of HA crystals.[20] Diphosphonates without the added hydroxyl group, such as MDP, can only undergo bidentate binding to bone. This prompted the development of hydroxymethylene diphosphonate (HMDP). Experimental work in animals has demonstrated that HMDP has a higher binding affinity for apatite crystals than EHDP or MDP.[21]

The structures of the various phosphate and diphosphonate ligands used to complex with Tc-99m for bone imaging are shown in Figure 13–2.

The primary Tc-99m agents used for bone imaging include complexes of PPi, etidronate (EHDP), medronate (MDP) and oxidronate (HMDP). Currently, Tc-99m PPi is almost exclusively used for myocardial infarct avid imaging and as a source of stannous ion for blood pool imaging. Its production and properties are discussed in Chapter 9, but it will be included here for comparison with the diphosphonates.

PRODUCTION AND PHYSICAL PROPERTIES OF Tc-99m BONE AGENTS

All of the Tc-99m bone agents are prepared by simply adding Tc-99m pertechnetate to a sterile kit containing a lyophilized mixture of stannous ion and the appropriate ligand shown in Figure 13–2. Kits are available from commercial pharmaceutical houses or can be prepared locally. Table 13–2 describes several bone kits.

After complexation with Tc-99m the product must be checked for the impurities Tc-99m pertechnetate and hydrolyzed–reduced colloid. This is easily accomplished using the standard saline and acetone (or methyl-ethyl ketone) thin-layer chromatography system previously described in Chapter 6. Formation of the colloidal impurity is favored if the tin content and the pH of the reaction mixture are too high. Liver uptake on clinical images has been observed when the colloidal impurity is significant. Although this is not a major problem with current bone kits, liver uptake was not uncommon when Tc-99m PPi was first introduced for bone imaging. The problem was corrected when the pH of the kit reaction mixture was maintained in the slightly acidic range (pH 4 to 6).

Other factors important to the clinical performance of a kit formulation include the proper ligand-to-tin ratio and the amount of bone agent injected, which affects tissue distribution and toxicity. Tofe and Francis[22] found that the optimum EHDP-to-stannous chloride weight ratio was between 5:1 and 50:1 based upon binding affinity to HA in vitro. Ratios at 12:1 and 50:1 gave the same biodistribution in

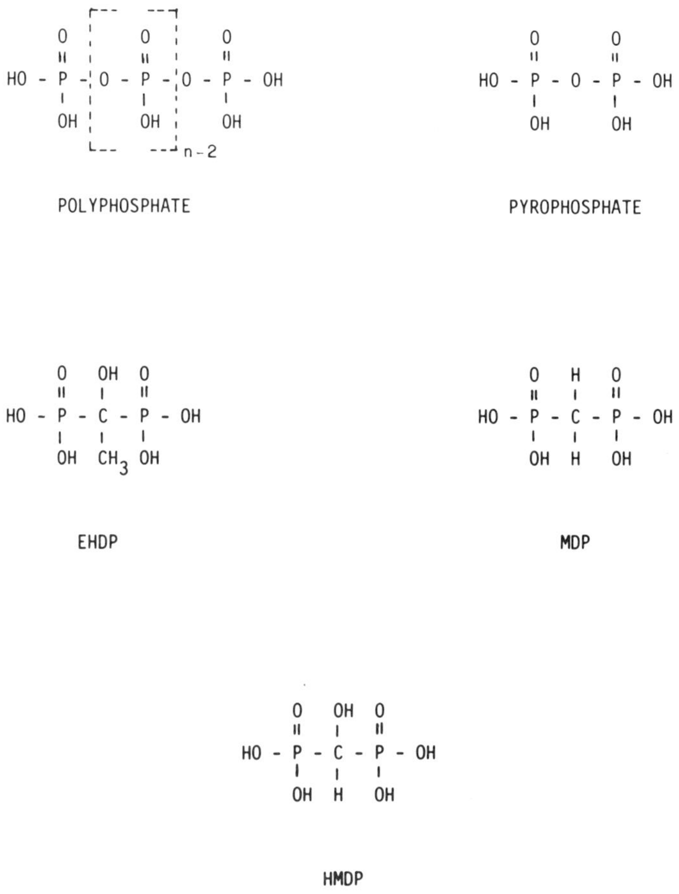

```
    O     O     O                         O       O
    ‖     ‖     ‖                         ‖       ‖
HO- P -O- P -O- P -OH                 HO- P - O - P -OH
    |     |     |                         |       |
    OH    OH    OH                        OH      OH
         └─ ─┘n-2

    POLYPHOSPHATE                         PYROPHOSPHATE


    O   OH  O                             O   H   O
    ‖   |   ‖                             ‖   |   ‖
HO- P - C - P -OH                     HO- P - C - P -OH
    |   |   |                             |   |   |
    OH  CH₃ OH                            OH  H   OH

       EHDP                                   MDP


                  O   OH  O
                  ‖   |   ‖
              HO- P - C - P -OH
                  |   |   |
                  OH  H   OH

                     HMDP
```

Figure 13-2. Chemical structures of ligands used to complex technetium for bone imaging.

animals. Subramanian et al[19] obtained optimal skeletal localization with MDP-to-tin ratios of 10:1 at doses between 0.01 and 0.5 mg MDP/kg body weight, with no significant difference in distribution. Bevan et al[23] found that the liver uptake of Tc-99m activity occurred when the Na_2HMDP load was above 0.1 mg/kg body weight in rats, guinea pigs, and dogs. These considerations were taken into account when formulating the HMDP kit for human use.

All of the Tc-99m bone complexes are fairly weak chelates and tend to degrade with time and produce pertechnetate impurity. This oxidative degradation is promoted by atmospheric and dissolved oxidants. It is also promoted by radiolytic decomposition reactions caused by radiation-induced free radicals. The latter problem is particularly significant when large amounts of radioactivity (200 to 300 mCi) are added to the bone kits. There are several ways to retard oxidation reactions in bone kits: increase the amount of stannous tin in the kit, remove oxygen from kits by nitrogen purging, or use antioxidants.

The effects of oxidative degradation in Tc-99m PPi kits before and after radiolabeling with Tc-99m has been reported.[24] Figure 13-3 and Table 13-3 illustrate that large quantities of Sn(II) are required to prevent oxidation of Tc-99m PPi; however, large amounts of Sn(II) in bone kits have been shown to interfere with the biodistri-

TABLE 13-2 KITS FOR PREPARING Tc-99m BONE-IMAGING AGENTS

Kit Manfacturer	Composition Component	Quantity		Maximum Tc-99m Activity	Expiration Time after Labeling	Kit Storage before Labeling	Kit Storage after Labeling
Pyrophosphate							
Mallinckrodt	$Na_4P_2O_7$	11.9 mg		100 mCi	6 hr	2–8°C	15–30°C
	$SnCl_2 \cdot 2\,H_2O$	3.2 mg	(min)				
		4.4 mg	(max)				
Dupont/NEN	$Na_4P_2O_7$	10.0 mg		200 mCi	6 hr	15–30°C	15–30°C
	$Na_3P_3O_9$	30.0 mg					
	$SnCl_2 \cdot 2\,H_2O$	0.95 mg	(min)				
		1.8 mg	(max)				
Squibb	$Na_4P_2O_7$	23.9 mg		75 mCi	6 hr	2–8°C	2–8°C
	SnF_2	0.4 mg	(min)				
		0.9 mg	(max)				
Medronate							
Mallinckrodt	Medronic acid	0.0 mg		200 mCi	6 hr	15–30°C	2–8°C
	$SnCl_2 \cdot 2\,H_2O$	0.8 mg	(min)				
		1.15 mg	(max)				
Dupont/NEN	Na_2 medronate	10.0 mg		300 mCi	6 hr	15–30°C	15–30°C
	$SnCl_2 \cdot 2\,H_2O$	0.5 mg	(min)				
		1.0 mg	(max)				
Squibb	Medronic acid	20.0 mg		150 mCi	6 hr	15–30°C	2–8°C
	SnF_2	0.33 mg					
	Ascorbic acid	1.0 mg					
Amersham	Na_2 medronate	15.6 mg		200 mCi	6 hr	2–25°C	15–25°C
	SnF_2	0.53 mg	(min)				
		0.93 mg	(max)				
Syncor	Medronic acid	10.0 mg		300 mCi	6 hr	15–30°C	15–30°C
	$SnCl_2 \cdot 2\,H_2O$	0.6 mg	(min)				
		1.1 mg	(max)				
Medi-Physics	Medronic acid	10.0 mg		—	6 hr	15–30°C	15–30°C
	$SnCl_2 \cdot 2\,H_2O$	0.17 mg	(min)				
		0.29 mg	(max)				
	Ascorbic acid	2.00 mg					
Oxidronate							
Mallinckrodt	Na_2 hydroxy medronate	2.0 mg		200 mCi	8 hr	15–30°C	15–30°C
	$SnCl_2$	0.16 mg					
	Gentisic acid	0.56 mg					

bution of pertechnetate during brain scans for up to 2 weeks after the administration of bone agents containing high levels of Sn(II).[25] Such clinical problems prompted the development of low-tin-containing bone kits, but this created a stability problem whereby Tc-99m complex degradation occurred over time with the production of free pertechnetate. Clinically the free pertechnetate manifests itself by visualization of the stomach and thyroid on bone images. Nitrogen gas purging of Tc-99m solutions and kits

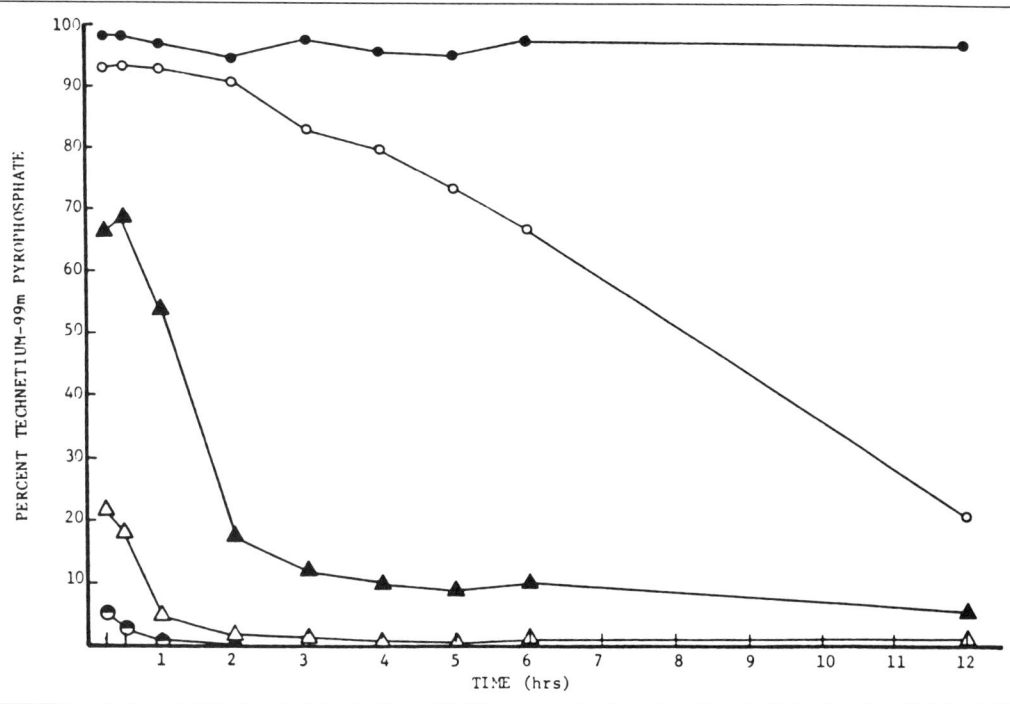

Figure 13-3. Effect of Sn: Tc molar ratio on the labeling efficiency and stability of Tc-99m PPi. Molar ratio legend: ◐, 10; △, 21; ▲, 52; ○, 209; ●, 2085. *(Data from Kowalsky RJ, et al, 1981, p 1722, with permission.[24])*

helps rid them of gaseous and dissolved oxygen, but it does not provide satisfactory protection against oxidation by radiation-induced free radicals as shown in Figure 13-4.

A significant solution to the problem of bone agent oxidation was created by the introduction of antioxidants in the kit formulation. Ascorbic acid[26] and gentisic acid[27] have been shown to be effective in maintaining the stability of low-tin Tc-99m diphosphonate preparations; however, only

TABLE 13-3. PERCENTAGE OF Tc-99m PERTECHNETATE IN SnPPi KITS CONTAINING VARIOUS AMOUNTS OF Sn(II) LABELED WITH 100 mCi Tc-99m

	Sn/Tc Molar Ratio (Sn(II) /Kit)				
Time (hr)	10 (5 μg)	20 (10 μg)	50 (25 μg)	200 (100 μg)	2000 (1000 μg)
0.25	94	78	33	6	2
1.00	99	95	42	7	2
3.00	100	98	87	13	2
6.00	100	99	90	31	3
12.00	100	100	95	79	3

(Data from Kowalsky RJ, et al, 1981, p 1722.[24])

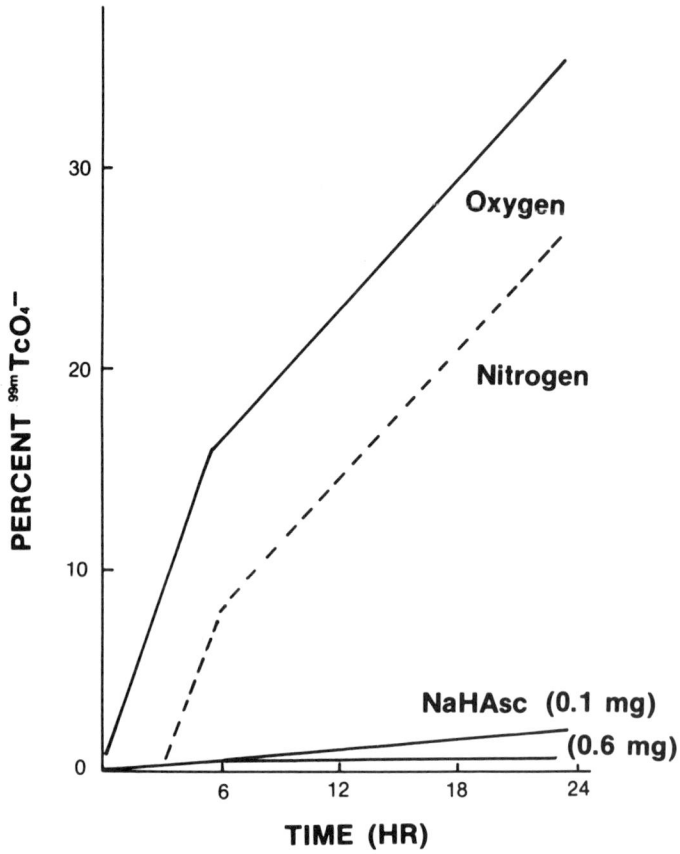

Figure 13-4. In vitro stability of Tc-99m Sn-HEDP without stabilizer (top two curves), with vials under an oxygen (air) and nitrogen atmosphere, and with stabilizer (0.1 mg and 0.6 mg sodium ascorbate, bottom two curves) under either an oxygen (air) or nitrogen atmosphere. (From Tofe AJ, et al, 1976, p 820, with permission.[26])

gentisic acid can be used in PPi kits. If ascorbic acid is used in PPi kits, it competes with PPi for reduced Tc-99m and forms a Tc-99m ascorbate complex that results in renal images.[28] The antioxidants act as free radical scavengers and produce their stabilizing effect by retarding the free radical reaction with the Tc-99m complex. Alkoxy (RO·) and peroxy (RO$_2$·) radicals can be stabilized by ascorbate through the transfer of an H atom from the ascorbate molecule to the free radical, yielding a resonance-stabilized and nonreactive molecule, RO$_2$H, according to Reaction 4-21 in Chapter 4. Elimination of the intermediate radical by the ascorbate (or gentisate) is believed to provide in vitro stability by inhibition of the slow oxidation of TcO$_2$ to TcO$_4^-$.[26]

CHEMICAL STRUCTURE OF Tc-99m COMPLEXES

Analytic work has been performed to identify the chemical structure of Tc-labeled phosphonate complexes.[29] The results indicate that Tc-99m diphosphonate (and presumably PPi, polyphosphate, etc.) are not single, well-defined, chemical species but are most probably mixtures of short- and long-chain polymers. The polymeric structure of $[Tc(OH)MDP^-]_n$ is characterized

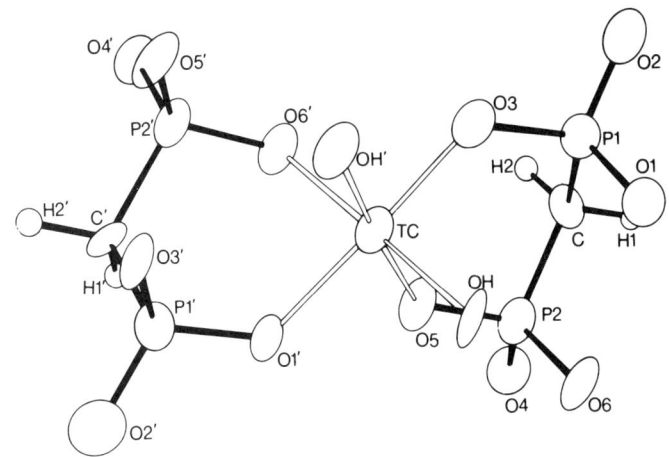

Figure 13-5. Perspective view of a portion of the [Tc(OH)(MDP)$^-$]$_n$ infinite polymer where MDP represents methylene diphosphonate in an unknown protonation state. Hydrogen atoms bonded to oxygen, lithium counterions, and waters of hydration have been omitted for clarity. (From Deutsch E, 1979, p 134, with permission.[29])

by technetium atoms bridged by MDP and OH ligands and MDP ligands in turn bridged by technetium atoms as shown in Figure 13-5.[29]

BIOLOGIC DISTRIBUTION AND COMPARISON OF BONE AGENTS

The biodistribution of Tc-99m bone agents has been compared in humans and animals.[19] After IV administration the agents are rapidly distributed in the body, and by 3 hours most of the activity is located in the blood, urine, and skeleton. The whole blood activity at this time is 8 percent for PPi, 5 percent for EHDP, and 3 percent for MDP. For PPi the blood activity is distributed between plasma protein (43 percent) and red blood cells (30 percent). The blood activity of the diphosphonates is primarily associated with protein, with no significant binding to red cells. Consequently, the blood clearance rates for EHDP and MDP are significantly faster than that of PPi. The most rapid rate is obtained with MDP as shown in Figure 13-6. The 3-hour urine accumulation in humans is 43 percent for PPi, 56 percent for EHDP, and 59 percent for MDP. The absolute average bone concentration of the diphosphonates has been shown to be 1.6 times higher than PPi in rabbits. No statistically significant difference is found between the bone concentration of EHDP and MDP.[19] In humans approximately 45 to 55 percent of the injected activity of EHDP or MDP localizes in bone within 3 hours.[14]

More recent comparisons have been made between the diphosphonates EHDP, MDP, and the newest agent HMDP. The blood clearance rate of HMDP is faster than EHDP and similar to MDP up to 3 hours after injection, but thereafter it is faster than MDP as shown in Figure 13-7.[23] In vitro and in vivo bone uptake experiments have demonstrated that HMDP has significantly higher bone affinity than EHDP and MDP.[30] Indirect whole body retention measurements made in humans demonstrate that HMDP has a 20 percent higher skeletal uptake than MDP.[31] Despite these differences, however, clinical comparisons between HMDP and EHDP[32] and MDP[33,34] have shown no significant difference in lesion detection between these agents. Scan quality of HMDP, as determined by bone-to-soft tissue ratio has been reported to be equivalent to or slightly better than EHDP.[32] Earlier comparisons made between MDP and PPi showed higher

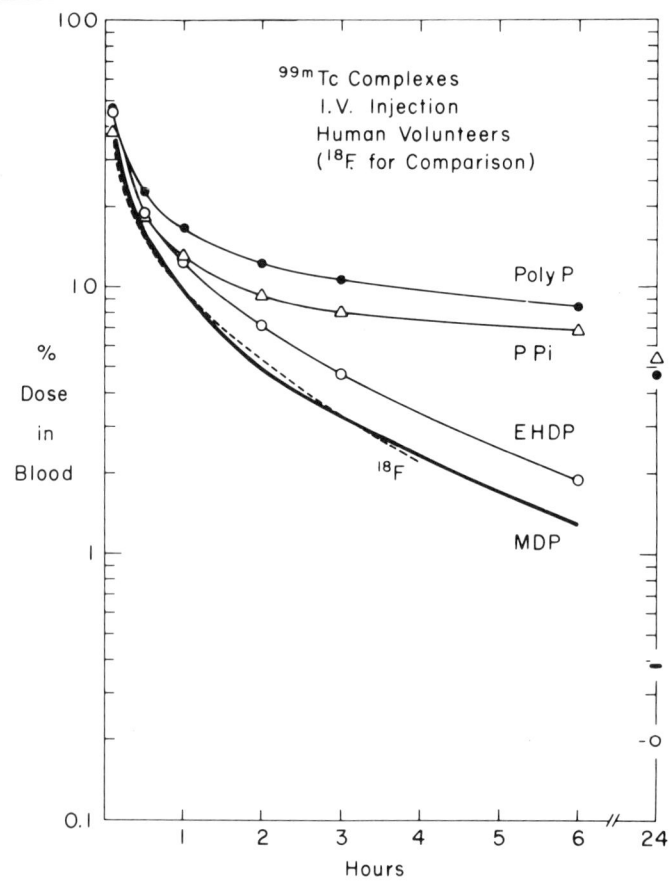

Figure 13-6. Blood clearance of MDP in humans compared with three other Tc-99m complexes and F-18 (corrected for physical decay). (From Subramanian G, et al, 1975, p 744, with permission.[19])

quality bone scans with MDP but no obvious difference in diagnostic sensitivity between the two agents.[35] In another comparison between MDP and EHDP there was no significant difference in lesion detection or scan quality although the lesion-to-normal bone ratio was higher with EHDP, indicating a higher uptake of EHDP in abnormal bone compared with normal bone.[36] This may be a function of its chemical structure and the surface of newly forming bone.

In summary, a series of Tc-99m bone agents have been developed since 1971. The first was STPP, then polyphosphate, followed by PPi, etidronate (EHDP), medronate (MDP) and finally oxidronate (HMDP). In general, each successive agent yielded improved scan quality because of a higher bone-to-soft tissue ratio. Although there was no significant difference in lesion detection with the last four agents, MDP and HMDP appear to be preferred because of their higher-quality, cleaner-looking bone images.

LOCALIZATION AND REACTION MECHANISMS OF BONE-IMAGING AGENTS

The effective detection of subtle abnormalities of bone, such as early metastatic lesions, by bone-seeking agents depends upon the stability of the Tc-99m ligand complex,

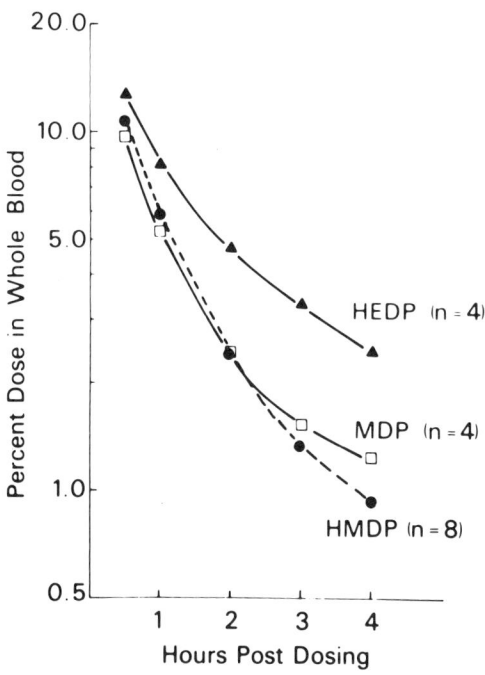

Figure 13-7. Blood clearance curves for Tc-99m HMDP, Tc-99m MDP, and Tc-99m HEDP in beagle dogs. (From Bevan J, et al, 1980, p 961, with permission.[23])

upon its ability to passively diffuse to the bone mineral surface, and upon the specific affinity of the ligand portion for the site of abnormal osseous metabolism.[30] Such an abnormal site is usually characterized by the deposition of amorphous calcium phosphate such as that found in embryonic and newly forming bone.[30]

The localization of a bone-imaging agent on bone surface depends, first, upon delivery of the agent to this site. This, in turn, is determined by such factors as having adequate blood supply and overcoming diffusional barriers between the blood and bone surfaces, which relates to the agent's ionic charge, molecular size, and binding to red cells and plasma proteins. Although bone uptake cannot occur without adequate blood flow to bone, vascularity alone does not account for the increased uptake of activity seen in bone lesions.[37] Of more interest, however, is understanding how bone agents interact and bind to bone, and factors important in this regard include the chemical composition of the bone surface as well as that of the bone-imaging agent itself.

The anion fluoride (F^-) reacts with bone by isomorphous exchange of fluoride for a hydroxyl group (OH^-) in HA. An additional fact that made F-18 a useful bone imaging agent was its high bone-to-background ratio resulting from its low protein binding (5 percent) and lack of red cell binding at physiologic pH.[38]

The Tc-labeled phosphate and phosphonate anionic complexes are believed to interact with bone by binding to Ca^{2+} ions in calcium HA crystals. Localization occurs primarily in the mineral phase of bone, with insignificant binding to the organic matrix of bone.[21] Appreciable adsorption can take place on free matrix provided that saturation with phosphonate is allowed to occur; however, in the absence of complete saturation, analogous with the usual imaging situation, Tc-99m diphosphonates bind exclusively to bone mineral.[21]

In vitro and in vivo experiments have shown that Tc-99m diphosphonate binds to ACP to a higher degree than to crystalline HA.[21,30] The exact reason for this is not known, but it forms the basis for detecting bone lesions because areas of increased osteogenic activity contain higher concentrations of ACP than normal mature bone. One hypothesis to explain why ACP binds bone agents to a higher degree than HA is that ACP contains newly forming apatite crystallites that have a crystal growing face with a chemical configuration of calcium ions best suited to bind to the oxygen atoms in the diphosphonate ligand.[21] As bone matures, this configuration is altered so that less uptake of bone agent occurs in mature bone.

The binding of Tc-99m complexes to bone also depends on the chemical structure of the ligand that complexes Tc-99m. The ligands EHDP, MDP, and HMDP are geminal diphosphonates, i.e., both phospho-

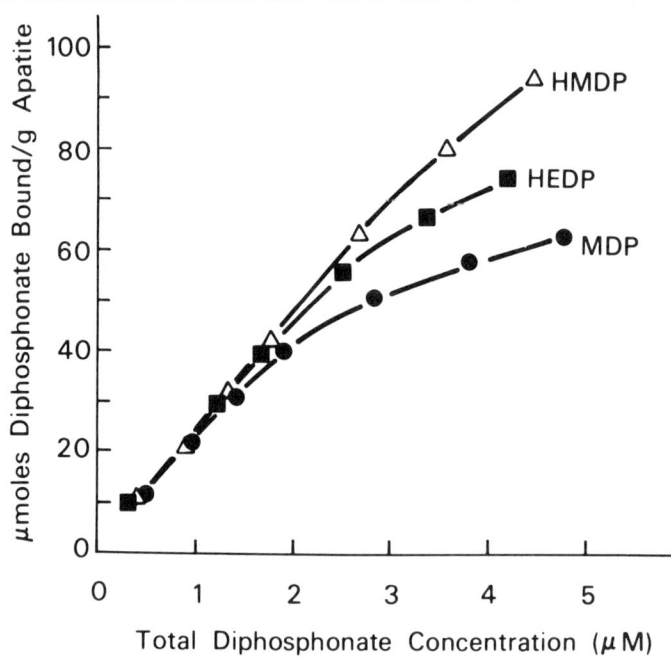

Figure 13-8. Adsorption of C-14 MDP, C-14 HEDP, and C-14 HMDP on crystalline HA. (From Francis MD, et al, 1979, p 609, with permission.[21])

nates are attached to the same carbon atom. This places the oxygen atoms on the phosphate groups at a distance and position conducive to binding with calcium in bone.[20] Additionally, the type of substitution at the two remaining sites on the central carbon atom can also influence the agent's binding to bone. Binding to calcium in bone is highest when one of these substituents is hydroxyl (OH) and the other is hydrogen (H) as in HMDP.[21] This is illustrated in Figure 13-8. The triangular face of the HMDP ligand allows an optimal tridentate binding of the ligand to the calcium atom in HA (through both geminal diphosphonate oxygens and the hydroxy group)[20] as shown in Figure 13-9. The same is theoretically true for EHDP; however, its binding to bone is less than HMDP perhaps because of stearic hindrance from the methyl group. The binding affinity for MDP is the lowest of these diphosphonate ligands because the hydroxy group is absent on the carbon atom and only bidentate binding to calcium is possible (through both geminal diphosphonate oxygens). One additonal factor that may contribute to the binding affinity of bone agents to bone is the relative solubilities of their calcium salts formed when they react at the bone surface. In this regard the decreasing order of solubility has been determined to be MDP > EHDP > HMDP $\geq$ PPi.[21]

RADIATION DOSE AND TOXICITY OF Tc-99m BONE AGENTS

Radiation dose estimates to selected organs for Tc-99m diphosphonates are listed in Table 13-4. The dose for the skeleton is an average adult dose that assumes uniform skeletal distribution; however, bone distribution is frequently nonuniform, having higher concentration in the vertebrae and ribs compared with long bones.[19] Additionally, bone activity has been shown to be two to three times higher in the epiphyseal region compared with the diaphysis in

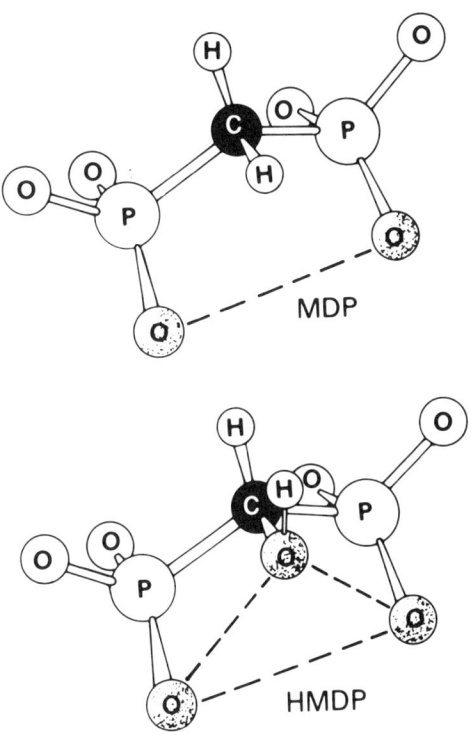

Figure 13-9. Comparison of HMDP and MDP structures. Phosphate oxygen atoms are shown unprotonated. Tridentate binding potential of hydroxylated molecules is emphasized in heavy print. *(From Bevan J, et al, 1980, p 961, with permission.[23])*

TABLE 13-4. RADIATION DOSE ESTIMATES FROM Tc-99m DIPHOSPHONATES

Organ	Radiation Dose (rad/15 mCi Administered)
Skeleton	0.53
Red marrow	0.42
Kidney	0.60
Bladder wall	
2-hr void	1.95
4.8-hr void	4.65
Ovaries	
4.8-hr void	0.26
Testes	
4.8-hr void	1.17

growing long bones of animals.[19] Clinically, this type of distribution is evident particularly in the pediatric patient where the growth plate has a much higher concentration than in the adult. The radiation dose to the pediatric growth plate may be six to eight times higher than in the adult skeleton.[39]

The critical organ for Tc-99m bone agents is the bladder wall because of the rapid urinary excretion. This radiation dose is reduced significantly if the radioactivity is administered with the bladder partially filled, if the patient is well hydrated, and if frequent voiding occurs. Generally, the radiation dose to all organs, except the bladder wall, is higher for Tc-99m PPi than for diphosphonates, chiefly because of the slower renal clearance of PPi.

No significant toxicity has been reported for Tc-99m bone agents at the dose normally administered. The usual dose range for Tc-99m PPi is 0.02 to 0.2 mg PPi/kg body weight and one fifth to half this dose for Tc-99m diphosphonate. The first level of toxicity is related to the complexing of bone agents with serum calcium. With PPi, tetany in rats is produced by 22 mg/kg and electrocardiographic (ECG) changes of hypocalcemia at 12 mg/kg IV doses.[40] If these doses are extrapolated to humans, the safety factor between a diagnostic injection and the lowest dose for minimally detectable hypocalcemia (by ECG) is 55.[19]

ALTERED BIODISTRIBUTION OF BONE-IMAGING AGENTS

Bone-imaging agents labeled with Tc-99m are relatively weak complexes and are subject to degradation in vitro and in vivo. The literature contains several reports of altered biodistribution of bone-imaging agents caused by drugs and treatment regimens. These reports are summarized by Hladik et al[41] and Lentle et al.[42]

Intense renal parenchymal uptake of bone agent has been reported in children who were treated with vincristine, doxorubicin, and cyclophosphamide, either alone or in combination. The mechanism of renal uptake is unknown. Long-term steroid therapy induces bone mineral depletion and has been shown to cause a generalized decrease in skeletal uptake of bone-imaging agents. Bilateral breast uptake of Tc-99m PPi has been reported in a man being treated with diethylstilbestrol for prostatic carcinoma. Several reports have demonstrated abnormal distribution and localization of Tc-99m bone agents because of iron. Localized activity has occurred at sites where intramuscular iron–dextran had been injected. This may be due to localized hyperemia or complexation of the bone agent with iron. Plasma iron overload has been associated with a decreased skeletal uptake of bone agents in several cases. Technetium diphosphonates have shown splenic uptake in sickle cell disease, which may be related to increased iron concentration. Increased liver uptake of Tc-diphosphonates has been shown to occur in cases of increased levels of plasma aluminum. This has also been documented with controlled animal experiments. A so called sickle sign, an area of diffuse activity around the calvarium, has been observed on bone scans in 56 percent of breast cancer patients receiving intensive cytotoxic therapy.

These examples are only some of the reported maldistributions. More detailed information may be found in the review article.[42,43] Although it is difficult to determine the exact causes for these maldistributions, it is important to be aware that they are not uncommon and may occur for many different reasons that may not be necessarily associated with the particular disease being evaluated by the bone scan.

Clinical Evaluation of Bone with Radiopharmaceuticals

RATIONALE

Indications for bone scanning include the workup for metastatic disease, osteomyelitis, avascular necrosis, trauma, metabolic disorders, and arthritic disease. The most common indication is the workup for metastatic disease. In the mid-1970s, the x-ray skeletal survey was replaced by the bone scan because of its 95 percent sensitivity in detecting metastatic disease to bone and because lesions could be detected an average of 6 months earlier than with x-ray examination. The reason for the latter lies in the fact that the bone scan demonstrates osseous remodeling, which must precede and is the cause of structural changes seen on the x-ray image.

Infectious processes, such as an area of inflammation with a drainage site, pose a particular problem clinically because of a distinct difference in the way they are treated. Cellulitis (soft-tissue infection) generally requires treatment with antibiotics for only a short period of time, whereas osteomyelitis is much more difficult to treat and usually requires expensive antibiotic therapy for 6 months or more. The differentiation, therefore, between cellulitis and cellulitis with underlying osteomyelitis is important to make. The bone scan is particularly useful because it will show increased osseous remodeling resulting from acute osteomyelitis several weeks before the anatomic changes are evident on x-ray examination. The bone scan generally documents the extent of osteomyelitis much better than the radiograph.

Avascular necrosis of bone is an uncommon disorder with debilitating consequences. It generally presents as atraumatic pain in a major joint, e.g., the hip. When it presents in a child, the pathway to the diagnosis nearly always includes a bone scan, again because the physiologic processes precede the anatomic changes. In this case the study shows an absence of tracer material in the femoral head when imaged early in the disease process. This is caused by occlusion of the nutrient artery blood supply, which passes through the marrow space of the femoral neck. So-called cold-spot imaging due to infarction can also occur in sickle cell disease and occasionally in osteomyelitis. Later in the course of avascular necrosis when collateral perfusion and repair processes are active, the preferred diagnostic method is marrow imaging with sulfur colloid.

Metabolic disorders such as Paget's disease are often discovered incidentally while doing a bone scan for other reasons. The bone scan has been used to document the extent of involvement with the disease and to evaluate the effect of therapy. Poor skeletal concentration of phosphate tracer is usually seen in scans of patients with osteoporosis or who have been bedridden and in a negative calcium balance. Myositis ossificans activity can be documented also.

Many of the forms of arthritic disease can be recognized by their distribution of involvement. Degenerative joint disease is nearly always seen on bone scans of older patients in the process of metastatic disease workup and occasionally presents a problem in differentiation from malignancy, necessitating spot radiographs to make a distinction. The diagnosis and activity of anklylosing spondylitis has been aided by sacroiliac bone agent imaging.

The indications in trauma include the early diagnosis of march or stress hairline fractures, the status of nonunion in longbone fractures, the activity of calcific bridging of elbow joints in burn patients, and looseness or infection of prosthetic joints or marrow space stabilizing rods, plates, or screws. Traumatic rib fractures are usually linear or in a curvilinear pattern if due to a crush injury.

PROCEDURE

In general, 15 mCi of the bone-scanning agent is injected IV and imaging accomplished 2 to 3 hours later. The patient should be encouraged to void carefully to avoid clothing contamination and frequently to minimize the bladder radiation dose. Pelvic views should be obtained soon after voiding to minimize bladder activity interference with visualization of the pelvic structures. Many centers routinely use a view in which the patient is seated on the detector collimator to separate the bladder from osseous pelvic structures. An extrarenal pelvis may masquerade as a rib lesion until a repeat image is obtained with the patient in a different position, e.g., seated, to change the location of the kidneys. Benign patellar pathology cannot be distinguished from femoral metaphyseal metastatic disease unless lateral views of the knees are obtained.

Better resolution can be obtained of most of the skeleton by simply making certain that the part to be examined is as close as possible to the collimator. In situations where the structure of interest is deeper or obscured by overlying skeleton, e.g., hips, spine, or the base of the skull, acquisition and display by emission computed tomography (ECT) techniques usually will improve delineation of structural detail.

A blood pool phase image may be helpful in documenting the extent of inflammation resulting from cellulitis. Inflammation increases vascularity, and if an image is obtained in the first few minutes after injection before much tracer has localized in kidneys or bone, this blood pool image will show the extent of the hypervascularity. Comparison should be made with the nor-

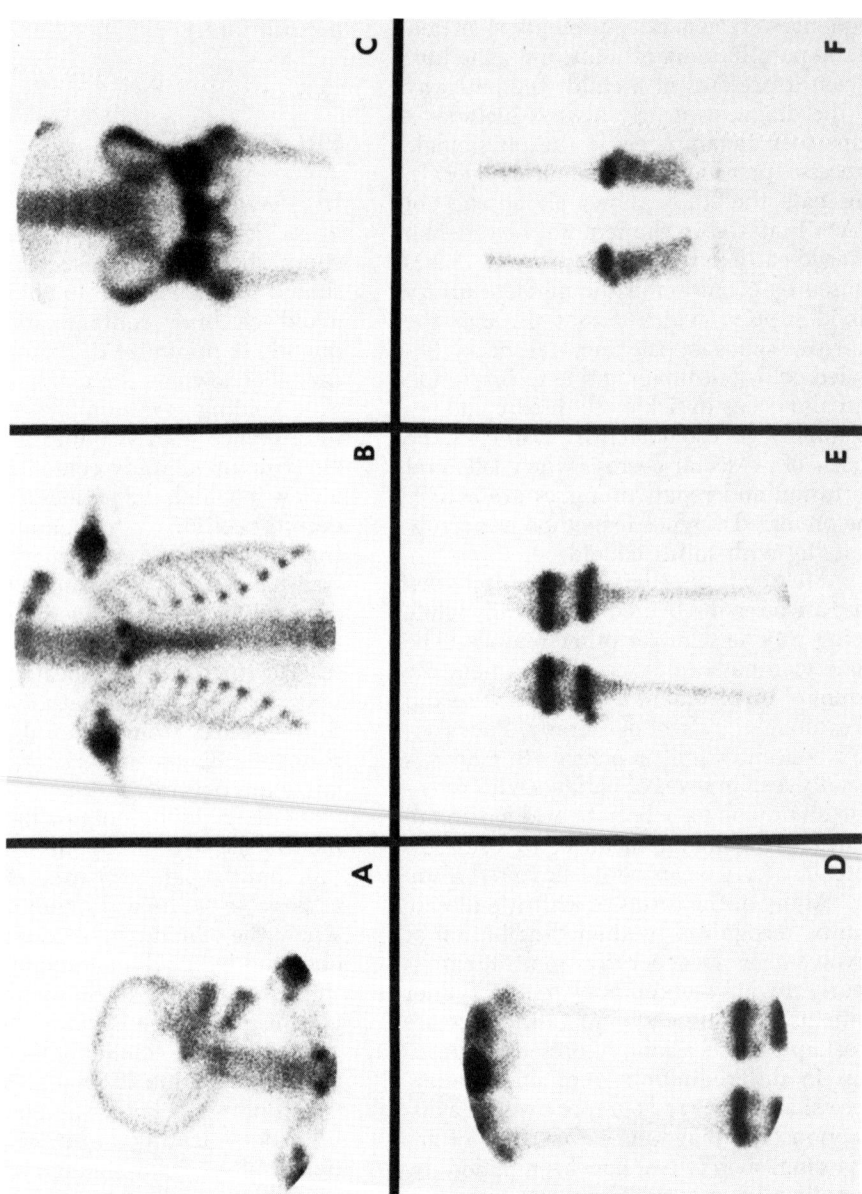

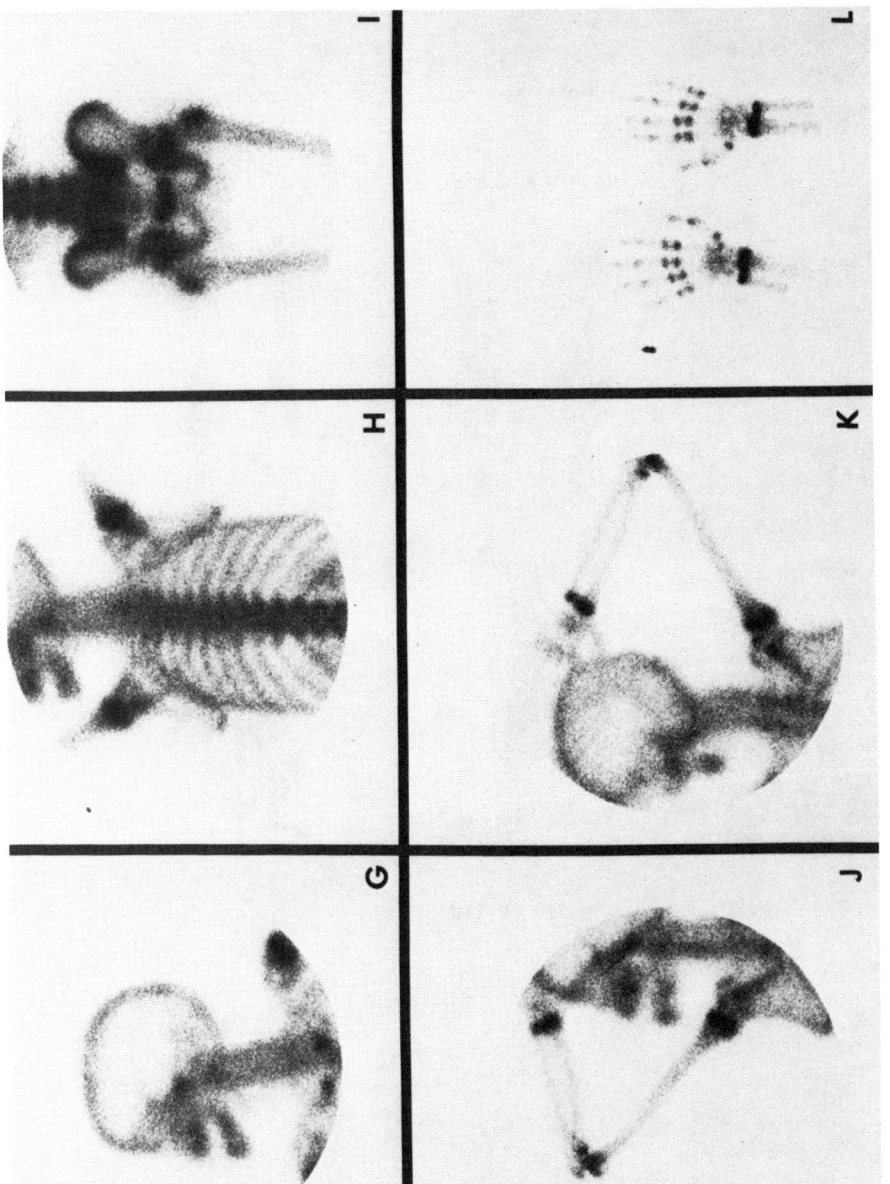

Figure 13-10. Normal bone scan in a 7-year-old child obtained 2 hours after the injection of 8 mCi of Tc-99m oxidronate. Panels **A** through **F** show a right lateral view of the head and anterior views of the thorax and abdomen, pelvis, and legs and feet. Panels **G** through **L** show the left lateral view of the head and posterior views of the thorax and abdomen, pelvis, arms and palmar view of the hands. Note the high concentration of activity in the epiphyseal regions, characteristically seen in pediatric patients.

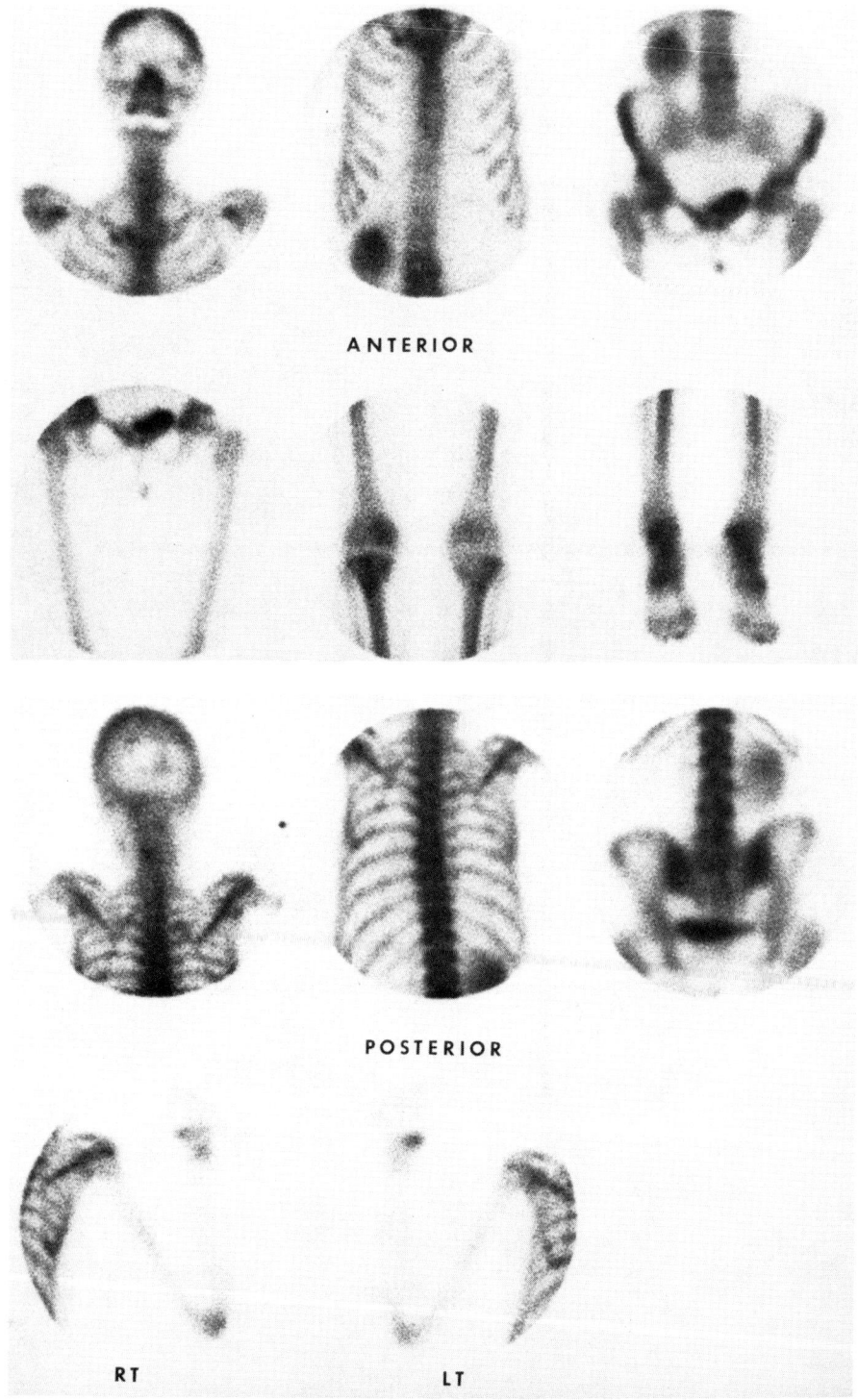

Figure 13-11. Bone scan in an adult obtained 3 hours after injection of 15 mCi of Tc-99m medronate. Note the absence of the left kidney. Bone tracers are excreted by the kidneys.

mal side. If, on the 2-hour delayed images, there is focally increased osseous remodeling present, then it is likely that the patient also has osteomyelitis.

PHARMACEUTICALS

The radiopharmaceuticals of choice for bone imaging are the diphosphonates EHDP, MDP, and HMDP. PPi has its place, not for bone imaging, but for myocardial infarct avid imaging and as the best commercially available source of stannous ion for red cell labeling in cardiac blood pool imaging (Table 13-2). Other bone agents will not have the same margin of safety for blood pool imaging because of their higher phosphate-to-tin ratios.

INTERPRETATION

The term osseous remodeling is virtually synonymous with bone scanning because the bone scan demonstrates physiologic processes (Figs. 13-10 and 13-11). The focal area of abnormally increased osseous remodeling, i.e., the area of hyperconcentration (hot spot) of the phosphate tracer, is what attracts the examiner's eye in viewing the images (Fig. 13-12). Diffusely increased concentration in the entire skeleton may be seen in patients with hyperparathyroidism, and this results from a generalized increase in osseous remodeling. Diffusely increased concentration in a limb, however, generally coincides with increased blood flow to the limb because of a tumor, arteriovenous malformation, or infection (Fig. 13-13). In this

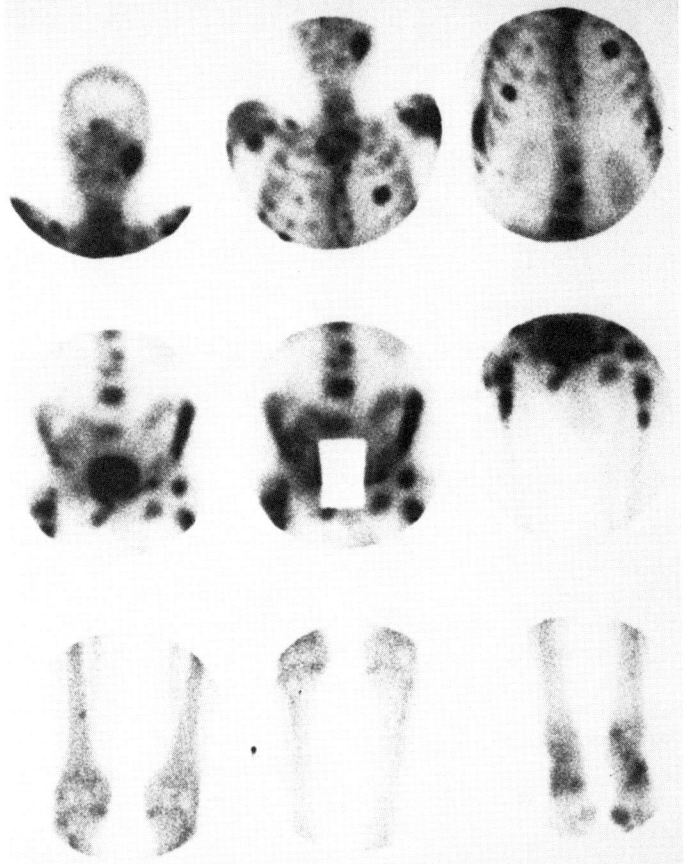

Figure 13-12. Abnormal bone scan in an 82-year-old man with metastatic prostate carcinoma. Multiple focal areas of increased uptake of Tc-99m medronate are seen in the axial skeleton and the extremities. **A.** Anterior view. *(continued)*

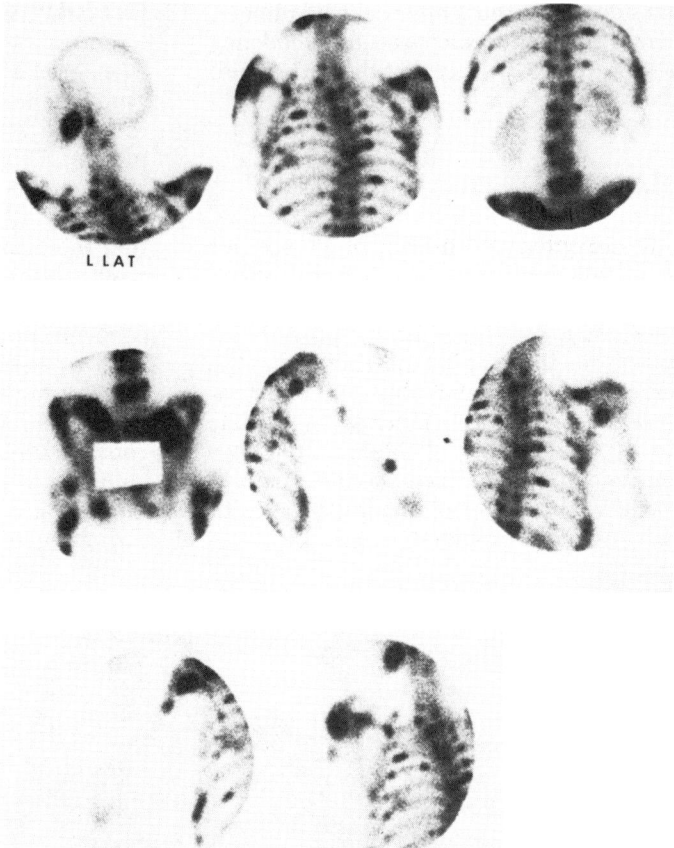

Figure 13-12. B. Posterior view.

case the bones of the affected limb are preferentially bathed in a greater amount of tracer. When diffusely increased soft-tissue concentration is seen, it generally indicates the presence of impaired venous drainage or edema in the limb.

In contrast to these are the cold areas seen with vasoocclusive disease (Fig. 13-14), metal prostheses, and the occasional site where tumor has replaced most of the bone. Often, cool areas or areas of mildly diminished phosphate concentration will be seen demarcating a site of external radiation therapy where osteocytes have been destroyed.

One should expect that increased osseous remodeling will continue after healing of a fracture, eradication of tumor metastases, or eradication of the infectious organism in osteomyelitis until the bone has achieved a strong, stable anatomic configuration. For this reason it is important to look primarily for new lesions in the serial bone scans of tumor patients.

Another agent must be used to resolve the question of the presence or absence of infection in patients with chronic osteomyelitis because increased osseous remodeling will continue for some time. Ga-67 citrate has been used traditionally for the evaluation of chronic osteomyelitis, though improved sensitivity and specificity may come from indium-111 white blood cells or ionic In-111 when the comparative investigations are completed[43] (Fig. 13-15).

In some instances it is helpful to use

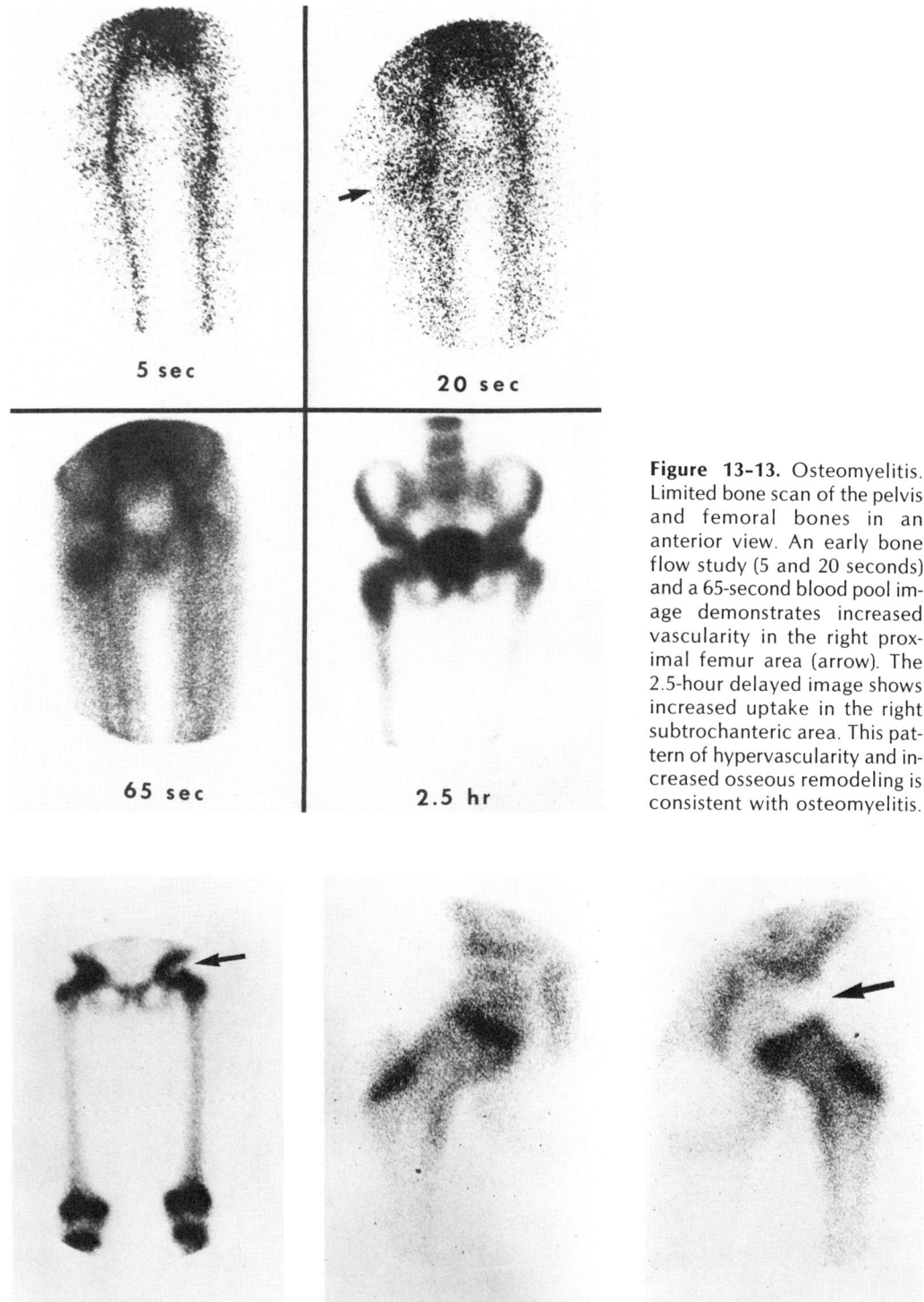

Figure 13-13. Osteomyelitis. Limited bone scan of the pelvis and femoral bones in an anterior view. An early bone flow study (5 and 20 seconds) and a 65-second blood pool image demonstrates increased vascularity in the right proximal femur area (arrow). The 2.5-hour delayed image shows increased uptake in the right subtrochanteric area. This pattern of hypervascularity and increased osseous remodeling is consistent with osteomyelitis.

Figure 13-14. Avascular necrosis. **A.** Anterior pelvis and thighs. **B.** Anterior right hip. **C.** Anterior left hip. Note the absence of tracer in the left femoral head and the increased concentration in the epiphyseal growth plates in this child.

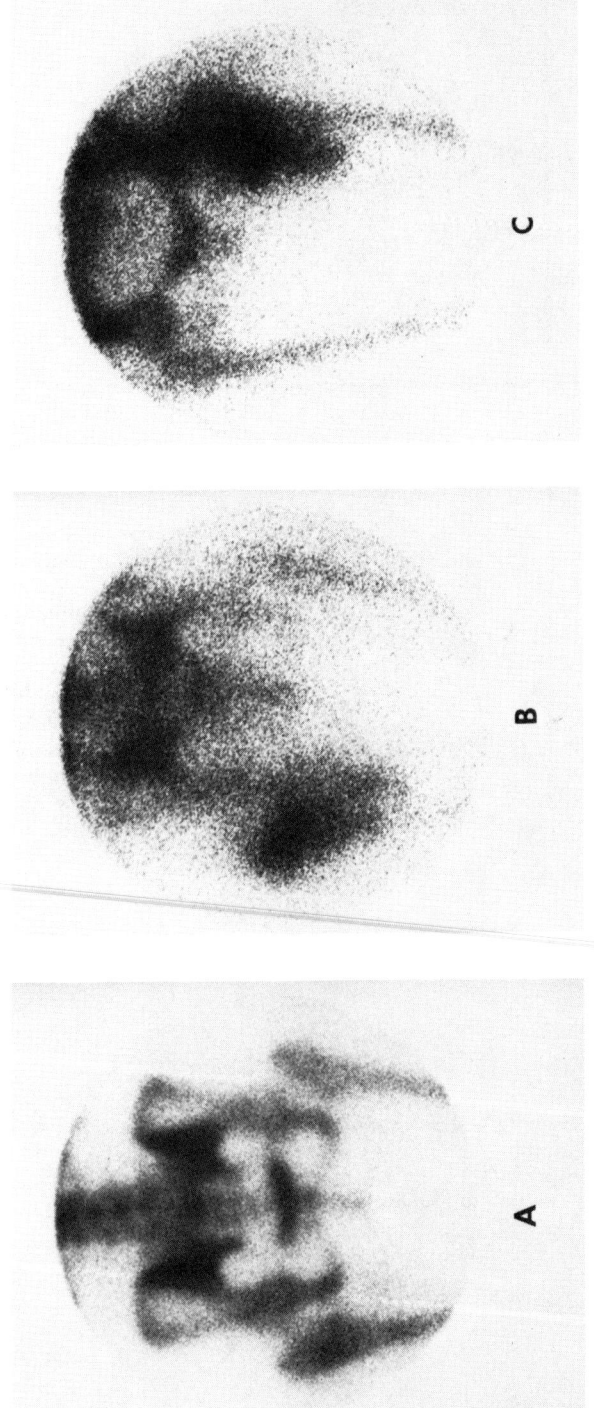

Figure 13-15. A. Posterior bone scan of the pelvic region with Tc-99m MDP demonstrating increased tracer uptake in the left proximal femur that was considered to be secondary to trauma or inflammatory disease. Further evaluation with a Ga-67 scan demonstrated increased tracer uptake in the proximal left femur and soft tissues of the left thigh on the 24-hour posterior image (**B**) and 48-hour anterior image (**C**). A psoas abscess was found at surgery.

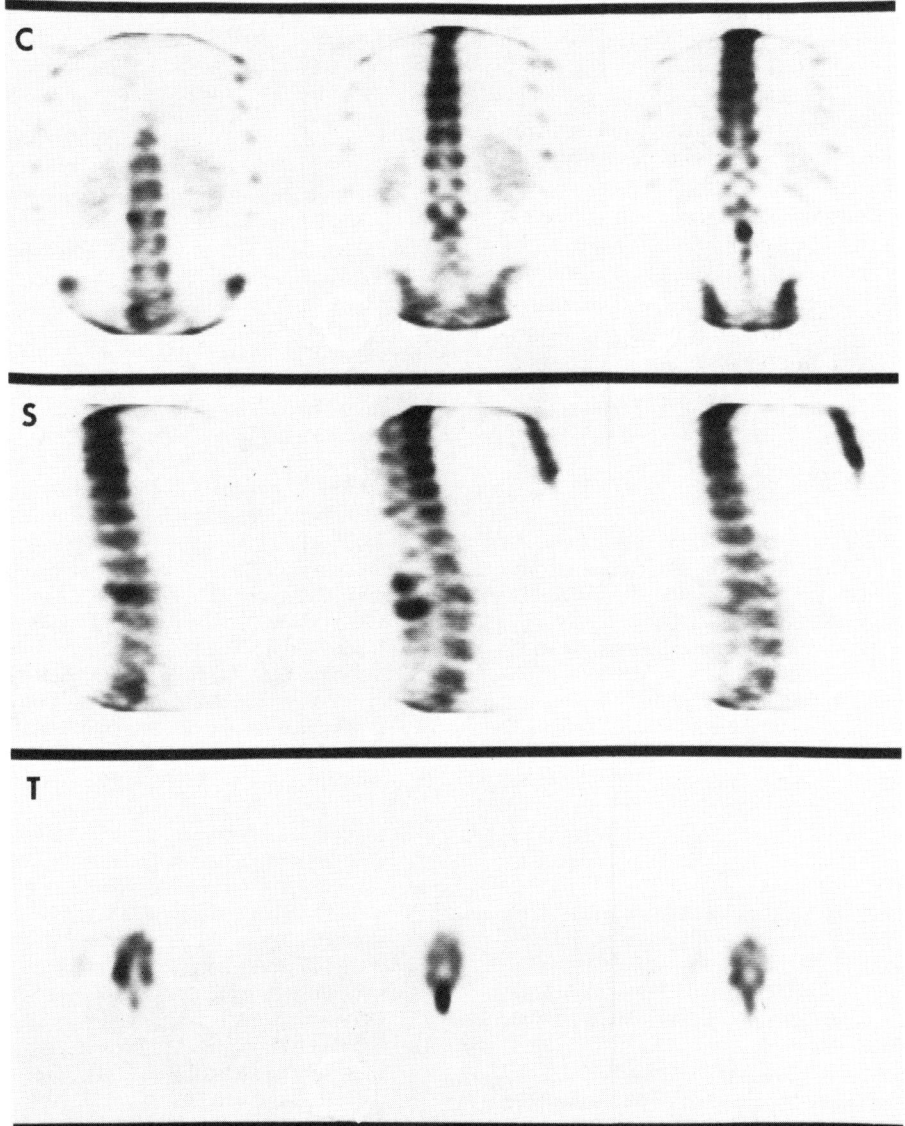

Figure 13-16. Bone SPECT coronal (C), sagittal (S), and transaxial (T) images demonstrating metastatic disease to the pedicle and posterior elements of the spine in a patient with lung cancer. SPECT 3-D definition allowed differentiation from arthritic disease.

single-photon emission computed tomography (SPECT) imaging to obtain a correct diagnosis, (Fig. 13–16).

Information from a bone scan is usually assimilated by one of two methods. One method is to integrate solitary findings on the bone scan with pertinent clinical information to formulate a differential diagnosis. This is best done with foreknowledge of the patient's clinical information so that the study can be properly tailored to answer the question. When a bone scan in a cancer patient shows a solitary lesion only, then a pertinent trauma history, x-rays, or both must be evaluated to determine the likelihood of benignancy or malignancy. The second method is to use pattern recognition as in the case of widespread metastatic disease to bone.

In summary, the bone scan renders a unique form of physiologic information by showing areas of increased osseous remodeling, absence of bone, and increased or absent blood flow and occupies a position of great importance among medical tests.

REFERENCES

1. Triffitt JT: The organic matrix of bone tissue. In Urist MR (ed): Fundamental and Clinical Bone Physiology. Philadelphia, Lippincott, 1980 pp 45–82
2. Neuman WF: Bone material and calcification mechanisms. In Urist MR (ed): Fundamental and Clinical Bone Physiology. Philadelphia, Lippincott, 1980, pp 83–107
3. Brown WE, Chow LC: Chemical properties of bone mineral. Ann Rev Mater Sci 6:213, 1976
4. Guyton AC: Textbook of Medical Physiology, 6th ed. Philadelphia, Saunders, 1981, pp 977 981
5. Dudley HC, Maddox GE, LaRuc HC: Studies of the metabolism of gallium. J Pharmacol Exp Ther 96:135, 1949
6. Edwards CL, Hayes RL: Tumor scanning with Ga-67 citrate. J Nucl Med 10:103, 1969
7. Charkes ND, Sklaroff DM: Early diagnosis of metastatic bone cancer of photoscanning with strontium-85. J Nucl Med 5:168, 1964
8. Gynning I, Langeland P, Lindberg S, et al: Localization with Sr-85 of spinal metastasis in mammary cancer and changes in uptake after hormone and roentgen therapy: A preliminary report. Acta Radiol 55:119, 1961
9. Meckelnburg RI: Clinical value of generator produced 87m-strontium. J Nucl Med 5:929, 1964
10. Blau M. Nagler W, Bender MA: Fluorine-18. A new isotope for bone scanning. J Nucl Med 3:332, 1962
11. Fels IG, Kaplan E, Greco J: Incorporation in vivo of P-32 from condensed phosphates. Proc Soc Exp Biol Med 100:53, 1959
12. Subramanian G, McAfee JG: A new complex of Tc-99m for skeletal imaging. Radiology 99:192, 1971
13. Subramanian G, McAfee JG, O'Mara RE, et al: Tc-99m polyphosphate PP_{46}: A new radiopharmaceutical for skeletal imaging. J Nucl Med 12:399, 1971
14. Davis MA, Jones AG: Comparison of Tc-99m labeled phosphate and phosphonate agents for skeletal imaging. Semin Nucl Med 6:19, 1976
15. Perez R, Cohen Y, Henry R, et al: A new radiopharmaceutical for Tc-99m bone scanning. J Nucl Med 13:788, 1972
16. Yano Y, McRae J. Van Dyke DC, et al: Technetium-99m labeled stannous ethane-1-hydroxyl-1, 1-diphosphonate: A new bone scanning agent. J Nucl Med 14:73, 1973
17. Castronovo FP, Callahan RJ: New bone scanning agent: Tc-99m-labeled 1-hydroxyethylidene-1, 1-disodium phosphonate. J Nucl Med 13:823, 1972
18. Subramanian G, McAfee JG, Blair RJ, et al: Tc-99m EHDP: A potential radiopharmaceutical for skeletal imaging. J Nucl Med 13:947, 1972
19. Subramanian G, McAfee JG, Blair RJ, et al: Technetium 99m methylene diphosphonate—A superior agent for skeletal imaging: Comparison with other technetium complexes. J Nucl Med 16:744, 1975
20. Barnett BL, Strickland LC: The crystal structure of disodium dihydrogen-1-hydroxyethylidene diphosphonate tetrahydrate: A bone growth regulator. Acta Cryst 35:1217, 1979
21. Francis MD, Tofe AJ, Benedict JJ, et al: Imaging the skeletal system. In Sorenson JA (ed): Radiopharmaceuticals II. New York, Society of Nuclear Medicine 1979, pp 603–614
22. Tofe AJ, Francis MD: Optimization of the ratio of stannous tin: ethane-1-hydroxy-1-diphosphonate for bone scanning with Tc-99m pertechnetate. J Nucl Med 15:69, 1974
23. Bevan J, Tofe AJ, Benedict JJ, et al: Tc-99m HMDP (hydroxymethylene diphosphonate): A radiopharmaceutical for skeletal and acute myocardial infarct imaging. 1. Synthesis and distribution in animals. J Nucl Med 21:961, 1980

24. Kowalsky RJ, Dalton DR: Technical problems associated with the production of technetium Tc-99m tin (II) pyrophosphate kits. Am J Hosp Pharm 38:1722, 1981
25. Chandler WM, Shuck LD: Abnormal technetium-99m pertechnetate imaging following stannous pyrophosphate bone imaging. J Nucl Med 16:518, 1975
26. Tofe AJ, Francis MD: In vitro stabilization of a low-tin bone-imaging agent (Tc-99m-Sn-HEDP) by ascorbic acid. J Nucl Med 17:820, 1976
27. Tofe AJ, Bevan JA, Fawzi MD, et al: Gentisic acid: A new stabilizer for low tin skeletal imaging agents: Concise communication. J Nucl Med 21:366, 1980
28. Ballinger J, Der M, Bowen B: Stabilization of Tc-99m pyrophosphate injection with gentisic acid: Eur J Nucl Med 6:153, 1981
29. Deutsch E: Inorganic radiopharmaceuticals. In Sorenson JA (ed): Radiopharmaceuticals II. New York, Society of Nuclear Medicine, 1979, pp 129–146
30. Francis MD, Ferguson DL, Tofe AJ, et al: Comparative evaluation of three diphosphonates: In vitro adsorption (C-14 labeled) and in vivo osteogenic uptake (Tc-99m complexed). J Nucl Med 21:1185, 1980
31. Fogelman I, Pearson DW, Bessent RG, et al: A comparison of skeletal uptake of three diphosphonates by whole body retention: Concise communication. J Nucl Med 22:880, 1981
32. Silberstein EB: A radiopharmaceutical and clinical comparison of Tc-99m-Sn-hydroxymethylene diphosphonate with Tc-99m-Sn-hydroxyethylidene diphosphonate. Radiology 136:747, 1980
33. Littlefield JL, Rudd TG: Tc-99m hydroxymethylene diphosphonate (HMDP) versus Tc-99m methylene diphosphonate (MDP): Biological and clinical comparison. Clin Nucl Med 5:10, 1980
34. Rosenthall L. Arzoumanian A, Damtew B, et al: A crossover study comparing Tc-99m labeled HMDP and MDP in patients. Clin Nucl Med 6:353, 1981
35. Rudd TG, Allen DR, Hartnett DE: Tc-99m methylene diphosphonate versus Tc-99m pyrophosphate: Biologic and clinical comparison. J Nucl Med 18:872, 1977
36. Fogelman I, Citrin DL, McKillop JH: A clinical comparison of Tc-99m HEDP and Tc-99m MDP in the detection of bone metastasis. J Nucl Med 20:98, 1979
37. Fogelman I: Skeletal uptake of diphosphonate: A review. Eur J Nucl Med 5:473, 1980
38. Jones AG, Francis MD, Davis MA: Bone scanning: Radionuclidic reaction mechanisms. Semin Nucl Med 6:3, 1976
39. Thomas SR, Gelfand MJ, Keriakes JG, et al: Dose to the metaphyseal growth complexes in children undergoing Tc-99m EHDP bone scans. Radiology 126:193, 1978
40. Stevenson JS, Eckelman WC, Sobocinski PZ, et al: The toxicity of Sn-pyrophosphate: Clinical manifestations prior to acute LD-50. J Nucl Med 15:252, 1974
41. Sayle BA, Balachandran S, Rogers CA: Indium-111 chloride imaging in patients with suspected abscesses: Concise communication. J Nucl Med 24:1114, 1983
42. Hladik WB III, Nigg KK, Rhodes BA: Drug-induced changes in the biologic distribution of radiopharmaceuticals. Semin Nucl Med 12:184, 1982
43. Lentle BC, Scott JR, Noujaim AA, et al: Iatrogenic alterations in radionuclide biodistributions. Semin Nucl Med 9:131, 1979

CHAPTER 14

Total Body Imaging: Gallium and Indium Radiopharmaceuticals

The previous chapters have focused on radiopharmaceuticals used to evaluate the major organ systems in the body. The general approach was to discuss systems from the head on downward ending with a chapter on bone, which looks at the total body skeleton. In this chapter we will discuss radiopharmaceuticals used in total-body soft-tissue imaging without regard for any particular organ system. In general, this involves tumor imaging and the detection of inflammatory and thrombotic processes. The major radionuclides used in this regard are gallium and indium, and the chapter will focus on the production and properties of their radiopharmaceuticals.

The chemistry of gallium and indium is similar. In some instances the radiopharmaceuticals of these nuclides have been used for similar purposes such as tumor and abscess localization, but this is not the rule. The most frequently used radionuclides, indium-111 and gallium-67, are cyclotron produced, have similar half-lives, and decay by electron capture to yield photons with useful imaging characteristics. Other radioisotopes of gallium and indium have achieved a place in nuclear medicine applications over the years, and they will also be discussed in this chapter.

GENERAL CHEMISTRY OF GALLIUM AND INDIUM

Gallium and indium are members of the group IIIA elements of the periodic table. They therefore have three valence electrons beyond the noble gas configuration and readily lose these electrons to assume the 3+ oxidation state. In acidic aqueous solution below pH 2, gallium and indium exist in the ionic form; however, when the pH is raised toward neutrality, these ions readily hydrolyze to form insoluble metal hydroxides that at tracer concentrations exist as radiocolloids. Gallium and indium ions complex with various ligands to form stable chelates in neutral aqueous solution. Chelating agents commonly used to stabilize these ions in vitro include citrate, edetate (EDTA), pentetate (DTPA) and 8-hydroxyquinoline (oxine). In vivo Ga^{3+} and In^{3+} will bind to certain proteins, most notably plasma transferrin. In this regard, these ions exhibit an in vivo chemistry similar to iron.

GALLIUM RADIOPHARMACEUTICALS

The development of gallium radiopharmaceuticals has an involved and interesting history. In a fashion similar to some of the drugs now used in traditional therapeutics, gallium's current applications in nuclear medicine have been achieved through a series of planned scientific investigations and serendipity. The reader is referred to an informative paper dealing with the chronology of gallium's rise to clinical use in nuclear medicine.[1]

Gallium was discovered in 1875. The high boiling point of elemental gallium suggested its use as a reactor coolant in nuclear submarines in the 1940s. This application eventually stimulated investigation into the toxicology of gallium whereupon biodistribution experiments in animals revealed that gallium localized to a significant degree in bone. The use of Ga-72 radiotracer in these studies led to the suggestion of its possible use in the diagnosis and treatment of metastatic bone disease. Clinical investigations soon ended with this nuclide, however, because of its poor decay properties and the inferior quality of detection equipment available at that time. Subsequent studies were performed using Ga-67 because of its more favorable physical properties. One significant finding during these investigations was that gallium's biodistribution could be altered if the administered radiotracer dose contained stable carrier gallium. Initial biodistribution studies in animals, before the Ga-67 studies, were conducted with low specific activity Ga-72, which was reactor produced according to the reaction $^{71}Ga(n,\gamma)^{72}Ga$. These studies, containing carrier Ga-71, demonstrated localization in bone in preference to soft tissue. Subsequent studies with cyclotron-produced carrier-free Ga-67, by the reaction $^{68}Zn(p,2n)^{67}Ga$, however, demonstrated a quite different pattern of biodistribution. Indeed, compared with Ga-72, the rate of uptake and degree of deposition of carrier-free Ga-67 in bone were decreased, localization in liver and other soft tissues was greatly enhanced, blood clearance was slower, and a complete reversal of the urinary and fecal excretion pattern occurred.[2] At the time of these early studies in 1953, however, nuclear medicine instrumentation had not yet achieved the necessary sophistication to produce good-quality diagnostic studies, and therefore clinical investigation was not pursued.

In 1961 the development of the Ge-68/Ga-68 generator at Brookhaven National Laboratory[3] stimulated a renewed interest in gallium as a bone-imaging agent. Studies at Oak Ridge in 1965 were initiated based on the speculation that the faster blood clearance and shorter half-life of Ga-68 compared with Sr-85 offered some advantage over the latter nuclide for bone imaging; however, the continued fear of chronic toxic effects of administering carrier gallium to achieve bone localization was still a concern. Additionally, the suboptimal annihilation radiation from positron-emitting Ga-68 eventually switched interest back to Ga-67 in 1968 because its physical properties were more compatible with gamma cameras and less carrier gallium was needed to obtain bone scans. Clinical studies were thus initiated with Ga-67 as a proposed bone-scanning agent at Oak Ridge. It was at this point in time that serendipity prevailed. The plan of investigation was that initial studies were to be conducted with carrier-free Ga-67 followed by studies with carrier-added gallium in the same patients. One of the first few studies with carrier-free Ga-67, however, showed intense localization of activity in the afflicted lymph nodes of a patient with Hodgkin's disease.[4] Because the original intent of the study was to detect bone lesions, this discovery quickly changed the course of investigation and eventually led to the use of Ga-67 citrate as one of the first radiopharmaceuticals for imaging soft-tissue tumors. Within a short period of time of this initial discovery, however, it was revealed that gallium localized also in inflammatory processes.[5,6]

This of course indicated that gallium was nonspecific for localizing soft-tissue tumors. This finding eventually led to its more widespread diagnostic use in abscess localization than in the detection of cancer. From the time of these initial clinical findings to the present, Ga-67 citrate has maintained a prominent position in routine diagnostic nuclear medicine studies, particularly for the localization of inflammatory foci in postoperative patients and in patients who present with fever of undetermined origin.[7]

Ga-67 Citrate Production

Ga-67 is produced in a cyclotron by bombarding a zinc metal target enriched with Zn-68 with 22- to 12-MeV protons according to the reaction $^{68}Zn(p,2n)^{67}Ga$. The irradiated target is dissolved in HCl and the gallium extracted with isopropyl ether while leaving the zinc and other impurities behind.[8] The gallium is backextracted from the ether into 0.2 M HCl, evaporated to dryness, and redissolved in 0.05 M HCl. The citrate complex is formed by adding the required amount of sodium citrate and raising the pH with sodium hydroxide. The chemical structure of the complex and its production are summarized in Figure 14-1.

Being an amphoteric element, gallium reacts as a metal at a low pH but forms the insoluble hydroxide when the pH is raised toward neutrality. At high pH gallium acts as a non-metal forming soluble gallate species. The degree of formation of the gallium citrate complex is a function of pH and citrate concentration.[9] These relationships are illustrated in Figure 14-2 A and B. Apparently, a competition exists between citrate and hydroxyl ions for gallium such that when the citrate concentration is low (less than 0.2 percent), successful chelation occurs only at low pH or when the pH is high (greater than 7) chelation occurs only at a high citrate concentration (greater than 1 percent).

The radiochemical purity of gallium citrate can be determined on Whatman No. 1 paper developed in pyridine, ethanol, water in a ratio 1:2:4.[9] The various radiochemical species evaluated are gallium citrate (Rf, 0.9) and the impurities gallate (Rf, 0.6) and gallium hydroxide (Rf, 0.0).

Physical Properties of Ga-67

Figure 14-3 illustrates the decay scheme for Ga-67. Being a proton-rich nuclide, Ga-67 decays by electron capture to stable zinc-67 with a transition energy of 1.001 MeV. Positron decay does not occur. The half-life of Ga-67 is 78.25 hours. The most prominent photon emissions and abundances are γ-2,

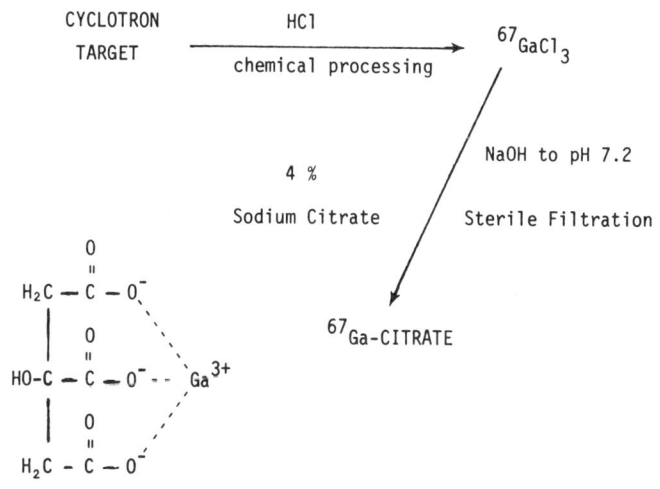

Figure 14-1. Schematic diagram of Ga-67 citrate production and structure of the complex.

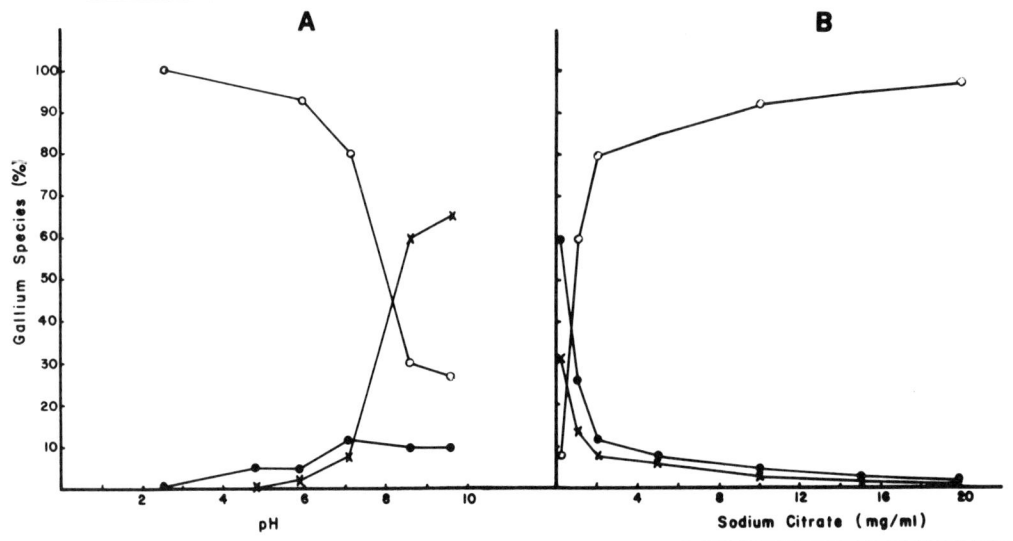

Figure 14-2. Percentage of gallium citrate (O), gallate (X), and gallium hydroxide (●) species as a function of pH at a sodium citrate concentration of 2 mg/ml (**A**) and as a function of the sodium citrate concentration at pH 7.1 (**B**). *(Data from Hnatowich DJ, et al, 1977, p. 925.[9])*

93 keV (38 percent); γ-3, 185 keV (24 percent); γ-5, 300 keV (16 percent); and γ-6, 394 keV (4 percent). The specific gamma ray constant for Ga-67 is 1.6 R/hr/mCi at 1 cm. The half-value layer in lead is 0.04 mm.

Biologic Distribution of Ga-67 Citrate

After intravenous (IV) administration of Ga-67 citrate, disappearance from the blood occurs at an exponential rate, and there appear to be three components: about 48 percent of the dose is removed quickly with a half-life of 30 minutes, 12 percent with a half-life of 4 hours, and 38 percent with a prolonged half-life of 38 hours. At 24, 48, and 72 hours about 20, 10 and 5 percent, respectively, of the administered Ga-67 citrate is still in the blood.[10] When Ga-67 citrate is introduced into the blood, the complex dissociates rapidly, and gallium binds to serum proteins, principally transferrin. Transferrin is a β-globulin present in the blood responsible for transporting iron. It has a molecular weight of 77,000 and is capable of binding two gallium ions per molecule of transferrin.[11] About 80 percent of the injected Ga-67 activity is protein bound.[9] The extent of protein binding depends on several factors. Large amounts of citrate have been shown to decrease protein binding in vitro, but in vivo the effect produced by the amount of citrate in the gallium dose is insignificant because of dilution in the serum.[9] A range of 5 to 500 mg of sodium citrate administered with Ga-67 has not altered its distribution significantly.[9] The degree to which transferrin binding sites are saturated influences gallium's binding and biodistribution. Metal ions that compete for transferrin-binding sites affect the rate of blood disappearance, tissue distribution, and whole-body retention of injected gallium. In general, when transferrin is saturated with iron or scandium, the blood and urinary clearance rates of gallium are more rapid, and gallium distribution shifts from soft tissue to bone. This alteration in tissue distribution is in turn accompanied by a greatly reduced body retention of Ga-67 as shown in Figure 14-4.[12]

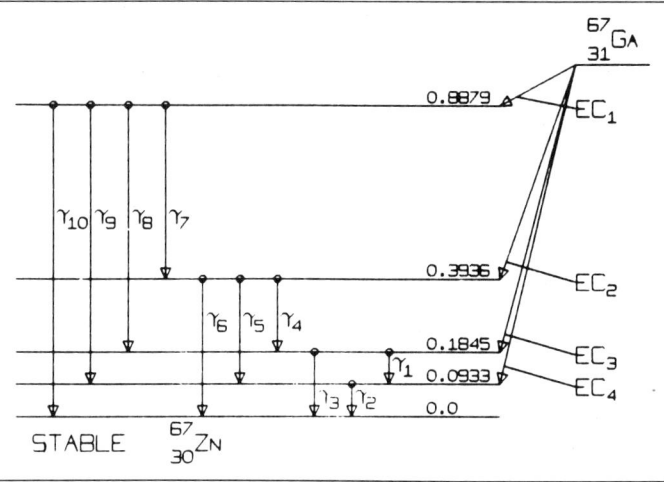

Figure 14-3. Decay scheme of Ga-67. *(From Dillman LT, Von der Lage FC: MIRD Pamphlet No. 10. New York, Society of Nuclear Medicine, 1975, with permission.)*

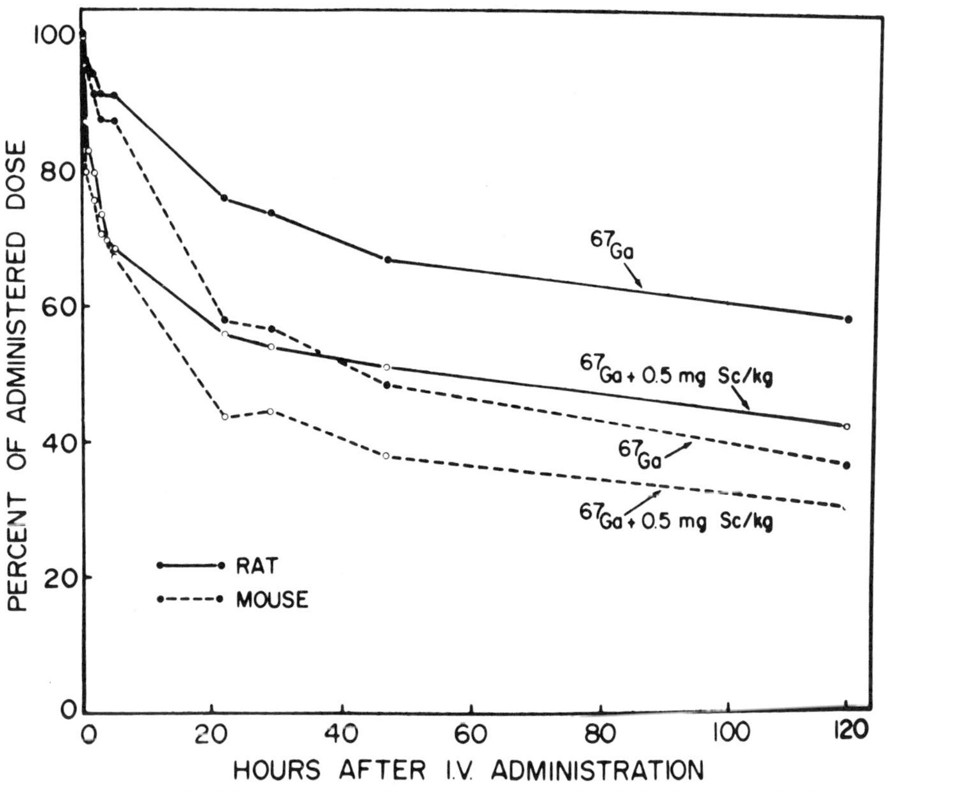

Figure 14-4. Effect of scandium administration on body retention of Ga-67 in the Fischer-344 rat and CD, 2F mouse. The points are means of measurements on four animals. *(From Hayes RL, et al, 1980, p 361, with permission.[12])*

Interestingly, in tumor-bearing animals under similar conditions of transferrin loading, gallium activity in tumors, as a fraction of the administered dose, is unchanged.[12,13] On the other hand, increasing Ga-67 protein binding through induction of anemia or by administration of apotransferrin produced the reverse effect, that is, soft-tissue activity increased, and tumor activity decreased.[13] This suggests that it is the unbound or loosely bound fraction of gallium in the blood that preferentially localizes in tumor and that the uptake by normal soft tissue is strongly promoted by its binding to transferrin.[13] The overall proposed scheme that summarizes gallium distribution from plasma compartments (bound and free) to various tissues, is shown in Figure 14-5.[13]

Gallium is excreted by the kidney, liver, and bowel. Approximately 15 to 25 percent of gallium is excreted in the urine within the first 24 hours after intravenous administration. Clearance from the body, thereafter, is slow, with the major route being the feces. By 7 days, 26 percent is eliminated in the urine, 9 percent is eliminated in feces, and 65 percent is retained and distributed within the plasma and body tissues.[14] Long-term retention studies demonstrate that the first component of excretion (17 percent) has a half-life of 30 hours and the long component (83 percent) has a half-life of 25 days.[15] This slowed excretion is the major reason for waiting 2 to 3 days after injection before imaging. The prolonged presence of bowel activity is a major disadvantage for using gallium to localize abdominal abscesses. Most of the colonic activity is within the bowel lumen, and therefore use of an evacuant or enema preparation has been advocated before imaging, albeit with limited success. A commonly used method of bowel preparation is the administration of laxatives, such as 15 mg of bisacodyl, orally each day starting on the day of injection of the radionuclide and continuing until imaging is completed. For postoperative scans, 12 ounces of citrate of magnesia is administered on the evening before the initial scan. Because gallium is secreted into the bowel, some activity is associated with intestinal mucosa. Consequently, incomplete removal of bowel activity should be expected by use of evacuants. For this reason it is felt by some practitioners that a normal diet with adequate roughage, to help denude the mucosa, is a satisfactory measure in removing bowel-associated gallium activity.

The principal organs in which gallium localizes are the adrenal glands, liver, spleen, kidney, skeleton, bone marrow, and bowel.[14,16] These data are summarized in Table 14-1. Kidney activity usually dissipates after 24 hours. Other sites that may demonstrate gallium uptake include lacrimal and nasopharyngeal tissues[17]; the breast, particularly under the physiologic stimulus of menarche; estrogenic and progestational agents or pregnancy[18]; and the salivary glands after radiation therapy induced sialadenitis.[19] One report demonstrated the localization of Ga-67 in the human placenta.[20] The high concentration of lactoferrin in many normal tissues is believed to be responsible for the localization of gallium in these tissues. Lactoferrin is a protein similar to transferrin that is capable of binding gallium. Both transferrin and lactoferrin are metabolized in the liver, thus

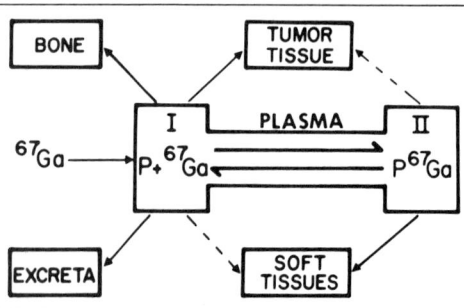

Figure 14-5. Proposed scheme of initial entry of Ga-67 into tumor and normal tissue. The solid lines indicate main pathways. This scheme does not take into account reverse processes and is intended to indicate only the overall movement of Ga-67 in the initial phase of its biodistribution after it enters the vascular compartment. *(From Hayes RL, et al, 1981, p 325, with permission.[13])*

TABLE 14-1. CONCENTRATION OF Ga-67 IN VARIOUS TISSUES

	% Administered Activity/kg	
Tissue	Mean	Range
Spleen	4.1	0.4–10.2
Kidney cortex	3.8	0.7–8.4
Adrenal	3.8	0.6–11.5
Marrow	3.6	0.7–9.9
Liver	2.8	0.6–5.2
Kidney	2.7	0.6–6.2
Bone	2.6	0.04–9.2
Kidney medulla	2.0	0.4–6.5
Jejunum	1.9	0.6–4.5
Colon	1.6	0.3–5.2

*Values are normalized to a body weight of 70 kg. Data are from autopsy tissue from patients who died at various times (3 hours to 23 days) after the Ga-67 dose.
(Data from Nelson B, et al, 1972, p. 92.[14])

offering a reasonable hypothesis for the liver concentration of gallium activity.

Whole body x-irradiation can alter the normal distribution of carrier-free Ga-67 citrate so as to produce increased excretion and bone deposition together with decreased soft-tissue uptake.[21] This pattern is similar to the effect produced by iron saturation of transferrin previously mentioned; indeed, the finding of elevated serum iron levels after irradiation of animals strongly suggests this mechanism.[13,22]

Mechanisms of Localization of Gallium in Tumors and Abscesses

Uptake of Ga-67 into transplanted animal tumors is mainly associated with viable rather than necrotic tissue.[23] Although recent experiments suggest that free or loosely bound gallium in the blood is the preferential form that enters tumor tissue, the exact mechanism involved is not known. Several mechanisms have been postulated including endocytosis of protein-bound gallium, diffusion resulting from hyperpermeability of tumor cell plasma membranes, or exchange of transferrin-bound Ga-67 with lactoferrin within tumor cells.[23] How gallium actually leaves the blood and enters the tumor cell is not clear, but some interesting postulates can be made if one considers gallium's chemistry. At physiologic pH, free or unchelated gallium theoretically undergoes hydrolysis to form the hydroxide $Ga(OH)_3$, which is a neutral species. Such neutral particles would thus encounter no charge barrier in diffusing through plasma cell membranes, particularly if tumor cell membranes are hyperpermeable. Once having entered the cytoplasmic fluid, the gallium particles could diffuse through lysosomal membranes. Once inside, the relatively high hydrogen ion concentration present in lysosomes could convert the neutral hydroxide particles into positively charged gallium ions that would resist backdiffusion because they could readily bind to lysosomal protein.[24]

Subcellular tissue fractionation studies have indeed shown gallium to be associated within lysosomes, whereas other studies show it to be localized in tumor tissue homogenates rather than with isolated cell organelles such as lysosomes. As Hayes points out,[23] however, this difference may be due to the technique of tissue preparation because lysosomes are quite fragile and may disrupt, releasing their gallium to the supernatant fraction of the homogenate. Still other studies have shown gallium to be bound in tumor tissue (hepatomas) to a 45,000 molecular weight macromolecule that has a much greater avidity for Ga-67 than does normal liver.[25]

The mechanism of localization of gallium at sites of inflammation is likewise unclear. It has been hypothesized that Ga-67 may bind to leukocytes that subsequently migrate to the inflammatory lesion or Ga-67 binds to leukocytes that have already localized in the lesion. Both mechanisms are possible. It is postulated that Ga-67 bound to transferrin passes into the leukocyte where it is bound to intracellular lactoferrin.[26] This mechanism is supported by the greater avidity of gallium for lactoferrin than for transferrin.[27] The presence of lactoferrin in high concentration in neutrophilic leukocytes and the presence of this protein in abscess fluid suggest that it plays some role in the process.[26] Because a variety of microorganisms take up gallium, it is also possible that the high local concentration of bacteria in the abscess is partly responsible for gallium localization.[28-30]

Additional experimental studies suggest that other intracellular iron-binding substances besides lactoferrin may also be responsible for Ga-67 localization in abscesses. Ferritin, the intracellular iron storage protein, and siderophores, iron-binding molecules synthesized by bacteria for assimilating iron, have been shown to have an affinity for Ga-67. Equilibrium dialysis experiments suggest that the relative affinities of Ga-67 for the various molecules are siderophores > ferritin > lactoferrin > transferrin.[31] These findings, along with studies demonstrating that indium chloride In-111, known to label plasma transferrin and to localize in abscesses,[32] suggest that Ga-67 is transported to an abscess bound to plasma transferrin and that translocation of Ga-67 to the abscess is mediated by the higher binding affinity of Ga-67 with bacterial siderophores, macrophage ferritin, and polymorphonuclear lactoferrin.[31]

Gallium Dosage Forms

Ga-67 citrate is supplied by several commercial manufacturers in single-dose or multiple-dose serum vials as a sterile, isotonic, pyrogen-free solution for injection. It is available in several activity sizes per vial, typically in 3 mCi, 6 mCi, and 12 mCi, in a concentration of 2 mCi/ml as carrier-free Ga-67 containing sodium citrate and benzyl alcohol as a preservative. It may be stored at room temperature with no special precautions except for protective lead shields. The recommended adult dose is 2 to 5 mCi intravenously.

Ga-67 citrate is the only dosage form routinely used in nuclear medicine and sold commercially. Ionic gallium, however, readily undergoes chemical modification into other chemical forms. Gallium can be hydrolyzed to form radiocolloids for reticuloendothelial system (RES) imaging and chelated to form stable chelates such as Ga-EDTA. Weak chelates such as gallium oxine can be used to label blood cellular elements. These chemical forms of Ga-67 are not routinely used because similar chemical forms labeled with more suitable radionuclides for diagnostic imaging are available.

The production and use of gallium radiopharmaceuticals other than the citrate complex have been pursued with more interest by investigators with the capability of positron emission tomography (PET). In this regard, Ga-68 is of most interest.

Ga-68 Radiopharmaceuticals

Interest in producing Ga-68 radiopharmaceuticals began with the development of the Ge-68/Ga-68 generator in 1961.[3] The 68-minute Ga-68 could be obtained on demand from its 287-day half-life radionuclide parent Ge-68. This early generator contained Ge-68 adsorbed onto alumina (Al_2O_3). The Ga-68 was eluted with 0.005 M EDTA at pH 7. The eluate contained the chelate Ga-68-EDTA. Presently, a similar generator is available for research applications from New England Nuclear Corporation.

The bond between Ga-68 and EDTA is quite strong, and the rate of dissociation is apparently quite slow under neutral pH conditions. Methods have been developed, however, to release Ga-68 bound to EDTA by using strong acid and ion-exchange resin so that other chemical forms can be prepared.[33] In view of the somewhat technical involvement of these procedures, a new Ge-68/Ga-68 generator based on solvent extraction has been developed.[34] This generator produces the Ga-68 oxine chelate. It is a labile complex that can be readily converted to other radiopharmaceuticals such as Ga-68 EDTA, Ga-68 colloid, and Ga-68-labeled blood cells.[34]

Ga-68, being a proton-rich nuclide with a transition energy of 2.92 MeV, decays by positron emission and electron capture to stable Zn-68. Its principal photon emissions are annihilation radiation of 511 keV (178 percent) and a gamma ray at 1.08 MeV (3.2 percent).

Ga-68 radiopharmaceuticals are not used in routine nuclear medicine and find most application in facilities that have PET capabilities.

Radiation Dosimetry of Gallium

The radiation absorbed dose to various organs from Ga-67 and Ga-68 are shown in Table 14–2. The critical organ is the large intestine. The radiation dose from Ga-68 is less than that from Ga-67 because of a shorter half-life, but not so appreciably less because of its positron decay.

Altered Biodistribution of Ga-67 Citrate

A number of drugs have been associated with altered biodistribution of gallium. These processes have been reviewed by Hladik et al[36] and Lentle et al.[37] The most noteworthy examples involve the influence that stable carrier gallium and other metal ions have on the distribution of tracer amounts of Ga-67. In general, gallium, scandium, and iron can saturate Ga-67 binding sites on plasma transferrin and cause increased urinary excretion of Ga-67 and a shift in localization from soft tissue to bone. Iron dextran has been shown to increase the abscess-to-muscle ratio in abscess-bearing rabbits only if it is administered after the Ga-67 dose. Coadministration of iron dextran with Ga-67 led to poorer ratios when compared with control animals. Post-administration of iron apparently allows Ga-67 to localize adequately in abscess sites but displaces it from plasma protein sites, thus leading to increased renal excretion. Similar results occur if deferoxamine is administered in lieu of iron dextrin, except that increased renal excretion is promoted by chelation of gallium with deferoxamine.

Chemotherapeutic agents have been observed to alter the biodistribution of radiogallium. Methotrexate simulates the effect of metal ions mentioned earlier, presumably through elevating serum iron levels by temporarily inhibiting incorporation of iron into erythrocytes. Chilton et al proposed that an increased number of gallium-binding sites in the serum are occupied by iron after administration of methotrexate.[38] Other drugs such as mechlorethamine and vincristine and irradiation also produce similar effects on Ga-67, perhaps through a similar mechanism.

Other drugs have been associated with maldistribution of radiogallium. The anticonvulsant drug phenytoin, which is known to initiate various alterations in lymphoid tissue, has been implicated in the lymphoma-like pattern of Ga-67 distribution in patients without lymphadenopathy who were receiving anticonvulsant therapy at the time of imaging.[36] Steroids are reported to suppress radiogallium localization in central nervous system (CNS) tumors,[39] presumably by decreasing interstitial fluid. Abnormal lung uptake of radiogallium has been seen in patients who were receiving cyclophosphamide, vincristine, busulfan, and bleomycin, drugs known to cause interstitial pulmonary fibrosis.

TABLE 14-2. RADIATION ABSORBED DOSE FROM Ga-67 and Ga-68 ADMINISTERED AS A SINGLE IV DOSE OF GALLIUM CITRATE

Tissue	(rad/mCi Injected)	
	Ga-67	Ga-68
Stomach	0.22	0.042
Small intestine	0.36	0.21
Upper large intestine	0.56	0.23
Lower large intestine	0.90	0.094
Ovaries	0.28	0.048
Testes	0.24	0.039
Kidneys	0.41	0.089
Liver	0.46	0.096
Marrow	0.58	0.10
Skeleton[a]	0.44	0.094
Spleen	0.53	0.13
Total body	0.26	0.052

[a]Skeleton, bone and marrow.
(Data from MIRD Report No. 2, 1973, p. 755.[35])

INDIUM RADIOPHARMACEUTICALS

In the early 1960s research efforts were directed toward the production of radiopharmaceuticals labeled with short-lived radionuclides to be able to administer larger amounts of activity. The intent was to improve image quality while at the same time reducing the radiation dose to the patient. One of the radionuclides investigated at that time was In-113m. It had several advantages: decay by isomeric transition, emission of a 390-keV gamma ray, 1.7-hour half-life, and availability from a generator as the daughter product of 115-day Sn-113 (Fig. 14-6). Elution from the Sn-113/In-113m generator with 0.05 M HCl yields an eluate of about pH 1.5 containing trivalent ionic indium, In^{3+}, and about 91 percent as the mono- and dichloro complexes $In(H_2O)_5Cl^{2+}$ and $In(H_2O)_4Cl_2^+$.[40] The cationic indium readily forms chelates, which is an advantage over Tc-99m, which must be reduced to a cationic species of lower valence before chelation occurs.

When the acidic eluate from the In-113m generator is injected intravenously, the indium quickly binds to plasma transferrin to form a blood pool agent. Early applications of In-113m transferrin were for brain imaging, cardiac blood pool studies, and localization of the placenta in the evaluation of placenta previa.[41-43]

Additional radiopharmaceuticals developed with radioindium were radiocolloids for RES imaging and macroaggregates for lung imaging.[44-47] The chloro complexes in the generator eluate readily hydrolyze at about pH 3; thus, the addition of a phosphate buffer to tracer concentrations of indium in the presence of gelatin stabilizer readily forms an indium phosphate colloid that can be used for RES imaging.[46,47] Macroaggregates for lung imaging can be made by incorporation of carrier indium chloride to form larger particles.[45] Initial experience with these indium

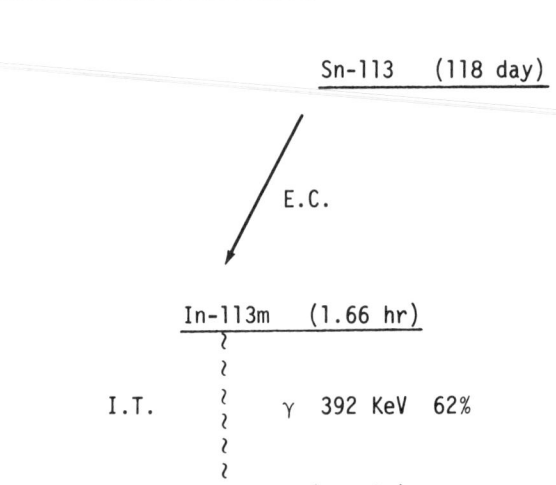

Figure 14-6. Schematic diagram of the decay process in the Sn-113/In-113 generator.

hydroxide aggregates in animals, however, demonstrated tissue toxicity that was associated with the indium. Subsequently, aggregates were prepared using ferric chloride as the carrier in which case the indium tracer coprecipitated with the iron hydroxide macroaggregates. These aggregates contained only trace amounts of indium and were found to be significantly less toxic and safe to use in clinical studies.

In 1967 a complex of In-113m DTPA was first reported for use in brain imaging.[41] This stable complex had the advantage over In-113m transferrin of more rapid blood clearance. Although the In-DTPA complex has a high stability constant ($k = 10^{28}$), its rate of formation is somewhat slow.[40] Above pH 3 the formation of insoluble indium hydroxide competes with and retards the formation of In-DTPA. Several methods have been used to prepare In-DTPA, but a simple effective technique is to add the acidic indium solution to a pH 4 solution of DTPA in the presence of acetate.[48] The rate of formation of indium acetate is quite rapid and prevents the formation of indium hydroxide as the pH is raised. The stability constant for In-acetate ($k = 10^3$), however, is such that ligand exchange can occur, which favors the eventual formation of In-DTPA.

During the years of their development the use of In-113m radiopharmaceuticals was primarily limited to larger research-type hospitals that had the expertise to prepare these agents. Although kit methods of preparation were eventually developed, their widespread general application in hospitals was not achieved. This was in part due to the simultaneous development of Tc-99m radiopharmaceuticals and kits since Tc-99m had more desirable decay properties for imaging with the gamma camera. One principal advantage of In-113m, however, was that it could be quite useful in regions of the world where routine delivery was a problem. In this regard, the 6-month shelf life of the Sn-113/In-113m generator was a desirable advantage.

The knowledge and experience gained with In-113m radiopharmaceuticals can be readily applied to other indium radionuclides having more favorable decay properties. One such nuclide is In-111. Of course, the same chemical forms developed with In-113m can be prepared with In-111 but with wider application.[49] The useful forms that have achieved the most interest in nuclear medicine are In-111 chloride, In-111 DTPA, and In-111 oxine-labeled blood cells.

Physical Properties of In-111

Figure 14-7 illustrates the decay scheme for In-111. As a proton-rich nuclide, In-111 decays by electron capture to stable cad-

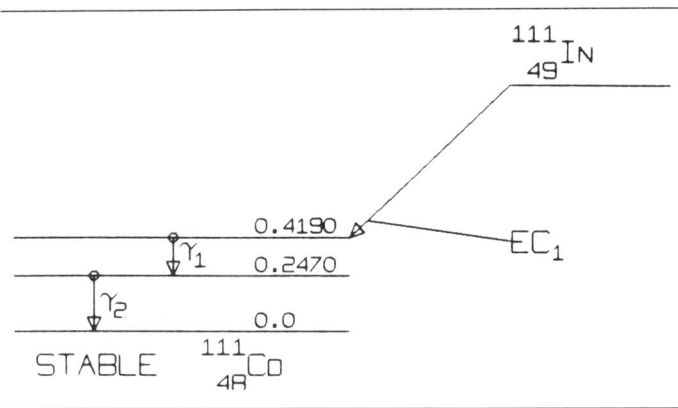

Figure 14-7. Decay scheme of In-111. *(From Dillman DT, Von der Lage FC: MIRD Pamphlet No. 10. New York, Society of Nuclear Medicine, 1975, with permission.)*

mium-111 with a transition energy of 0.863 MeV. Positron decay does not occur. The half-life of In-111 is 2.81 days. The most prominent photon energies and abundances are γ-1, 172 keV (91 percent); and γ-2, 247 keV (94 percent). The specific gamma ray constant for In-111 is 3.3 R/hr/mCi at 1 cm, and the half-value layer in lead is 0.021 cm.

In-111 Chloride

In-111 is produced in a cyclotron by bombarding a cadmium metal target with 22- to 12-MeV protons according to the nuclear reaction[112] $Cd(p,2n)^{111}$ In.[50] The irradiated target is dissolved in concentrated acid and subjected to several dissolution and extraction steps to remove iron and other impurities. The final HCl extracts are washed with isopropyl ether, evaporated to dryness, and dissolved in a desired volume of sterile, pyrogen-free 0.05 M HCl.[51]

In-111 chloride shares the same biologic properties after IV administration as those mentioned previously for In-113m chloride. Its usefulness, however, has been primarily as a starting material for the preparation of other radiopharmaceuticals because indium readily forms stable coordination complexes with many ligands. The direct intravenous administration of In-111 chloride has been used in the past to image the distribution of red marrow, but this has not achieved widespread clinical application. A recent report, however, has demonstrated its potential usefulness in the detection of abscesses.[32] The limited experience with In-111 chloride in this application, compared with In-111 leukocytes, demands that more extensive investigation and clinical confirmation of its specificity and predictive value be made.

In-111 DTPA

The DTPA complex with indium is prepared by adding high-purity In-111 chloride to about 2 ml of 0.05 M acetate buffer at pH 4 to 5. About 5 to 20 mg of DTPA is added and the pH adjusted to 5. The mixture is heated for 15 minutes in a boiling water bath to effect complexation. It is then cooled and purified by passing through a Sephadex G-25 column using 0.001 M DTPA in a saline eluant. The main impurity is hydrolyzed indium, which will either emerge in the void volume or remain on the column depending on particle size. Radiochemical purity is determined on Whatman No. 1 paper in 0.01 M DTPA in a saline solvent. The Rf for the DTPA complex is 0.8; hydrolyzed indium remains at the origin. The chemical structure of In-DTPA is shown in Figure 14–8.

Biologic Properties of In-111 DTPA. The biologic distribution of In-111 DTPA depends on its mode of administration. After IV administration In-111 DTPA is distributed and excreted similarly to Tc-99m DTPA, and the kinetics of its distribution are described in Chapter 12. In general, it leaves the plasma quickly and is distributed into the extracellular space and into the urine by glomerular filtration. Approximately 50 percent of the injected dose is in the urine by 1 hour, and only 4 to 5 percent remains in the body by 24 hours. The complex is quite stable and is excreted unchanged.

When administered intrathecally for cisternography it is transported in the cerebrospinal fluid (CSF) from the lumbar subarachnoid space to the basal cisterns and achieves peak concentration there by 4 hours. From this point it traverses around the hemispheres to the parasagittal region and is absorbed into the blood through the arachnoid villi. Greater detail of In-111 DTPA kinetics in the CSF can be found in Chapter 7.

In-111 Labeled Leukocytes

A great deal of interest has been generated over the past few years in the development of In-111 labeled blood cellular elements. Most of this interest has been directed toward the use of In-111 leukocytes for abscess localization. Before describing the preparation and properties of this diagnostic agent, a brief review of leukocyte proper-

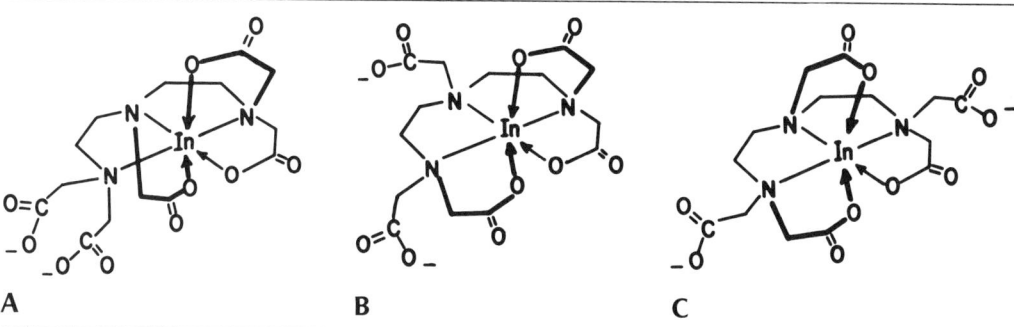

Figure 14-8. Possible structural configurations of In-DTPA in radiopharmaceutical solutions. An equilibrium mixture of various species (**A**, **B**, and **C**) may be present depending on pH, metal and ligand concentrations, competing ions, and reaction kinetics. The arrows emphasize that oxygen carries a negative charge.

ties and the inflammatory response will be made.

Leukocytes and the Inflammatory Process. The adult human has approximately 7000 white blood cells (WBC) per mm^3 of blood. These WBCs comprise polymorphonuclear neutrophils (62 percent), eosinophils (2.3 percent), and basophils (0.4 percent), collectively called polys. Because of the granular appearance of their cytoplasm they are also called granulocytes. The remaining WBCs are monocytes (5.3 percent) and lymphocytes (30 percent).

The life span of WBCs in the blood is limited to the time necessary for their transport from their sites of production in bone marrow or lymphoid tissue to the areas of the body where they are needed. The life span of polys once released from marrow is normally 6 to 8 hours circulating in the blood and 2 to 3 days within the tissues. During serious infection this time is shortened to only a few hours because the polys proceed rapidly to the infected area. Monocytes also have a short life in blood but may exist in the tissues as macrophages for months. Lymphocytes can have a prolonged life span, many having a lifetime of 100 to 300 days or even years. They cyclically enter the blood along with the drainage of lymph from lymph nodes, remain in blood a few hours, enter tissues by diapedesis, and then reenter the lymph, whereupon they return to the blood.

It is mainly the neutrophils and monocytes, however, that are involved in the inflammatory response to invading microorganisms.

An inflammatory response may be caused by localized injury resulting from any noxious stimulus or to a seemingly innocuous stimulus.[52] The first case may be characterized by bacterial infection or death of tissue, and the inflammatory reaction would include invasion by leukocytes and other cells at the site where the microcirculation survives. In the second case the reaction is characterized by the fact that the inflammatory response itself is the cause of tissue damage. Rheumatic and allergic diseases fall into this category.

Probably the most important cause of inflammation is bacterial invasion of the tissues; however, other types of injury such as thermal, chemical, or trauma induce a similar pattern of inflammatory reaction. This reaction is characterized by a vascular response that has associated with it a fluid phase and a cellular phase.

After the initial injury large quantities of histamine, bradykinin, and serotonin are liberated by the damaged tissue into the surrounding fluids. These substances cause localized increased blood flow and capillary permeability that allows large quantities of fluid and proteins to leak into the tissues producing localized edema. This constitutes the fluid phase. The presence of fibrinogen in the fluid produces a coagulation and clot formation that serves to "wall off" the injured area to delay the spread of bacteria and toxic products.

The cellular phase of the inflammatory response involves three stages. The first stage involves phagocytic activity by macrophages already present in the tissue, but their number is limited. The second stage is characterized by neutrophilia, sometimes referred to as leukocytosis. In this stage a large increase in circulating neutrophils occurs in the blood, stimulated by the release of chemical substances in the inflamed tissues. The number of neutrophils in the blood can increase to 15,000 to 25,000 per mm^3 within a few hours after the onset of inflammation. The neutrophils migrate to the inflamed area and enter the tissue by diapedesis through the porous capillary walls. The bacterial toxins and cellular products attract the neutrophils (chemotaxis) and cause them to adhere to the inflamed tissue, whereupon they exert their phagocytic function engulfing bacteria and cellular debris. The third stage is a slower but longer-lasting response in the defense against infection. In this stage monocytes released from the marrow migrate to the injured area and over a period of 8 to 12 hours undergo a marked degree of swelling and develop increased quantities of lysosomes. These mature monocytes then act as efficient macrophages, moving with ameboid-like motion to inflamed areas to engulf and digest bacteria and cellular products. Leukocytes eventually die and collect in the area to form pus.

An abscess is a localized area of pus and destroyed tissue formed by the inflammatory response. It usually contains pathogenic bacteria, and if untreated, can become life threatening or lead to extended periods of morbidity and hospitalization. The localization of an abscess is often a difficult clinical problem. Because an abscess is a focal accumulation of leukocytes, it is logical to radiolabel leukocytes with gamma-emitting radionuclides that can be detected externally with a gamma camera.

Methods for Radiolabeling Leukocytes. Several attempts have been made to successfully label leukocytes for abscess detection. These methods have been reviewed and studied extensively by McAfee and Thakur[53,54] who examined both soluble and particulate agents for labeling phagocytic leukocytes. Their study identified several problems with the use of radionuclide particles for labeling leukocytes, the principal one involving the difficulty in separating surface adherent and free particles from those engulfed by the cells. Investigation of soluble labeling agents demonstrated that only nonpolar, lipid-soluble chelates labeled cells to a significant degree. Although some of these chelates eluted from the cell, In-111 oxine remained bound to the cells as an effective label; however, because all types of blood cells are labeled with indium oxine, it is necessary to separate and isolate the blood cellular elements before radiolabeling to achieve a specific cell label. The labeling of leukocytes requires the preparation of In-111 oxine, which is then incubated with leukocytes that have been previously separated from whole blood. There are a number of technical problems that have been identified with this whole process, some of which have been solved whereas others have been mitigated to an acceptable degree. These problems with leukocyte labeling will be addressed in the subsequent discussion and include the following: (1) loss of protective plasma proteins during labeling, (2) morphologic changes in cells caused by ethanol, (3) oxine toxicity, (4) trace metal (Zn, Fe, Cd, Cu) interference with indium oxine labeling, (5) mechanical damage to cells during centrifugation, and (6) problems with complete cell separation in whole blood.

Although In-111 oxine has achieved the most attention in leukocyte labeling, other complexes of indium have been used to label cells.[55,56] Acetylacetone and tropolone form 3:1 ligand-to-metal complexes with indium; they also have a nonpolar lipophilic character capable of penetrating cell membranes. The advantage claimed for use of these complexes is that they are water soluble as opposed to the ethanol-based oxine complex. Use of these water-soluble complexes suggests a decreased chance of inducing cell toxicity from ethanol or oxine, although studies indicate that neither cell viability, structure, nor function of polymorphonucleocytes (PMNs) is significantly altered by the standard labeling procedure, namely, 2 to 5 μCi In-111 per million PMNs; 0.1 to 1.0 μg oxine per million cells (1 to 10 μg/ml of cell suspension); and 1.2 to 4 mg ethanol per milliliter of suspension.[57] Ethanol concentrations of up to 80 mg per million PMNs and radioactivity of up to 29 μCi per million PMNs have shown no appreciable effects on random migration and chemotaxis. Both of these parameters of cell viability, however, are significantly reduced at oxine concentrations of 10 μg or more per million PMNs, and at 25 μg oxine per million PMNs random migration is reduced to 20 percent and chemotaxis to 8 percent of the control values.[57]

McAfee and Thakur chose to use the indium oxine complex over indium acetylacetone because the latter complex tended to elute from leukocytes and demonstrated a higher degree of erythrocyte labeling.[53] Although successful claims have been made for the use of these three complexes for labeling cells, the choice of which one to use remains somewhat controversial.[58,59] A commercial indium oxine solution free of ethanol is available for labeling leukocytes and platelets[60] and contains 50 μg oxine/ml dissolved in HEPES–saline buffer with polysorbate 80.

Higher labeling yields are achieved with the lipophilic indium complexes if cells are labeled in the absence of plasma, but cell viability may be affected. Labeling yields are significantly lower in the presence of plasma because indium dissociates from the weaker complexes in favor of the more tightly bound indium transferrin. For these reasons a compromise is made by some investigators to concentrate the cells to be labeled in the presence of a small amount of plasma.[56] In this way the large number of cells can more effectively compete with plasma transferrin for the indium complex while at the same time providing greater protection of cell viability. This technique has been used more in the labeling of platelets than of leukocytes. Experience has demonstrated satisfactory clinical utility with leukocytes labeled with indium oxine in the absence of plasma, and this appears to be the method of choice.

In-111 Oxine. In-111 oxine (8-hydroxyquinoline) is a 1:3 indium-to-oxine neutral complex whose structure is shown in Figure 14–9. Its preparation is based upon the method described by Thakur et al.[61] The glassware used should be scrupulously cleaned in acid and rinsed in triple-distilled water to remove all traces of metal ions (Fe, Cd, Cu) that may interfere with the formation of the indium oxine complex.[62] To form the complex approximately 1 mCi of In-111-chloride is added to an equal volume of sterile water and 200 μl of 0.3 M acetate buffer at pH 5.0. Fifty micrograms of ox-

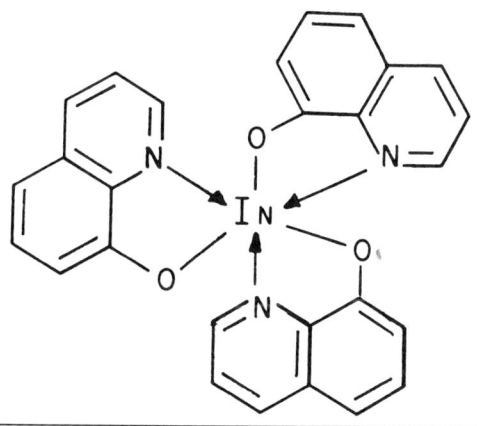

Figure 14–9. Structure of indium oxine.

ine in ethanol (1 mg oxine/1 ml absolute ethanol) is added and mixed. The complex forms immediately and is extracted into an equal volume of chloroform or methylene chloride. The chloroform layer is removed and evaporated to dryness in a 60 °C water bath over a stream of nitrogen gas to facilitate evaporation. The dried chelate of In-111 oxine is dissolved in 100 μl of ethanol and diluted to 500 μl with normal saline.

Alternatively, In-111 oxine that is not prepared as just described can be purchased from commercial suppliers ready for use in cell labeling.

Leukocyte Separation and Labeling. An important consideration in the labeling of leukocytes with indium is the method of separation and isolation of leukocytes from whole blood. Because red cells and platelets are also labeled with indium oxine and have longer survival in the circulation, it is important that as many of these cellular components be removed as possible. Additionally, it is necessary to maintain leukocyte viability if adequate abscess localization is to be achieved in vivo. Although in vitro testing of labeled leukocytes had demonstrated no significant damage to these cells, in vivo distribution studies show otherwise, with significant localization of labeled cells in the lung, liver, and spleen.[61] These cells should therefore be handled gently with as few manipulations as possible. Additionally, it should be pointed out that all separation and labeling procedures be conducted in a sterile air environment in a laminar air flow hood.

Several techniques have been used to separate leukocytes from whole blood.[63] The most popular method is gravity sedimentation. Accordingly, whole blood is allowed to stand at room temperature to allow the red cells to settle out. In some instances a sedimenting agent such as hydroxyethyl starch[64] or methylcellulose[65] is used. The former agent is preferred because it is Food and Drug Administration (FDA) approved for human use. These agents promote aggregation of red cells thus speeding up their settling rate. The sedimenting agent is omitted by some investigators in patients with leukocytosis who have an elevated sedimentation rate.[66] Additionally, cells that undergo the trauma of further purification have decreased viability.[67] In the earlier development stages of leukocyte labeling, more rigorous techniques were used to separate red cells and platelets from white cells. Methods were even used to isolate neutrophils from monocytes and lymphocytes. The current approach to cell labeling, however, accepts a level of erythrocyte and platelet contamination in the final product that is considered to be too low a concentration to interfere with the nuclear physician's ability to diagnose a marginal true positive in cases of suspected abscess.[68] The small amount (approximately 5 percent) of red cells in the product gives it a pink hue but presents little disadvantage in the labeling process because of the high concentration of white cells.

Several methods have been reported in the literature for preparing In-111 leukocytes. A typical method used will now be described to illustrate the basic technique. This method is summarized in Figure 14–10.

1. Collect 30 to 50 ml of venous blood in a 60-ml syringe with a 19-gauge needle and 1 ml of 1000 U/ml preservative-free heparin.
2. Remove any blood from the syringe tip, clamp the syringe to a ring stand in a laminar air flow hood with the needle end up, and allow the red cells to settle for 45 to 60 minutes. About 5 ml of 6 percent hetastarch may be added to speed up the settling rate.
3. After settling, the upper layer, the leukocyte-rich plasma (LRP) containing 50 to 70 percent of the leukocyte content of whole blood, can be demarcated from the lower red cell layer.
4. Place a 19-gauge butterfly set on the syringe and slowly express the LRP (slightly pink colored) into sterile plastic tubes, collecting 20 to 25 ml.

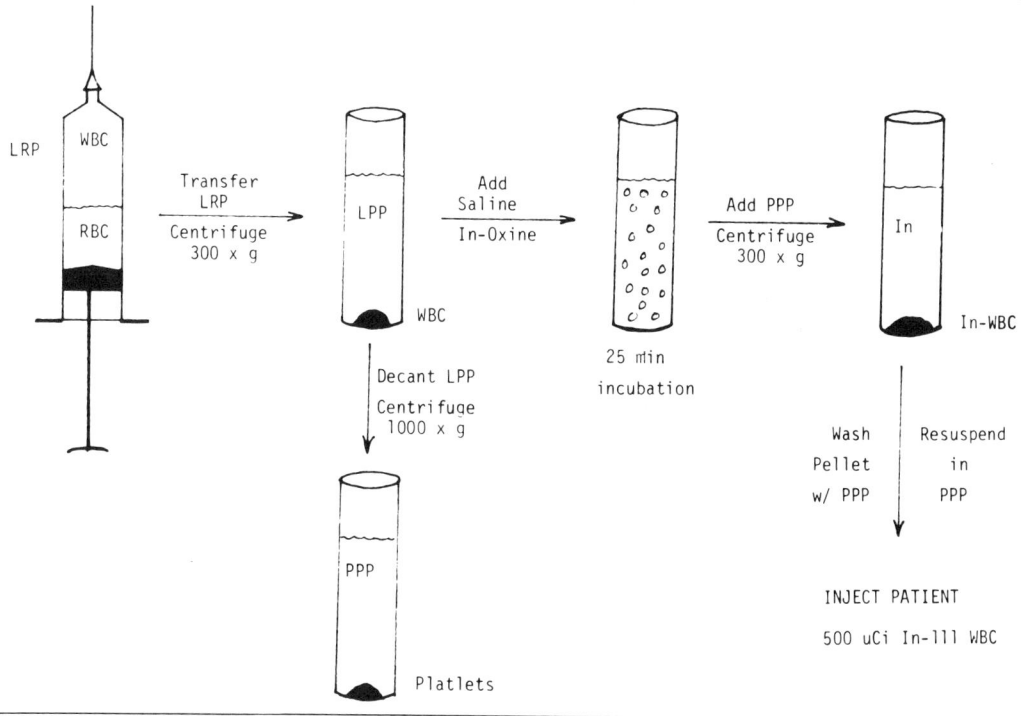

Figure 14-10. Diagram depicting the various steps involved in the preparation of In-111 oxine labeled leukocytes.

5. Spin the LRP in a centrifuge at 300 g for 5 minutes to obtain a leukocyte pellet.
6. Draw off the leukocyte-poor plasma (LPP) and transfer it to fresh plastic tubes. Centrifuge at 1000 g for 15 minutes to separate the platelets. Draw off the platelet-poor plasma (PPP) and save for future use.
7. Resuspend the leukocyte button from step 5 in 5 ml normal saline. Mix gently to disperse the cells.
8. Add dropwise 0.5 to 1.0 mCi In-111 oxine to the leukocyte suspension. Mix gently and incubate at room temperature (approximately 25°C) for 20 minutes.
9. After incubation add 5 ml PPP (from step 7) to the cell suspension. The plasma transferrin in PPP will bind up any indium not labeled to the leukocytes.
10. Centrifuge this cell–plasma mixture at 300 g for 5 minutes. Draw off the supernatant and place into a test tube.
11. Gently layer 2 ml PPP on to the labeled white cells without disturbing the button. Remove this PPP and add it to the supernatant from step 10.
12. Resuspend the labeled white cells in 5 ml PPP.
13. Determine labeling yield by radioassay of the In-111 activity in the tubes from step 12 and steps 10 and 11.

Labeling Efficiency and Viability of In-111 Labeled Leukocytes. The fraction of In-111 activity that is associated with leukocytes after labeling varies and depends, in part, on the concentration of cells and the amount of plasma present in the labeling mixture. Thakur et al showed that the labeling yield of leukocytes increased linearly from approximately 35 to 75 percent as the number of cells increased from 3.6×10^6 to 1.3×10^7, respectively.[61] Using an average of 10^8 cells, Goodwin et al achieved a labeling efficiency of 84 ± 9 percent, and in patients with white counts above $15,000/mm^3$ in peripheral blood, it was usually 90 percent or more.[69] Coleman et al reported a 34 percent labeling efficiency in dilute plasma compared with 87 percent in saline.[66] Normal adult whole blood contains 7000 white cells per cubic millimeter or $7 \times 10^6/ml$.

The effects of labeling on leukocyte viability in vitro and in vivo have been measured. As mentioned previously, in vitro testing has shown no significant effects resulting from typical labeling conditions.[57] Cell recovery, as measured by the percentage of administered dose associated with the white cells circulating in the blood after reinjection of labeled leukocytes, has given some measure of in vivo behavior. Disappearance half-times have also been measured and these data summarized.[70] The highest recovery and best disappearance half-time of labeled leukocytes in humans using tritiated thymidine has been 58 percent and 7.6 hours, respectively. The remaining 42 percent is assumed to be in the marginated pool and does not contribute to the blood samples withdrawn. The recovery using DFP-32 labeled granulocytes has been 40 to 50 percent and the disappearance half-time 5.4 hours. With In-111 oxine-labeled granulocytes, the intravascular recovery is 30 percent, and the disappearance half-time is 5.0 hours. Thakur et al found a disappearance half-time of 7.5 hours by using a mixed population of leukocytes.[67] Goodwin et al obtained a 7.1-hour half-time and a recovery of 38 percent.[69] The recovery of In-111 leukocytes is thus less than that obtained by tritiated thymidine and DFP-32-labeled leukocytes, and the disappearance half-time is similar. This discrepancy may be due to temporary sequestration of In-111 leukocytes in tissue with subsequent release (i.e., from lung), contamination with red cells or platelets that have a longer circulation time, or reutilization of In-111 by blood components.

Mechanism of Leukocyte Labeling with In-111 Oxine. Indium forms a saturated complex with oxine that is neutral and lipid soluble and capable of penetrating plasma cell membranes. The estimated stability constant of the indium–oxine complex is quite low (1×10^{10}) relative to indium complexes with other substances such as transferrin (1×10^{30}).[61] The labeling mechanism of indium oxine with leukocytes has been examined in vitro.[71] These studies indicate that greater than 95 percent of indium oxine is taken up by neutrophils within 15 minutes' incubation at room temperature. When the labeled cells are incubated in either plasma or saline for 2 hours, less than 1 percent of the indium activity elutes from the cells. Some of the oxine, however, does elute from the cell and quite quickly reaches a maximum in 5 minutes. The indium activity is distributed within the cystosol fraction of the cell bound to several components of varying molecular weight. Only about 3 percent of the indium activity is still bound to oxine.

These data suggest that the indium oxine complex efficiently penetrates the neutrophil membrane, whereupon the indium is displaced from oxine by intracellular components with higher binding affinities for the indium. Some of the released oxine readily diffuses out of the cell, but the indium remains within the cell because of its tight association with larger molecular weight substances. These processes are summarized in Figure 14–11.

Biologic Distribution and Radiation Dosimetry of In-111 Labeled Leukocytes. Factors that primarily influence the tissue distribution and blood clearance of In-111 leukocytes in humans include the method of

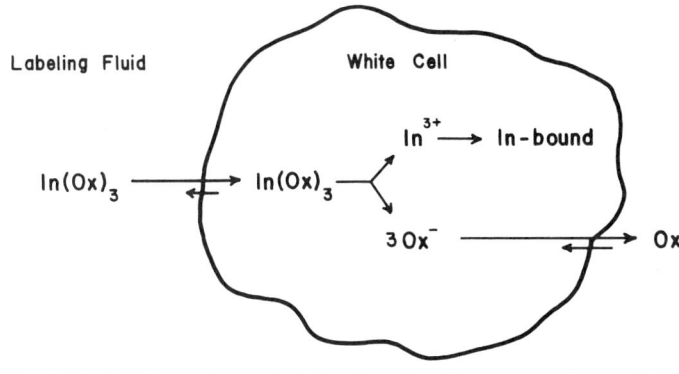

Figure 14-11. Diagram illustrating the proposed mechanism involved in the labeling of leukocytes with indium oxine.

cell labeling and the pathologic condition of the patient. In general, after intravenous injection, activity is immediately distributed throughout the lung where it remains transiently. Half of this lung activity clears within 15 minutes and is no longer present by 4 hours.[67] Activity is distributed subsequently to the spleen, liver, and bone marrow, and the concentration of activity in these organs remains essentially unchanged for up to 48 hours except for the physical decay of In-111.[67] Urinary excretion is essentially insignificant. The blood clearance half-time appears to be influenced by the method of cell separation. Leukocytes separated by gravity sedimentation and containing about 5 percent red cells have the longest half-time, ranging from 12 to 21 hours. When red cells are removed by hypotonic lysis, the half-time is decreased to 7.5 hours. If cells are purified further by Ficoll–sodium metrizoate gradient separation to obtain pure neutrophils, the half-time is shortened to 4.5 hours. This is caused by cell damage during separation because cell viability decreased to 45 percent compared with 75 percent viability of mixed cells.[67]

Estimated measurements of organ concentration of indium activity varies. Thakur et al reported that 25 to 50 percent of the administered dose is distributed in the spleen, liver, and bone marrow, with the amount varying according to method of cell labeling and patient condition.[67] Goodwin et al estimated that about 20 percent of the administered dose localized in the spleen, 20 percent in the liver, and 60 percent in the bone marrow regardless of whether the patients were normal or had abscesses.[72] Based upon this distribution the radiation dose estimates from 500 μCi of In-111 leukocytes are as follows: liver, 1.4 rad; spleen, 8.5 rad; and bone marrow, 2.3 rad.[72]

Localization of inflammatory sites may be visible at 4 hours, but diagnostic evaluation is routinely made at 18 to 24 hours after dose administration of 200 to 500 μCi. When In-111 leukocytes and Ga-67 citrate were compared by simultaneous injection into dogs with chemical or bacterial abscesses, a much higher abscess-to-muscle activity ratio was obtained with leukocytes (3000:1) than Ga-67 (72:1) for bacterial abscesses.[73]

Radiation Dose to Lymphocytes. Soon after the development of In-111-labeled leukocytes, attention was directed toward the real possibility of mutagenic effects developing from labeled lymphocytes.[74] This concern was founded in the fact that lymphocytes, which constitute 20 to 30 percent of the leukocyte population, are also labeled and are, by nature, more susceptible to radiation damage than any other circulating blood cells. Additionally, lymphocytes are long-living cells and may after years undergo malignant transformations in the body as a result of genetic aberrations induced by absorbed radiation. Lymphocytes play many critical roles in the immune system, and differentiated cells may carry immunologic memory for many years. Upon interaction with specific antigens, these cells undergo transformation, or blastogenesis, dividing into more cells with the same specific function including replication of DNA.[75] The information on this subject has been reviewed and summarized by Thakur and McAfee.[75] Their review points out that a number of factors contribute to the incidence of chromosome aberrations in lymphocytes such as an increase in age, drugs, radiation, and toxic environmental chemicals found in food, air, and water. With regard to the influence of cell labeling, limited studies[74] have demonstrated that at a concentration of 30 µCi of In-111 per 100 million lymphocytes, 54 percent of cells become abnormal, and at 80 to 90 µCi per 100 million cells, 90 to 92 percent were abnormal, equivalent to changes produced by 200 rad of x-radiation. At 150 µCi per 100 million lymphocytes, although 93 percent of the cells had abnormal chromosomes, their proliferative capacity in cultures was reduced only 50 percent. This does not mean, however, as Thakur et al point out, that in vitro proliferation can be equated to malignant transformation in vivo. At 300 µCi per 100 million cells, all lymphocytes were abnormal. Typical In-111 oxine labeling procedures involve the use of 500 µCi per 100 million leukocytes (containing 20 to 30 million lymphocytes), and therefore it is expected that all of these labeled lymphocytes will be abnormal. Under these conditions, In-111 lymphocytes should receive 8750 rad based on radiation dose estimates,[75] which is an excessive dose for lymphocyte killing.[76] Other substantiating studies have shown that lymphocytes receiving 300 to 380 rad during extracorporeal shunt irradiation of blood before renal transplantation had a mean residence time in the blood of only 2 minutes.[75]

Based upon these data it was concluded that chromosome damage occurs in lymphocytes labeled with radionuclides but that it was relatively insignificant compared with damage induced by other environmental causes and that the risk from lymphoid malignancy is small.[75] Furthermore, under the usual radiolabeling conditions with In-111 in mixed leukocyte preparations, the lymphocytes that are labeled are killed by the radiation and therefore pose no long-term risk.

In-111 LABELED PLATELETS

With the recognition of the importance of platelets in thrombosis and atherogenesis, there has been increasing interest in methods for radiolabeling and studying platelet behavior in vivo, particularly for localizing sites of actively forming thrombi.

Platelet Formation and Function

Platelets are round or oval disks about 2 µm in diameter. They are fragments of megakaryocytes formed in the bone marrow that disintegrate into platelets. The platelets are released into the blood and have a normal concentration between 200,000 and 400,000 per cubic millimeter.

Platelets circulate freely in the blood, but when they come into contact with a damaged vascular surface, they change their character. Collagen fibers in the vessel wall stimulate platelets and cause them to swell and become sticky. The platelets stick to the collagen fibers and secrete large quantities of adenosine diphosphate (ADP) and enzymes that cause the formation of thromboxane A in the plasma. These substances activate other platelets and cause them to stick to the damaged vessel also. A platelet plug forms that becomes the site for the coagulation process to occur, involving clotting factors, thrombin, and a fibrin clot.

Platelet Labeling

There are several reported methods for separating platelets from whole blood and labeling them with In-111.[77-80] Platelets are extremely sensitive to physical trauma, and their separation from whole blood must be done with care to maintain their viability. The anticoagulant used most frequently is acid-citrate-dextrose (ACD) solution in a ratio of six parts whole blood to one part ACD to give a final pH of about 6.5. This is optimal for handling platelets because aggregation is inhibited at an acidic pH.[77] Heparin should not be used to anticoagulate blood because it promotes platelet aggregation.

Before labeling platelets with In-111 the radiolabel used was chromium-51. Chromium is an unsatisfactory label, however, because of its poor decay properties and a low labeling efficiency (6 to 12 percent) which necessitates using a large volume of blood (200 to 500 ml) for labeling.[80] In-111, on the other hand, labels platelets with high efficiency (generally greater than 75 percent), requires only 50 ml of whole blood, and has adequate decay properties for thrombus detection[78] and for studying platelet kinetics in vivo.[80]

Several of the concerns mentioned previously in the discussion of In-111 leukocyte labeling are also important with platelet labeling. Most investigators believe that removal of all plasma by washing the platelet button is essential to ensure high labeling efficiency. There is generally good preservation of both in vivo and in vitro platelet function after platelet labeling in plasma-free media.[81] Others, however, believe that labeling in plasma is essential for consistent preservation of platelet function[78,82] and that labeling efficiency, albeit reduced, is still adequate (27 to 67 percent). Adequate time must be allowed for high labeling efficiency (typically 15 to 20 minutes) because the transfer of the indium–oxine complex into the platelets occurs by passive diffusion.[77] Finally, there is controversy regarding the type of ligand used to complex In-111: oxine, acetylacetone, or tropolone. The available data suggest that there is little difference in toxicity to platelets between the first two agents[83] and that the use of tropolone appears to be satisfactory also but requires further investigation.[79] The labeled platelets appear to be viable, and very little elution of indium occurs either in vivo or in vitro.[81] Moreover, In-111 is not released by stimuli sufficient to degranulate the labeled platelets.[81] In vivo recovery with In-111 is consistently higher than with Cr-51, and reutilization appears to be nil.[80] Figure 14–12 is a detailed flow chart of a method for labeling platelets with In-111 oxine.[77]

Use of In-111 Labeled Platelets

The principal use of In-111 labeled platelets has been for measuring platelet kinetics, investigating platelet–vessel wall interactions in vivo, and detecting deep venous thrombosis. The latter has particular interest in nuclear medicine although the clinical investigations to date have not been very encouraging.[77] Fresh venous thrombi have been imaged reliably with In-111 platelets as early as 4 hours after tracer injection, although 24 hours is the optimal imaging time. The detection of pulmonary emboli has been disappointing. It appears that old emboli and anticoagulant therapy are responsible for the poor detection rate. Lack of sensitivity in detecting formed thrombi appears to be the major limitation to clinical application of In-111 platelets.

Radiation Dose from In-111 Labeled Platelets

The most significant radiation exposure from In-111 platelets is to the spleen as a result of the prompt localization of 20 to 30 percent of radiolabeled platelets in this organ. The average radiation dose to the spleen is 26 rad/mCi, with a reported range of 24.6 to 33.6 rad.[77] For this reason the usual adult dose is limited to 500 µCi for the detection of venous thrombosis. Kinetic studies, however, require only 10 to 50 µCi.

I. COMPLEX FORMATION

a. 0.5–1.0 mCi In-111 chloride
  +
  50 µg oxine in 50 µl absolute ethanol
  +
  4 ml ACD:saline (1:7 V/V)

b. Adjust to pH 6.5

II. CITRATED PLASMA

a. 18 ml whole blood
  +
  2 ml 3.8% sodium citrate

b. Centrifuge at 180 x g for 15 min

c. Withdraw supernatant

d. Centrifuge at 1800 x g for 7 min

e. Withdraw and save supernatant

III. CELL SEPARATION AND LABELING

50 ml whole blood + ACD (6:1 V/V)

1
a. Centrifuge at 180 x g for 15 min
b. Remove supernatant
c. Discard red cells and white cells

Platelet-rich plasma

2
a. Centrifuge at 1800 x g for 7 min
b. Withdraw and save PPP
c. Wash with 4 ml ACD:saline to remove contaminating plasma
d. Centrifuge at 1800 x g for 7 min
e. Discard wash solution

Platelet Button

3
a. Add In-111 oxine complex from step Ib
b. Incubate 20 min at room temperature
c. Centrifuge at 1800 x g for 7 min
d. Withdraw supernatant

Labeled Platelets

4
a. Wash with 4 ml PPP from step 2b to remove loosely bound In-111
b. Centrifuge at 1800 x g for 7 min
c. Withdraw supernatant
d. Resuspend in 4 ml citrated plasma from step IIe

Labeled Platelet Injectate

Figure 14-12. Flow sheet diagram illustrating the labeling of platelets with indium-oxine. (From Cunningham DA, et al, 1982, p 143, with permission.[77])

Clinical Total Body Imaging

INTRODUCTION

Clinically, total-body imaging has been practiced for many years. For the most part, clinical indications have not changed, rather, indications have been added as new pharmaceutical uses and labeling techniques have developed. The basic clinical indications covered in this chapter are the detection and localization of malignancy and inflammation. Osseous changes, metastatic thyroid malignancy, marrow RES and erythropoiesis, and right-to-left vascular shunting are covered in the bone, thyroid, liver, and heart chapters respectively. The newest total body imaging indication is for monoclonal antibody localization.

GA-67 IMAGING

CLINICAL RATIONALE

The most common indication for Ga-67 imaging is now in the workup of the fever of unknown origin (FUO). Very often the FUO is found to be due to an occult abscess; however, not infrequently the cause is found to be a primary infection, e.g., a pneumonia, an infected wound, or an occult malignancy.

Malignancy is the next most common indication. Ga-67 was originally approved for use in humans on the basis of its efficacy for detection and staging of Hodgkin's and non-Hodgkin's lymphoma and lung cancer. Ga-67 is particularly useful for suspected lymphoma recurrence (Fig. 14-13). Its usefulness in the workup of other malignancies has been well documented; however, the use of x-ray computed tomography has foreshadowed the use of Ga-67 in many of these indications.

PROCEDURE

After the IV injection of Ga-67 citrate, early blood-phase images obtained at 1 to 24 hours may give the first evidence of an inflammatory lesion with its associated hypervascularity. At 48 hours the earliest optimum inflammatory lesion or malignancy concentration has usually been reached, and total-body images should be obtained. Images at 72 to 120 hours are generally obtained to follow the progress of Ga-67 concentrated in the bowel contents to differentiate that from abnormal concentrations in inflammation or malignancy. If at all possible, at least three of the four photon peaks should be imaged with a medium-energy collimator on a large field-of-view gamma camera.

PHARMACEUTICALS

The preferred form of Ga-67 is the citrate. Dosage may vary from 2 to 5 mCi IV for the adult patient and occasionally up to 8 mCi for malignancies or recurrent malignancies where the lesions are expected to be very small or single-photon emission computed tomography (SPECT) imaging techniques are used.

INTERPRETATION

Normally Ga-67 citrate is seen concentrating in the skeleton, liver, spleen, bowel, and bladder (Fig. 14-14). Occasionally it will also be seen in the lacrimal and salivary secretory glands, the breasts, and the kidneys. Concentration in the kidneys beyond 24 hours postinjection is abnormal. Kidney concentration bears explanation based on whether it is diffuse or focal and the patient's clinical condition. Breast concentra-

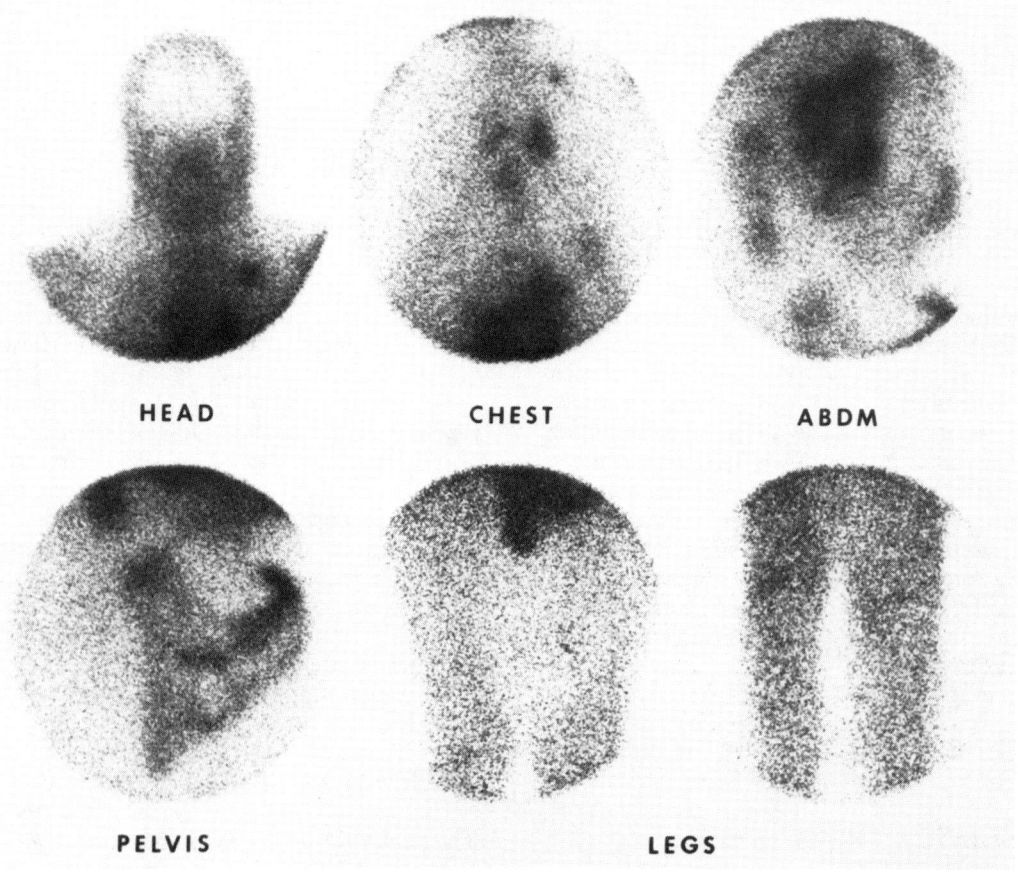

Figure 14-13. Lymphoma. Multiple areas of increased uptake are seen in the mediastinum and abdomen on this 24-hour gallium scan.

tion may be seen at menarche, with oral contraceptives or other female hormonal therapy, during pregnancy, and during postpartum lactation. Asymmetry bears explanation. Lacrimal or salivary concentration is usually due to a pathologic process.

Abscesses of a large size will usually show hypervascularity on the blood-phase images and intense concentration on the 48-hour or more images. Occult abscess as a cause of FUO may be localized with Ga-67 (Fig. 14–15). Malignant tumors and particularly small, deep metastases may be difficult to see on planar imaging. SPECT imaging has been advantageous for the latter. Hepatomas, which appeared as photon-deficient areas on Tc-99m sulfur colloid imaging, will appear to isoconcentrate or hyperconcentrate Ga-67 compared with the rest of the liver. Moreover, the difficulties with planar imaging in distinguishing bowel content concentration from abnormal foci in the abdomen or pelvis may be greatly alleviated by SPECT imaging of this area at 48 hours postinjection. SPECT images, under these circumstances, may precisely define the locations of concentration of Ga-67 to bowel lumen or nonlumen, e.g., pancreas, kidney, peritoneum, etc. (Fig. 14–16).

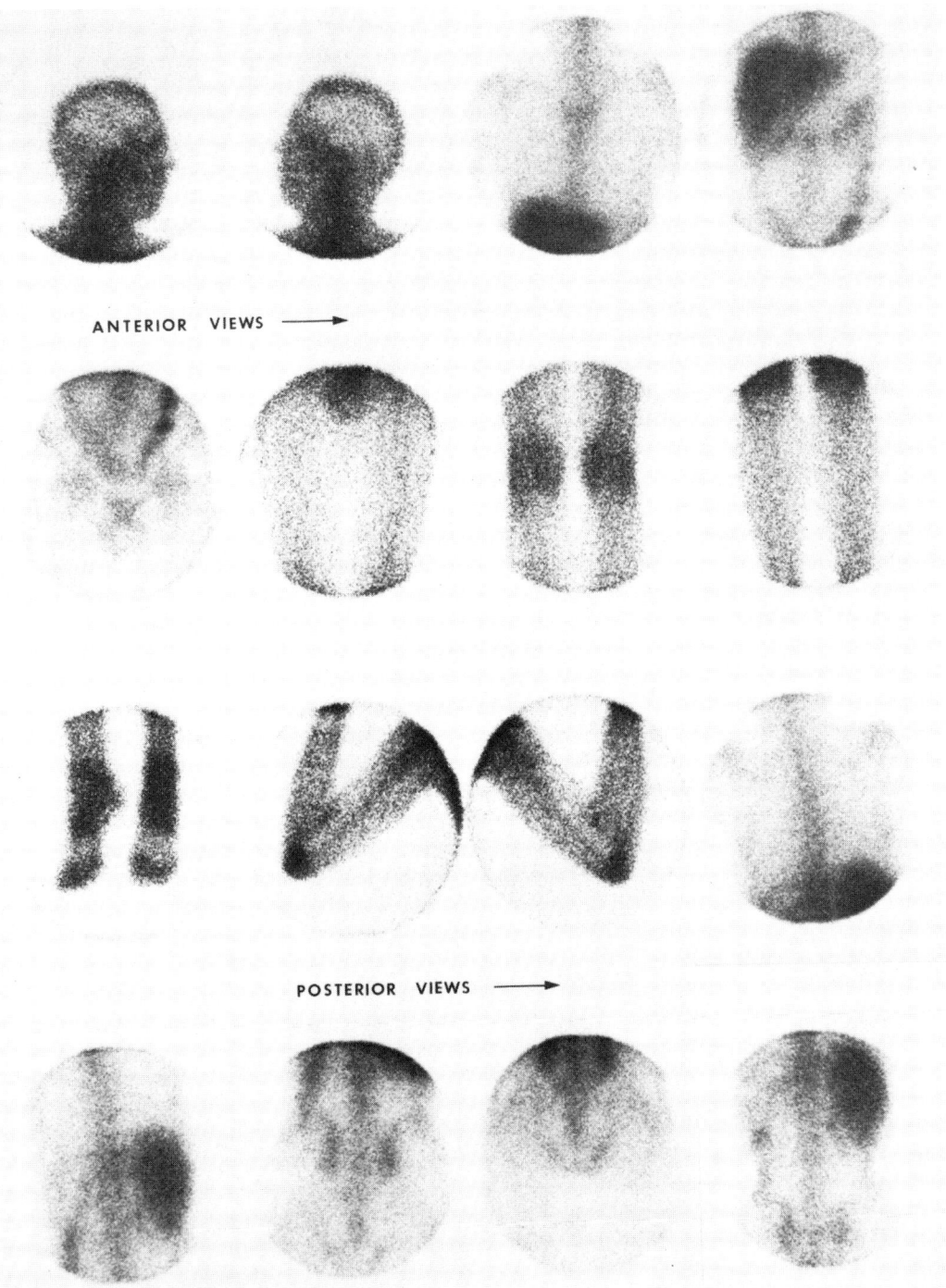

Figure 14-14. Normal gallium scan obtained 72 hours after intravenous administration of 3 mCi of Ga-67 citrate.

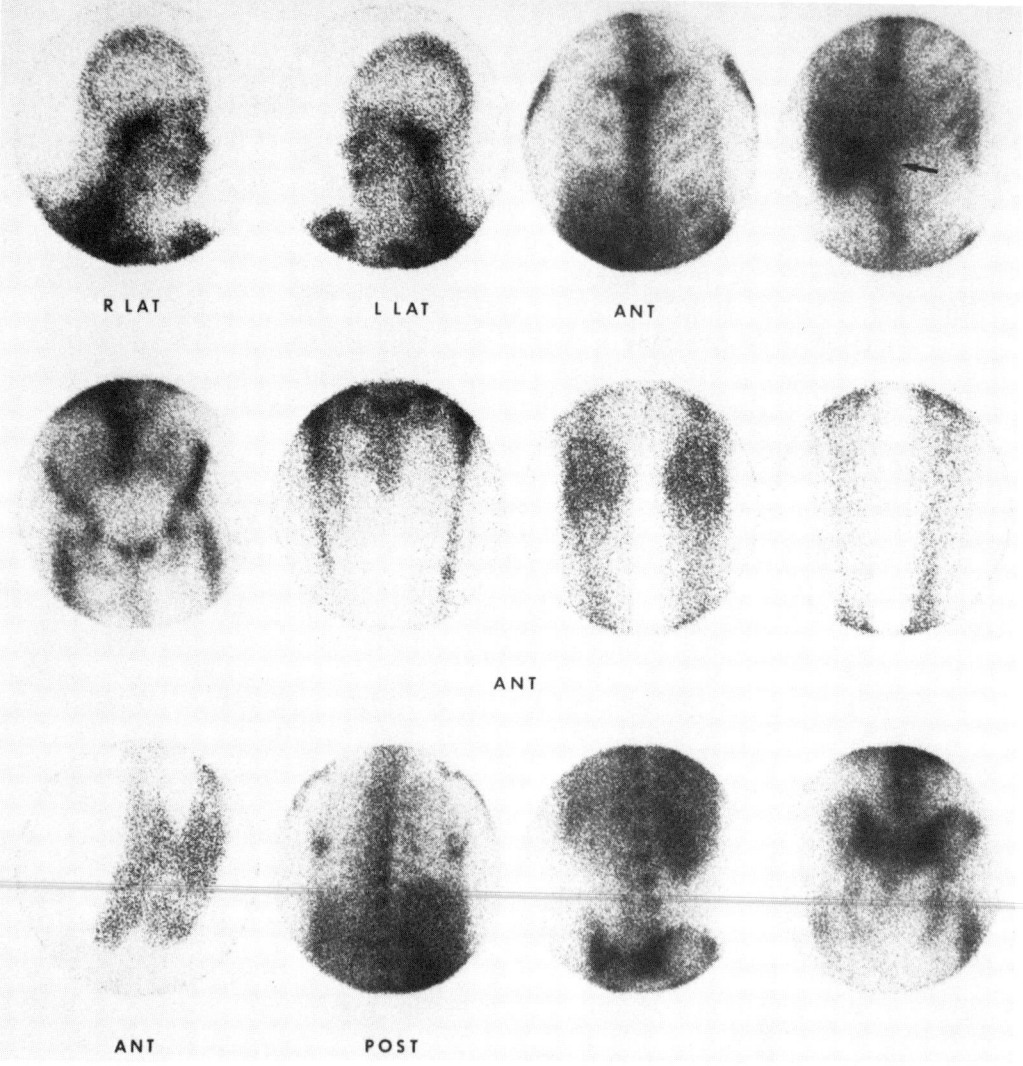

Figure 14-15. Occult abscess localized in the subhepatic region of the abdomen (arrow) 48 hours after injection of 3 mCi of Ga-67 citrate in a patient in whom a persistent fever developed 3 weeks after abdominal surgery.

IN-111 LEUKOCYTE IMAGING

CLINICAL RATIONALE

The major indication for the use of In-111 labeled leukocytes is the investigation of the FUO. In-111 labeled leukocytes have the advantage in the abdomen and pelvis of having no normal bowel concentration, thereby making it easier to see an abnormal focus of concentration with planar imaging (Fig. 14-17).

PROCEDURE

The cell labeling procedure for In-111 has been described previously in this chapter.

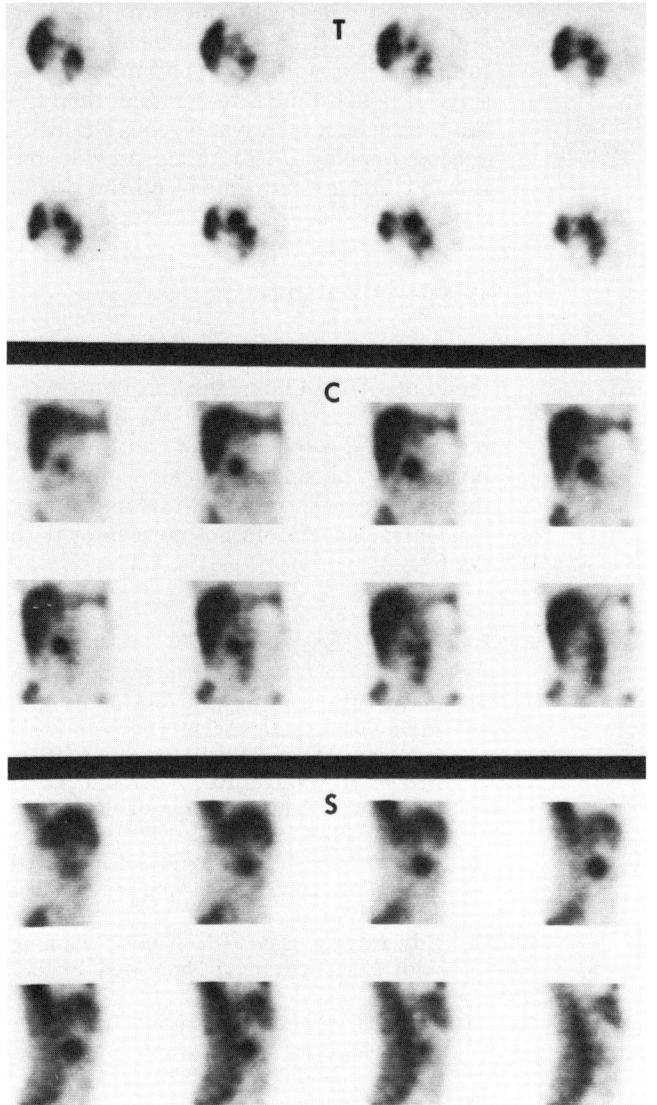

Figure 14-16. Gallium SPECT transaxial (T), coronal (C), and sagittal (S) arrays demonstrating an absess in the head of the pancreas. SPECT 3-D definition allowed the differentiation of the pancreatic focus from bowel activity.

After the IV administration of 200 to 500 μCi of In-111 leukocytes, imaging may take place from 4 to 48 hour later. Imaging before 4 hours may lend confusion because of incomplete clearance of In-111 leukocytes from lung tissue. The optimum imaging time seems to be 18 to 24 hours after IV administration using both photo peaks and a medium-energy collimator. SPECT imaging with In-111 leukocytes is usually fraught with difficulties in interpretation because of the microcurie amounts used and the consequently low scintillation statistics in the image data obtained.

PHARMACEUTICALS

In-113m could be used for labeling leukocytes; however, its decay properties make the choice of In-111 more favorable except in remote locations where there is de-

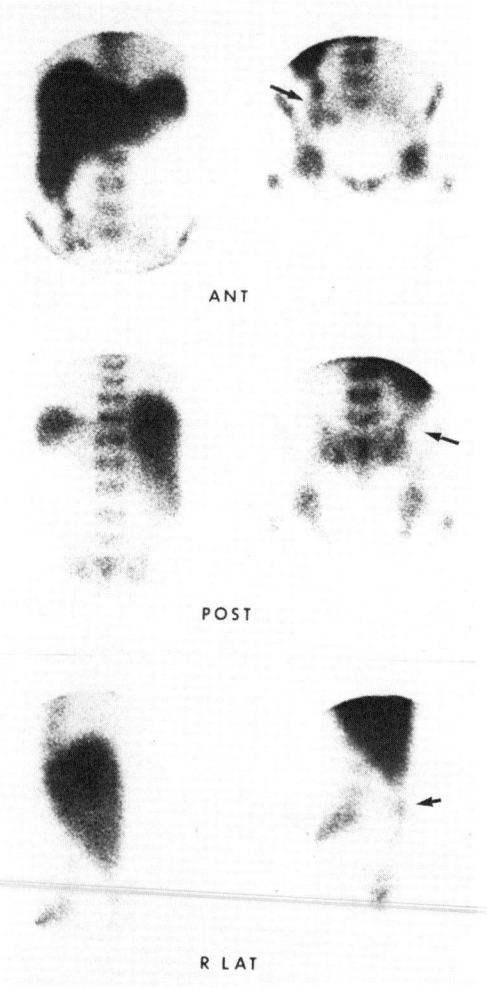

Figure 14-17. Abdominal abscess localized (arrow) 24 hours after injection of 500 μCi of In-111 oxine-labeled autologous leukocytes.

tion. Also, a technique for labeling leukocytes with Tc-99m has been reported preliminarily, with very good imaging results. If bench time is reasonable, then the latter may be most advantageous clinically because imaging at 1 to 2 hours provides the shortest turnaround time of all the procedures discussed.

INTERPRETATION

In-111 leukocytes concentrate initially in the lungs. After 4 hours the lung concentration is no longer present, and the In-111 will be seen in the spleen, liver, and marrow normally. The spleen appears to have the maximum concentration. Bowel and kidney concentrations should not be seen as with Ga-67.

REFERENCES

1. Hayes RL: The medical use of gallium radionuclides: A brief history with some comments. Semin Nucl Med 8:183, 1978
2. Bruner HD, Hayes RL, Perkinson JD Jr: Preliminary data on gallium-67. Radiology 62:602, 1953
3. Greene MW, Tucker WD: An improved gallium-68 cow. Int J Appl Radiat Isot 12:62, 1961
4. Edwards Cl, Hayes RL: Tumor scanning with Ga-67 citrate. J Nucl Med 10:103, 1969
5. Bell EG, O'Mara RE, Henry CA, et al: Non-neoplastic localization of Ga-67 citrate. J Nucl Med 12:338, 1971
6. Lavender JP, Lowe J, Barker JR: Gallium-67 citrate scanning in neoplastic and inflammatory lesions. Br J Radiol 44:361, 1971
7. Staab EV, McCartney WH: Role of gallium-67 in inflammatory disease. Semin Nucl Med 8:219, 1978
8. Brown LC: Chemical processing of cyclotron-produced Ga-67. Int J Appl Radiat Isot 22:710, 1971
9. Hnatowich DJ, Kulprathipanja S, Beh R: The importance of pH and citrate concentration on the in vitro and in vivo behavior of radiogallium. Int J Appl Radiat Isot 28:925, 1977

pendence on long-lived generators because of a lack of fast air transportation of radiopharmaceuticals.

Preliminary reports in the literature have suggested that ionic In-111 chloride may be as useful as In-111 leukocytes in inflammatory processes, particularly in osteomyelitis. This offers the advantage of little or no bench preparation time and diminished chances of bacterial contamina-

10. Larson SM: Mechanisms of localization of gallium-67 in tumors. Semin Nucl Med 8:193, 1978
11. Larson SM, Allen DR, Rasey JS, et al: Kinetics of binding of carrier-free Ga-67 to human transferrin. J Nucl Med 19:1245, 1978
12. Hayes RL, Byrd BL, Rafter JJ, et al: The effect of scandium on the tissue distribution of Ga-67 in normal and tumor-bearing rodents. J Nucl Med 21:361, 1980
13. Hayes RL, Rafter JJ, Byrd BL, et al: Studies of the in vivo entry of Ga-67 into normal and malignant tissue. J Nucl Med 22:325, 1981
14. Nelson B, Hayes RL, Edwards CL, et al: Distribution of gallium in human tissues after intravenous administration. J Nucl Med 13:92, 1972
15. Watson EE, Cloutier RJ, Gibbs WD: Whole-body retention of Ga-67 citrate. J Nucl Med 14:840, 1973
16. Larson SM, Hoffer PB: Normal patterns of localization. In Hoffer PB, Bekerman C, Henkin RE (ed): Gallium-67 Imaging. New York, Wiley, 1978, p 23
17. Mishkin FS, Maynard WP: Lacrimal gland accumulation of Ga-67. J Nucl Med 15:630, 1975
18. Larson SM, Schall GL: Gallium-67 concentration in human breast milk. JAMA 218:257, 1971
19. Bekerman C, Hoffer PB: Salivary gland uptake of GA-67 citrate following radiation therapy. J Nucl Med 17:685, 1976
20. Newman RA, Gallagher JG, Clements JP, et al: Demonstration of Ga-67 localization in human placenta. J Nucl Med 19:504, 1978
21. Fletcher JW, Herbig FK, Donati RM: Ga-67 citrate distribution following whole-body irradiation or chemotherapy. Radiology 117:709, 1975
22. Bradley WP, Alderson PO, Eckelman WC, et al: Decreased tumor uptake of gallium-67 in animals after whole-body irradiation. J Nucl Med 19:204, 1978
23. Hayes RL: The tissue distribution of gallium radionuclides. J Nucl Med 18:740, 1977
24. Hayes RL: Chemistry and radiochemistry of metal-ion nuclides commonly employed in radiopharmaceuticals. In Heindel ND, Burns HD, Honda T, Brady LW (ed): The Chemistry of Radiopharmaceuticals. New York, Masson Pub, 1977, p 155
25. Brown DH, Byrd BL, Carlton JE, et al: A quantitative study of the subcellular localization of Ga-67. Cancer Res 36:956, 1976
26. Hoffer PB: Mechanisms of localization. In Hoffer PB, Bekerman C, Henkin Re (eds): Gallium-67 Imaging. New York, Wiley, 1978, p 3
27. Hoffer PB, Huberty JP, Hassan KB: The relative binding affinity of gallium-67 for lactoferrin and transferrin. J Nucl Med 18:619, 1977
28. Tsan MF, Chen WY, Scheffel U, et al: Mechanism of gallium localization in inflammatory lesions. J Nucl Med 18:619, 1977
29. Tsan M, Chen W, Scheffel U, et al: Studies on gallium accumulation in inflammatory lesions: Gallium uptake by human polymorphonuclear leukocytes. J Nucl Med 19:36, 1978
30. Menon S, Wagner H, Tsan M: Studies on the gallium accumulation in inflammatory lesions: Uptake by *Staphylococcus aureus*: Concise communication. J Nucl Med 19:44, 1978
31. Weiner RE, Schreiber GJ, Hoffer PB, et al. Compounds which mediate gallium-67 transfer from lactoferrin to ferritin. J. Nucl Med 26:908, 1985
32. Sayle BA, Balachandran S, Rogers CA: Indium-111 chloride imaging in patients with suspected abscesses: Concise communication. J Nucl Med 24:1114, 1983
33. Hnatowich DJ: A method for the preparation and quality control of Ga-68 radiopharmaceuticals. J Nucl Med 16:764, 1975
34. Ehrhardt GJ, Welch MJ: A new germanium-68/gallium-68 generator. J Nucl Med 19:925, 1978
35. MIRD Report No. 2: Summary of current radiation dose estimates to humans from Ga-66, Ga-67, Ga-68, and Ga-72 citrate. J Nucl Med 14:755, 1973
36. Hladik WB III, Nigg KK, Rhodes BA: Drug-induced changes in the biologic distribution of radiopharmaceuticals. Semin Nucl Med 12:184, 1982
37. Lentle BC, Scott R, Noujaim AA: Iatrogenic alterations in the biodistribution of radiotracers. J Nucl Med 19:743, 1978
38. Chilton HM, Witcofski RL, Watson NE Jr, et al: Alteration of Ga-67 distribution in tumor-bearing mice following treatment with methotrexate: Concise communication. J Nucl Med 22:1064, 1981

39. Waxman AD, Beldon JR, Richli W, et al: Steroid induced suppression of gallium uptake in tumors of the central nervous system: Concise communication. J Nucl Med 19:480, 1978
40. Welch MJ, Welch TJ: Solution chemistry of carrier-free indium. In Subramanian G, Rhodes B, Cooper JF, Sodd VJ (eds): Radiopharmaceuticals. New York, Society of Nuclear Medicine, 1975, p 73
41. Stern HS, Goodwin DA, Scheffel U, et al: In-113m for blood pool and brain scanning. Nucleonics 25:62, 1967
42. Stern HS, Goodwin DA, Wagner HN: Cardiac and placental scanning with indium-113m. J Nucl Med 8:351, 1967
43. Potchen EJ, Adatepe M, Welch M, et al: Indium-113m for visualizing body organs. JAMA 205:208, 1968
44. Adatepe MH, Welch M, Archer E, et al: The laboratory preparation of indium-labeled compounds. J Nucl Med 9:426, 1968
45. Stern HS, Goodwin DA, Wagner HN Jr, et al: In-113m as a short-lived isotope for lung scanning. Nucleonics 24:57, 1966
46. Goodwin DA, Stern HS, Wagner HN Jr, et al: In-113m colloid: A new radiopharmaceutical for liver scanning. Nucleonics 24:65, 1966
47. Cooper JF, Wagner HN Jr: Preparation and control of In-113m radiopharmaceuticals. In Radiopharmaceuticals from Generator-Produced Radionuclides. Vienna, IAEA, 1971, p 83
48. Hill T, Welch MJ, Adatepe M, et al: A simplified method for the preparation of indium-DTPA brain scanning agent. J Nucl Med 11:28, 1970
49. Goodwin DA, Menzimer D, Del Castilho R: A dual-spectrometer system for high-efficiency imaging of multi-gamma–emitting nuclides with the anger camera. J Nucl Med 11:221, 1970
50. Lamb JF: Commercial production of radioisotopes for nuclear medicine, 1970–1980. IEEE Transaction on Nuclear Science, Vol NS-28, No. 2, pp 1916–1920, 1982
51. Brown LC, Beets AL: Cyclotron production of carrier-free indium-111. Int J Appl Radiat Isot 23:57, 1972
52. Spector WG, Willoughby DA: The inflammatory response. Bact Rev 27:117, 1963
53. McAfee JG, Thakur ML: Survey of radioactive agents for in vitro labeling of phagocytic leukocytes. I. Soluble agents. J Nucl Med 17:480, 1976
54. McAfee JG, Thakur ML: Survey of radioactive agents for in vitro labeling of phagocyte leukocytes. II. Particles. J Nucl Med 17:487, 1976
55. Sinn H, Silvester DJ: Simplified cell labeling with indium-111 acetylacetone. Br J Radiol 52:758, 1979
56. Danpure HJ, Osman S, Brady F: The labeling of blood cells in plasma with In-111 tropolonate. Br J Radiol 55:247, 1982
57. Zakhireh B, Thakur ML, Malech HL, et al: Indium-111–labeled human polymorphonuclear leukocytes: Viability, random migration, chemotaxis, bactericidal capacity, and ultrastructure. J Nucl Med 20:741, 1979
58. Hawker RJ, Hall CE, Gunson BK: Re: Indium-111 tropolone versus oxine. J Nucl Med 24:367, 1983
59. Dewanjee MD: Reply. J Nucl Med 24:368, 1983
60. Package Insert: Indium In-111 oxine solution, radiochemical for cell labeling. Amersham Corporation, Arlington Heights, Ill.
61. Thakur ML, Coleman RE, Welch MJ: Indium-111–labeled leukocytes for the localization of abscesses: Preparation, analysis, tissue distribution, and comparison with gallium-67 citrate in dogs. J Lab Clin Med 82:217, 1977
62. Goodwin DA, Bushberg JT, Doherty PW, et al: Indium-111 labeled autologous platelets for location of vascular thrombi in humans. J Nucl Med 19:626, 1978
63. McAfee JG: Techniques of harvesting platelets and neutrophils and labeling them with indium-111 oxine. In Thakur ML, Gottschalk A (eds): Indium-111 Labeled Neutrophils, Platelets, and Lymphocytes. New York, Trivirum, 1981, p 51
64. Roy AJ, Franklin A, Simmons WB: A method for separation of granulocytes from normal human blood using hydroxyethyl starch. Prep Biochem 1:197, 1971
65. Boyum A: Isolation of leukocytes from human blood. Further observations. Methylcellulose, dextran and ficoll as erythrocyte aggregating agents. Scand J Clin Lab Invest 21 (Suppl 97): 37, 1968
66. Coleman RE, Welch DM, Baker, et al: Clinical experience using indium-111 labeled leukocytes. In Gottschalk A (eds): Indium-111 Labeled Neutrophils, Platelets, and Lymphocytes. Thakur ML, New York, Trivirum, 1981, p 103
67. Thakur ML, Lavender JP, Arnot RN, et al:

Indium-111 labeled autologous leukocytes in man. J Nucl Med 18:1012, 1977
68. Gobuty AH, Kim EE, Lazarre C: Technologic, clinical, and basic science considerations for In-111-oxine–labeled leukocyte studies. Teaching editorial. J Nucl Med Tech 11:190, 1983
69. Goodwin DA, Doherty PW, McDougall IR: Clinical use of indium-111 labeled white cells: An analysis of 312 cases. In Thakur ML, Gottschalk A (eds): Indium-111 Labeled Neutrophils, Platelets, and Lymphocytes. New York, Trivirum, 1981, p 131
70. Coleman RE: Radiolabeled leukocytes. In Freeman LM, Weissmann HS, (eds): Nuclear Medicine Annual. New York, Raven Press, 1982, p 119
71. Thakur ML, Segal AW, Louis L, et al: Indium-111–labeled cellular blood components: Mechanism of labeling and intracellular location in human neutrophils. J Nucl Med 18:1020, 1977
72. Goodwin DA, Finston RA, Smith SI: The distribution and dosimetry of In-111 labeled leukocytes and platelets in humans. In Watson EE, Schafke-Stelson AT, Coffey JL, Cloutier RJ (eds): The Third International Radiopharmaceutical Dosimetry Symposium. US Department of Health and Human Services, 1981, p 88
73. McAfee JG, Gagne GM, Subramanian G, et al: Distribution of leukocytes labeled with In-111 oxine in dogs with acute inflammatory lesions. J Nucl Med 21:1059, 1980
74. ten Berge RJM, Natarajan AT, Hardeman MR, et al: Labeling with indium-111 has detrimental effects on human lymphocytes: Concise communication. J Nucl Med 24:615, 1983
75. Thakur ML, McAfee JG: The significance of chromosomal aberrations in indium-111–labeled lymphocytes. J Nucl Med 25:922, 1984
76. Segal AW, Detrix P, Garcia R, et al: Indium-111 labeling of leukocytes: A detrimental effect on neutrophil and lymphocyte function and an improved method of cell labeling. J Nucl Med 19:1238, 1978
77. Cunningham DA, Siegel BA: Radiolabeled platelets. In Freeman LM, Weissman HS (eds): Nuclear Medicine Annual 1982. New York, Raven Press, 1982, p 143
78. Goodwin DA, Bushberg JT, Doherty PW et al: Indium-111–labeled autologous platelets for location of vascular thrombi in humans. J Nucl Med 19:626, 1978
79. Dewanjee MK, Rao SA, Didisheim P: Indium-111 tropolone, a new high-affinity platelet label: Preparation and evaluation of labeling parameters. J Nucl Med 22:981, 1981
80. Heaton WA, Davis HH, Welch MJ, et al: Indium-111: A new radionuclide label for studying human platelet kinetics. Br J Haematol 42:613, 1979
81. Joist JH, Baker RK, Thakur ML, et al: Indium-111–labeled human platelets: Uptake and loss of label and in vivo function of labeled platelets. J Lab Clin Med 92:829, 1978
82. Scheffel U, Tsan M, McIntyre PA: Labeling of human platelets with In-111-8 hydroxyquinoline. J Nucl Med 20:524, 1979
83. Mathias CJ, Heaton WA, Welch MJ, et al: Comparison of In-111 oxine and In-acetylacetone for the labeling of cells: In vivo and in vitro biological testing. Int J Appl Radiat Isot 32:651, 1981

CHAPTER 15

In Vivo Function Studies

In vivo function studies are performed to determine to what extent an organ or system is functioning in the body. It is with these types of studies that the term *tracer* finds its niche. A simple definition of a tracer is a species that follows or outlines something else, the tracee.[1] In nuclear medicine, in vivo function studies are accomplished by measuring the absorption, dilution, concentration, or excretion of a radioactive tracer in the body. The labeled tracer species (radiopharmaceutical) must act the same way as the nonlabeled species (tracee) in the system of interest, and its behavior must be representative of the whole population of the species. Although the tracer may be made of the same chemical substance as the tracee, this is not essential. The tracer must only act like the tracee. In addition, the tracer must not interfere with the process being studied.

Tracers that are commonly used in biomedical studies may be divided into three categories: contrast material (dyes), nonradioactive (stable) isotopes, and radioactive isotopes. In this chapter we will discuss some of the important and routine applications of radioisotopic tracers in nuclear medicine for in vivo function studies.

Before we begin the discussion of individual procedures some consideration will be given to specific terminology of interest; accordingly, the following considerations should be noted[2]: A *compartment* is an anatomic, physiologic, chemical, or physical subdivision of a system throughout which the ratio of the concentration of tracer-to-tracee is uniform. A system may be mono- or multicompartmental. For example, the distribution of albumin within the body may be subdivided into intravascular and extravascular compartments.

A *space* is an apparent volume throughout which the tracer is distributed and is obtained by dividing the amount of retained tracer by the concentration of the tracer at the sampling site. In essence, space measurement is the application of the principle of isotope dilution analysis, which will be discussed later on. It is important to realize that determination of a space yields only an apparent volume of distribution of the tracer, which may change with time. For example, in the measurement of plasma volume using radiolabeled albumin, the plasma space measured will change (increase) with the time of measurement because albumin leaks slowly from the intravascular space.

A *pool* is defined as the total amount

of substance in a space. For example, the intravascular albumin pool equals the concentration of albumin times the albumin space; in numbers, 2450 ml × 0.045 g/ml = 110.25 g.

BLOOD VOLUME MEASUREMENT

Blood consists of a fluid fraction (plasma) and formed elements that can be differentiated into red cells (erythrocytes), white cells (leukocytes), and platelets (thrombocytes). Each microliter of adult human blood contains an average of about 5×10^6 red cells, 7×10^3 white cells, and 3×10^5 platelets. Most of the cellular volume is comprised of erythrocytes, however, because of the abundance of red cells in relation to white cells and because of the small size of platelets. When anticoagulated whole blood is centrifuged, it is separated into a volume of packed cells and supernatant plasma. The volume of packed erythrocytes expressed as a percentage of the whole blood sample is called the hematocrit. It normally averages 45 percent; therefore, the supernatant plasma expressed as a percentage of the whole blood is 55 percent and is called the plasmacrit.

Theoretically one could determine the whole blood volume from either the hematocrit or the plasmacrit and a measurement of either the red cell or the plasma volume as follows:

$$\text{Whole blood volume} = \frac{\text{Red cell volume}}{\text{Hematocrit}} \text{ or } \frac{\text{Plasma volume}}{\text{Plasmacrit}}$$

There is some error associated with such a measurement, however, because of differences between the peripheral venous hematocrit and the mean whole-body hematocrit. The mean whole-body hematocrit is calculated from independent measurements of the red cell volume and the plasma volume as follows:

$$\text{Mean whole-body hematocrit} = \frac{\text{Red cell volume}}{\text{Red cell volume} + \text{Plasma volume}}$$

The peripheral venous hematocrit is determined by centrifuging a sample of blood obtained from an arm vein. Its value is somewhat higher than the mean whole-body hematocrit because the cell concentration is higher in blood vessels of small diameter having a slower blood flow rate. Additionally, the volume of plasma between the packed cells in the hematocrit tube contributes to the error. In general, the mean whole-body hematocrit is about 91 percent of the peripheral hematocrit. Because of these sources of error it has been found best to measure the red cell volume and the plasma volume independently and add them together to arrive at a more accurate determination of whole blood volume.

Principle of Blood Volume Measurement

The measurement of whole blood volume is based on the principle of isotope dilution analysis. In this method of volume determination a radioactive tracer of known volume (V_1) and concentration (C_1) is added to an unknown volume (V_2). The tracer is allowed to mix in the system for a period of time to achieve equilibrium (uniform distribution of tracer), whereupon a sample is removed for analysis of the new tracer concentration (C_2). Refer to Figure 15-1. The unknown volume is then calculated from the following equation:

$$V_2 = \frac{C_1 V_1}{C_2} \quad (15\text{-}1)$$

An accurate determination of blood volume is predicated on the requirement (1) that the tracer not degrade in or leak significantly from the compartment during the time of measurement and (2) that the volume of tracer added is insignificantly small compared with the volume of the compartment being measured.

In the measurement of whole blood

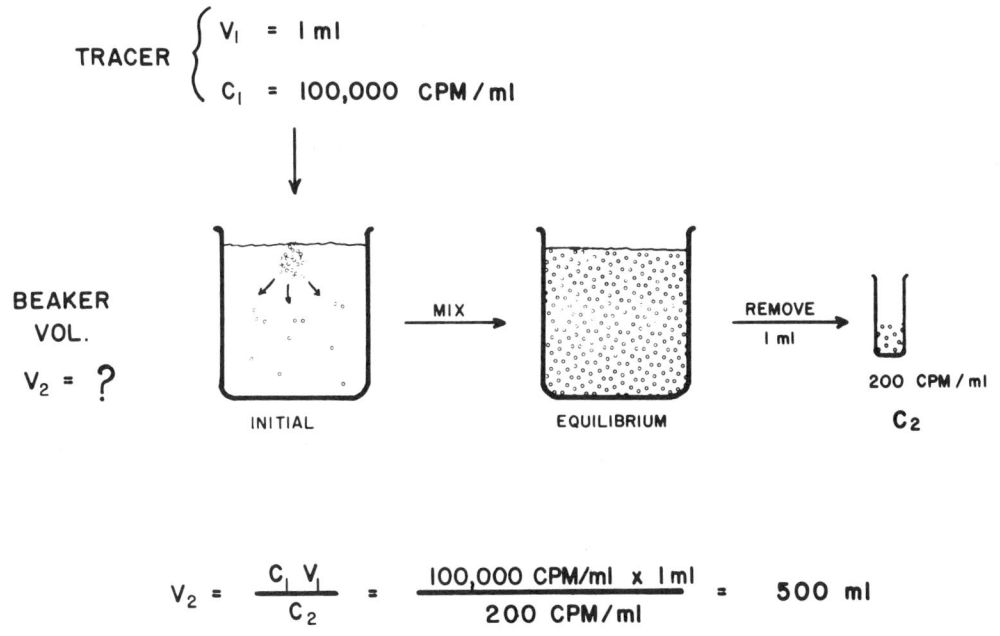

Figure 15-1. Determination of the unknown volume of a compartment (beaker) using the principle of isotope dilution analysis.

volume two compartments are measured using isotope dilution analysis: the red cell compartment (volume) and the plasma compartment (volume).

Red Cell Volume

The red cell volume is routinely measured by labeling a sample of autologous red cells with radioactive chromium-51. An accurate volume of Cr-51 red cells of known concentration (μCi or cpm per ml) is injected intravenously into the patient and allowed to reach equilibrium (usually 15 to 30 minutes). At this time a sample of blood is removed from a site other than the injection site. Samples are counted in a scintillation well counter, corrected for background count, and expressed as counts per minute per milliliter. By using isotope dilution Equation 15-1 the red cell volume is then calculated as follows:

$$\text{Red cell volume (ml)} = \frac{\text{Injected Cr-51 RBC cpm}}{\text{Removed Cr-51 RBC cpm/ml}}$$

With this method the Cr-51-labeled cells do not readily leak from the red cell compartment, and although Cr-51 activity does elute from the cells at about 1 percent per day, this does not significantly affect the results of the study, which is completed in less than 1 hour.

The following example will illustrate a routine procedure for labeling red cells with Cr-51. Forty milliliters of patient whole blood is mixed with 8 ml of an acid-citrate-dextrose (ACD) solution in a syringe. Fourteen milliliters of this anticoagulated mixture is used to prepare background RBC and plasma samples. The remaining 34 ml is added to the vented, empty ACD bottle followed by 150 μCi of sodium chromate

Cr-51. This mixture is allowed to incubate for 20 to 30 minutes with gentle mixing every 5 minutes. During the labeling reaction, chromate anion, $^{51}CrO_4^{2-}$ penetrates the red cell membrane and is reduced intracellularly to chromic ion, $^{51}Cr^{3+}$, which becomes bound to hemoglobin.[3-5] The maximum amount of chromium that labels red cells is less than 0.5 µg/ml of red cells and is nontoxic to the cells. Labeling efficiency is about 90 percent. At the end of incubation the blood is either centrifuged to separate the labeled cells from the unlabeled plasma activity, or alternatively ascorbic acid (100 mg) is added to the blood–chromate mixture and incubated for 5 minutes. The latter method is preferred by some investigators because it spares the cells from centrifuge and manipulation trauma. The ascorbic acid reduces the unlabeled chromate ion to chromic ion, which prevents the in vivo labeling of red cells when the labeled blood mixture is reinjected. When the ascorbic acid method is used, however, plasma activity must be subtracted from whole blood measurements in the final analysis because chromic ion labels plasma protein. The labeling method is shown in Figure 15-2.

When the labeling procedure is completed, 1 ml of tagged blood is diluted to 100 ml with water. This 1:100 dilution is used to determine the total activity injected into the patient because the tagged blood is too "hot" to count in a scintillation counter. After this, 20 ml of labeled blood (equivalent to 8 ml of packed red cells if the hematocrit is 0.40) containing about 80 µCi of Cr-51 activity is injected intravenously into the patient. After a 30-minute time period to allow for adequate mixing, a 15-ml sample of blood is removed from the opposite arm into a heparinized syringe to determine the new activity concentration.

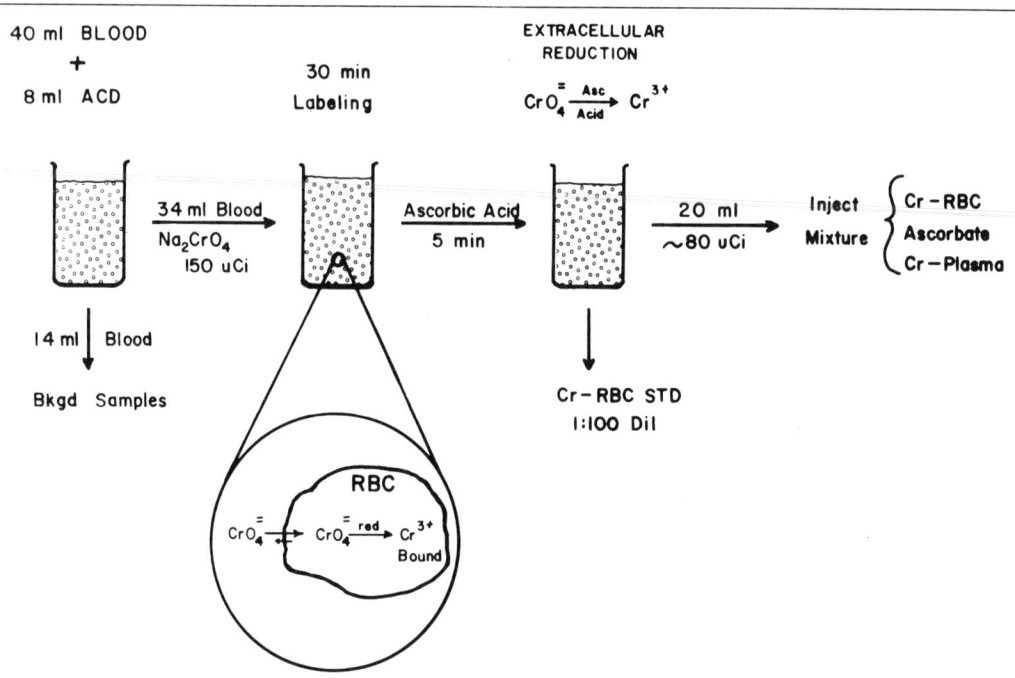

Figure 15-2. Diagram illustrating the technique of labeling RBCs with sodium chromate Cr-51 for use in determining the red cell volume.

Several manipulations are required, and minor adjustments are made for hematocrit differences and background counts as previously described to obtain a final result. The reader is referred to standard nuclear medicine texts for detailed procedures.[6,7] The following values from a typical patient study will serve to illustrate the calculation and normal values for the red cell volume. A detailed worksheet is shown in Figure 15-3.

C_1 = 2,673,594 net cpm/ml packed Cr-51 RBC injected

(Note: C_1 obtained by counting 1 ml of a 1:100 whole blood dilution multiplying by 100, and subtracting plasma counts to get packed cell counts)

- V_1 = 8 ml packed Cr-51 RBC injected (20 ml whole blood × 0.4 hematocrit)
- C_2 = 11,753 net cpm/ml packed RBC removed at 30 minutes
- V_2 = Unknown red cell volume in the patient
- $V_2 = \dfrac{(2{,}673{,}594 \text{ cpm/ml})(8 \text{ ml})}{11{,}753 \text{ cpm/ml}}$
  = 1820 ml

The value is usually reported as ml/kg body weight; thus for a 66.8-kg patient the result in this case is 1820 ml/66.8 kg or 27.2 ml/kg. The normal range is 25 to 30 ml/kg.

Cr-51 Sodium Chromate

The physical properties of Cr-51 were described in detail in Chapter 2. Briefly reviewed here, Cr-51 decays by electron capture with a 27.7-day half-life emitting a 320-keV gamma ray with a 9 percent abundance. The long half-life gives this radiopharmaceutical an extended shelf life in the nuclear pharmacy so that it is available when needed. The low photon abundance is a deterrent from using Cr-51 as an imaging radionuclide, but it is satisfactory for studies that involve in vitro scintillation counting.

Cr-51 is produced in a nuclear reactor by irradiating stable chromium metal or oxide enriched (80 to 90 percent) in Cr-50, in a high neutron flux for about 4 weeks according to the reaction $^{50}Cr(n,\gamma)^{51}Cr$.[8] The irradiated material is dissolved in hydrochloric acid, and the chromic chloride formed is oxidized to chromate.

Sodium chromate Cr-51, $Na_2{}^{51}CrO_4$, is available as a clear, colorless sterile solution adjusted to pH 7.5 to 8.5. The specific activity is not less than 10 mCi/mg of sodium chromate at the end of expiration, which is 4 months from the date of manufacture. The radiochemical purity is not less than 90 percent as sodium chromate, which is determined by paper chromatography.[9] The presence of excess chromic impurity, $^{51}Cr^{3+}$, must be limited because it does not label the red cells. Sodium chromate Cr-51 injection is available from commercial suppliers in various sizes, usually 0.25-mCi and 1.0-mCi vials.

Cr-51 is also available as the radiochemical chromic chloride, $^{51}CrCl_3$, for other labeling purposes. As Cr-51 EDTA it has been used to determine the glomerular filtration rate.

Plasma Volume

The measurement of plasma volume is accomplished using radioiodinated human serum albumin labeled with I-125 (I-125 HSA). A known amount of I-125 HSA activity, usually 5 to 10 μCi, is injected intravenously and allowed to reach equilibrium in the body (about 15 minutes). A sample of blood is then removed from a site other than the injection site. After analysis in a scintillation counter the plasma volume is calculated from the total activity injected and the concentration of activity per milliliter of plasma in the 15-minute sample using the isotope dilution formula:

$$\text{Plasma volume (ml)} = \frac{\text{Injected cpm I-125 HSA}}{\text{Removed cpm/ml I-125 HSA}}$$

When measuring plasma volume with I-125 HSA one must pay particular attention to the methodology used because albumin slowly leaks from the intravascular space into the extravascular space. If one observes the intravascular concentration of

RED CELL VOLUME / MASS WORKSHEET (Na$_2$^{51}CrO$_4$)

Patient's Name: _____ Unit #: _____ Date: _____

Height: __71__ In. Weight: __147__ Lbs. __66.8__ KG Sex: __M__ Age: __22__

Dose: uCi(Na$_2$^{51}CrO$_4$) __80__ Volume Inj: __20__ ml Std Dilution Factors: WB __1:100__
Pl __1:25__

Counting Vol.: __2__ ml Counting Time: __10__ min.

Microhematocrits: Standard Hct   = __0.35__ x 0.96 = __0.34__ Corrected (Hct$_S$)
Standard Plasmacrit = __0.66__ (1.0 - Corrected Std Hct) (Pct$_S$)
30" Sample Hct   = __0.42__ x 0.96 = __0.40__ Corrected (Hct$_V$)
30" Sample Plasmacrit = __0.60__ (1.0 - 30" Corrected Sample Hct) (Pct$_V$)

	Total Counts	Net Counts (Tot Cts - BKG)	Corr Net Cts (Net Cts x DF)	Symbol
STD WB	61343	WB BKG / 57123	DF = 100 / 5,712,300	(WB$_S$)
STD Plasma	26552	Pl BKG / 22128	DF = 25 / 553,200	(Pl$_S$)
30" Pt WB	28143	WB BKG / 23923	DF = 1 / 23,923	(WB$_P$)
30" Pt Plasma	5119	Pl BKG / 695	DF = 1 / 695	(Pl$_P$)
WB BKG	4220		DF = 1	
Plasma BKG	4424		DF = 1	

Calculation Formula:

$$\text{RBC Volume in Ml.} = \frac{[WB_S - (Pl_S \times Pct_S)] \times \text{Vol Inj} \times Hct_V}{WB_P - (Pl_P \times Pct_V)}$$

$$\frac{[5,712,300 - (\overbrace{553,200 \times 0.66}^{365,112})] \times 20 \times 0.40}{23,923 - (\underbrace{695 \times 0.60}_{417})} = \frac{(42,777,504)}{(23,506)} = 1820 \text{ ml RBC Volume}$$

__27.2__ ml/kg RBC Mass

Results:

Determined RBC Vol = __1820__ ml

Determined RBC Mass = __27.2__ ml/kg (Normal: 25-30 ml/kg)

Predicted WB Vol   = _____ (Chart)

Predicted RBC Vol   = _____ (Predicted WB Vol x 0.4)

Figure 15-3. Red cell volume worksheet.

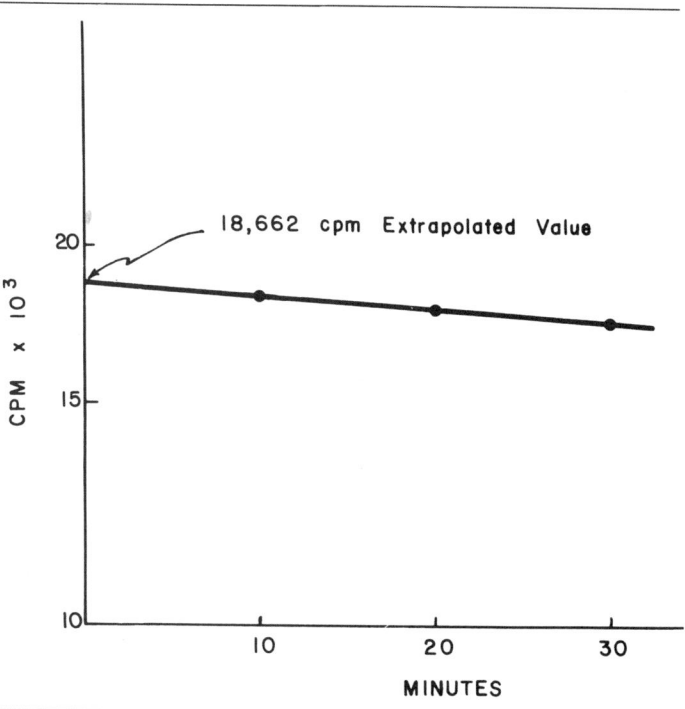

Figure 15-4. Graphic method for determining the zero-time concentration of I-125 HSA in the analysis of plasma volume by extrapolation of 10-, 20-, and 30-minute samples.

I-125 HSA activity over a prolonged period of time (several hours), one can thus see the volume of distribution (actually the albumin space) increase as more and more of the albumin leaves the intravascular space. For practical purposes a 15-minute albumin space has been accepted to be representative of the plasma volume. A more accurate method, however, is to measure plasma activity at two or three sampling times after injection of the dose. A plot of the log of sample activity against time is then extrapolated back to zero time to obtain the true activity concentration (Fig. 15-4).

The following example will illustrate the procedure for measuring plasma volume. An intravenous line is started with a butterfly-type infusion set, and a 5-ml sample of blood is obtained for background measurements. After this the content of a unit-dose syringe containing 5 to 10 μCi of I-125 HSA is injected intravenously in the opposite arm while noting the exact time.

From the previous arm 5-ml samples of blood are removed into heparinized syringes at 10, 20, and 30 minutes from the initial injection time. These samples and the background samples are centrifuged, and the net activity per milliliter of plasma is determined after assay in a scintillation counter. The net sample activity is plotted on semilog paper and extrapolated to zero time to obtain the plasma concentration (C_0) of the I-125 HSA at that time (Fig. 15-4). Alternatively the C_0 plasma concentration can be calculated from the following equation if the second sample is taken at exactly twice the time of the first sample (10 and 20 minutes or 15 and 30 minutes). This method is easier and more accurate than interpolation of plotted data.

$$\text{Zero time count}^* \ (C_0) = \frac{(C_1)^2}{C_2}$$

* Derivation of this equation can be found in Figure 15-5.

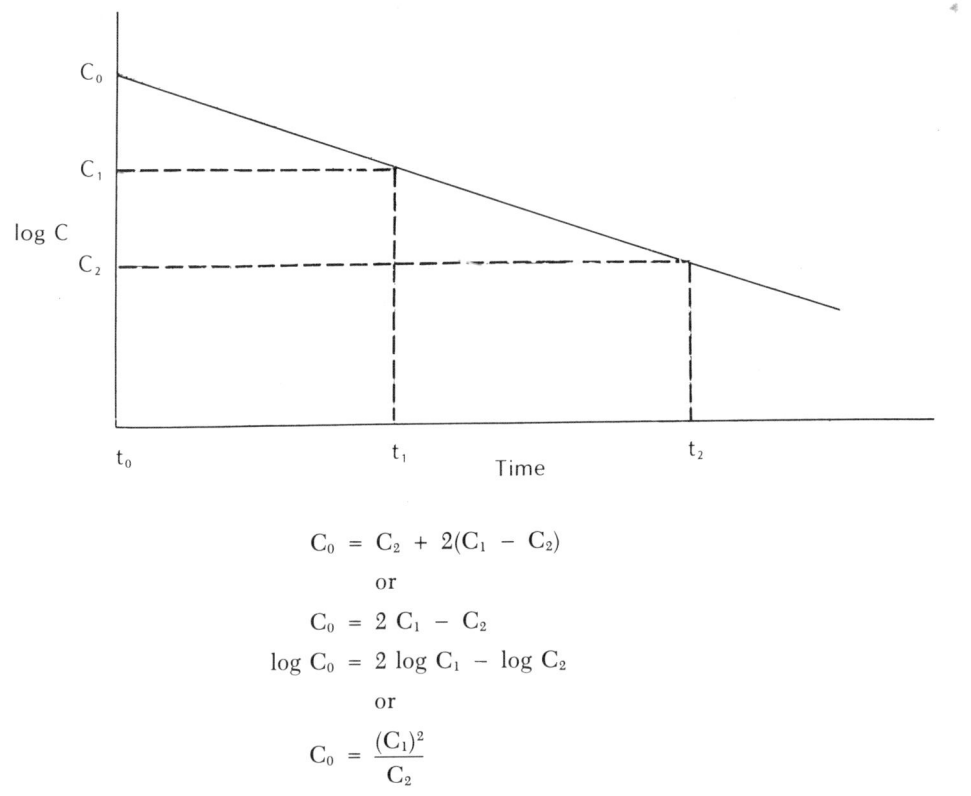

Figure 15-5. Derivation of the simplified equation for determining C_0 in plasma volume analysis. Assumptions: First-order rate of I-125 HSA loss from plasma compartment and t_2 equals $2 \times t_1$.

The total activity of I-125 HSA injected initially is determined from the assay of a standard dilution of the injected dose. This standard dilution is either supplied with the I-125 HSA syringes purchased commercially, or it can be prepared beforehand from another I-125 HSA syringe from the same lot. The standard dilution is usually 1:1000 of the injected dose in a volume of 4 ml; thus, 1 ml of dilution represents one four-thousandth of the injected dose. The following values from a typical patient study will serve to illustrate the calculation and normal values for plasma volume. A detailed worksheet is shown in Figure 15-6.

- Net cpm/ml of 1:1000 standard I-125 HSA = 12,603

- C_1 (10 min) net cpm/ml = 18,246
- C_2 (20 min) net cpm/ml = 17,839
- C_3 (30 min) net cpm/ml = 17,441
- C_0 (0 min) net cpm/ml = $\dfrac{(18,246)^2}{17,839}$ = 18,662

- Plasma volume (ml) = $\dfrac{\left(\dfrac{\text{Net cpm}}{\text{standard}}\right)\left(\dfrac{\text{dilution}}{\text{factor}}\right)}{C_0, \text{cpm/ml}}$

  = $\dfrac{(12,603 \text{ cpm})(4000)}{18,662 \text{ cpm/ml}}$

  = 2701

For a patient weight of 65.8 kg the plasma volume is 2701 ml/65.8 kg or 41 ml/kg. The

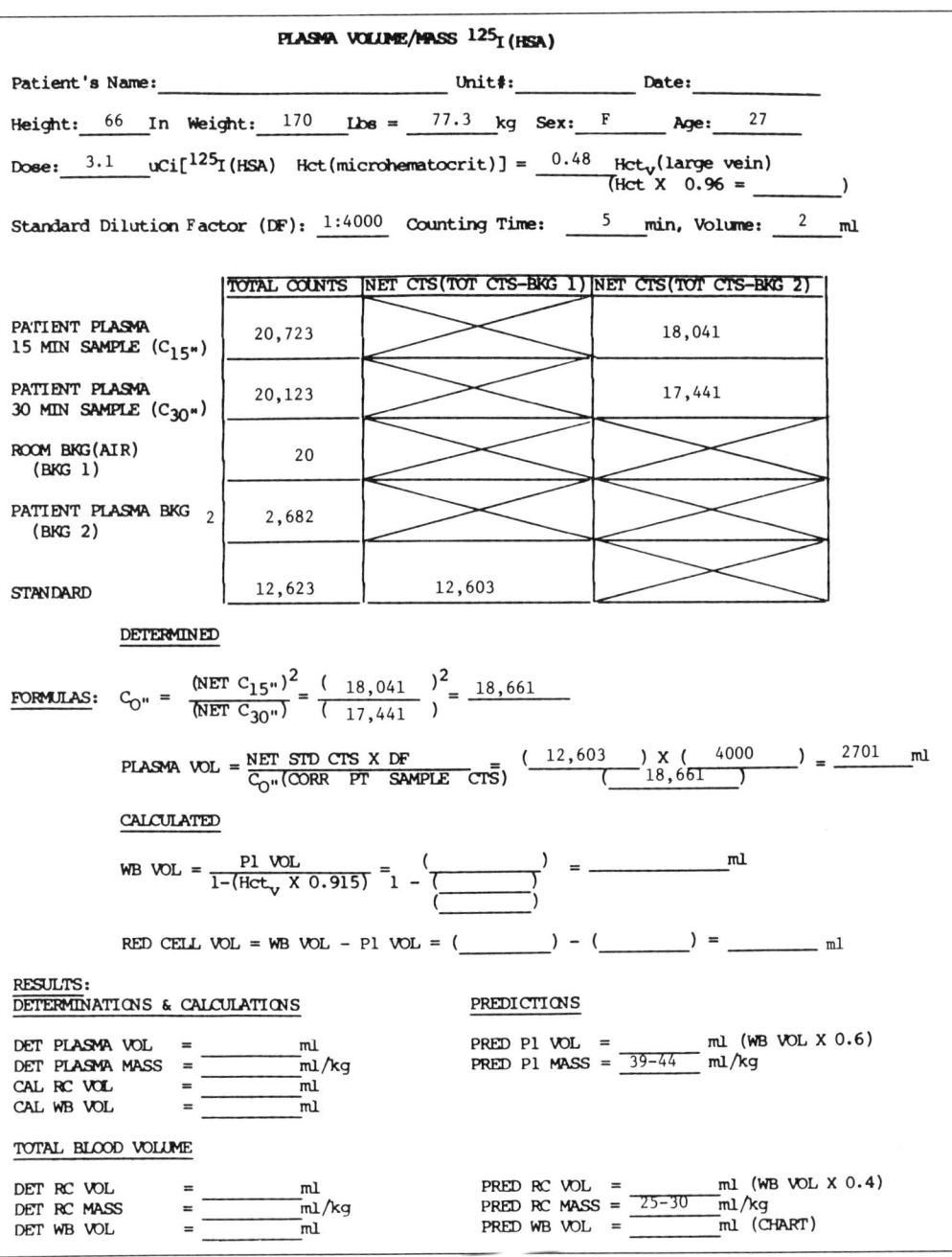

Figure 15-6. Plasma volume worksheet.

normal range for plasma volume is 39 to 44 ml/kg.

The physical properties of I-125 were described in detail in Chapter 8. Briefly reviewed here, I-125 decays by electron capture with a 60-day half-life emitting a 35-KeV gamma (7 percent) and 27-keV x-rays (115 percent) from its excited daughter Te-125. The long half-life gives I-125 HSA an extended shelf life in the nuclear pharmacy. The low-energy photons from I-125 decay are not ideally suited for imaging studies but are quite satisfactory for in vitro counting with the scintillation well counter.

I-125 HSA is prepared by mild iodination (see Methods, Chapter 4) of normal serum albumin so as to introduce not more than one atom of iodine per molecule of albumin. This precaution is taken so as not to denature the albumin and cause it to lose its normal physiologic behavior. The radioiodine becomes covalently bound in the 3 and 5 positions in the ring of the tyrosyl residues in the protein molecule as shown below:

Iodine will label histidyl residues also, but to a lesser extent. The iodine is firmly bound and only released by metabolism of the protein or through radiolytic decomposition. Radiolytic decomposition is minimal with the I-125 label, and the expiration date is not later than 120 days from the date of iodination. If I-131 is labeled to albumin, radiolytic decomposition is accelerated because of the beta radiation. Its expiration date is 30 days. The radiochemical purity of I-125 HSA is not less than 97 percent of the I-125 bound to HSA as determined by paper chromatography.[9] The product is available commercially as a sterile solution, clear to slightly amber in color and adjusted to pH 7.0 to 8.5. Because I-125 HSA is a biologic product without preservative, it should be stored at 2 to 8°C. I-125 HSA is available with specific activities of 1 μCi/mg of albumin in 100-μCi multidose vials and 8.5 μCi/mg of albumin in 500-μCi multidose vials or in single-dose syringes containing 10 μCi.

Combined Red Cell–Plasma Volume Measurement

Frequently, for convenience the Cr-51 RBC volume and I-125 HSA plasma volume studies are performed simultaneously rather than as separate studies. When this approach is taken, the I-125 HSA is injected first, and samples of blood for plasma volume measurement are obtained while the red cells are being labeled with sodium chromate Cr-51. Typically, 15-minute and 30-minute blood samples are taken. After the 30-minute sample is obtained for the plasma volume, the tagged Cr-51 RBCs are injected, and 30 minutes later a sample of blood is obtained for the RBC volume determination. Although the blood sample used for the red cell volume measurement will contain both Cr-51 and I-125, the I-125 counts can be easily discriminated from the Cr-51 counts with scintillation spectrometer because the I-125 photon energies (27 to 30 keV) are much lower than that of Cr-51 (320 keV). The calculations involved in determining the whole blood volume are the same as those previously described.

RED CELL SURVIVAL

The study of the survival of red cells in the circulation adds significant diagnostic information regarding the spheres of blood transfusion and hemolytic anemia. Measurement of the rate of loss of transfused blood provides a means of establishing compatibility and suitability of donor blood. In hemolytic anemias, red cell survival studies may provide an insight into both the rate and the mechanism of hemolysis. In general, a shortened half-time of the disappearance of labeled red cells from the circulation supports the diagnosis of intravascular hemolysis or hypersplenism. Because the spleen is the normal site for red cell destruction, a splenic sequestration study will also yield useful information. In general, the normal spleen-to-liver ratio of activity from Cr-51-labeled red cells is 1:1. In cases of hypersplenism it is greater than 2:1. Increased liver activity is indicative of intravascular hemolysis.

The most significant of the early nonradioisotopic methods for measuring red cell survival was the differential agglutination technique.[10] In this technique, the survival of transfused cells in the circulation of a recipient is studied, with donor cells being distinguished from recipient cells on the basis of their agglutinability (direct method) or inagglutinability (indirect method) by appropriate antisera. The elimination of the transfused cells was then monitored by red cell counting. Although refinements in this technique were developed, the principal disadvantage of these immunologic techniques was that they were not applicable to the study of patients' red cells in their own circulation.

An important advance in the technology of red cell survival determination in patients was the application of radiotracer techniques. In this method the patient's own blood, as well as donor blood, can be labeled with a radionuclide and the survival of cells in the circulation monitored by radioactive counting methods.

Cohort and Random Labeling of Red Cells

Radionuclide methods of labeling red cells may be divided into two groups, namely, cohort labeling and random labeling. In *cohort labeling*, the radiotracer is incorporated into cells as they are newly formed, and the survival of this group or cohort of cells of similar age is studied by monitoring their passage into and subsequent removal from the circulation. In *random labeling*, cells are labeled in such a way that the age distribution of the labeled sample of cells reflects the age distribution of the parent population. Survival is studied by monitoring the disappearance of the labeled sample from the circulation.

Although cohort labeling is the ideal method for studying red cell survival, it requires that labeling be confined to the shortest possible time period, that the label remain within the cell throughout its life span, and that there be no reutilization of the label after destruction of the cell. Because no radiolabel meets all of these requirements, cohort labeling is not used routinely. The radiolabel used in cohort labeling such as C-14-labeled glycine and Fe-59 fail the last criterion because they are reutilized by the red cell. More detail regarding cohort and random labeling can be found elsewhere.[11]

Of the random labels for red cells Cr-51 as sodium chromate and P-32 as diisopropyl phosphorofluoridate (DFP-32) are the most satisfactory agents. DFP-32 produces an irreversible label when cells are labeled in vivo or in vitro. The intravenous route is usually used, and red cell labeling yields are around 35 percent of the administered dose. Because leukocytes and platelets are labeled also, the red cells must be washed free of these components before counting. Red cell survival studies using the in vivo DFP-32 label demonstrate a mean red cell life span of 120 days.[12] The primary disadvantage of using DFP-32 is the requirement of liquid scintillation counting and the problems associated with quench correction for colored solutions.

The advantages of Cr-51 for red cell survival are that labeling is simple and convenient, the label is not reutilized, and external gamma counting can be performed with in vitro samples and for in vivo detection to localize areas of red cell sequestration in the body. The latter is an important aspect for assessing the relative roles of different sites of red cell destruction in known cases of hemolytic anemia. One disadvantage is that Cr-51 elutes from the cells in vivo at an exponential rate of 1 percent per day,[13] which requires that correction factors be applied to obtain clinically satisfactory approximations of the mean red cell life span.

Red Cell Survival Method

The procedure of red cell survival is useful for measuring the life span of red cells in patients with known or suspected hemolytic anemia. Survival is determined by monitoring the disappearance from the circulation of red cells labeled with Cr-51. The disappearance in normal subjects measured by this method occurs with a half-time of around 30 days.[6] This value is about twice the normal rate of removal by red cell destruction alone, which occurs at about 1 percent per day for senescent red cells. The increased rate with Cr-51 RBCs is due to an additional 1 percent loss per day from elution of the Cr-51 label. Consequently, Cr-51 survival data bear no simple relationship to the mean cell life span, which is the parameter required in clinical practice. If, however, as recommended by the International Committee for Standardization in Hematology, the Cr-51 survival data are corrected for Cr-51 elution and the patient is in a steady state of red cell production and destruction during the course of study, then the corrected half-time value obtained is a measure of red cell destruction only. Furthermore, multiplying this corrected half-time value by 1.443 gives the mean life of red cell survival.

The procedure may be summarized as follows, with greater detail found elsewhere.[14] Autologous red cells are labeled with Cr-51 as described previously under red cell volume determination. This method conforms to the recommended methods established for labeling red cells with Cr-51.[14] Labeled blood is then injected into the patient. On day 1 after injection a sample of blood is withdrawn, and the net count rate in the red cells is determined. This procedure is repeated three times per week for 2 weeks. The percentage of red cell activity of the day 1 sample present in each subsequent sample is determined as follows:

$$\% \text{ labeled red cells} = \frac{\text{Sample net cpm of red cells}}{\text{Day 1 net cpm of red cells}} \times 100$$

These data are then corrected for Cr-51 decay and elution[14] and plotted on semilog graph paper. The mean cell life span is calculated as the reciprocal of the slope of the line plotted, or 1.443 times the half-time (Fig. 15-7). The normal mean cell life span by this method has been determined to be 115 days.[14]

In Vivo Cross Match

The use of a shortened version of the Cr-51 red cell survival study may be used as a test of recipient–donor cross match incompatibility.[14] This test is useful and indicated in certain patient populations as follows: (1) when serologic tests suggest that all donors are incompatible; (2) when cold antibodies are present, active in vitro at 30°C or higher, and a nonreacting donor cannot be found; and (3) when the recipient has had an unexplained hemolytic transfusion reaction and requires a further transfusion.

In this test 0.5 ml of red cells from the "least incompatible" donor is labeled with 20 μCi of sodium chromate Cr-51 and washed three times with saline to remove unbound activity. After injection of labeled red cells into the recipient patient, 10-ml blood samples are removed from the opposite arm at 3-, 10-, and 60-minute intervals. Whole blood and plasma activity are determined for each sample.

Interpretation of compatibility is made as follows. When compatible red cells have been injected, the counting rate of the 60-minute sample is, on the average, about 99 percent of the 3-minute sample. Acceptable limits of compatibility for the individual case, however, are 94 to 104 percent owing to errors of measurement. Additionally, donor cells may be transfused in ex-

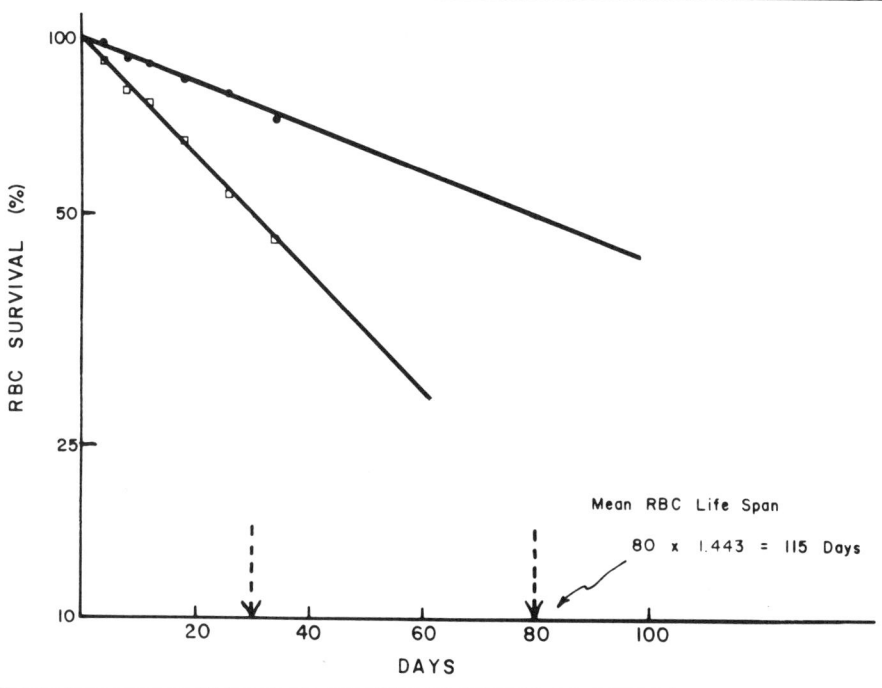

Figure 15-7. Determination of the mean red cell life span from the in vivo survival of Cr-51-labeled RBCs: □, survival related to red cell destruction and Cr-51 elution; ●, survival related to red cell destruction only, corrected for Cr-51 elution.

treme urgency if the compatibility test demonstrates not more than 5 percent of the injected radioactivity in the plasma in the 10-minute and 60-minute samples and red cell survival at 60 minutes is not less than 70 percent.[14]

Radiation Dose from Cr-51 Red Blood Cells

The estimated radiation absorbed dose to an average patient (70 kg) from an intravenous injection of a maximum dose of 200 μCi of Cr-51 is as follows:

Tissue	rad/200 μCi
Blood	0.20
Spleen	2.64
Testes	0.066
Ovaries	0.066
Whole body	0.005

TESTS FOR VITAMIN B_{12} DEFICIENCY

Vitamin B_{12} (cyanocobalamin) is an essential nutrient for all cells of the body because it is required for the synthesis of DNA.[15] Lack of this vitamin therefore causes failure of nuclear maturation and division of cells. Because tissues that produce RBCs are among the most rapidly proliferating in the body, a lack of vitamin B_{12} inhibits the rate of RBC production especially. This is manifested, in part, by adult erythrocytes, which have flimsy membranes and are large, oval, and irregularly shaped instead of the usual biconcave disk. Such cells have a normal amount of hemoglobin and are quite capable of carrying oxygen, but their fragility causes them to have a short life span, measured in weeks rather than months as for normal cells. B_{12} deficiency thus causes maturation failure in the process of erythropoiesis.

The most common cause of maturation failure is not the lack of B_{12} in the diet but the failure to absorb it from the gastrointestinal tract. This often occurs in the disease called pernicious anemia in which the basic disorder is a failure of the gastric mucosa to secrete a substance called intrinsic factor. Intrinsic factor is a glycoprotein secreted by the parietal cells of the gastric glands that combines with the B_{12} in food and makes the vitamin available for absorption from the intestine in the following way: first, the intrinsic factor binds tightly with B_{12} and in this bound state, the vitamin is protected from digestion by gastrointestinal enzymes. Second, the B_{12} intrinsic factor complex becomes bound to specific receptor sites on the brush-border membranes of the mucosal cells in the ileum. Third, from this site the complex is transported into the cells by pinocytosis, and within about 4 hours the B_{12} is released into the blood. Without intrinsic factor the vitamin is destroyed and cannot be absorbed. Fourth, in the blood B_{12} is bound to a plasma β-globulin, transcobalamin II, which transports it to the tissues, primarily the liver, where it is stored. It is slowly released from the liver when needed by the body. The normal amount needed for maturation of red cells is about 1 µg per day, and the normal amount stored in the liver is about 1000 µg. This scenario of vitamin B_{12} absorption and distribution is shown in Figure 15-8.

Besides the lack of intrinsic factor as a cause for vitamin B_{12} deficiency, any number of intestinal diseases or defects can interfere with the absorption of the B_{12}–intrinsic factor complex.[16] Antibodies to intrinsic factor or to the B_{12}–intrinsic factor complex may play a role in impaired uptake by the ileal cells. Bacterial overgrowth or certain intestinal parasites can prevent an adequate supply of vitamin B_{12} from reaching the ileum. Additionally, any damage to

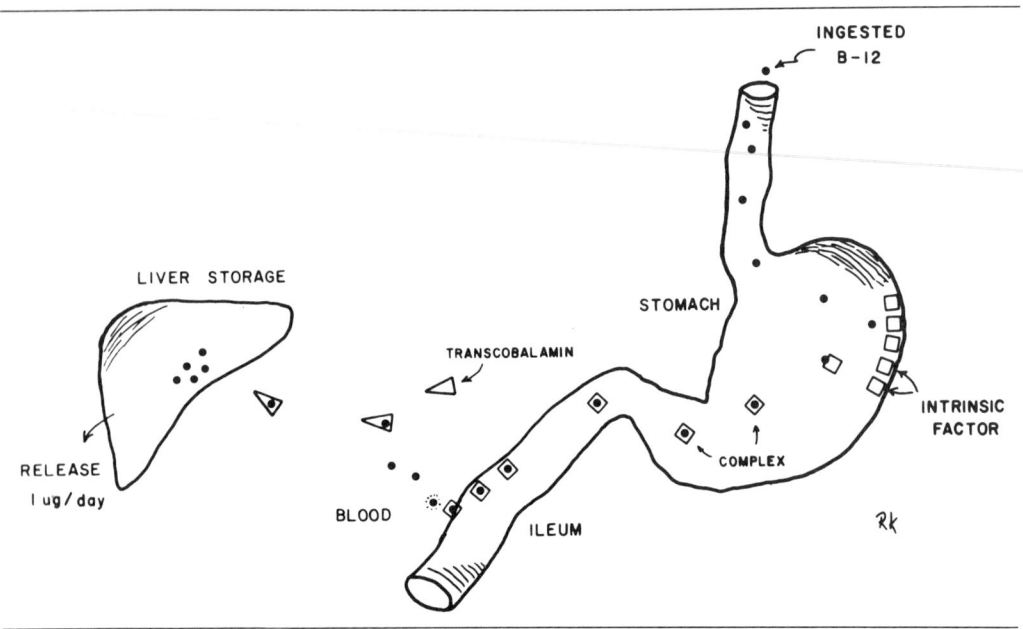

Figure 15-8. Schematic diagram illustrating the pathways of vitamin B_{12} metabolism. See the text for an explanation.

ileal mucosal cells by disease or surgical procedures can interfere with absorption. Finally, pure vegetarianism may be a cause because B_{12} is found only in animal protein.

Normal individuals have plasma concentrations of B_{12} between 200 and 900 pg/ml, whereas a deficiency state is usually present whenever the value falls below 200 pg/ml.[16] The serum level of B_{12} is usually measured using a competitive protein-binding radioassay that uses purified intrinsic factor as a binder for Co-57-labeled B_{12} and patient B_{12}.

Once the diagnosis of B_{12} deficiency is made through a combination of clinical signs and symptoms and a demonstration of a low serum B_{12} level, the question arises as to whether the B_{12} deficiency is due to a lack of intrinsic factor or to ileal dysfunction. A number of methods have been used to measure the absorption of B_{12} from the gastrointestinal tract, all using radioactive B_{12} labeled with Co-57, Co-58, or Co-60. The properties of these isotopes are listed in Table 15-1. In principle, the radioactive B_{12} is given orally, and absorption or lack of absorption is determined by measuring samples of blood, stool, or urine by scintillation counting. In the blood-sampling method,[17] plasma activity levels are measured at selected time intervals, with the maximum peak obtained in 8 to 12 hours. In the stool sampling method,[18] fecal excretion of nonabsorbed radioactive B_{12} is measured for 7 days and subtracted from the amount administered to obtain the quantity absorbed. With the urinary excretion method (Schilling test), the fraction of the administered dose excreted in the 24-hour urine is measured.[19] Of these methods the Schilling test is most often used.

Schilling Test

In the traditional Schilling test a patient who has fasted for at least 8 hours is administered an oral dose of radiolabeled B_{12} containing about 0.5 µCi of Co-57 and between 0.5 and 1.0 µg of vitamin. It is important that the amount of vitamin be physiologic, no more than might be present in a normal meal, because quantities above this level might be absorbed by mechanisms not dependent on intrinsic factor.[20] Within 2 hours after the oral dose, 1000 µg of stable B_{12} is administered intramuscularly as a flushing dose. This amount of vitamin will temporarily saturate B_{12}-binding sites in the tissues to enable a significant fraction of the radioactive dose that is absorbed into the blood to be excreted in the urine. A 24-hour urine that must be complete is collected and the volume measured accurately. Equal volumes of urine and a Co-57 standard, representing 20 percent of the administered dose, are counted in a scintillation counter, and the fraction of the dose excreted is calculated as follows:

$$\% \text{ Co-57 } B_{12} \text{ dose excreted} = \frac{\text{Net counts in urine}}{\text{Net counts in standard} \times 5} \times 100$$

In normal subjects greater than 7 percent of the dose is excreted in 24 hours. A value less than 7 percent excreted is indicative of absorption abnormality. The procedure just described is known as the Schilling test I.

TABLE 15-1. PROPERTIES OF COBALT RADIONUCLIDES

Nuclide	Decay Mode	$T_{1/2}$	Photon Energy (%)	R/mCi-hr at 1 cm	HVL (Pb)
Co-57	EC	270 d	122 keV (86%)	1.0	0.20 mm
			136 keV (10%)		
Co-58	EC	71.3 d	811 keV (99%)	5.5	9.0 mm
	β^+		511 keV (31%)		
Co-60	β^-	5.26 yr	1.17 MeV (100%)	13.2	12 mm
			1.33 MeV (100%)		

If the percent dose excreted is less than 7 percent, a Schilling test II is performed. Within 3 to 5 days of the first test a repeat test is administered that includes a 60-mg capsule of intrinsic factor along with another dose of Co-57 B_{12}. Under these test conditions, if the patient has pernicious anemia or total gastrectomy, the 24-hour urine excretion will become normal. If some other malabsorption problem exists, however, no change will be observed. If such a continued low value is related to increased bacterial competition in the gastrointestinal tract, a repeat study following a course of oral broad-spectrum antibiotics is indicated. If such diseases are the cause of malabsorption, urinary excretion will then become normal.

One weakness in this technique lies in the dependence on a complete 24-hour urine collection. Maximal excretion of B_{12} occurs between 8 and 12 hours after the oral dose, and loss of specimen during this time may produce a falsely low result in a normal subject. Erroneously low results may also occur in subjects with delayed urinary excretion such as patients with renal failure. It is therefore wise to procure two separate 24-hour urine collections in succession. Patients whose initial low 24-hour excretion rate was due to renal disease will readily be uncovered by this method, and if there is a gross discrepancy between the urine volumes collected during the first and second day, one can suspect that significant loss of urine did occur.

An alternative approach to performing the sequential Schilling test I and II, as just described, is to use the dual-isotope technique.[21] A version of this originally reported technique is available in a commercial kit (Dicopac, Amersham/Searle). The kit provides unit test doses for two to five patients. Each test dose consists of one capsule (0.5 μCi per 0.25 μg) of Co-57-labeled cyanocobalamin (bound to intrinsic factor), one capsule (0.8 μCi per 0.25 μg) of Co-58-labeled cyanocobalamin (without intrinsic factor), and one ampule of unlabeled cyanocobalamin (1000 μg) for intramuscular injection. One vial each of Co-57 standard and Co-58 standard are also included in the kit. With this method both capsules of radioactive B_{12} are administered simultaneously by mouth followed within 2 hours by 1000 μg of unlabeled B_{12} intramuscularly. After the 24-hour urine is collected and measured, an aliquot is taken for counting. The urine sample and the Co-57 and Co-58 standards are counted using dual-isotope counting techniques. Because of the different photon energies of Co-57 (122 keV) and Co-58 (811 keV), a correction for spilldown of Co-58 counts in the Co-57 window must be made. The data obtained are then used to calculate the percent excretion of each radionuclide and the ratio of the percent excretion of Co-57 to the percent excretion of Co-58. Typical values for various patient conditions are listed in Table 15-2.

The advantage of this dual-isotope method is that Schilling test I and II can be accomplished in a single test in 24 hours. Additionally, a complete urine collection is

TABLE 15-2. RESULTS OF 24-HOUR URINE EXCRETIONS AND Co-57/Co-58 RATIOS WITH DICOPAC

	Percent Excreted, Mean Values (Usual Range)		
Diagnosis	Co-57 B_{12} + IF	Co-58 B_{12}	Ratio of Co-57/Co-58
Normals	18 (10–42)	18 (10–40)	0.7–1.3
Pernicious anemia and certain gastric lesions	9 (6–12)	3 (0–7)	>1.7
Malabsorption syndromes	<6	<6	0.7–1.3

(Data from Package insert, Dicopac kit, 1978.[29])

not absolutely necessary because the ratio of excreted activity of the two isotopes is independent of volume excreted. If ileal malabsorption is suspected, however, the absolute volume of the 24-hour urine is needed because an accurate assessment of the percentage of the administered dose excreted is required. It is recommended, however, that an accurate and complete urine collection be obtained with the dual-isotope test because a more reliable interpretation of results occurs if both the percent dose excreted and ratios are known.

In the dual-isotope kit the intrinsic factor bound to the Co-57 B_{12} is obtained from human gastric juice. This is an advantage over hog intrinsic factor, which is routinely used in the single-isotope Schilling test. Hog intrinsic factor has at times demonstrated variable potency that can invalidate a Schilling test II. Additionally, some patients may have taken vitamins containing hog intrinsic factor in the past and have developed antibodies to this foreign protein. Consequently, they will not be able to absorb B_{12} bound to hog intrinsic factor but will have no difficulty absorbing it when bound to human intrinsic factor.

The dual-isotope test has been evaluated by several investigators.[22-24] These reports offer a word of caution that some patients exhibit Co-57/Co-58 excretion ratios that fall into a "gray zone," i.e., ratios between 1.3 and 1.7 that are not clearly normal nor clearly abnormal. One of these studies[23] found that the excretion range of the free vitamin (Co-58) seen in patients with proven pernicious anemia was greatly increased and nearly overlapped with that seen in patients with normal B_{12} absorption. This result was thought to be due to some in vivo exchange of vitamin B_{12} on intrinsic factor present in the capsules administered. To circumvent this possibility their recommendation was to administer the Co-58 capsule without intrinsic factor first, followed in 2 hours by a Co-57 capsule with intrinsic factor.[23] The manufacturer of the kit, however, recommends giving the capsules simultaneously, that being the conditions under which the kit was developed, tested, and approved for routine use.

Radiolabeled Cyanocobalamin

The primary cobalt radionuclides used to label cyanocobalamin for use in nuclear medicine have been Co-57, Co-58, and Co-60. The properties of these nuclides are presented in Table 15-1. Co-60 is produced in a nuclear reactor by neutron irradiation of stable cobalt according to the reaction $^{59}Co(n,\gamma)^{60}Co$. Co-60 has the longest half-life, most energetic photons, and produces the highest radiation dose. It is no longer routinely used. Co-58 is generally prepared by neutron irradiation of a nickel target according to the reaction $^{58}Ni(n,p)^{58}Co$. The irradiated target materials, namely, nickel metal, oxides, or carbonate, are dissolved in concentrated acids and the Co-58 nuclide isolated by ion-exchange and solvent extraction methods.[25] Co-57 is produced in a cyclotron by four simultaneous proton-induced reactions on a nickel target electroplated on a copper target holder.[26] The reactions are as follows:

$^{58}Ni(p,2p)^{57}Co$

$^{58}Ni(p,2p)^{57}Ni \xrightarrow{37\ hr} {}^{57}Co$

$^{58}Ni(p,2n)^{57}Cu \longrightarrow {}^{57}Ni \xrightarrow{37\ hr} {}^{57}Co$

$^{58}Ni(p,\alpha)^{57}Co$

After bombardment the nickel target is stripped from the copper with concentrated HCl, isolated on an ion exchange resin, and eluted with 6 M HCl.

Cyanocobalamin is a water-soluble compound that crystallizes as small red needles. Its solutions are cherry red in color. Cyanocobalamin is a cobalt coordination complex in which the cobalt is trivalent and has a coordination number of six. The complex is neutral, and its structure is shown in Figure 15-9. The cyanide group coordinated to the cobalt is not a part of the true vitamin but rather is an artifact caused by isolation of the vitamin on charcoal; in the liver the ligand is 5´-deoxyadenosyl anion instead of cyanide.[27] By strict organic chemical definition, however, because cya-

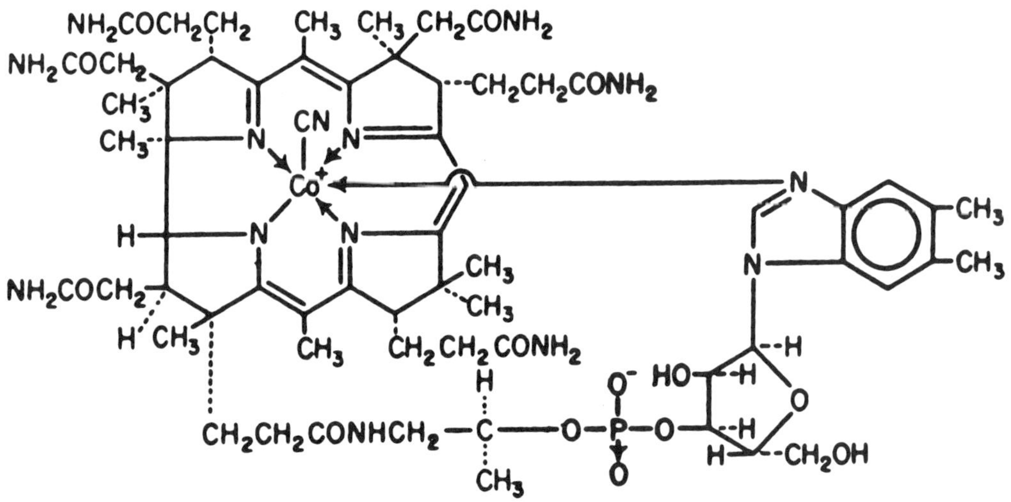

Figure 15-9. Chemical structure of vitamin B_{12} (cyanocobalamin).

nide was the first form of the vitamin to be isolated, cyanocobalamin is vitamin B_{12}.

Cyanocobalamin labeled with cobalt radionuclides is prepared biosynthetically by fermentation of the microorganism *Streptomyces griseus* grown in a nutrient medium containing the appropriate cobalt radionuclide salt and isolating the cobalamins.[28] The resulting product is an isotopic label in which a portion of the cobalamin molecules contains radioactive cobalt. The Co-57- and Co-60-labeled vitamins are available in capsules and oral solution. They are required to have a specific activity not less than 0.5 μCi/μg of cyanocobalamin.[9] Capsules contain between 0.5 and 1.0 μCi, which is the usual adult dose. Cyanocobalamin is degraded by heat, light, and alkaline solutions. Preparations should therefore be stored in a cool, dark place, and solutions should have a pH between 4.0 and 5.5 and contain a suitable preservative.[9] The radiochemical purity of radiocyanocobalamin as determined by paper chromatography is not less than 95 percent.[9] Co-58 cyanocobalamin is prepared in Europe and is available as an oral solution at pH 4 to 6 containing a preservative. It has the same storage conditions as the Co-57 and Co-60 preparations. A capsular form is available in the Dicopac kit previously described.

Radiation Absorbed Dose

The radiation absorbed dose to various organs after the coadministration of one 0.5-μCi capsule of Co-57 and one 0.8-μCi capsule of Co-58 in the dual-isotope study is as follows[29]:

Tissue	Normal (rad)	Pernicious Anemia (rad)
Liver	0.205	0.095
Stomach	0.00031	0.00046
Intestine	0.00343	0.0092
Testes	0.01	0.00297
Ovaries	0.0133	0.0054
Whole body	0.017	0.0072

THYROID UPTAKE STUDY

The radioactive iodine uptake (RAIU) study is a classic in vivo function study based on the physiologic incorporation of radioactive iodine into the thyroid gland to determine

FERROKINETIC STUDIES

The availability of ferrous citrate and other salts containing Fe-59 as a radioisotopic label has provided a physiologic tracer for studying iron metabolism and diseases of the hematopoietic system. Fe-59 is produced in a nuclear reactor by neutron irradiation of a ferric oxide target enriched in Fe-58 according to the reaction $^{58}Fe(n, \gamma)^{59}Fe$. The irradiated target is then dissolved in HCl, reduced to the ferrous state, and neutralized with NaOH in the presence of sodium citrate, which yields ferrous citrate containing Fe-59. Fe-59 undergoes β^- decay with a half-life of 44.5 days to form stable Co-59. Excited states of Co-59 formed during the decay process emit gamma rays with principal energies and abundances of 1.10 MeV (55 percent) and 1.29 MeV (44 percent). These energetic photons are used in some diagnostic studies for external counting. The specific gamma ray constant for Fe-59 is 6.4 R/hr/mCi at 1 cm. The half-value layer is 1.1 cm of Pb.

Ferrous citrate Fe-59 injection is a sterile solution of ferrous iron complexed with citrate ion. The structure of the complex is shown in Figure 15-10. The solution is made isotonic with sodium chloride. It may contain bacteriostatic agents such as benzyl alcohol and reducing agents such as ascorbic acid to preserve the ferrous valence state. The pH is between 5 and 7. Its specific activity is not less than 5 mCi/mg ferrous citrate on the date of manufacture. It is available commercially in multidose vials of 125-μCi and 250-μCi amounts.

Iron Metabolism

A simplified scheme of iron metabolism is shown in Figure 15-11. This scheme demonstrates that iron entering the plasma is bound to transferrin, a β-globulin, which loosely binds and transports iron to the tissues and bone marrow. In the tissues, pri-

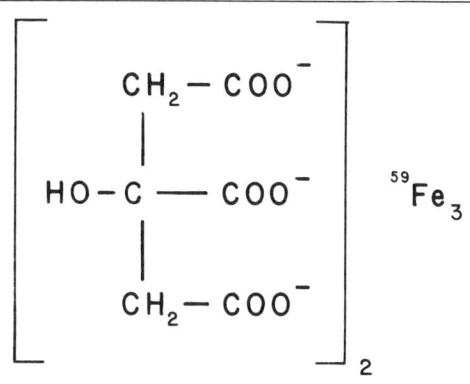

Figure 15-10. Chemical structure of ferrous citrate Fe-59.

marily the liver, iron is stored mostly as ferritin, a readily exchangeable form of storage iron, and smaller amounts of insoluble hemosiderin. In bone marrow the iron is synthesized into hemoglobin within the red blood cells. When the senescent red cells are eventually destroyed, the released hemoglobin is phagocytosed by the reticuloendothelial system (RES) and metabolized. The freed iron is released to the plasma for eventual reutilization by the tissues. The heme portion of hemoglobin is converted by the RES to bilirubin, which is eventually excreted in the bile.

Studies with Ferrous Citrate Fe-59

Although ferrous citrate Fe-59 is not used frequently in nuclear medicine, it is occasionally used for determining various ferrokinetic measurements in the study of iron metabolism. Some of the more common studies include the measurement of plasma iron clearance, plasma iron turnover rate (PITR), and iron utilization.

Plasma Iron Clearance

In this study an intravenous injection of 10 μCi of ferrous citrate Fe-59 is made. From the opposite arm 10-ml samples of blood are removed at various times and centrifuged and the plasma radioactivity counted in a scintillation well counter. The net count per minute per sample is plotted on semilog

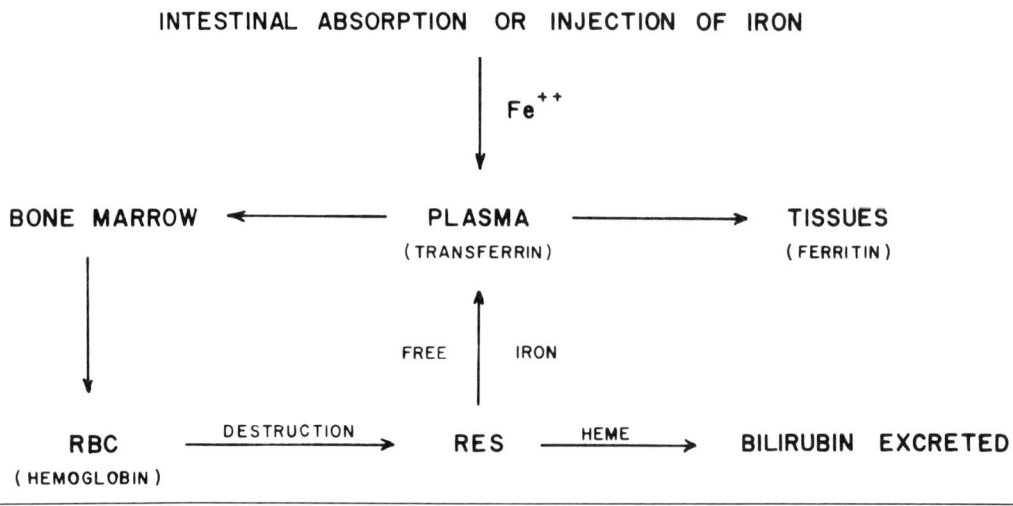

Figure 15-11. Simplified scheme of iron metabolism. See the text for an explanation.

paper to determine the half-time of clearance from the blood (Fig. 15–12). Normal subjects will demonstrate a plasma clearance half-time of 90 ± 30 minutes. Patients with conditions such as hemolytic anemia, polycythemia, and iron deficiency anemia often reveal clearance half-times of less than 60 minutes. Conversely, patients with aplastic anemia, myelofibrosis, and hemochromatosis generally display half-times greater than 120 minutes. Under ordinary circumstances when body iron stores are normal, the rate of clearance is proportional to the rate of erythropoiesis. Erroneous interpretation of rapid or slow clearance rates, however, might occur if the level of plasma iron is not taken into account. A more effective measurement, therefore, is the plasma iron turnover rate.

Plasma Iron Turnover Rate

The plasma iron turnover rate (PITR) supplements the plasma clearance study. Because the results of the clearance study may be influenced by the iron levels of the plasma, it becomes advantageous to know whether a reduced clearance time is due to decreased body iron storage, such as in iron deficiency anemia, or from increased iron turnover, as in hemolytic anemia, polycythemia, or blood loss. The PITR test can be used in this differentiation. The PITR is calculated from the following equation.

$$\text{PITR (mg/24 hr)} = \frac{0.693 \times \text{plasma iron (mg/ml)} \times \text{plasma volume (ml)} \times 24}{T_{1/2} \text{ plasma iron clearance}}$$

A plasma volume determination is required, and the plasma iron concentration must be obtained from the chemistry laboratory. The normal range for PITR is 27 to 42 mg per 24 hours. It can be expected to be prolonged in aplastic anemia and hemochromatosis.

The PITR does not differentiate between iron clearance to erythroid or non-erythroid tissue and therefore can be a misleading guide to the state of erythropoiesis if most of the iron is distributed to non-erythroid tissue.

Iron Utilization

To obtain a better handle on the function of bone marrow, the fraction of administered radioiron incorporated into the RBCs

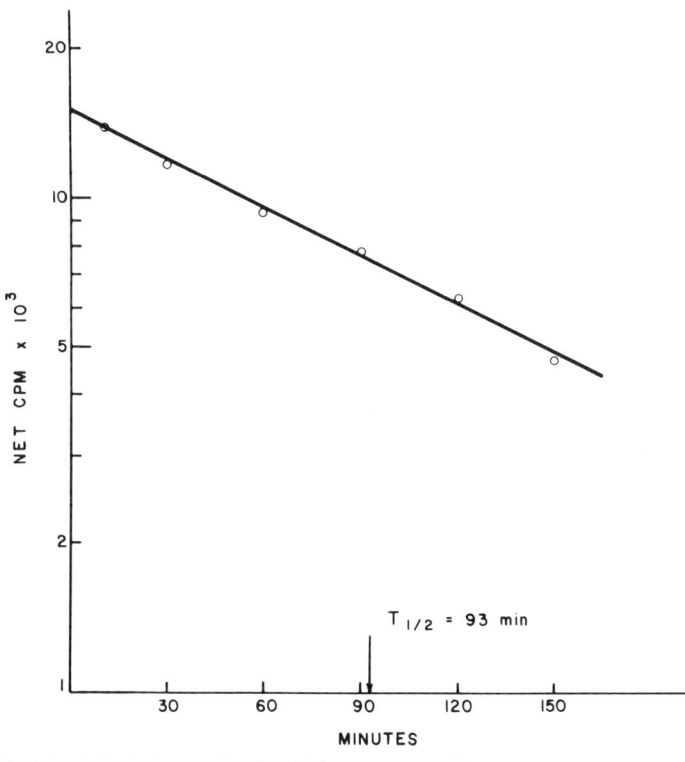

Figure 15-12. Determination of the plasma clearance half-time for Fe-59.

can be measured. This can be obtained with the same dose of Fe-59 used for the plasma clearance and PITR studies. Serial 3- to 5-ml samples of heparinized blood are obtained every other day for 10 to 14 days. The percent utilization can then be determined by the following equation:

$$\% \text{ utilization} = \frac{\frac{\text{cpm/ml}}{\text{whole blood}} \times \frac{\text{blood}}{\text{volume}} \times 100}{\text{cpm injected}}$$

Normally 80 to 90 percent of the injected Fe-59 that is cleared by erythroid tissue reappears in the circulating red cells within 7 to 10 days. In diseases such as iron deficiency anemia, hemolytic anemia, polycythemia, and blood loss the percent utilization may approach 100 percent in only 3 or 4 days. Other disorders such as hypoplastic anemia, pernicious anemia, myeloid metaplasia, and uremia may cause retarded utilization rates. Greater detail regarding the studies of iron clearance, PITR, and iron utilization can be found elsewhere.[6,30,31]

Radiation Dose from Fe-59

The estimated absorbed radiation dose to an average patient (70 kg) from an intravenous injection of a maximum dose of 10 μCi of Fe-59 as ferrous citrate is as follows[32]:

Tissue	rads/10 μCi
Liver	0.29
Kidneys	0.45
Spleen	0.58
Bone marrow	0.65
Testes	0.34
Ovaries	0.33
Whole body	0.23

REFERENCES

1. Welch TJC, Potchen EJ, Welch MJ: Fundamentals of the Tracer Method. Philadelphia, Saunders, 1972
2. Brownell GL, Berman M, Robertson JS: Nomenclature for tracer kinetics. Int J Appl Radiat Isot 19:249, 1968
3. Gray SJ, Sterling K: The tagging of red cells and plasma proteins with radioactive chromium. J Clin Invest 29:1604, 1950
4. Pearson HA: The binding of Cr-51 to hemoglobin. I. In vitro studies. Blood 22:218, 1963
5. Ebaugh FG, Samuels AJ, Dobrowlski P, et al: The site of the CrO_4^- hemoglobin bond as determined by starch electrophoresis and chromatography. Fed Proc 20:70, 1961
6. Albert SN, Sodee DB: In vivo and in vitro studies of hemopoietic production and components. In Sodee DB, Early PJ (eds): Mosby's Manual of Nuclear Medicine Procedures, 3rd ed. St Louis C.V. Mosby, 1981, p 269
7. Arnold JE: Blood volume. In Gottschalk A, Potchen EJ (eds): Diagnostic Nuclear Medicine. Baltimore, Williams & Wilkins, 1976, p 130
8. Radioisotope Production and Quality Control, Technical Report No. 128. Vienna, IAEA, 1971
9. US Pharmacopeia XXI, National Formulary XVI. Rockville, Md, US Pharmacopeial Convention, 1985
10. Ashby W: The determination of the length of life of transfused blood corpuscles in man. J Exp Med 29:267, 1919
11. Bentley SA: Red cell survival studies reinterpreted. Clin Haematol 6:601, 1977
12. Cohen JA, Warringa MGPJ: The fate of P-32 labeled di-isopropyl fluorophosphate in the human body and its use as a labeling agent in the study of the turnover of blood plasma and red cells. J Clin Invest 33:459, 1954
13. Ebaugh FG Jr, Emerson CP, Ross JF: The use of radioactive chromium-51 as an erythrocyte tagging agent for the determination of red cell survival in vivo. J Clin Invest 32:1260, 1953
14. Recommended methods for radioisotope red-cell survival studies: A report by the International Committee for Standardization in Hematology panel on diagnostic applications of radioisotopes in hematology. Br J Haematol 21:241, 1971
15. Guyton AC: Textbook of Medical Physiology, 6th ed. Philadelphia, Saunders, 1981, p 59
16. Hillman RS: Vitamin B-12, folic acid, and the treatment of megaloblastic anemias. In Gilman AG, Goodman LS, Gilman A (eds): The Pharmacological Basis of Therapeutics, 6th ed. New York, Macmillan, 1980, p 1331
17. Nelp WB, McAfee JG, Wagner HN Jr: Single measurement of plasma radioactive vitamin B-12 as a test for pernicious anemia. J Lab Clin Med 61:158, 1963
18. Heinle RW, Welch AD, Scharf V, et al: Studies of excretion (and absorption) of Co-60 labeled vitamin B-12 in pernicious anemia. Trans Assoc Am Physicians 65:214, 1952
19. Schilling RF: Intrinsic factor studies. II. The effect of gastric juice on the urinary excretion of radioactivity after the oral administration of radioactive vitamin B-12. J Lab Clin Med 42:860, 1953
20. McIntyre PA: The blood and blood-forming organ. In Wagner HN Jr (ed): Nuclear Medicine—A Hospital Text. New York, HP Publ, 1975, p 185
21. Katz JH, Dimase J, Donaldson RM Jr: Simultaneous administration of gastric juice bound and free radioactive cyanocobalamin. Rapid procedure for differentiating between intrinsic factor deficiency and other causes of vitamin B-12 malabsorption. J Lab Clin Med 61:266, 1963
22. Domstad PA, Choy YC, Kim EE, et al: Reliability of the dual-isotope Schilling test for the diagnosis of pernicious anemia or malabsorption syndrome. Am J Clin Pathol 75:723, 1981
23. Briedis, D, McIntyre PA, Judisch J, et al: An evaluation of a dual-isotope method for the measurement of vitamin B-12 absorption. J Nucl Med 14:135, 1973
24. Pathy MS, Kirkman S, Malloy MJ: An evaluation of simultaneously administered free and intrinsic factor bound radioactive cyanocobalamin in the diagnosis of pernicious anemia in the elderly. J Clin Pathol 32:244, 1979
25. Radioisotope Production and Quality Control: Technical Reports Series No. 128. Vienna, IAEA, 1971, p 151
26. Hupf HB: Production and purification of radionuclides. In Tubis M, Wolf W (eds):

Radiopharmacy. New York, Wiley 1976, p 225
27. Kline OL, Boehne JW: Vitamins and other nutrients. In Osol A, Hoover JE (eds): Remington's Pharmaceutical Sciences, 14th ed. Easton, Pa, Mack Publ Co., 1970, p 1011
28. Rosenblum C: Production and metabolism of cobalt-labeled cyanocobalamin. In Andrews GA, Kniseley RM, Wagner HN Jr (eds): Radioactive Pharmaceuticals. Oak Ridge, Tenn, US Atomic Energy Commission, 1966, p 455
29. Package insert, Dicopac kit: Arlington Heights, Ill, Amersham Corp, 1978
30. Maynard CD: Clinical Nuclear Medicine. Philadelphia, Lea & Febiger, 1971
31. Friedman BI: Radionuclide studies associated with abnormalities of iron. In Rothfeld B (ed): Nuclear Medicine in Vitro. Philadelphia, Lippincott, 1974, p 85
32. Package insert, Ferrous Citrate Fe-59 Injection. St Louis, Mallinckrodt Diagnostics, 1980

CHAPTER 16

In Vitro Radioassay Tests

In vitro radioassay tests in nuclear medicine involve the use of radioactive material to measure various substances present in the blood such as hormones, biochemicals, and drugs. Because these substances are often present in very low concentrations, the use of radiation detection methods provides the analytic sensitivity required for accurate measurement. In vitro radioassay tests require only a sample of patient's blood for analysis. No radioactivity is administered to the patient.

PRINCIPLE OF RADIOASSAY TESTS

In principle radioassay tests are based upon competitive binding between a binding agent (B) and a labeled (S*) and unlabeled (S) form of the substrate to be measured as described by the following set of equations:

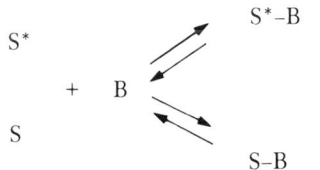

Under these circumstances, if S and S* have equal affinity for B and the amounts of S* and B are fixed, the amount of S*–B complex formed will be inversely related to the amount of S present. In general, S represents the unknown amount of substance in the blood that is to be measured and S* is the radioactive form of the substance. S* and B are supplied as reagents with the test kit. The binder B is either a protein or an antibody that binds specifically with the substance to be measured. When B is a protein, the radioassay test is called a competitive protein-binding assay; when B is an antibody with specific reactivity for S antigen, the test is called a radio-immunoassay (RIA). The majority of in vitro radioassay tests performed in nuclear medicine are radioimmunoassays.

The underlying goal of any competitive binding assay, such as RIA, is to measure the amount of unlabeled antigen (drug, hormone, or other substance) in the blood after it reacts with antibody. The techniques used to accomplish this task may be divided into two categories based on the type of kinetics used: (1) equilibrium or one-stage assays and (2) nonequilibrium or sequential assays. In a one-stage assay the labeled and unlabeled antigen and antibody are incubated together for a defined period of time sufficient to approximate equilibrium conditions. Under these circumstances the labeled and unlabeled antigen compete for the limited amount of antibody present. The law of mass action is operational, and the antigen in higher concentration has the competitive advantage for binding with antibody. In a sequential assay, the unlabeled antigen is allowed to react with an excess of antibody first so that essentially all of the antigen is bound. In a subsequent step, labeled antigen is added to bind with unreacted antibody. With either technique the antibody-bound antigen is separated and counted. The amount of radioactivity counted will be inversely proportional to the amount of unlabeled antigen in the blood sample. Standard curves are used to determine the actual amount of unlabeled antigen in the blood.

RADIOIMMUNOASSAY

RIA was first developed in the mid-1950s by Berson and Yalow to measure serum levels of insulin.[1] During their work studying the role of insulin in diabetes they noted that treated diabetics carried antibodies to insulin. Subsequently, they demonstrated that these antibodies could bind radiolabeled insulin, and the science of radioimmunoassay had begun.

Antibodies have several characteristics that make them uniquely suitable for analytic purposes.[2] First, antibodies can be manufactured against a wide diversity of antigens. Even small molecules that are not immunogenic themselves (haptens) elicit an immune response when coupled to a larger "carrier" molecule. Second, antibodies are specific for the immunizing antigen; thus, when analyzing a complex solution such as serum, antibodies discriminate between the various antigens in solution and combine only with those antigens against which they are specifically directed. That specificity is not absolute, however, and cross-reactions with structurally similar antigens must be considered when designing a RIA procedure. Third, the high affinity of antibodies for antigens allow them to combine rapidly and firmly, thus providing high sensitivity in RIA procedures. Finally, antibodies are stable molecules that can be stored for years without losing their potency.

Antibody Production

Developing an antibody with high affinity and specificity for the substance to be measured is a crucial step in the development of a RIA method. A substance must be immunogenic if antibodies are to be developed against it. The factors determining immunogenicity include molecular weight, chemical composition, and molecular charge and configuration. Proteins with molecular weights greater than 5000 daltons are usually immunogenic whereas those with molecular weights less than 1000 are generally poor immunogens. Many hapten subtances such as steroids, hormones such as thyroxine, and most drugs must thus be conjugated to a carrier to render them immunogenic. Some typical examples are shown in Table 16–1. The conjugation between hapten and carrier is crucial and must be accomplished in a manner that leaves the immunogenic portion of the hapten exposed for antibody production.

The most common animal species used for antibody production include rabbits, guinea pigs, goats, and sheep. The antigenic substance or hapten–carrier conjugate is injected into the animal. Most immunization schedules use a relatively large antigen dose for primary immunization (0.2 to 1.5 mg/kg) followed by booster injections every 2 to 4 weeks using antigen concentrations from 5 to 50 percent of the priming dose.[2] Immunizations are usually done by intradermal, subcutaneous, or intramuscular injection. Animals can be bled 7 to 100 days after booster injections and their serum tested for antibody. When optimal conditions are reached, the antibody is then isolated and purified for use in development of the RIA procedure. Antibody is then tested for binding affinity with antigen to

TABLE 16-1. HAPTEN–CARRIER CONJUGATES FOR ANTIBODY PRODUCTION

Hapten	Carrier	Animal Species
Digoxin	Human serum albumin	Rabbit
Aldosterone	Bovine serum albumin	Sheep
Cortisol	Bovine serum albumin	Rabbit
Insulin	None	Guinea pig
Thyroxine (T_4)	Thyroglobulin	Rabbit
Triiodothyronine (T_3)	Thyroglobulin	Rabbit
Vitamin B_{12}	Bovine serum albumin	Rabbit

(Data from Howard PL, et al, 1980.[2])

ascertain the binding force or avidity between these species. Affinity is related to the sensitivity that may be obtained in the assay. Antibody specificity refers to the ability of specific antibodies to discriminate between two structurally similar molecules. Specificity testing will establish the degree to which cross-reacting antigens will interfere with the assay.

Antigen–Antibody Separation Methods

Once the antibody characteristics are optimized, a method of separating antibody-bound antigen from free antigen must be developed to make the RIA kit an easy-to-use method of analysis. Ideally, a separation system would instantly and totally separate bound and free antigen with a minimal effect on the results of the assay, being unaffected by pH, volume, ionic strength, time, temperature, and other factors. No system can fulfill all these requirements. Over the years of RIA development several separation methods have been used. Some of the methods used include electrophoresis, chromatography, filtration, salting out, adsorption, immunoprecipitation, and immunosorption.[2] The first four methods are traditional physicochemical methods that are not routinely used in modern RIA methods because of their time-consuming and complex nature. Adsorption methods rely mostly on the binding of free antigen to activated charcoal, with separation being effected by centrifugation and decantation of bound antigen. In general, charcoal adsorption methods are inexpensive, rapid, and simple. Immunoprecipitation is a double-antibody technique whereby the soluble antigen–antibody complex is separated from free antigen by precipitation of the antigen–antibody complex by the addition of a second antibody that has specificity for it. Immunosorption is a solid-phase system whereby the antibody is immobilized onto insoluble materials such as starch, glass, cellulose, acrylamide gels, and plastics, to name a few. A common method is to bond antibody to the bottom inner surface of the plastic tube used in the assay system. These methods allow for a variety of separation techniques.

Some of the substrates (antigens–haptens) for which commercial RIA tests have been developed include thyroid-stimulating hormone (TSH), carcinoembryonic antigen (CEA), cortisol, digoxin, estriol, ferritin, folate, gastrin, hepatitis-associated antigen (HAA), human chorionic gonadotropin (HCG), insulin, renin, thyroxine (T_4), and triiodothyronine (T_3).

To illustrate the methodology involved in RIA, single-stage RIA based on immunosorption as a separation method (T_4 RIA) and sequential RIA based on immunoprecipitation as a separation method (TSH RIA) will be discussed. Detailed procedures for other RIA procedures are supplied with each kit, and more complete discussion of RIA methods can be found elsewhere.[2-5]

THYROXINE RIA

The status of thyroid function is commonly evaluated by measurement of serum levels of the thyroid hormone, L-thyroxine (T_4). Greater than 99.95 percent of circulatory T_4 serves as a metabolically inert reservoir because it is transported in serum bound primarily to thyroxine-binding globulin (TBG) (60 percent), and secondarily, to thyroxine-binding prealbumin (30 percent) and albumin (10 percent).[5] A great deal of evidence indicates that the unbound or free fraction (FT_4), which is less than 0.05 percent of the total circulating T_4, is the physiologically active form. Additionally, FT_4 is the major precursor to triiodothyronine (T_3).

Several tests are available to measure the total T_4 in the serum. A typical procedure will be used to illustrate the methodology of immunosorbant RIA.[6]

Total Thyroxine Determination

In the total T_4 determination, T_4 (bound to serum protein) and FT_4 are measured together. T_4 must be displaced from its serum-binding proteins so that it can react with antibody. This can be accomplished using agents such as ANS (8-anilino-1-naphthalene sulfonic acid) and salicylate in the buffer solution. Serum samples from the subject containing unknown amounts of T_4 are incubated with I-125 T_4 and ANS–salicylate buffer in antibody-coated tubes. During this time the labeled and unlabeled T_4 compete for a limited number of binding sites of antibody, which is immobilized on the lower inner wall of the tube. After equilibrium is achieved the contents of the tube are aspirated and the tube counted. The amount of radioactivity (labeled T_4) bound in the tube will be inversely related to the concentration of T_4 in the serum sample.

Standards of T_4 serum are subjected to the same procedure as patient samples and a standard curve is plotted. Unknown values of T_4 in the patient's serum are obtained from the standard curve by interpolation. The stepwise procedure for the test is illustrated in Figure 16–1. Typical data for the total T_4 assay are shown in Table 16–2 and Figure 16–2. The normal range of total T_4 levels in serum is 4.5 to 11.5 µg/dl.

THYROID-STIMULATING HORMONE RADIOIMMUNOASSAY

Thyroid stimulating hormone (TSH) is produced by specific thyrotropic cells of the anterior pituitary gland. Its only known physiologic function is to stimulate production and secretion of the thyroid hormones (T_4) and (T_3) by the thyroid gland. TSH is a glycoprotein hormone with a molecular weight of approximately 28,000

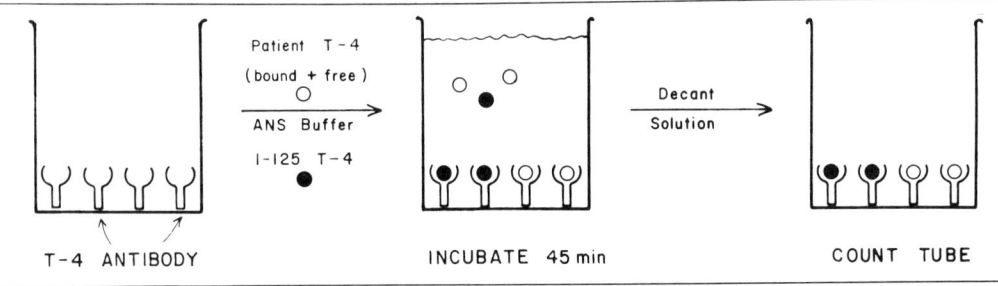

Figure 16–1. Stepwise procedure for the total T_4 RIA illustrating a method of immunosorbant RIA.

TABLE 16-2. TYPICAL STANDARD AND PATIENT DATA FOR THE T_4 ASSAY

Sample No.	T_4 Serum	Concentration (μg/dl)	cpm Bound
1, 2	Standard	1	24,984
			24,202
3, 4	Standard	4	17,512
			16,993
5, 6	Standard	8	11,327
			11,181
7, 8	Standard	12	8,644
			8,349
9, 10	Standard	20	5,959
			5,643
11, 12	[a]Patient X	6.8	12,735
		6.7	12,770
13, 14	[b]Patient Y	11.2	8,837
		11.7	8,586

[a]Average T_4 concentration, 6.8 μg/dl.
[b]Average T_4 concentration, 11.4 μg/dl.
(Data for Tables 16-2 and 16-3 from Instruction manual: Gamma Coat I-125 Free/Total T-4 Radioimmunoassay Kit, Clinical Assays, 1984.[6])

are useful in evaluating thyroid disease, particularly hypothyroidism.

Thyroid-Stimulating Hormone Test Procedure

A typical sequential-type assay for TSH based on immunoprecipitation will be described. Serum samples from the subject containing unknown amounts of TSH are incubated with TSH antibody. During this first incubation, essentially all of the TSH is bound to the antibody. In the second step, TSH labeled with I-125 is added to the mixture. During the second incubation the labeled TSH binds to the unreacted binding sites on the antibody. In the third step, a precipitating antibody (goat antirabbit antiserum) is added to the mixture. This antibody combines with the antibody of the initial TSH-antibody complex, which causes it to precipitate. After centrifugation, the free labeled TSH is decanted, and the labeled precipitate is counted. The amount of radioactivity in the precipitate is inversely proportional to the amount of TSH in the serum sample. Standard TSH samples are also run simultaneously with patient samples, and a standard curve is plotted. Unknown values of TSH are inter-

daltons. It is present in the circulation as the intact molecule and is not bound to any plasma protein. Serum TSH concentrations

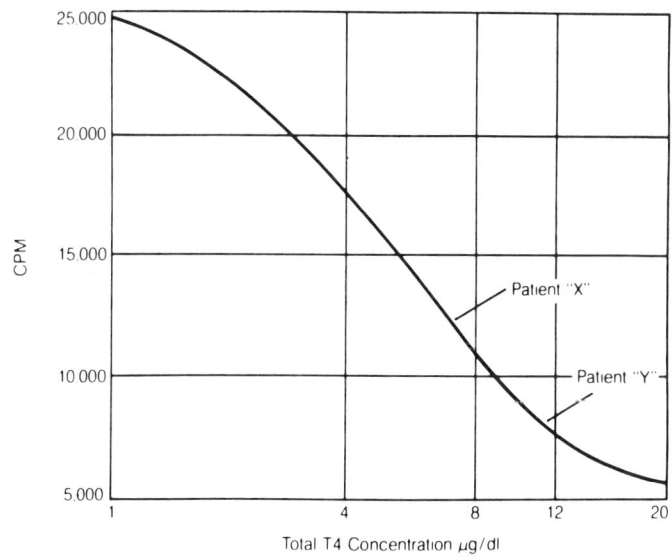

Figure 16-2. Typical standard curve for the total T_4 RIA. (From Instruction manual: Gamma Coat I-125 Free/Total T-4 Radioimmunoassay Kit, Clinical Assays, 1984, with permission.[6])

TABLE 16-3. TYPICAL STANDARD AND PATIENT DATA FOR THE TSH ASSAY

Sample No.	Sample Content	Net cpm	B/B_0 (%)	TSH ($\mu U/ml$)
1	Zero-standard (B_0)	15,650	100.0	0
2	Standard serum A	14,134	90.4	1.5
3	Standard serum B	11,826	75.6	4.0
4	Standard serum C	8200	52.4	10.0
5	Standard, serum D	5319	34.0	20.0
6	Standard serum E	2817	18.0	50.0
7	Patient X	9650	61.7[a]	7.6[b]

[a] $\dfrac{(B)\ 9650}{(B_0)\ 15650} \times 100 = 61.7\%$

[b] Interpolated from Figure 16-5.

polated from the standard curve. The concentration of TSH in the standards is shown in Table 16-3. The stepwise procedure is summarized in Figure 16-3. All samples and standards are run in duplicate. As shown in Table 16-3, sample number 1, the zero standard, represents the amount of radioactivity in the final precipitate when no "cold" TSH is present. It is designated as B_0. Standards (samples 2 through 6) and patient samples, designated as B, will contain an amount of radioactivity less than B_0 and inversely proportional to the amount of "cold" TSH present in the sample. The percent of tracer bound in each standard and patient sample is calculated as $B/B_0 \times 100$. Typical results are shown in Table 16-3.

The percent trace binding ($B/B_0 \times 100$) for each standard sample is plotted against the log of the TSH concentration to obtain the standard curve shown in Figure 16-4. Because such curves are often sigmoid

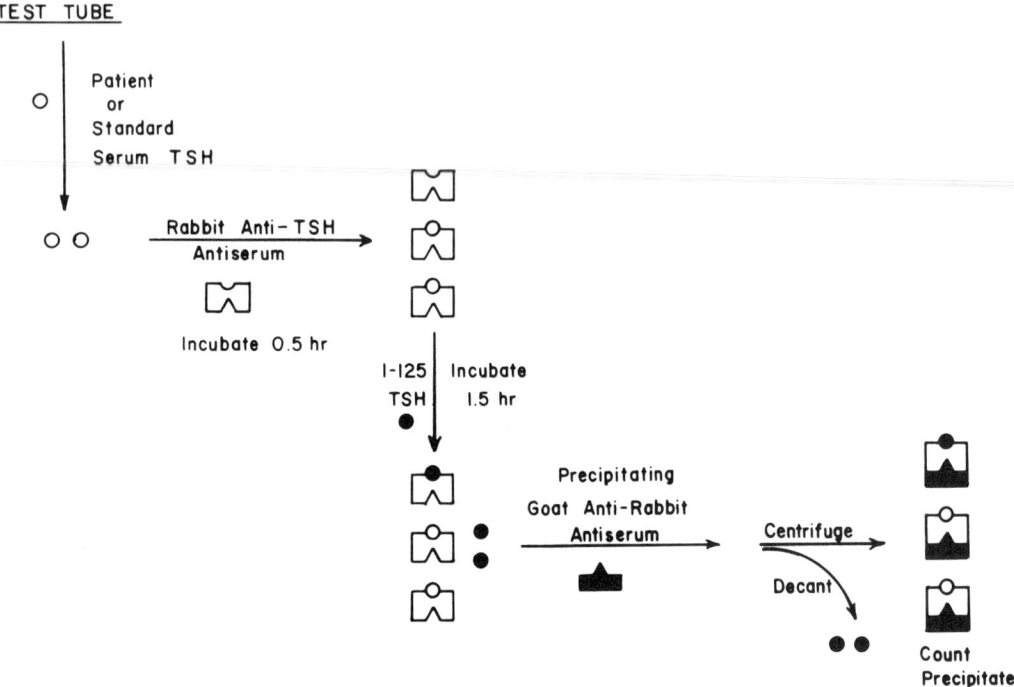

Figure 16-3. Stepwise procedure for the TSH RIA illustrating a method of immunoprecipitation RIA.

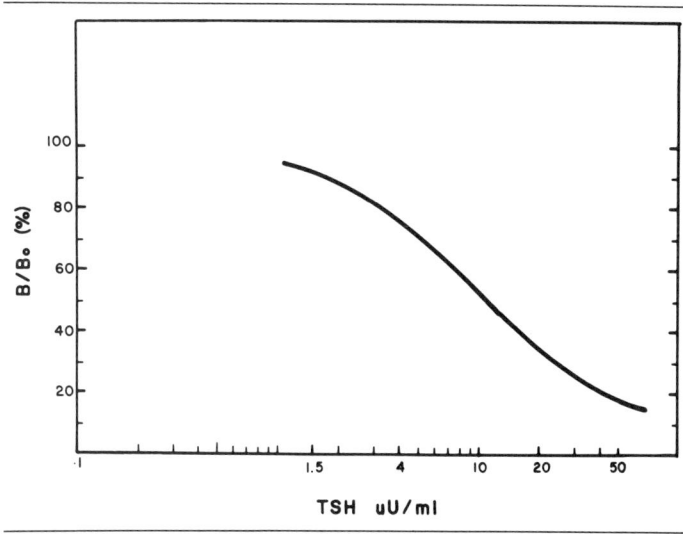

Figure 16-4. Sigmoidal standard curve for the TSH RIA (semilog plot).

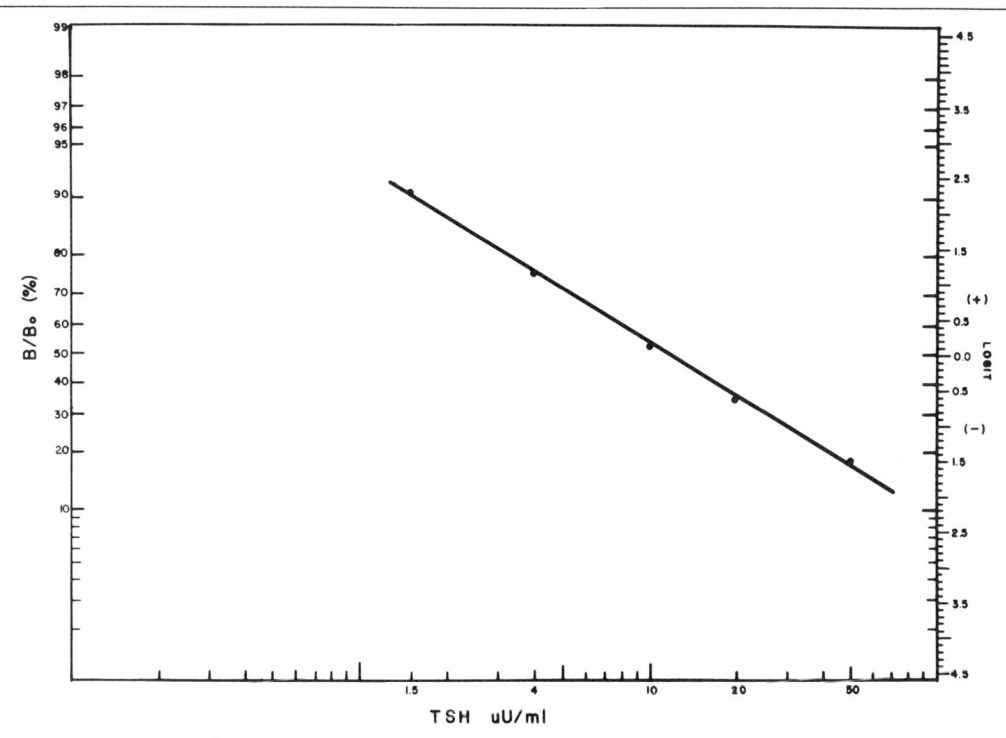

Figure 16-5. Linear standard curve for the TSH RIA (logit-log plot).

shaped, it is common to linearize the curve by plotting the logistic transformation (logit) of $B/B_0 \times 100$ against the log of the TSH concentration. The logit of Y is defined as

$$\text{Logit}(Y) = \ln\left(\frac{Y}{1-Y}\right)$$

If we choose Y as the fraction of trace binding (B/B_0), then

$$\text{Logit } B/B_0 = \frac{B/B_0}{1 - B/B_0}$$

If B/B_0 is expressed as a percentage then

$$\text{Logit } B/B_0 = \frac{B/B_0}{100 - B/B_0}$$

A logit–log standard curve of the data from Figure 16–4 is shown in Figure 16–5. It is much easier to interpolate the TSH concentration from the percent trace binding data using a linear standard curve. As shown in Table 16–3, a patient specimen exhibiting a 61.7 percent trace binding corresponds to a TSH concentration of 7.6 μU/ml. The normal range of TSH values in euthyroid subjects is 1.3 to 5.9 μU/ml. The reader is referred to standard texts and individual test monographs for more detailed procedures and interpretation of these tests and other specific RIA tests.

REFERENCES

1. Berson SA, Yalow RS: Quantitative aspects of the reaction between insulin and insulin-binding antibody. J Clin Invest 38:1996, 1959
2. Howard PL, Trainer TD: Radionuclides in Clinical Chemistry. Boston, Little, Brown, 1980
3. Zetner A: Principles of competitive binding assays (saturation analyses) I, equilibrium techniques. Clin Chem 19:699, 1973
4. Zetner A, Duly PE: Principles of competitive binding assays (saturation analyses) II, sequential saturation. Clin Chem 20:5, 1974
5. Hayes RL, Goswitz FA, Murphy BE (eds): Radioisotopes in Medicine: In Vitro Studies. AEC Symposium Series 13. Oakridge, Tenn, USAEC, 1968
6. Instruction manual: Gamma Coat I-125 Free/Total T-4 Radioimmunoassay Kit, Clinical Assays, Cambridge, Mass, Travenol-Genentech Diagnostics, 1984

CHAPTER 17

Miscellaneous Radiopharmaceuticals and Applications

This chapter will cover useful applications of radiopharmaceuticals previously discussed in other chapters and those agents that are important in nuclear medicine but either are used infrequently, do not fit into any of the major organ systems, or have mainly investigational applications.

GASTROINTESTINAL STUDIES

Several useful procedures have been developed to evaluate the gastrointestinal (GI) system with radiopharmaceuticals. Some of the more significant procedures are the GI bleeding study, the gastroesophageal reflux study, the gastric emptying study, and the detection of Meckel's diverticulum.

Detection of Gastrointestinal Bleeding

Successful management of acute GI bleeding may depend upon accurate localization of the bleeding site. Most GI bleeding occurs intermittently. This presents a problem to the clinician in effectively using invasive diagnostic methods such as angiography. Angiography relies on extravasation of radiographic contrast material for bleeding-site detection and therefore requires active bleeding at the time the study is performed. Because such procedures are associated with significant morbidity and mortality, other methods have been sought to identify GI bleeding.

Scintigraphic methods to localize sites of GI bleeding using radiopharmaceuticals have been developed. The radiopharmaceuticals that have evolved as most clinically useful can be categorized into two groups: (1) agents that are rapidly extracted from the circulation and (2) agents that remain in the circulation for a prolonged period of time. In the former group is Tc-99m sulfur colloid (Tc-SC), and the latter, Tc-99m red blood cells (Tc-RBCs).

Considerable controversy appears to exist regarding which of these radiopharmaceuticals is the agent of choice.[1-3] Ideally, one would like a significant fraction of the intravenously adminstered activity to extravasate into the bleeding site and remain fixed there, with the remaining fraction in the blood being rapidly excreted from the body. This would provide high target-to-background ratios and detection sensitivity. Neither Tc-SC nor Tc-RBCs meet these stringent requirements. Tc-SC has the capacity to produce scans with the least amount of background activity in the lower two thirds of the abdomen because the colloid particles are efficiently removed from the blood by the reticuloendothelial system (RES).

There are two apparent limitations with the use of Tc-SC. First, the accumulation of activity in the liver and spleen may obscure bleeding sites in these areas of the abdomen. Second, with rapid blood clearance, active bleeding must be occurring at the time of dose administration, otherwise extravasation of tracer activity into the bleeding site is not likely to occur. With a blood clearance half-time of 2 to 3 minutes, Tc-SC is essentially cleared within 12 to 15 minutes after injection. Because bleeding is often intermittent by nature, detection of bleeding sites with Tc-SC is more likely to occur if multiple, sequential injections are given at 15-minute intervals while imaging.

Proponents of Tc-RBCs for detecting GI bleeding argue that intermittent bleeding is more likely to be detected if the radiotracer remains in the circulation for a prolonged period of time from which it is able to extravasate when active bleeding occurs. The prolonged blood clearance of in vitro labeled Tc-RBCs ($T_{1/2}$ = 29 hours) is an advantage in this regard. The disadvantage of this technique is a higher body background. The latter has not appeared to interfere significantly with the detection of bleeding sites by those who prefer this method.

One attempt at a compromise between the two agents is to heat damage the Tc-RBCs slightly before injection.[4] Under such circumstances the Tc-RBCs exhibit a blood clearance half-time of about 10 minutes, which allows more time for uptake into bleeding sites and eventual removal from the blood by the spleen with decreased background activity. This method is more demanding technically and has not been extensively evaluated in humans.

An important consideration with radiopharmaceuticals used for the detection of GI bleeding is the presence of free pertechnetate. Because pertechnetate is secreted by the gastric mucosal cells into the bowel lumen, significant activity in the bowel contents may lead to false-positive scans. Free pertechnetate is probably of more concern with the use of Tc-RBCs than with Tc-SC,[1] particularly during prolonged studies.[2] Free pertechnetate is usually less than 5 percent in Tc-SC preparations but should be checked using radiochromatography before use, especially if the product is several hours old. Greater potential exists for free pertechnetate in Tc-RBCs, depending on the method of preparation. The in vivo method of labeling has the highest potential for free pertechnetate (approximately 30 percent) and is least satisfactory for GI bleed studies, often requiring nasogastric suction to remove pertechnetate in the stomach.[5] The modified in vivo method[6] is an improvment (less than 10 percent pertechnetate), but the in vitro method[7] of labeling is probably the first choice (less than 5 percent pertechnetate) even though it is less convenient than the other methods. The inconvenience, however, is outweighed by a decidedly superior study.

The significant properties of Tc-SC and Tc-RBCs are listed in Table 17-1. In general, it appears that Tc-SC is the favored agent if active bleeding is occurring at the time of study, whereas Tc-RBCs are more desirable if the bleeding status is unknown and when a prolonged study is anticipated. Evidence acquired from a comparative study of the two agents in the same patient is in favor of Tc-RBCs.[3] This study compared Tc-SC by single injection of 10 mCi followed by image acquisition for 15 to 20 minutes. This phase was followed immediately by injection of 15 to 25 mCi of Tc-RBCs (prepared by the in vitro method) with imaging for 90 minutes. Continuous 1-minute computer-acquired images were made along with 5-minute scintiphotos in each phase of the study. Of 100 patients studies, 41 had active bleeding, 38 of which were accurately identified by Tc-RBCs. Only five cases were identified by Tc-SC, and in no instance did Tc-SC demonstrate active hemorrhage that was not subsequently identified by Tc-RBCs. The detection rate

TABLE 17-1. PROPERTIES OF Tc-SC and Tc-RBC RELATED TO THE DETECTION OF GI BLEED STUDIES

Tc-99m SC
Fast blood clearance
High target-to-background ratio
Active bleeding required at time of dosing for bleed detection
Multiple injections required for prolonged studies (intermittent bleeding)
Less likelihood of highly vascular structures to interfere with bleed detection
Readily available, easy to prepare (about 15 min)
Pertechnetate impurity not significant

Tc-99m RBCs
Slow blood clearance
Low target-to-background ratio
Active bleeding not required at time of dosing
Single injection, prolonged study possible for detecting intermittent bleeding
Frequent sequential imaging required to identify bleeding site versus translocated activity
Techniques of preparation require about 30 min
In vitro kit currently under IND status
Pertechnetate impurity may be significant

---

with Tc-SC probably would have been higher in this study if multiple sequential injections of Tc-SC had been made. In this study 83 percent of all active hemorrhage cases were identified in 90 minutes of continuous imaging. Another study using Tc-RBCs (modified in vivo method) reported that 55 percent of the positive studies were detected within 4 hours of dosing and 90 percent by 14 hours.[2] The delay in achieving a high detection rate in the latter study was probably due to a less frequent interval of imaging than that of the previous study.

The importance of continuous imaging in the detection of GI bleeding should be emphasized because of its intermittent nature.[1,2] Additionally, if delayed scintigraphy is required, sequential imaging is mandatory to differentiate radiotracer activity that has moved from the site of hemorrhage by peristalsis from activity extravasating at the actual bleeding site. In general, in the detection of GI bleeding, a positive bleeding site is identified as an area demonstrating increasing activity or translocation of activity over time as opposed to nonbleeding sites that are visualized as fixed, unchanging activity. Figures 17-1, 17-2, and 17-3 illustrate the detection of GI bleeding with Tc-SC and Tc-RBCs.

Gastroesophageal Reflux Study

Nonradionuclidic techniques to evaluate gastroesophageal reflux have been noted to be inconvenient, indirect, and in some instances insensitive.[8,9] The radionuclide gastroesophageal reflux study has been reported to be a sensitive, noninvasive test that is able to detect reflux in 90 percent of symptomatic patients.[8] Additionally, the study permits quantitation of the extent of reflux into the esophagus and can be extended to detect pulmonary aspiration of gastric contents.[10,11]

The procedure is well tolerated in children. Tc-99m SC (200 µCi) is administered orally in 30 ml of apple juice followed by additional juice or formula until the patient is sated. Abdominal pressure measurements are performed as will be described using a blood pressure cuff in small children to demonstrate reflux. The value of the radionuclide gastric reflux study has been demonstrated in children where an 80 percent detection rate was found in subjects previously documented by other acid reflux methods.[12]

Gastroesophageal reflux is a common problem in infants and children but also occurs in adults. It frequently leads to respiratory complications, presumably resulting from aspiration of gastric contents.[10]

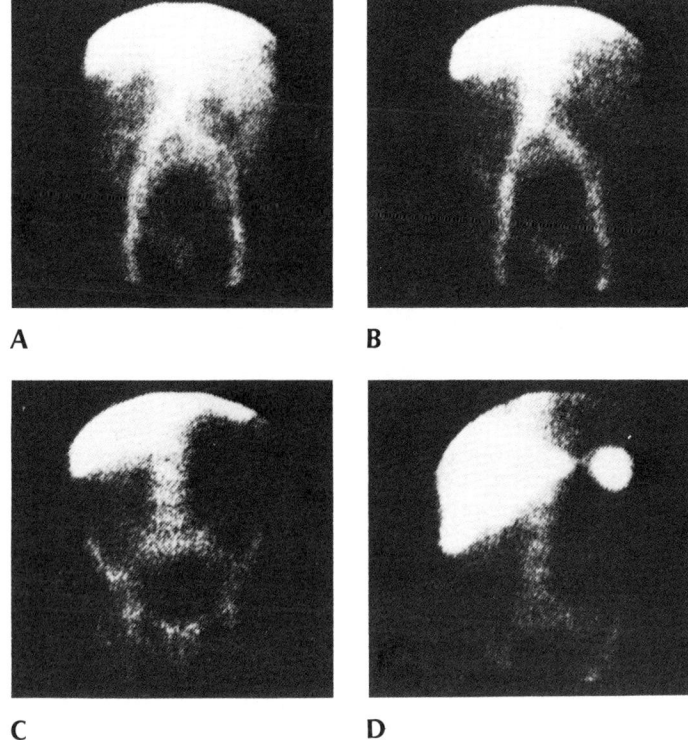

Figure 17-1. Detection of GI bleeding: normal scan, no hemorrhage. These images demonstrate the sequence of findings after the administration of Tc-99m SC. **A.** Immediately after the injection of the radiopharmaceutical, significant activity is visualized in the major vessels, and high background is noted in the rest of the abdomen. There is also early visualization of the liver and the spleen. **B, C.** Within minutes, the major vessel and background activities are significantly diminished. There is gradual visualization of the bone marrow of the spine, pelvis, and proximal femurs. **D.** The final image is a left anterior oblique view of the upper abdomen that shows the space between the left lobe of the liver and the spleen. (From Alavi A, 1982, p 126, with permission.[1])

The reflux study can be extended to detect pulmonary aspiration as a consequence of the gastroesophageal reflux and has been shown to be more sensitive than conventional nonradionuclide procedures.[11] Although the clinical value of a radionuclide technique for detecting lung aspiration is recognized, more experience must be gained in this area to establish sensitivity and specificity.

The radionuclide gastroesophageal reflux study in adults is quite simple and can be performed in a short period of time.[9] In principle the test is as follows: a patient who has fasted overnight is administered an oral dose of 300 μCi of Tc-99m SC in a mixture of 150 ml of orange juice and 150 ml of 0.1 N hydrochloric acid. After 10 to 15 minutes the patient is imaged in the anterior upright position against the collimator of a gamma camera. Normally, no activity is seen above the stomach. Visible esophageal activity above the stomach is abnormal and represents reflux or incomplete clearance of swallowed tracer in subjects with disorders of esophageal motility. In the latter case, if residual activity cannot be washed out with 15 to 30 ml of water, then the study should be repeated with intubation for administration of the tracer and fluid. If no activity is seen in the esophagus, the patient is fitted with an abdominal binder and placed supine under the gamma camera. Pressure is applied in increments of 20 mm Hg while taking 30-second images at each increment until 100 mm Hg is reached.

Gastroesophageal reflux can be quantitated using the following formula:

$$R = \frac{E_t - E_b}{G_o} \times 100$$

where

- R = gastroesophageal reflux percentage
- E_t = esophageal counts at time t when reflux is maximal
- E_b = esophageal background counts
- G_o = gastric counts at the beginning of the study

computer regions of interest.[9] Studies using this method have demonstrated a mean value for reflux in normal subjects of 2.7 ± 0.3 percent, with an upper limit of 3 to 4 percent that begins to overlap the lower range of values in reflux patients.[8] Quantitative reflux in symptomatic subjects ranges from 3.4 to 45.6 percent, with a mean value of 11.7 ± 1.8 percent.[8] Figures 17-4 and 17-5 illustrate, respectively, a typical scintigraphic image and reflux index values for normal and previously documented reflux subjects.

Technetium sulfur colloid is used in gastroesophageal reflux studies because it is insoluble in gastric juices. Significant amounts of soluble technetium pertechnetate are undesirable because its systemic absorption may contribute to increased background activity in the esophageal region. The reason for performing the test with patients in the supine position is to induce more frequent episodes of reflux in that position as opposed to the standing position. An acid liquid meal tends to aggravate reflux because an acid load in the stomach appears to delay gastric emptying and lower the resting lower esophageal sphincter pressure gradient.[9]

Gastric Emptying Studies

Radionuclide gastric emptying studies measure the rate of removal of radiolabeled liquids and solids from the stomach. Such studies provide a noninvasive method of evaluating gastric physiology. Under normal conditions liquids clear faster than solids. Although such studies of gastric emptying are relatively simple to perform, accurate quantitation requires that attention be given to several aspects of the study[13]:

1. Radionuclide markers must have high labeling efficiency and remain stable in vivo during the study.
2. Meal size and composition should be standardized.
3. A standard patient position and posture should be maintained for times of imaging.
4. Correction techniques should be applied when needed to compensate for radio-

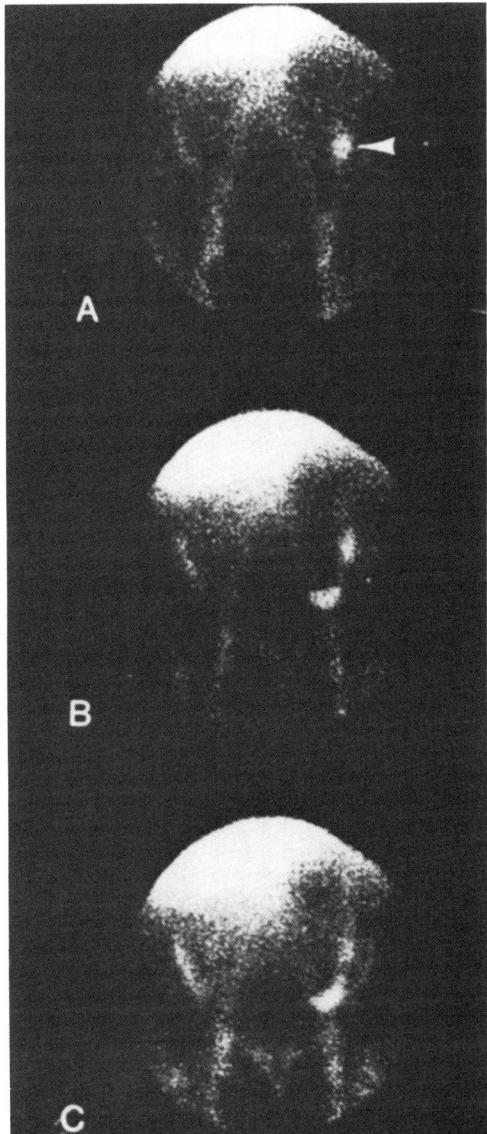

Figure 17-2. Detection of GI bleeding: slow rate of sigmoid bleed. A. Within a few minutes of IV administration of Tc-99m SC the scan shows evidence of extravasation in the left lower area. B, C. Later the activity moves along the iliac crest corresponding to the direction of the sigmoid colon. (From Alavi A, 1982, p 126, with permission.[1])

The respective amounts of activity in the esophagus, stomach, and background are determined by counting activity within

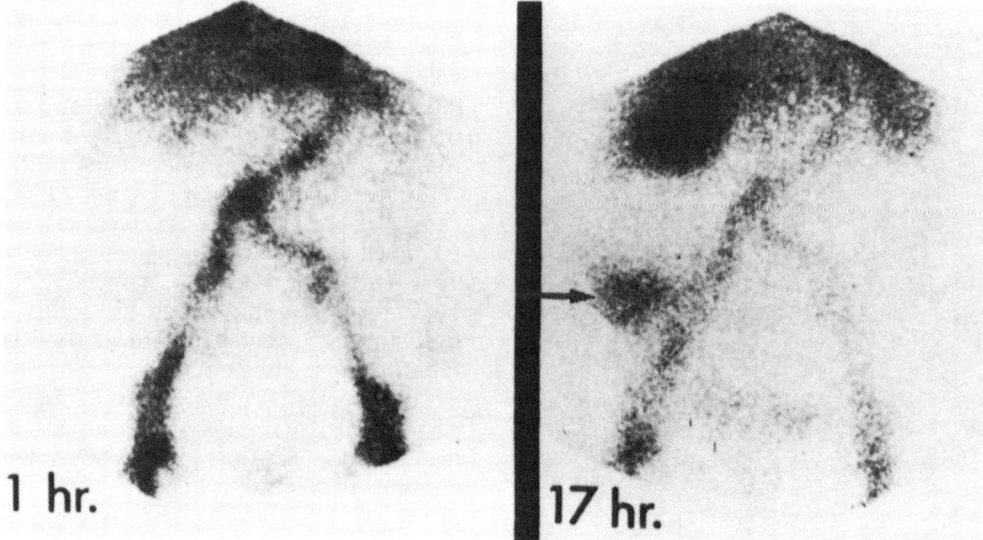

Figure 17-3. Detection of GI bleeding with Tc-99m RBCs. Anterior abdominal scintiscan in an elderly patient with melena. An initial scintiscan at 1 hour is normal. At 17 hours an abnormal focal collection is noted in the cecum (arrow). Surgery confirmed a bleeding cecal carcinoma. *(From Winzelberg GG, et al, 1982, p 139, with permission.[2])*

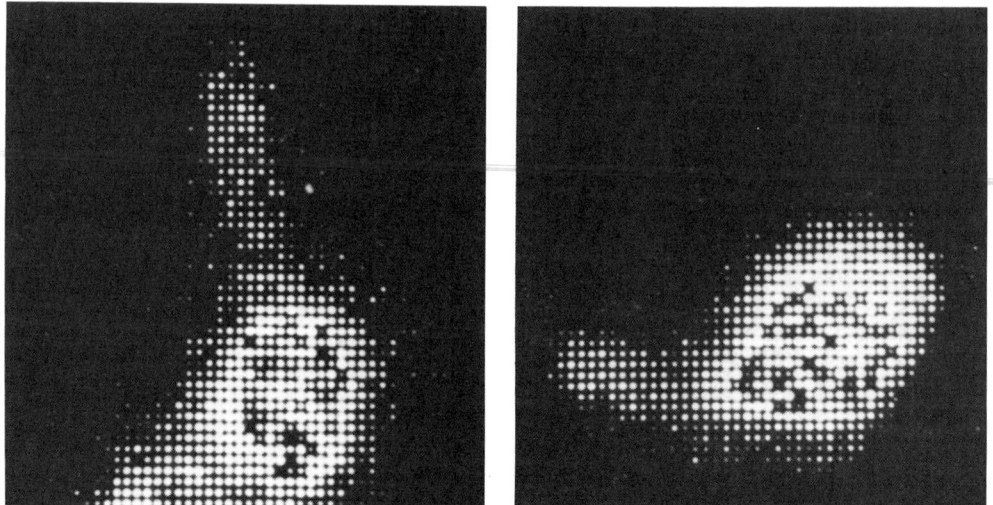

Figure 17-4. Gastroesophageal scintigraphy displayed on an oscilloscope of a data processor. **A.** This study demonstrates reflux above the stomach into the esophagus. **B.** In an asymptomatic normal volunteer, this demonstrates gastric activity and filling of the pylorus, but no reflux cephalad. *(From Malmud LS, et al, 1982, p 104, with permission.[9])*

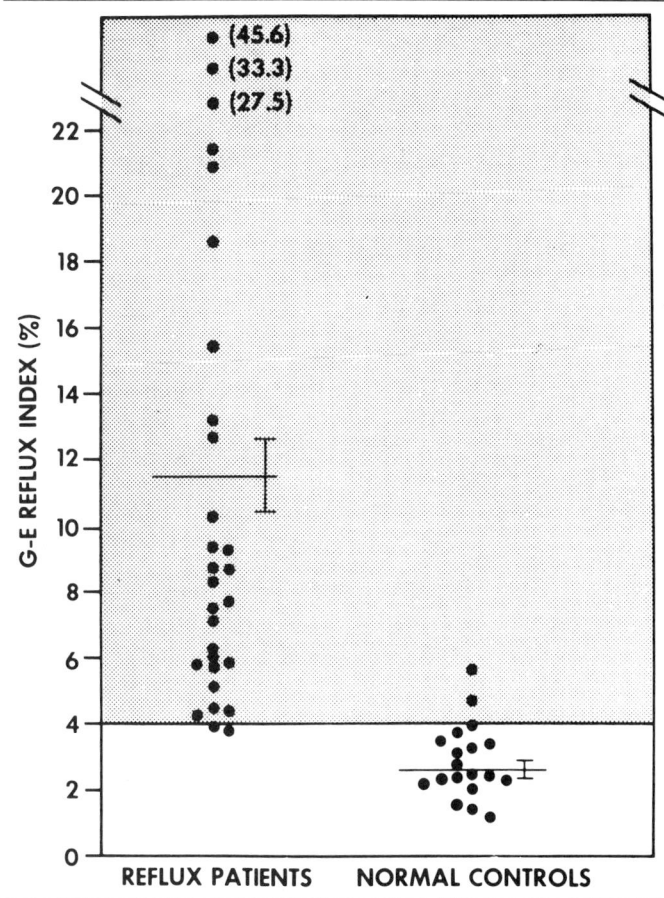

Figure 17-5. Gastroesophageal reflux index in all patients with reflux and normal subjects studied. Each point represents the percent maximal gastroesophageal reflux index of a single patient. Gastroesophageal reflux was visualized at a reflux index at or above 4 percent. (From Fisher RS, et al, 1976, p 305, copyright 1976, the Williams & Wilkins Co, with permission.[8])

nuclide decay, multiple radionuclide interference, geometry changes, septal penetration, and scatter from high-energy gamma rays.

Radiopharmaceuticals for Gastric Emptying. The ideal tracer should not be absorbed through nor bound to the gastric mucosa, should have no effect on gastric emptying, and should mix evenly with ingested food. The two types of radionuclide markers used for gastric emptying studies are liquid markers and solid markers. Liquid markers are soluble radiopharmaceuticals that are miscible with aqueous liquids and will trace the movement of liquids from the stomach. They must be nonabsorbable and stable. Commonly used liquid markers include DTPA labeled with Tc-99m, In-111 or In-113m and Tc-99m SC. Tc-99m pertechnetate is not used because it is secreted by the mucous cells of the gastric glands. Solid food markers are radionuclides bound to a solid food such as chicken liver, scrambled eggs, egg whites, or oatmeal.

Various techniques have been developed to bind radionuclides to solid food. A most important factor is that the label remain bound to the solid during the course of the study, otherwise gastric emptying of solids will be erroneously shortened because of leaching of the radionuclide into stomach fluids. Attempts to incorporate soluble agents such as radiolabeled DTPA into solid food have failed because of significant leaching.[14] The best label of solid food is achieved by injecting Tc-SC into a live chicken, whereby the colloid is incorporated into Kupffer's cells. The chicken is then killed and the liver cooked, chopped, and administered with a solid meal. Although leaching is minimal with this method (2 to 3 percent), other techniques have been used that are more convenient.[15,16] These include injecting Tc-SC into fresh raw chicken liver cubes, mixing with fresh liver cubes followed by cooking, or mixing Tc-SC or macroaggregates of albumin (MAA) with eggs, which are then scrambled and cooked. When compared with the in vivo labeled chicken liver method, these in vitro methods are more convenient but produce a greater degree of leaching (10 to 15 percent) when incubated in gastric juice for 3 hours.[15]

Another method used is to bind Tc-99m to an inert resin, which is then incorporated into oatmeal.[17] In this method 1 to 2 mCi of Tc-99m pertechnetate is incubated for 10 minutes with 0.5 g of Chelex-100 cation-exchange resin previously treated with stannous pyrophosphate. The mean labeling efficiency is 98.5 percent. The labeled resin is stable in vitro, in simulated gastric fluid and intestinal fluid, and upon heating in a boiling water bath. In vivo decomposition is insignificant. A meal for gastric emptying studies is prepared by mixing 1 mCi of labeled resin with one packet of instant oatmeal and 100 ml of hot milk. Studies have shown that the resin remains uniformly mixed with the oatmeal with minimal separation.

Procedure. To obtain meaningful results one must establish a standard protocol for performing gastric emptying studies. The size of the meal and its composition will affect emptying rates. Liquids empty from the stomach monoexponentially with time and at a faster rate than solids, which tend to empty at a constant rate,[13,15] being restricted by the action of the pylorus. The emptying rate is also influenced by the type of food and the amount. In general, large meals and high-calorie meals empty more slowly.

Although gastric emptying studies have been performed using only a liquid marker, experience has shown that studies are more informative if the test meal contains both a liquid marker and a solid marker because some patients demonstrate disparate emptying of solids and liquids. If a mixed solid and liquid meal is given to a patient using only a liquid marker such as Tc-99m DTPA, the patient may demonstrate normal emptying of the liquid while actually retaining solids abnormally.[13] Solid food, being more difficult for the stomach to empty, should be the labeled material if only one radionuclide is to be used.[13]

A recommended procedure is to administer a meal size of 300 g consisting of equal parts of solid and liquid food materials. A stable solid phase could be a beef stew meal labeled with 600 µCi of Tc-99m SC-labeled liver pâté, and the liquid phase could be labeled with 100 µCi of In-111 DTPA. Imaging of Tc-99m and then In-111 (247 keV) photopeaks is made with a 360- to 400-keV collimator. If the Tc-99m:In-111 activity ratio is 6:1 or greater, downscatter of In-111 counts into the Tc-99m window is minimized, otherwise downscatter correction may be necessary, depending on the properties of the camera and collimator. Images are obtained for 60 seconds at 15- to 30-minute intervals in a consistent position, either upright or supine until greater than 50 percent of the solid-phase emptying occurs in both the anterior and posterior views.[17] Computer-stored images may be analyzed correctly for decay and downscatter. The geometric mean (anterior count × posterior count)$^{1/2}$ may be determined from anterior and posterior computer images to correct for variations in tissue depth and attenuation.[13] These corrections are most important in obese patients and when large meals are administered. The activity in each image, expressed as a percentage of the initial activity in the field of view, is plotted versus time to determine the gastric emptying half-time. The normal mean half-times for a 300-g meal based on geometric mean data analysis are 38 minutes for a liquid meal and 77 minutes for a solid meal.[18]

These values vary in normal subjects depending on the size and composition of the meal. Short half-times are seen in dumping syndrome and prolonged half-times in gastric ulcers, pyloric obstruction, vagotomy, and malignancies.

Meckel's Diverticulum

Meckel's diverticulum is the most frequent congenital malformation of the GI tract in humans. It is found in 1 to 2 percent of persons and most commonly in children, although it has been diagnosed at every age from birth onward. The diverticulum is usually situated 30 to 90 cm proximal to the ileocecal valve. It may vary in size up to about 30 cm in length, but it is usually about the size of a small finger (3 to 5 cm). It is a true diverticulum containing all layers of the bowel wall (mucosal, serosal, and muscle layer); however, about 50 percent of diverticula contain heterotopic tissue, namely, gastric or duodenal mucosa or pancreatic tissue.[19] In most cases it is gastric mucosa.

The most common symptom of Meckel's diverticulum is rectal bleeding that results from peptic ulceration of the bowel by acid secreted from the gastric mucosa in the diverticulum.[20] Those cases that appear clinically usually do so before the age of 2 years.

The difficulty in diagnosing Meckel's diverticula with conventional radiologic methods and the frequent presence of gastric mucosa in them lead to the use of Tc-99m pertechnetate for scintigraphic localization. Tc-99m pertechnetate is a logical choice because it concentrates in the mucous cells of the gastric mucosa. The use of Tc-99m pertechnetate has demonstrated a sensitivity of 85 percent and a specificity of 95 percent in cases of surgically proven Meckel's diverticula with ectopic mucosa.[21,22] The procedure will not directly detect diverticula that do not contain gastric mucosa.

The technique involves IV administration of 30 to 100 μCi/kg of Tc-99m pertechnetate followed by serial anterior images with the patient's right side tilted upwards about 30 degrees (to sequester gastric secretions) made at 5- to 10-minute intervals for at least 1 hour. Other views may be needed to localize the sites of activity. Perchlorate diminishes gastric uptake and should be withheld until the study is complete. A Meckel's diverticulum often appears within 10 to 30 minutes after injection and coincides with the peak visualization of activity within the stomach. A Meckel's diverticulum usually appears as a single discrete area of activity most commonly located in the right lower quadrant and may change position with maneuvers that shift the gut.[22] Figure 17-6 illustrates a positive scan for Meckel's diverticulum.

Gastrointestinal Protein Loss

Under normal circumstances large amounts of protein (approximately 100 g) enter the GI tract daily as a result of digestive secretory processes; however, this protein is largely reabsorbed after intestinal catabolism. Protein-losing enteropathy (PLE) is characterized by an excessive protein loss in the stool. Several diseases that produce inflammation and ulceration of the GI tract may be the cause of excessive protein loss.

Several radiolabeled substances have been used to measure protein loss in the stool.[23] The ideal agent should be firmly bound to a plasma protein and not excreted in the urine. It should be excreted into the intestinal tract only through abnormal leakage sites and not be readsorbed from the intestinal tract. Iodine-131 albumin was one of the first agents used to study PLE; however, it has the disadvantage of being catabolized in the gut with reabsorption of the free radioiodide label. Studies using Cr-51 albumin and chromic chloride have shown that the Cr-51 label is recovered virtually completely from the stool after oral administration.[24,25] After intravenous administration of Cr-51 albumin or chromic chloride, significant stool radioactivity implies intestinal plasma exudation. As a result, Cr-51 as chromic chloride or albumin has become the agent of choice for the assessment of GI protein loss.

After IV injection, Cr-51 chromic

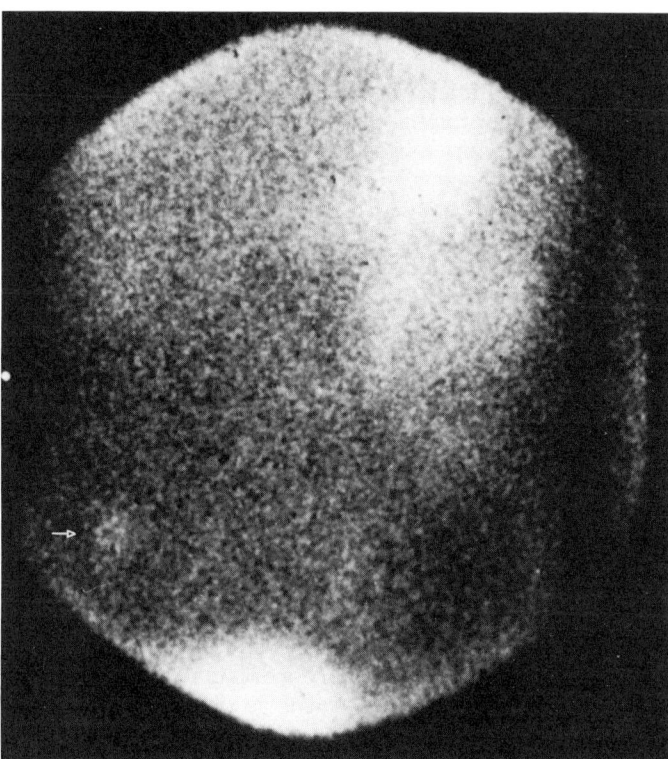

Figure 17-6. Meckel's diverticulum (*arrow*) seen as a persistent area of localized activity in the right lower quadrant 30 minutes after IV injection of 5 mCi of Tc-99m sodium pertechnetate. The diagnosis was confirmed after surgical resection of the ileum.

chloride labels plasma transferrin. In normal subjects less than 1 percent of intravenously administered Cr-51 chromic chloride or albumin is recovered in a 4-day stool collection.[24] Recovery of Cr-51 albumin in a 3-day urine collection is 13 percent, compared with 60 percent for chromic chloride. For this reason, Cr-51 albumin is the preferred agent by some investigators because there is less of a problem with urine contamination of stool samples that may lead to erroneous test results.

If chromic chloride is used it must be prepared carefully since it adheres tenaciously to glass. The loss can be minimized by maintaining solution pH at or below 4 and using plastic or siliconized glass containers.

Test Procedure. A dose of 0.25 to 0.5 µCi per pound of body weight is administered intravenously. All stools passed during the next 4 days are collected. Multiple containers may be needed for some patients because of the large volume of liquid stool (e.g., Crohn's disease). Empty metal paint cans containing 10 ml phenol preservative are satisfactory. Each sample is adjusted to a standard weight with water and assayed for radioactivity using a gamma scintillation spectrometer. A standard of the dose administered and a background sample are prepared in a similar manner and radioassayed. The percentage of the dose excreted in the cumulative 4-day stool sample is calculated. Normal subjects excrete 1 percent or less of the administered dose in 4 days. Patients with PLE excrete 2 to 40 percent of the dose.

Care must be taken to instruct subjects not to contaminate stool samples with urine.

Salivary Gland Imaging

The salivary glands consist of the parotid, submandibular, and sublingual glands. The epithelial cells of these glands produce saliva and have concentrating mechanisms for the group VII anions, including iodide and its analogues pertechnetate, thiocyanate, and perchlorate. The glands are innervated by the autonomic nervous system. Stimulation of gland function and saliva production occurs by parasympathetic stimulation by food or drugs such as pilocarpine, whereas sympathetic stimulation decreases function. Anticholinergics such as atropine cause decreased saliva production and "dry mouth."

Salivary gland imaging is usually performed with Tc-99m pertechnetate. Although anatomic lesions in the glands are not readily detected, imaging with pertechnetate does provide a unique and sensitive means for investigating salivary gland physiologic function and its derangement.[26] In general, the study involves injecting 10 mCi of Tc-99m pertechnetate intravenously and taking images at 1- to 5-second intervals. A 5-minute image is made and compared with the thyroid activity. Salivary gland and thyroid gland activity should be approximately equal. A normal image shows the parotids and submandibular glands. Concentration in the sublinguals is similar to plasma concentration, and they are not visualized. A second image is made after the patient sucks on a lemon or tart lemon candy for 5 minutes. Normally functioning parotid glands will demonstrate almost complete discharge of their activity after salivary gland stimulation.

A number of conditions can be evaluated with salivary gland imaging and include detection of reduced salivary gland trapping and excretory capacity in subclinical stages of lupus erythematosus, sarcoidosis, and abnormalities in gland concentration and discharge in parotitis.[26,27]

DACRYOCYSTOGRAPHY

Radionuclide dacryocystography is a useful method for acquiring physiologic information concerning nasolacrimal drainage. It is not useful for gaining anatomic information, which is best acquired by contrast dacryocystography.[28]

The radionuclide technique involves placing a small drop of Tc-99m pertechnetate onto the conjunctiva near the lateral canthus. A 1-ml tuberculin syringe fitted with a 21-, 23-, or 25-gauge needle protected by a special holder can be used to place 50 to 150 μCi (100 μCi average) of activity in a volume of 10 to 35 μl into the eye.[29] The needle size depends on the pertechnetate concentration. The normal human lacrimal fluid volume is 7 μl, but up to 30 μl can be added without overflow provided the subject does not blink.[30] The normal eye is done first to familiarize the patient with the procedure and provide a normal control for comparison. A specially constructed pinhole collimator with a 1-mm aperture is used and gives the best balance between resolution and sensitivity.[28] After drop placement serial scintigrams are obtained every 30 seconds for 5 minutes. The normal transit time from the conjunctiva to the nasolacrimal sac is less than 1.5 minutes.[28] Longer times indicate delay and provide a sensitive means for detecting obstruction to drainage. Partial obstruction can be demonstrated with a negative Valsalva's maneuver (pinching the nostrils while attempting to draw in air). Figure 17–7 illustrates a radionuclide dacryocystogram demonstrating normal and abnormal drainage in the same patient.

The radiation dose to the lens of a normally draining eye is estimated at 14 to 21 mrad/100 to 150 μCi dose, whereas in total obstruction the worst case would be 400 to 600 mrad.[31]

DETECTION OF DEEP VENOUS THROMBOSIS

The three classic underlying causes of venous thrombosis are circulation abnormalities such as venous stasis, blood vessel abnormalities resulting from trauma, and blood coagulation abnormalities resulting in hypercoagulability. Thrombosis of deep veins of the lower extremities is the most common source of pulmonary emboli. Because pulmonary embolization can be fatal, deep venous thrombosis (DVT) is a serious condition; therefore, early detection of this

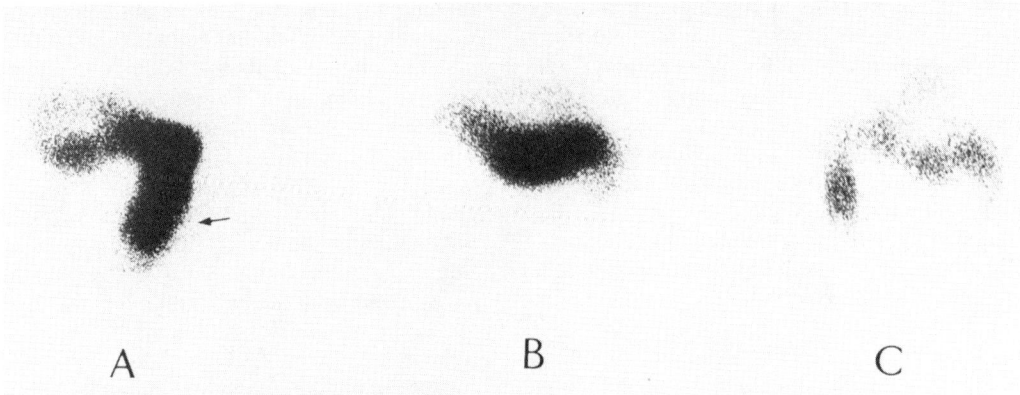

Figure 17-7. Dacryocystogram obtained with a pinhole collimator and scintillation camera after instillation of 100 μCi of Tc-99m sodium pertechnetate into the eye. **A.** The right eye exhibits normal drainage into the lacrimal sac (arrow). **B.** The left eye demonstrates a lack of drainage under normal conditions, but drainage into the lacrimal sac is induced (**C**) after a negative Valsalva's maneuver, which indicates a stenotic condition rather than complete obstruction.

condition with prompt treatment is an important measure in reducing the risks associated with pulmonary embolism. Unfortunately, DVT is manifest clinically in less than 50 percent of cases with lethal embolism.[32] Frequently pulmonary embolism is the initial clinical event that indicates the presence of DVT.

Several methods are available to aid in the diagnosis of DVT. Radiographic contrast venography is the standard test by which others are compared. It is highly sensitive and specific for this condition but is painful, may induce thrombophlebitis, and is not readily repeatable. Other tests include Doppler ultrasound, impedance plethysmography, radionuclide venography, radiolabeled fibrinogen imaging, and the I-125 fibrinogen uptake study. The underlying causes of DVT and the methods for detection have been reviewed and compared.[23]

I-125 Fibrinogen Uptake Study

The I-125 fibrinogen uptake study was developed after the introduction of I-125 fibrinogen in the mid 1960s.[33,34] Investigational studies established its sensitivity in the detection of DVT.[35,36]

The primary indications for the I-125 fibrinogen uptake study are as follows:

1. Preoperative major orthopedic surgery
2. Detection of thrombus formation concomitant with myocardial infarction, pulmonary disease, and malignant disease
3. Medical conditions predisposing to thromboembolism
4. Patients presenting with pulmonary emboli, with or without DVT

The study is based on the principle of fibrinogen conversion to fibrin, which is incorporated into the actively forming thrombus.

The technique involves IV administration of 100 μCi of I-125 fibrinogen into an arm vein. Injection should not be made nor blood samples obtained from the legs. Before initial monitoring, the patient should be marked for counting. Marks should be made over the precordium and on the legs with a waterproof pen, and marks should not be removed during the monitoring procedure to ensure monitoring of the same position each day. The precordium is marked over the fourth intercostal space 3 inches to the left of the sternum for determination of heart blood pool activity. This point serves as a 100 percent reference count to which individual leg counts are compared. Leg markings are made in 2-inch intervals extending from the middle of the inguinal ligament down the thigh, following the femoral vein to the posterior portion of the knee, and then following the wide portion of the calf and extending to a point just posterior to the internal malleolus of the ankle (Fig. 17–8).

Counts are made over each mark using a hand-held portable scintillation counter (see Chapter 2, Fig. 2–37), which should be calibrated each day with a reference source to assure proper operation. Monitoring of marked areas begins at 1 to 3 hours after injection of the I-125 fibrinogen, and daily counts are made thereafter for 5 to 7 days. Beyond this time a repeat injection of I-125 fibrinogen is necessary because of decreased circulating activity. The legs are elevated 20 degrees and kept straight at the knees to facilitate counting and to reduce venous pooling and background activity. The precordial area is monitored first and the rate meter set to read 100 percent. A stabilized meter reading over each leg mark will then give a direct reading as a percentage of precordial counts. The results of each count are plotted on graph paper for interpretation (Fig. 17–9).

Normal studies show a gradual decrease in percent recordings from the inguinal ligament down to the ankle, often with a slight increase over the knee. Abnormal studies show an increase of 20 percent or greater calculated as a percentage of precordial counts compared with the corresponding position on the opposite leg or compared with adjacent positions on the same leg, with persistance of these counts for the next 24 hours. Upper thigh counts are often high because of bladder activity, femoral vein blood activity, or urine contamination on the leg.

Of those patients with active thrombophlebitis at the time of injection, 98 percent will show active localization of I-125 fibrinogen activity by 24 hours.[37] The method is not specific for fibrinogen deposition in thrombophlebitis, however, because other causes of fibrinogen deposition or pooling such as arthritis, cellulitis, edema, recent tendon or muscle injury, burn, hematoma, Baker's cyst, and marked varicosities will give positive tests.[23] The technique is most sensitive in the calf and least sensitive in the thigh. The combination of a positive fibrinogen uptake study and impedance plethysmogram, or either of these being positive alone, provides as sensitive an indication as contrast venography for deciding when to institute therapy for thromboembolic disease.[23] Less than 2 percent of the patients in whom both of these tests are negative will, if untreated, have thromboembolic events, whereas the false-positive rate compared with venography is about 5 percent.[38]

To prevent uptake of I-125 by the thyroid gland from metabolized fibrinogen, 100 mg of iodine daily should be given either as 130 mg of potassium iodide, 0.13 ml (SSKI), or 0.8 ml Lugol's solution given orally 24 hours before injection of the I-125 fibrinogen and continued daily for at least 10 days. More expeditiously, 100 mg of sodium iodide may be given intravenously 1 hour before injection to block the thyroid. Sodium or potassium perchlorate may be used in patients sensitive to iodine.

Radioiodinated fibrinogen is prepared by the iodine monochloride method or the Chloramine-T method of radioiodination. Various labels have been used including I-131 and I-123 for imaging studies. I-125 fibrinogen is supplied as a freeze-dried product containing approximately 1 mg fibrinogen and 150 μCi of I-125 on the calibration date. It is reconstituted with sterile water for injection just before use.

The risk of hepatitis after the use of this product is small because each batch of I-125 fibrinogen is prepared from a single patient who has previously undergone a rigorous physical exam and whose blood has been tested for hepatitis-associated antigen.

The radiation absorbed dose to various body organs is shown in Table 17–2.

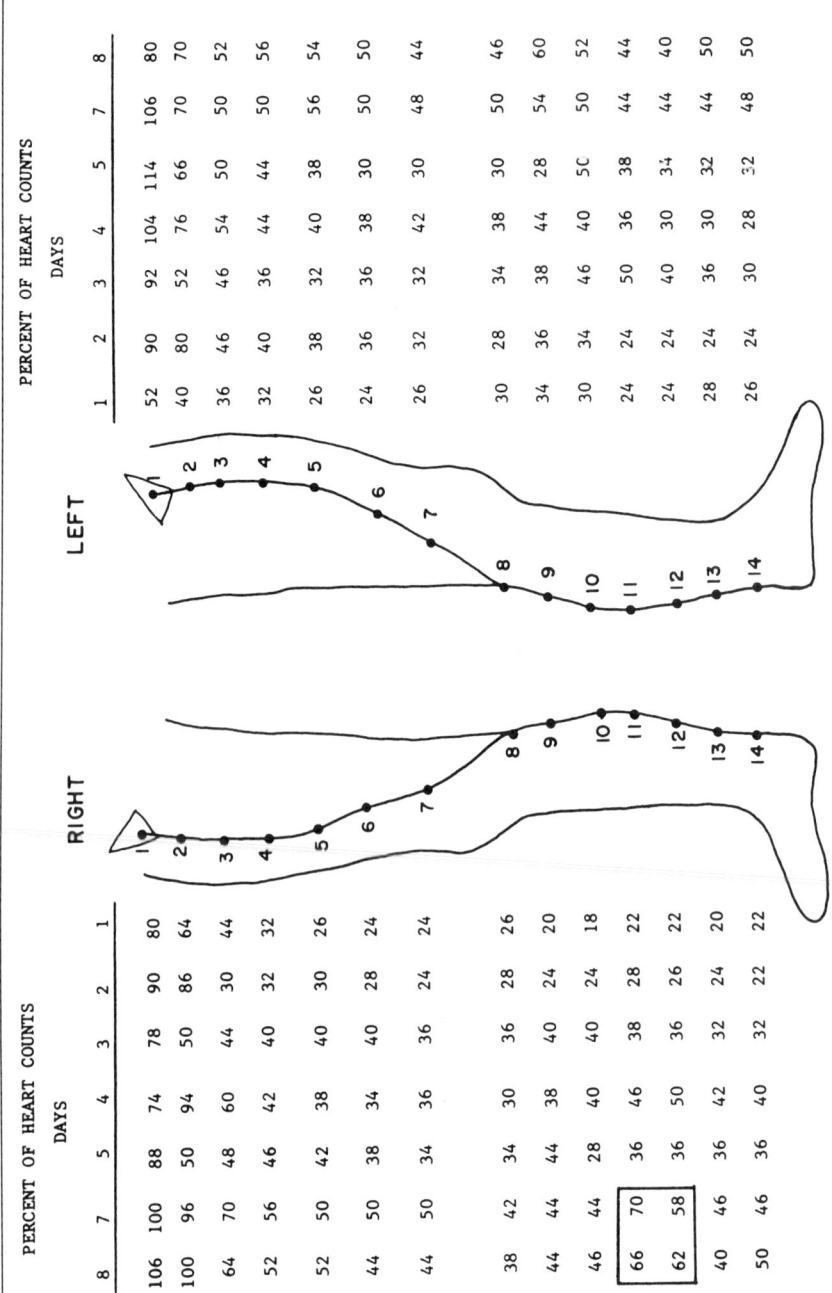

Figure 17-8. Leg positions marked for counting with a scintillation probe during an I-125 fibrinogen uptake test. Right and left leg uptakes are counted in an elevated position. Numbers for each leg mark represent the percentage of probe count taken over the heart on various days after injection of 100 μCi of I-125 fibrinogen. Note the dramatic rise in counts (greater than 20 percent) for the right leg on days 7 and 8, which indicate thrombus formation in the right calf.

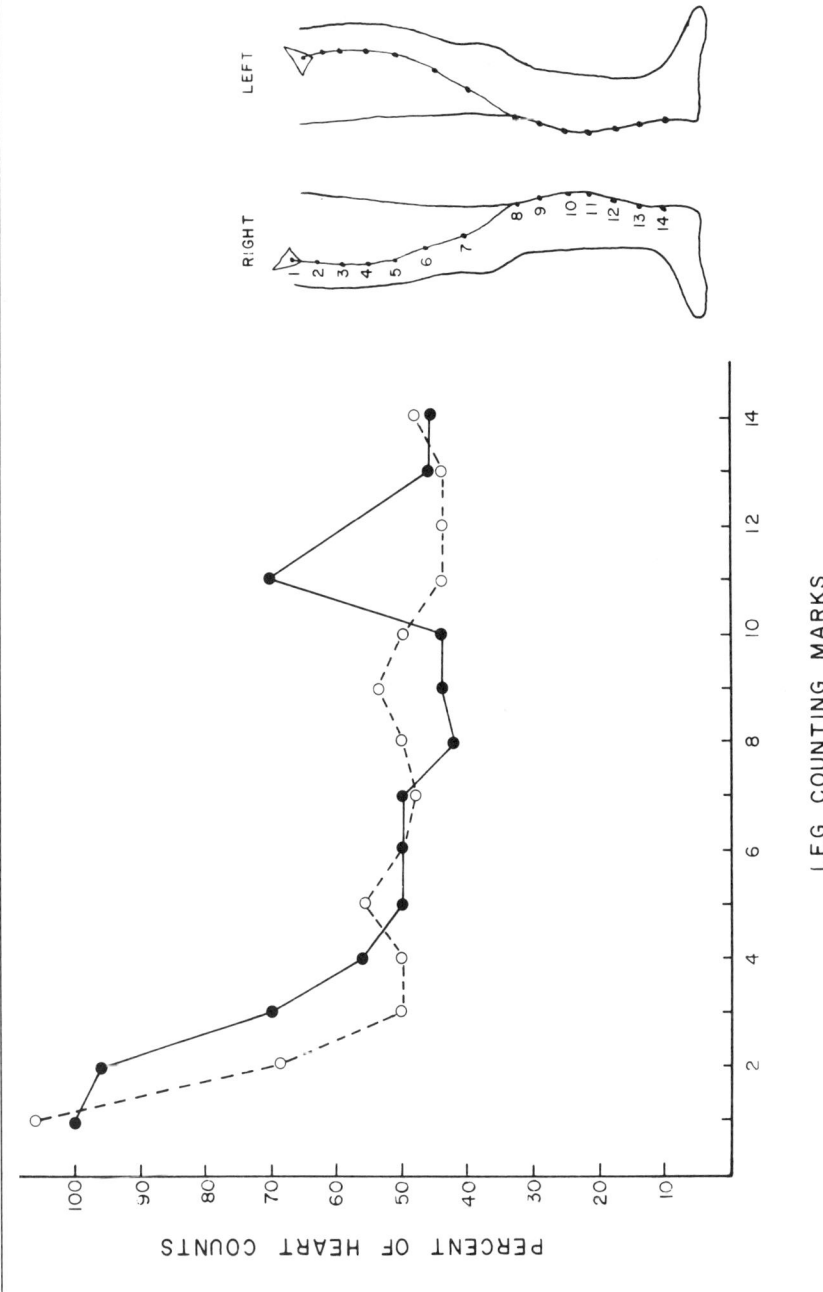

Figure 17-9. I-125 fibrinogen uptake test: plotted data for day 7 demonstrating the presence of a thrombus in the right calf. Data are taken from Figure 17-8. Legend: ●— — —●, right leg; ○ – ○ – ○, left leg.

TABLE 17-2. RADIATION DOSE FROM I-125 FIBRINOGEN

Organ	Dose (rad/100 μCi) Administered
Thyroid	
(Unblocked)	1.3
(Blocked)	0.02
Stomach wall	0.13
Kidneys	0.06
Liver	0.08
Lungs	0.04
Testes	0.027
Ovaries	0.028
Whole body	0.02

LYMPH NODE SCANNING

The lymphatic system has been studied by contrast lymphography after injection of radiographic contrast material (ethiodized oil) into cannulated lymphatic vessels. This procedure is technically difficult and may result in complications such as embolism and contrast reaction. By comparison, radionuclide lymphoscintigraphy with radiocolloids has proved to be technically more facile, with minimal complications and excellent correlations with contrast lymphography.[39,40] Additionally, the radiocolloid technique does not require lymph vessel cannulation. Consequently, radionuclide lymphoscintigraphy has provided a means to evaluate lymphatic drainage in previously inaccessible areas. A fair amount of investigative and clinical work has focused on internal mammary lymphoscintigraphy because of the accessibility of radiocolloids to the parasternal lymph nodes after subcostal injection. Details of this technique are described by Ege.[41]

A number of radiocolloid preparations have been investigated for use in lymphoscintigraphy. The clinical efficacy of these agents is highly dependent on colloid particle size and stability. A uniform dispersion of small articles (less than 100 nm) is necessary for the colloid to translocate from the interstitial injection site to the lymphatic channels and nodes. Large particles (500 to 2000 nm) remain trapped at the injection site and are unsatisfactory.[41] Larger particles will migrate through the lymphatics after direct intralymphatic injection, but this precludes the advantage of interstitial administration.

Gold-198 was the first colloid shown to be taken up by the lymph nodes after interstitial injection[42] and later found application in lymphoscintigraphy.[39,40] Its particle size was in the range of 5 to 50 nm. Its main disadvantage was the high radiation dose for diagnostic use.

Several technetium agents have been developed for lymphoscintigraphy. The more important ones are Tc-99m-labeled sulfur colloid, stannous phytate, and antimony sulfide. Sulfur colloid produced by the thiosulfate kit method is unsatisfactory because of inadequate migration from the injection site. This has been ascribed to the relatively large particle size range (100 to 1000 nm).[43] Sulfur colloid produced by the hydrogen sulfide method produces smaller particles (less than 100 nm) and satisfactory lymph node scans[44]; however, the method of preparation is technically cumbersome.

Tc-99m antimony sulfide colloid currently appears to be the agent of choice for lymphoscintigraphy. It has a small particle size (3 to 30 nm),[45] is readily prepared from a kit, and yields satisfactory lymphatic scans. Tc-99m stannous phytate forms an in vivo colloid of about the same size as antimony sulfide[46] but has been found to be inferior to the latter in clinical studies.[46,47] Tc-99m antimony sulfide allows visualization of a greater number of more intense lymph nodes, better delineation of the total length of the internal mammary lymph node chain, and more consistent visualization of supraclavicular nodes.[47]

Tc-99m Antimony Sulfide Colloid

Preformed antimony sulfide kits are prepared as follows[46]: 1 percent antimony potassium tartrate solution is added to a saturated solution of hydrogen sulfide in boiling water, which results in a deep red-orange colored mixture. Polyvinylpyrolidone, 3.5 percent (molecular weight, 40,000) is added as a stabilizer. Residual hydrogen sulfide is removed by bubbling nitrogen gas through the solution for about 30 minutes and is ensured by a negative test with lead acetate paper. The product is sterile filtered through a 0.22-μm membrane into presterilized vials, each to contain 3 ml of an antimony sulfide solution, equivalent to 2.35 mg Sb_2S_3. Alternatively, a commercial kit can be purchased.

Technetium labeling is accomplished by adding 3 ml of sodium pertechnetate and 0.2 ml of 1 N HCl to the kit followed by incubation for 30 minutes in a boiling water bath. Buffer is then added to bring the final pH to between 6 and 7.

For internal mammary lymphoscintigraphy the usual dose is 500 μCi injected into the subcostal interstitial space in a volume of 0.3 ml.[41,45] Under these conditions the estimated radiation dose at the injection site is 90 rad.

ADRENAL GLAND IMAGING AGENTS

The body has two adrenal glands, each weighing about 5 g. They are situated normally in the upper pole region of each kidney. The right adrenal gland is roughly triangular shaped whereas the left adrenal is somewhat crescent shaped. Each adrenal gland is divided into two major zones that produce important hormone substances. The adrenal cortex (outer zone) is responsible for producing the mineralocorticoids, the primary one being aldosterone, and the glucocorticoids, primarily cortisol. The cortex also produces androgenic hormones. The adrenal medulla (inner zone) produces epinephrine and norepinephrine, the pressor amines that are associated with stimulation of the sympathetic nervous system.

Radiopharmaceutical agents have been developed to image the adrenal cortex and the adrenal medulla on the basis of knowledge of the normal biochemical processes that occur in the gland.

Adrenal Cortical Imaging Agents

Cholesterol is the principal precursor substance in the production of the adrenocortical steroids. This fact led to the development of carbon-14-labeled cholesterol and radiolabeled cholesterol analogues to study cholesterol tissue distribution, particularly within the adrenal gland. Two of the radiolabeled analogues have achieved clinical usefulness for imaging the adrenal cortex in the evaluation of adrenal gland disease; these are 19-iodocholesterol I-131 (NM-145)[5] and 6-β-iodomethyl-19-norcholesterol I-131 (NP-59).[9]

Radioiodinated 19-iodocholesterol is prepared by isotope exchange between "cold"iodocholesterol and radioiodine.[48] The C-19 position in the cholesterol molecule was selected as the site of iodination because synthetic methods for iodinating this position were known and the presence of an iodine atom at this site was thought to produce minimal steric interference with cholesterol's biochemical interactions.[48] Experimental studies in dogs demonstrated that C-14 cholesterol and I-125 19-iodocholesterol had similar tissue distribution, with the latter demonstrating an adrenal-to-liver ratio as high as 168:1[49] Using 19-iodocholesterol labeled with I-131, Beierwaltes et al reported the first satisfactory visualization of both adrenal glands in a patient with Cushing's syndrome.[50]

In the course of study with NM-145 it was discovered that an impurity found in the synthesis of NM-145 had an adrenal gland uptake between 5 and 50 times that of NM-145.[51] The compound isolated was NP-59.[52] The chemical structures of cholesterol and these iodinated analogues are shown in Figure 17–10. A higher adrenal uptake with no concomitant increase in background activity produced higher target-to-background ratios with NP-59 and shortened the dose-to-imaging time from 5 days for NM-145 to 3 days for NP-59.[53,54]

Currently the agent of choice for adrenocortical imaging is NP-59. It is formulated in aqueous saline that contains 1.6 percent Tween 80 and 6.6 percent

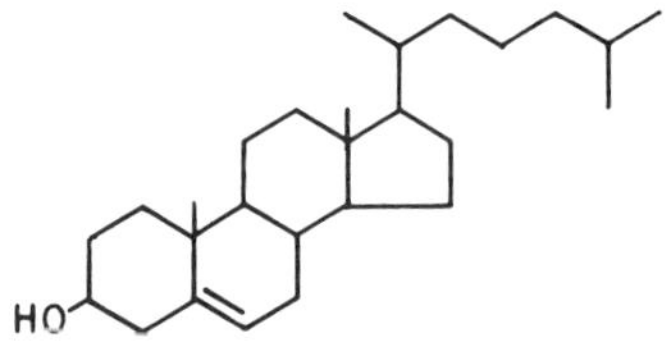

Figure 17-10. Chemical structures of cholesterol, NM-145, and NP-59.

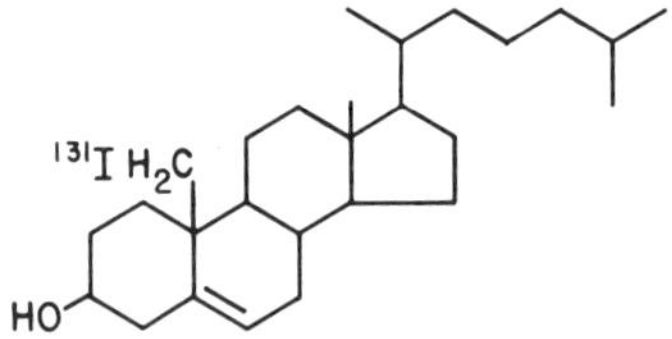

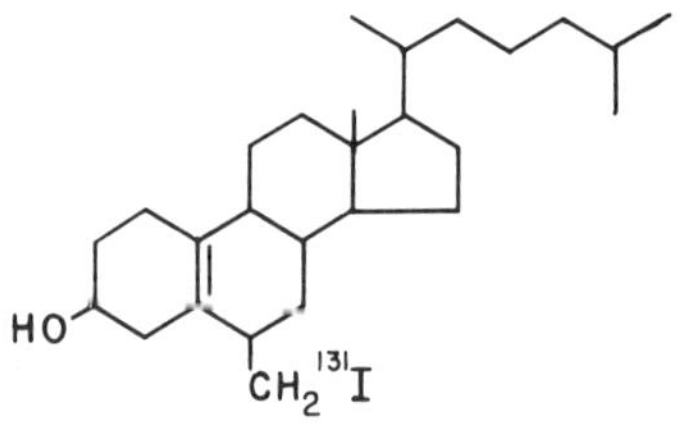

When clinical studies are done, patients must receive 100 mg of iodine (0.8 ml Lugol's solution or 0.13 ml SSKI) per day 2 days before and for 2 weeks after injection of the dose to protect the thyroid gland from unbound iodide in the dose and from that released during the drug's metabolism in the body.

Both NM-145 and NP-59 appear to be taken up by the adrenals along with cholesterol. They are firmly bound in the adrenal gland and are believed to act as enzyme inhibitors. The long residence time in the adrenals allows for an extended imaging time (2 to 3 weeks) if needed. A number of conditions affecting the adrenal gland such as Cushing's syndrome, primary aldosteronism, hyperandrogenism, adrenal masses, hypofunction, and others have been studied with NM-145 and NP-59 and are reviewed in the literature.[55]

Because of the prolonged retention of NM-145 and NP-59 in the adrenal gland the radiation dose is quite high, being estimated at 27 rad/mCi. The usual activity administered per study is 1 to 2 mCi intravenously, with imaging begun 3 to 6 days later to allow background activity to subside.[53]

Efforts to develop adrenocortical imaging agents with a shorter dose-to-imaging time interval and with lower radiation dose using an I-123 label have met with limited success. Noteworthy are the adrenal enzyme inhibitors metyrapol, the alcohol derivative of metyrapone, and the phenethylamine derivative, SKF-12185. Although tritiated metyrapol achieved high adrenal uptake within 1 to 2 hours in the dog, a gamma-emitting radioiodine derivative showed a fourfold lower uptake. SKF-12185 surprisingly showed higher uptake in the adrenal cortex after radioiodination. Its percent uptake in the adrenals at 1 to 2 hours is equivalent to that of NM-145 at 2 days.[51]

Adrenal Medullary Imaging Agents

The role that the adrenal medulla plays in the synthesis and storage of catecholamines has led to various approaches in developing radionuclide imaging agents specific for the

ethanol to keep the cholesterol in solution.[52] The product undergoes rapid deiodination unless stored at 0 to 5°C where it is stable for 2 weeks. Up to 20 percent deiodination may occur within 4 days' storage at room temperature.[52] Radiochemical purity can be determined using TLC–silica gel (Eastman) in 100 percent chloroform.[51] In this system the Rf of NP-59 is 0.4; free radioiodide Rf, 0.0; and NM-145 impurity Rf, 0.3.

adrenal medulla. One approach was to radiolabel dopamine[56] and its analogues.[57] Dopamine is the immediate precursor to norepinephrine, which is synthesized in the chromaffin cells of the adrenal medulla. Dopamine has been labeled with carbon-11, and although it has shown high adrenal medullary concentration, technical requirements for its production have precluded routine use for adrenal imaging. A sulfur 35-labeled sulfonanilide analogue of dopamine that demonstrates adrenal uptake has been prepared, but efforts to incorporate a gamma-emitting label were not successful.[57]

A second approach involved preparing radiolabeled compounds known to have an affinity for adrenergic nerves and therefore also an affinity for the adrenal medullary chromaffin cells. Several I-125-labeled analogues of the antiadrenergic agent bretylium have been developed, but in vivo experiments have been met with limited success in adrenal imaging.[58]

The search for antihypertensive agents that would selectively block the sympathetic nervous system without concomitantly blocking the parasympathetic system led to the development of the first two agents with such action: bretylium tosylate and guanethidine sulfate. Medicinal chemists then chose to combine the benzyl portion of bretylium with the guanidine moiety of guanethidine to produce a series of benzylguanidine compounds with potent antiadrenergic activity.[59] The ability to halogenate the aromatic ring in benzylguanidines led Wieland et al to investigate radioiodinated benzylguanidines labeled at the *ortho*-, *meta*-, and *para*-positions as potential adrenal medulla-imaging agents[60] (Fig. 17–11). The *meta*- and *para*-isomers showed the highest adrenal medullary concentration in dogs. Further studies in monkeys and dogs demonstrated that the *meta*-isomer was superior for imaging by virtue of its resistance to in vivo deiodination and its lower concentration in the liver, which improved the target-to-nontarget activity ratio.[61] Subcellular tissue distribution studies with homogenized dog adrenal medullary tissue demonstrated that I-125 *meta*-iodobenzylguanidine (MIBG) was associated with the fraction that contains the chromaffin catecholamine storage granules.

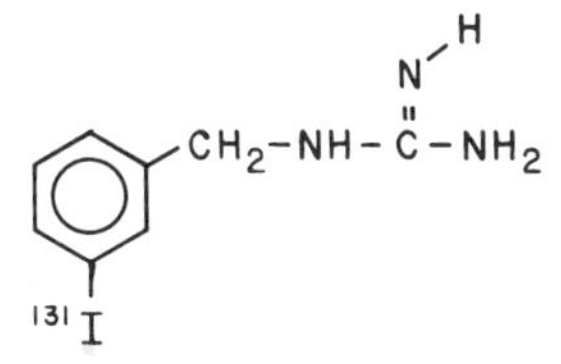

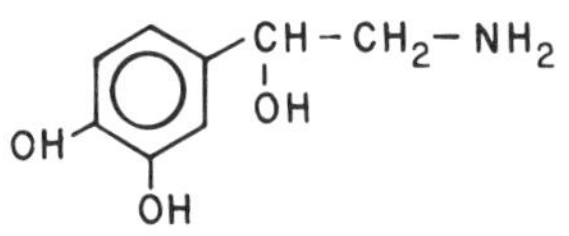

Figure 17–11. Chemical structures of *meta*-iodobenzylguanidine (MIBG) and norepinephrine.

Drug interventional studies have provided some evidence regarding the mechanism of localization of MIBG. Reserpine is a drug known to inhibit the uptake of norepinephrine by chromaffin granules and to deplete stores of catecholamines in the adrenal medulla.[62] When reserpine was administered to dogs previously injected with I-131 MIBG, the adrenal medullary activity was depleted approximately 90 percent by 3 days so that adrenal gland images could not be obtained.[61] The marked depletion of the I-131 MIBG from the dog adrenal medulla by reserpine suggests that norepinephrine and MIBG share a common storage mechanism in the adrenal medulla.[61] This dramatic effect of reserpine has led to the suggestion that it may become a useful clinical tool for lowering the radiation dose to the adrenal gland from I-131 MIBG.

Iodine-131 MIBG has been shown to be of great value in localizing pheochromocytomas within the adrenal glands and in extraadrenal tumors.[63] Pheochromocytomas are functional medullary neoplasms, usually benign, that produce sustained hypertension. Diagnosis of pheochromocytomas is based on the fact that these tumors synthesize and store large quantities of catecholamines that can be measured in the plasma and urine as metabolites. Localization of the tumor, however, is sometimes difficult, particularly those found in extraadrenal tissue.

Adrenal imaging is performed in 1 to 3 days after intravenous injection of 0.5 mCi of I-131 MIBG. Lugol's solution, 0.8 ml per day, is given orally 1 day before injection and 4 days afterward to block thyroid uptake of I-131.[63] Radioactivity localizes in the heart soon after injection because of its rich adrenergic innervation, but heart activity is gone by 24 hours. One to 2 days after injection radioactivity is seen in the urinary bladder and less distinctly in the liver and spleen. Normal adrenal glands are not visualized. Pheochromocytomas are readily visualized, and uptake in them is not impaired by therapeutic amounts of phenoxybenzamine or propranolol, drugs used to control the hypertensive episodes and cardiac effects caused by pheochromocytoma.[61]

The calculated radiation dose estimates from I-131-MIBG are shown in Table 17-3.

PHOSPHORUS-32 THERAPY

P-32 is a pure beta emitter with a half-life of 14.3 days. It decays to stable S-32. The maximum beta particle energy is 1.7 MeV with an average beta energy of 0.69 MeV, which gives maximum and average ranges in tissue of 8 and 3 mm, respectively. The decay scheme for P-32 is shown in Figure 2-8, Chapter 2.

There are two P-32 radiopharmaceu-

TABLE 17-3. RADIATION DOSE FROM I-131 MIBG

Organ	Dose (rad/0.5 mCi Administered)
Adrenal (normal)	17.5
Liver	0.2
Spleen	0.8
Ovaries	0.5
Bladder	3.9
Whole body	0.11

(Data from Sisson JC, et al, 1981, p 12.[63])

tical products available for therapeutic use in radiation therapy: sodium phosphate P-32 and chromic phosphate P-32. Although each agent is labeled with P-32, each has unique properties and applications.

Sodium Phosphate P-32

Sodium phosphate P-32 is a clear, colorless solution of the soluble sodium phosphate salts. It is prepared by simple titration of *ortho*-radiophoshoric acid with sodium hydroxide to form the sodium salts. Because phosphoric acid has three acid dissociation constants, the salts formed will depend on the final solution pH. The US Pharmacopeia (USP) states the chemical form of the radiopharmaceutical as dibasic sodium phosphate (Na_2HPO_4) at a final pH of 5.0 to 6.0; however, at this pH the salt is greater than 90 percent monobasic sodium phosphate (NaH_2PO_4). For example, using the Henderson–Hasselbalch equation, at pH 5.5 the ratio of monobasic-to-dibasic salt is 51:1.

Sodium phosphate P-32 is administered orally or intravenously for treatment of polycythemia vera. Because absorption from the GI tract is incomplete and variable between patients, the intravenous route is recommended. The Polycythemia Vera Study Group[64] recommends an initial dose of 2.3 mCi/m^2 body surface area and not to exceed 5 mCi. This is usually sufficient to produce a remission. If remission does not occur in 3 months, the dose should be increased by 25 percent. Another increase by 25 percent, but not exceeding 7 mCi, may be tried as a third dose after a period of another 3 months. Retreatment is usually restricted for 6 months thereafter.

When soluble radiophosphate enters the miscible body phosphate pool, it is concentrated by rapidly proliferating tissue. Its use in polycythemia vera and other bone marrow diseases is based on the fact that blood cell precursors in the bone marrow divide and proliferate rapidly in health and even more so in these diseases. The radionuclide selectively concentrates in the mitotically active cells of the bone marrow and in trabecular and cortical bone.[64] The radiation dose to the bone marrow has been estimated to be 24 rad/mCi divided between marrow (13 rad), trabecular bone (10 rad) and cortical bone (1 rad).[65]

Chromic Phosphate P-32

Chromic phosphate P-32 is a grayish-green colored suspension of insoluble colloidal chromic phosphate ($Cr^{32}PO_4$) in 30 percent dextrose. A commercially prepared product is available. It is prepared by mixing chromic nitrate solution with radiophosphoric acid. The resulting precipitate of chromic phosphate is dried in an oven and reduced to a particle size of 1 μm or less in a ball mill.[66] The colloidal-sized particles are suspended in a suitable vehicle.

Chromic phosphate P-32 is used as a neoplastic suppressant for palliative treatment of pleural and peritoneal effusions. For this use it has replaced colloidal Au-198, a beta–gamma emitter. Because P-32 emits only beta radiation (exept for bremsstrahlung), the hazard to personnel is greatly reduced.* Additionally, the dose delivered per millicurie during an effective half-life is about ten times greater for P-32 than for Au-198.[64] Relatively smaller doses of P-32 can therefore be used. The dosage range for intraperitoneal instillation is 10 to 20 mCi, and for intrapleural instillation it is 6 to 12 mCi. The chromic phosphate may be dispersed in 30 to 50 ml of sterile saline before instillation. A patent route of instillation may be ascertained before P-32 administration by introducing Tc-99m SC and observing the cavitary distribution with a gamma camera.

The colloidal particles of chromic phosphate P-32 are engulfed by floating macrophages and eventually by fixed tissue macrophages lining the wall of the serous cavity. The beta radiation causes fibrosis of the mesothelium and small blood vessels, which leads to a reduced fluid production.[68]

PARATHYROID IMAGING

A satisfactory parathyroid imaging agent has been sought for many years. Cobalt-57 cyanocobalamin, Se-75 selenomethionine, I-131 toluidine blue, Cs-131, and Ga-67 citrate have been tried without lastingly impressive results. In the early 1980s, about the same time Tl-201 was being investigated for the differentiation of cold thyroid nodules seen on Tc-99m pertechnetate scans, it was discovered that hyperplastic parathyroid tissue concentrated Tl-201. The thyroid also concentrated Tl-201, so a way of substracting the thyroid gland image was devised by subtracting a Tc-99m pertechnetate image from a Tl-201 image using computer image matrix subtraction. In fact, the subtraction often seems unnecessary because the configurations of the two images are different enough to provide strong clues to the location of parathyroid adenomas. When the parathyroid tissue underlies thyroid tissue, the value of computer image matrix subtraction becomes more apparent.

Technically, the study is accomplished most expediently for the patient and with best visual results when the Tc-99m pertechnetate image is obtained first. It is important to include the entire neck and up-

---

* One should be aware that a significant fraction of the very energetic beta particles from P-32 (1.7 MeV max) may penetrate a plastic syringe and deposit a high radiation dose to the hands. A dose of 4.5 rad can be delivered to the finger held for 30 seconds in contact with a syringe containing 10 mCi of P-32 in a 5-ml volume.[67]

per half of the mediastinum in the search field and that the patient not be allowed to move until all images have been obtained. After the pertechnetate thyroid image is stored as a matrix in the computer, a 75-keV downscatter image from Tc-99m is also stored. Tl-201 is injected and Tl-201 75-keV images obtained. The Tc-99m 140-keV and 75-keV downscatter images are of 5-minutes duration each. The Tl-201 75-keV image is acquired as an accumulation of 1-minute images for 25 minutes so that part of these may be discarded if patient motion occurs. During processing the technetium downscatter image matrix is subtracted from the Tl-201 cumulative image. The Tc-99m 140-keV image is then subtracted serially until the enlarged or hyperplastic parathyroid tissue becomes apparent in the image. Usually 2 mCi of each tracer are used for this procedure.

Some authors have found that parathyroid tissue of less than 5 mm in diameter is only rarely visualized.[69] Secondary hyperparathyroidism may give misleading results by not showing all the hyperplastic tissue.[70] Thyroid adenomas may be nonfunctional with pertechnetate and functional with Tl-201. Primary and tertiary (progressive secondary hyperplasia that has become autonomous) parathyroid adenomas are generally visualized well with this technique (Fig. 17–12). This imaging technique is of greatest value to the surgeons who often must hunt extensively for abnormal tissue. It is of particularly great value when a second surgical approach must be made through scarred tissue.

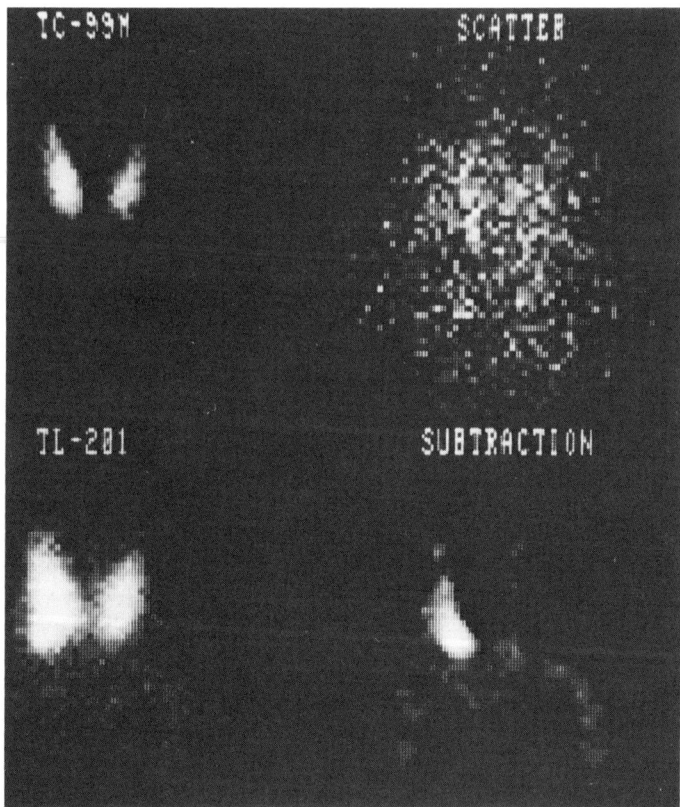

Figure 17-12. Parathyroid imaging using a subtraction technique. The technetium pertechnetate image was subtracted from the thallium image to demonstrate the location of the parathyroid adenoma.

SKIN BLOOD FLOW MEASUREMENT

Xenon-133 is an inert diffusible tracer. It diffuses so freely between tissue and the capillary blood that diffusion equilibrium is practically maintained. Because Xe-133 is not diffusion limited, the rate of removal from its tissue injection site will be proportional to the rate of blood flow, i.e., it is a flow-limited tracer.

Xe-133 dissolved in saline and injected intradermally has been used successfully to measure skin blood flow[71] and to estimate the level of amputation.[72]

After intradermal injection of Xe-133 in saline, the washout of radioactivity is biexponential. The first component of the washout is influenced by trauma from the injection, which causes a slight overestimation of the blood flow, whereas the second component underestimates the blood flow because of backdiffusion of Xe-133, which is taken up by subcutaneous fat.

Daly et al[71] have developed a method of quantitatively measuring skin perfusion from data obtained from the first portion of the biexponential curve. Their method involves injection 0.05 ml of Xe-133 in saline intradermally. The washout of activity is monitored over the area for 10 minutes at four frames per minute with a scintillation camera and computer to generate time–activity curves. The rate constant for xenon washout during the first 6 minutes is determined from a least-squares fit for a monoexponential function. The blood flow rate is determined by inserting the rate constant into the Schmidt–Kety equation as follows:

$$F = \frac{100 \cdot \lambda \cdot K}{P}$$

Where

- F = blood perfusion (ml/min/100 g tissue)
- λ = tissue-to-blood partition coefficient (0.7)
- K = rate constant for Xe-133 washout ($0.693/T_{1/2}$)
- P = specific gravity of skin (1.05)

Mean skin blood perfusion rates (ml/min/100 g) on the anterior surface of the lower legs determined in normal male volunteers varied with the position of injection and ranged from 8.9 at a point 10 cm above the knee to 14.3 at the ankle. Malone et al[72] found that when preoperative skin blood flow rates exceeded 2.2 ml/min/100 g tissue, 95 percent (70/74) of lower extremity amputations healed primarily, thus providing accurate objective information for determining the optimum amputation level.

Xe-133 in saline is available commercially in a prefilled Carpule for injection or in a multidose serum vial.

MONOCLONAL ANTIBODIES

Site-specific localization of radiotracers with high affinity and avidity for tumors is a continuing goal in nuclear medicine. The discovery of a technique of producing large quantities of highly purified monoclonal antibodies that can be radiolabeled has brought us one giant step closer to that goal. Although the current techniques are far from perfected, they hold high promise for success.[73]

In a typical immunologic response an antibody or immunoglobulin is capable of recognizing the shape of a particular site (determinant) on an antigen, thereby forming an antigen–antibody complex that neutralizes the antigen. To develop antibodies an organism must be subjected to an antigenic challenge. The spleens of animals and humans produce B lymphocytes that can differentiate into antibody-producing plasma cells after exposure to foreign substances. A foreign substance may contain several different antigens, and each antigen may contain several different determinants. Each determinant can stimulate one or more B lymphocytes whose plasma cells produce a specific antibody to a specific determinant. After immunization with a foreign substance, the host recipient will

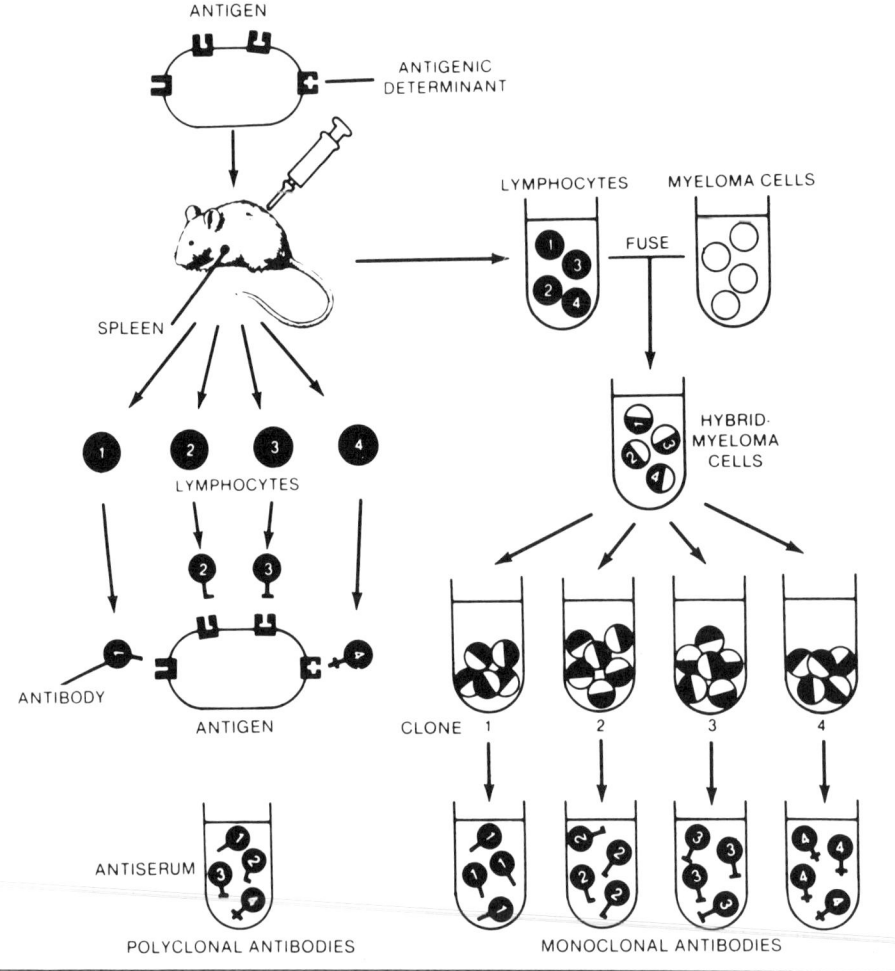

Figure 17-13. Injection of antigen into a mouse or other higher animal elicits a heterogeneous antibody response because of the stimulation of several B lymphocytes by various determinants on the antigen, which results in polyclonal antibodies in the serum (left). If sensitized lymphocytes are removed from the spleen of an immunized animal and induced to fuse with myeloma cells, individual hybrid cells can be cloned, each producing monoclonal antibodies to a single antigenic determinant (right). (From Keenan AM, et al, 1985, p 531, with permission.[76])

thus produce a diverse number of antibodies (polyclonal antibodies). If, however, one could select a single lymphocyte and culture it in vitro, the single cell's progeny, or clone, would produce antibody specific for a single antigenic determinant, i.e., a monoclonal antibody (Fig. 17-13).

In 1975 Kohler and Milstein developed a method of producing monoclonal antibodies in vitro by fusing splenic lymphocytes from immunized mice with mouse myeloma cells. The result was clones of hybrid cells called hybridomas.[74] Because antigenically stimulated lymphocytes will not survive alone in cell culture and myeloma cells cannot be induced to secrete antigen-specific antibodies, the advantage of hybridomas is that the "cells express both the lymphocyte's property of specific-antibody production and the immortal character of the myeloma cells."[75]

Hybridomas usually produce IgG immunoglobulin. Immunoglobulin molecules are Y-shaped structures comprised of two long (heavy or H) chains and two short (light or L) chains of amino acids linked together by disulfide bridges (Fig. 17–14). The variable region of the molecule controls antibody specificity for antigens whereas the constant region is responsible for various functions such as binding of complement, transport across membranes, and binding to membranes.

Although all the antibody a hybridoma clone secretes is genetically derived from a single cell, it is not a monoclonal antibody in the immunologic sense because each cell of the clone has some chromosomes from the myeloma cell parent and some from the spleen cell parent. As a result, the hybridoma antibody is frequently a mix of H and L chains of both parent cells. Because the aim is to find a clone with only H and L chains of the specifically immune spleen cell, hundreds of fusions and reclonings may be required before a single hybrid that secretes the desired antibody is formed (Fig. 17–15). Once the desired clone is found, it can be frozen for long-term storage. At any time thereafter a sample of the clone can be injected into animals of the same strain as those that provided the original cells for fusing. The animals will develop tumors that secrete the specific monoclonal antibody in high concentration within their serum. Alternatively, a clone can be grown in mass culture, and the antibody can be harvested from the medium.

Radiolabeling of whole antibodies and antibody fragments has been accomplished with various radionuclides by using different techniques.[76] Mild iodination of tyrosine moieties with I-123, I-125, and I-131 is the most common radiolabel. In

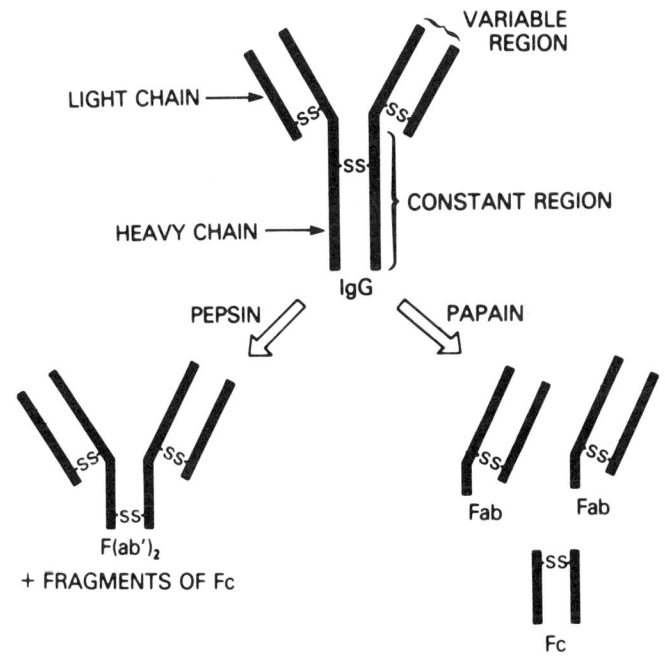

Figure 17-14. Immunoglobulin G molecules consist of two heavy and two light protein chains held together by disulfide bonds. Two variable regions can bind to specific antigenic sites, and the constant region interacts with the host immune system. Enzymatic digestion with pepsin removes part of constant region to produce an F (ab')₂ fragment, whereas papain splits the molecule into an Fc fragment and two Fab fragments. (From Keenan AM, et al, 1985, p 531, with permission.[76])

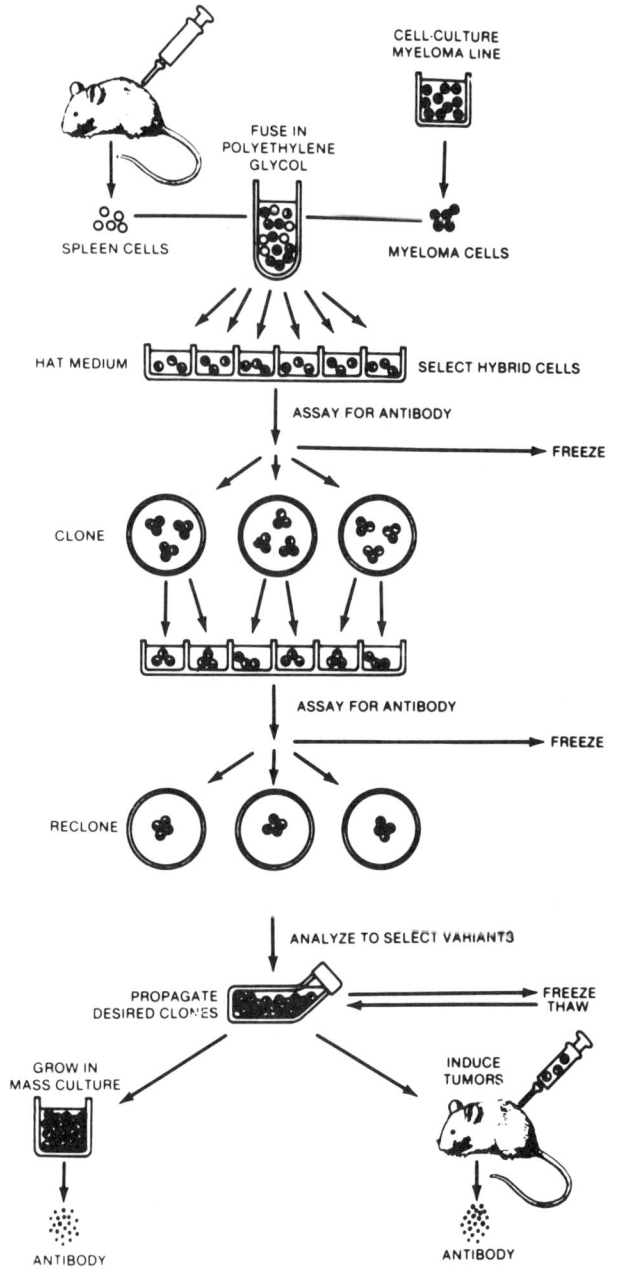

Figure 17-15. Fusion of antigen-stimulated spleen cells with myeloma cells in polyethylene glycol results in hybrid cells that can be cloned in hypoxanthene-aminopterin-thymidine (HAT) medium. Those clones that generate immunoglobulin are further propagated, and those producing antibodies to the desired antigen are selected to find the variant that produces antibody with the desired specificity and binding properties. Hybridomas can be maintained in mass culture or mouse ascites, and clones at any stage of development can be frozen for later use. (From Keenan AM, et al, 1985, p 531, with permission.[76])

another technique antibody–DTPA conjugates can be made and then labeled with In-111 or less successfully with Tc-99m. Radiolabeling antibody with the alpha emitter Bi-212 and the beta emitter Cu-64 have been investigated for therapeutic application.

Because most antibodies are of animal origin, allergic reactions in humans have developed. To counter this problem, enzymatic cleavage of the heavy chain is done to produce antibody fragments. Papain digestion cleaves the allergenic Fc portion and leaves two Fab (antigen binding) fragments. Pepsin digestion cleaves a fragment of the Fc portion below the disulfide bridge and leaves the Fab fragments bound together as the divalent $F(ab')_2$ fragment. The monovalent Fab fragments have weaker binding to cell-bound antigen than the whole antibody. The $F(ab')_2$ fragments have the avidity of divalent binding without the immunogenicity of the Fc region, which may be an advantage over whole antibody or Fab fragments.

The diagnosis and treatment of tumors with antibodies requires antibodies to be developed to tumor-specific antigens that are expressed on tumor cell surfaces. Monoclonal antibodies under clinical investigation have been developed toward antigens associated with cancer of the colon, breast, ovary, lung, and liver and melanoma and lymphoproliferative disorders.

REFERENCES

1. Alavi A: Detection of gastrointestinal bleeding with Tc-99m sulfur colloid. Semin Nucl Med 12:126, 1982
2. Winzelberg GG, McKusick KA, Froelich JW, et al: Detection of gastrointestinal bleeding with Tc-99m labeled red blood cells. Semin Nucl Med 12:139, 1982
3. Bunker S, Lull R, Tanasescu D, et al: Scintigraphy of gastrointestinal hemorrhage: Superiority of Tc-99m red blood cells over Tc-99m sulfur colloid. Am J Roentgen 143:543, 1984
4. Som P, Oster Z, Atkins H, et al: Detection of gastrointestinal blood loss with Tc-99m labeled, heat-treated red blood cells. Radiology 138:207, 1981
5. Winzelberg G, McKusick K, Strauss H, et al: Evaluation of gastrointestinal bleeding by red blood cells labeled in vivo with technetium-99m. J Nucl Med 20:1080, 1979
6. Callahan RJ, Froelich JW, McKusick KA, et al: A modified method for the in vivo labeling of red blood cells with Tc-99m: Concise communication. J Nucl Med 23:315, 1982
7. Bunker SR, Brown JM, McAuley RJ, et al: Detection of gastrointestinal bleeding sites: Use of in vivo technetium Tc-99m labeled RBCs. JAMA 247:789, 1982
8. Fisher RS, Malmud LS, Roberts GS, et al: Gastroesophageal (GE) scintiscanning to detect and quantitate GE reflux. Gastroenterology 70:301, 1976
9. Malmud LS, Fisher RS: Radionuclide studies of esophageal transit and gastroesophageal reflux. Semin Nucl Med 12:104, 1982
10. Chernow B, Johnson LF, Janowitz WR, et al: Pulmonary aspiration as a consequence of gastroesophageal reflux. Dig Dis Sci 24:839, 1979
11. Heyman S, Kirkpatrick JA, Winton HS; et al: An improved radionuclide method for the diagnosis of gastroesophageal reflux and aspiration in children (milk scan). Radiology 131:279, 1979
12. Rudd TG, Christie DL: Demonstration of gastroesophageal reflux in children by radionuclide gastroesophagography. Radiology 131:483, 1979
13. Christian PE, Datz FL, Sorenson JA, et al: Technical factors in gastric emptying studies: Teaching editorial. J Nucl Med 24:264, 1983
14. Kroop HS, Long WB, Alavi A, et al: Effect of water and fat on gastric emptying of solid meals. Gastroenterology 77:997, 1979
15. Malmud LS, Fisher RS, Knight LC, et al: Scintigraphic evaluation of gastric emptying. Semin Nucl Med 12:116, 1982
16. Meyer JH, MacGregor IL, Guellar R, et al: Tc-99m tagged chicken liver as a marker of solid food in the human stomach. Dig Dis Sci 21:296, 1976
17. Wirth N, Swanson D, Shapiro B, et al: A conveniently prepared Tc-99m resin for semi-solid gastric emptying studies. J Nucl Med 24:511, 1983
18. Christian PE, Moore JG, Sorenson JA, et al: Effects of meal size and correction technique on gastric emptying time: Studies with two tracers and opposed detectors. J Nucl Med 21:883, 1980
19. Anderson WAD, Scatti TM: Synopsis of Pathology. St Louis, C.V. Mosby, 1968, p 638
20. Kilpatrick ZM: Scanning in diagnosis of Meckel's diverticulum. Hosp Pract 9:131, 1974
21. Sfakianakis GN, Conway JJ: Detection of ectopic gastric mucosa in Meckel's diver-

21. ticulum and in other aberrations by scintigraphy: I. Pathophysiology and 10 year experience. J Nucl Med 22:647, 1981
22. Sfakianakis GN, Conway JJ: Detection of ectopic gastric mucosa in Meckel's diverticulum and in other aberrations by scintigraphy: II. Indications and methods—A 10 year expericnce. J Nucl Med 22:732, 1981
23. Stanley MM, Cerniak G; Protein-losing enteropathy. In Rothfeld B (ed): Nuclear Medicine In Vitro. Philadelphia, Lippincott, 1974, p 341
24. Mabry CC, Greenlaw RH, DeVore WD: Measurements of gastrointestinal loss of plasma albumin: A clinical and laboratory evaluation of chromium-51 labeled albumin. J Nucl Med 6:93, 1965
25. Rubini ME, Sheehy TW, Johnson CR: Exudative enteropathy 1. A Comparative study of Cr-51 chloride and I-131 PVP. J Lab Clin Med 58:892, 1961
26. Mishkin FS, Freeman LM: Miscellaneous applications of radionuclide imaging. In Clinical Radionuclide Imaging, 3rd ed. Orlando, Fla, Grune & Stratton, 1984, Vol 2, p 1365
27. Miskin F: Radionuclide salivary gland imaging. Semin Nucl Med 11:258, 1981
28. Brown M, El Gammal TAM, Luxenberg MN, et al: The value, limitations, and applications of nuclear dacryocystography. Semin Nucl Med 11:250, 1981
29. Brizel HE, Sheils WC, Brown M: The effects of radiotherapy on the nasolacrimal system as evaluated by dacryoscintigraphy. Radiology 116:373, 1975
30. Mishima S, Gasset A, Klyce SD, et al: Determination of tear volume and tear flow. Invest Ophthalmol 5:264, 1966
31. Robertson JS, Brown ML, Colvard DM: Radiation absorbed dose to the lens in dacryoscintigraphy with pertechnetate. Radiology 113:747, 1979
32. Sevitt S, Gallagher N: Venous thrombosis and pulmonary embolism. Br J Surg 48:475, 1961
33. Atkins P, Hawkins LA: Detection of venous thrombosis in the legs. Lancet 2:117, 1965
34. Kakkar VV: The diagnosis of deep vein thrombosis using the I-125 labeled fibrinogen test. Arch Surg 104:152, 1972
35. Flanc C, Kakkar VV, Clarke MB: The detection of venous thrombosis of the legs using I-125 labeled fibrinogen. Br J Surg 55:742, 1968
36. Kakkar VV, Nicolaides AN, Penny JTG, et al: I-125 labeled fibrinogen test adapted for routine screening for deep vein thrombosis. Lancet 1:540, 1970
37. DeNardo GL, DeNardo SJ, Barnett CA, et al: Assessment of conventional criteria for the early diagnosis of thrombophlebitis with I-125 fibrinogen uptake test. Radiology 125:765, 1977
38. Hull R, Hirsh J, Sackett DL, et al: Replacement of venography in suspected venous thrombosis by impedance plethysmography and I-125 fibrinogen leg scanning. A less invasive approach. Ann Intern Med 94:12, 1981
39. Kazem I, Antioniades J, Brady LW, et al: Clinical evaluation of lymph node scanning utilizing colloidal gold 198. Radiology 90:908, 1966
40. Herting SE, Fredricksen PB, Jagt F, et al: Lymph node scanning with radioactive gold. Acta Radiol 16:359, 1970
41. Ege GN: Internal mammary lymphoscintigraphy: The rationale, technique, interpretation and clinical application: A review. Radiology 118:101, 1976
42. Sherman AL, Ter-Pogossian M: Lymph node concentration of radioactive colloidal gold following interstitial injection. Cancer 6:1238, 1953
43. Warbick A, Eye GN, Henkelman RM, et al: An evaluation of radiocolloid size technique. J Nucl Med 18:827, 1977
44. Dunson GL, Thrall JH, Stevenson JS, et al: Tc-99m minicolloid for radionuclide lymphoscintigraphy. Radiology 109:387, 1973
45. Ege GN, Warbick-Cerone A, Bronskill MJ: Radiocolloid Internal Mammary Lymphoscintigraphy. Toronto, Princess Margaret Hospital, Monograph, 1979
46. Ege GN, Warbick A: Lymphoscintigraphy: A comparison of Tc-99 antimony sulfide colloid and Tc-99m stannous phytate. Br J Radiol 52:124, 1979
47. Kaplan WD, Davis MA, Rose CM: A comparison of two technetium-99m–labeled radiopharmaceuticals for lymphoscintigraphy: Concise communication. J Nucl Med 20:933, 1979
48. Counsell RE, Ice RD: The design of organ-imaging radiopharmaceuticals. In Ariens EJ (ed): Medicinal Chemistry—A Series of Monographs—Volume VI. New York, Academic Press, 1975, pp 172–249
49. Blair RS, Beierwaltes WH, Lieberman LM,

et al: Radiolabeled cholesterol as an adrenal scanning agent. J Nucl Med 12:176, 1971
50. Beierwaltes WH, Lieberman LM, Ansari AN, et al: Visualization of human adrenal glands in vivo by scintillation scanning. JAMA 216:275, 1971
51. Beierwaltes WH, Wieland DW, Yu T, et al: Adrenal imaging agents: Rationale, synthesis, formulation and metabolism. Semin Nucl Med 8:5, 1978
52. Sarkar SD, Beierwaltes WH, Ice RD, et al: A new and superior adrenal scanning agent, NP-59. J Nucl Med 16:1038, 1975
53. Gross MD, Thrall JH, Beierwaltes WH: The adrenal scan: A current status report on radiotracers, dosimetry and clinical utility. In Freeman LM, Weissmann HS (eds): Nuclear Medicine Annual 1980. New York, Raven Press, 1980, p 127
54. Sarkar SD, Cohen EL, Beierwaltes WH, et al: A new and superior adrenal imaging agent, NP-59: Evaluation in humans. J Clin Endocrinol Metab 45:353, 1977
55. Thrall JH, Frietas JE, Beierwaltes WH: Adrenal scintigraphy. Semin Nucl Med 8:23, 1978
56. Fowler JS, Wolf AP, Christman RD, et al: Carrier-free C-11 labeled catecholamines. In Subramanian G, Rhodes BA, Cooper JF, Sodd VJ (eds): Radiopharmaceuticals. New York, Society of Nuclear Medicine, 1975, p 196
57. Ice RD, Wieland DM, Beierwaltes WH, et al: Concentration of dopamine analogs in the adrenal medulla. J Nucl Med 16:1147, 1975
58. Wieland DM, Swanson DP, Brown LE, et al: Imaging the adrenal medulla with an I-131 labeled antiadrenergic agent. J Nucl Med 20:155, 1979
59. Short JH, Darby TD: Sympathetic nervous system blocking agents III. Derivations of benzylguanidine. J Med Chem 10:833, 1967
60. Wieland DM, Wu JJ, Brown LE, et al: Radiolabeled adrenergic neuron-blocking agents: Adrenomedullary imaging with I-131 iodobenzylguanidine. J Nucl Med 21:349, 1980
61. Wieland DM, Brown LE, Tobes MC, et al: Imaging the primate adrenal medulla with I-123 and I-131 *meta*-iodo-benzylguanidine: Concise communication J Nucl Med 22:358, 1981
62. Weiner N: Drugs that inhibit adrenergic nerves and block adrenergic receptors. In Gilman AG, Goodman LS, Gilman A (eds): The Pharmacological Basis of Therapeutics, 6th ed. New York, Macmillan, 1980, p 202
63. Sisson JC, Fragen MD, Volk TW, et al: Scintigraphic localization of pheochromocytoma. N Engl J Med 305:12, 1981
64. Chaudhuri TK: Role of P-32 in polycythemia vera and leukemia. In Spencer RP (ed): Therapy in Nuclear Medicine. New York, Grune & Stratton, 1978, p 223
65. Spiers FW, Beddoe AH, King SD, et al: The absorbed dose to bone marrow in the treatment of polycythemia vera by P-32. Br J Radiol 49:133, 1976
66. Morton ME: Colloidal chromic radiophosphate in high yields for radiotherapy. Nucleonics 10:92, 1952
67. Henson PW: Radiation dose to the skin in contact with unshielded syringes containing radioactive substances. Br J Radiol 46:972, 1973
68. Hazra TA, Howell R: Uses of beta emitters for intracavitary therapy. In Spencer RP (ed): Therapy in Nuclear Medicine. New York, Grune & Stratton, 1978, p 307
69. Ferlin G, Borsato N, Camerani M, et al: New perspectives in localizing enlarged parathyroids by technetium–thallium subtraction scan. J Nucl Med 24:438, 1983
70. Young AE, Gaunt JI, Croft DN, et al: Location of parathyroid adenomas by thallium-201 and technetium-99m subtraction scanning. Br Med J 286:1384, 1983
71. Daly MJ, Henry RC: Quantitative measurement of skin perfusion with xenon-133. J Nucl Med 21:156, 1980
72. Malone JM, Leal JM, Moore WS, et al: The "gold standard" for amputation level selection: Xenon-133 clearance. J Surg Res 30:449, 1981
73. Larson SM: Radiolabeled monoclonal antitumor antibodies in diagnosis and therapy. J Nucl Med 26:538, 1985
74. Kohler G, Milstein C: Continuous culture of fused cells secreting antibody of predefined specificity. Nature 256:495, 1975
75. Milstein C: Monoclonal antibodies. Sci Am 243:66, 1980
76. Keenan AM, Harbert JC, Larson SM: Monoclonal antibodies in nuclear medicine. J Nucl Med 26:531, 1985

CHAPTER 18

Licensing, Regulatory Control, and Radiation Safety

Radiopharmaceuticals are radioactive prescription drugs. They are regulated currently by two federal agencies, namely, the Food and Drug Administration (FDA) and the Nuclear Regulatory Commission (NRC). The NRC may delegate its authority to radiation control agencies within the various states. Before considering the regulation of radioactive drugs per se, a historical sketch of drug regulations in general will be presented.

DRUG REGULATIONS: HISTORICAL

The Food and Drugs Act of 1906 was signed into law as a result of unscrupulous manufacturing practices, adulterated foods and drugs, and unfounded claims of therapeutic effectiveness of patent medicines. This act prohibited interstate sales of misbranded and adulterated foods and drugs and heralded the establishment of the FDA in 1931. The act did not require premarket testing of drugs to determine safety. Revisions in the 1906 act culminated in passage by Congress of the Federal Food, Drug, and Cosmetic Act of 1938 when 107 people died after ingesting sulfanilamide elixir formulated with diethylene glycol, a substance toxic to humans. The 1938 act required premarket testing of new drugs to establish their safety.

In 1962 the Kefauver–Harris Amendment to the act was enacted, which increased federal control over the methods of production and testing of drugs before their release for sale to the public. Emotional impetus for passage of this amendment came from another tragedy. Relying on the 1938 law, an FDA medical officer, Dr. Frances Kelsey, had blocked release of the drug thalidomide on the US market because of unexplained side effects. The subsequent discovery in Germany that thousands of deformed infants had been born to mothers who took the supposedly safe sleeping pill during pregnancy caused Congress to vote in strong new drug controls in 1962. Most important of the many changes was the requirement that the effectiveness of new drugs, as well as safety, be established by "substantial evidence" before approval for marketing. The amendment also introduced several new concepts, most importantly new drug investigational procedures and approval of a new drug application (NDA) before marketing.

INVESTIGATIONAL NEW DRUG PROCEDURES

Simply stated, a new drug may be a new entity that requires proof of safety and efficacy for its intended use (i.e., an investigational drug) or one newly released for use that has recently been shown to be safe and efficacious (i.e., a drug with NDA approval). A new drug may also be a new dosage form or route of administration of an old drug, or an old drug being used for a new purpose. Situations regarding the latter occur occasionally in nuclear medicine.

Before 1962, there was no requirement that the FDA be notified that drugs were being tested in humans. In compliance with the 1962 amendment however, a new drug, i.e., one without an approved NDA, that is intended for investigational use in human subjects may not enter into interstate distribution unless a responsible individual (physician) or a pharmaceutical firm sponsors scientific studies with the drug and obtains an approved notice of claimed investigational exemption for a new drug (IND). It is submitted on forms FDA 1571 *Notice of Claimed Investigational Exemption for a New Drug*, FDA 1572 *Statement of the Investigator (Clinical Pharmacology)*, and FDA 1573 *Statement of the Investigator (Clinical Trials)*.

IND procedures include preclinical studies in animals to define a drug's safety rather than efficacy. For radiopharmaceuticals this would entail characterization of radiochemical and radionuclidic impurities as well as biodistribution, metabolism, and excretion patterns of the drug to determine its toxicity and estimate its radiation dosimetry.

Clinical studies in humans occur in three phases. Phase I involves initial carefully controlled studies in a limited number of individuals to determine absorption, distribution, metabolism, excretion, toxicity, preferred route of administration, and safe dosage range. Phase II studies are conducted on a limited number of subjects for a specific disease to provide further evidence of safety and initial evidence of diagnostic or therapeutic efficacy. Phase III studies, known as clinical trials, are intended to assess the drug's safety, effectiveness, and most desirable dosage for the treatment or diagnosis of a specific disease in a large group of subjects by several independent investigators. Risk-versus-benefit assessment is also made during this phase.

Upon completion of all studies in each phase, the sponsor of the new drug (the drug company) submits supporting data to the FDA in an NDA which must be approved before the drug can be sold for routine use.

PHYSICIAN-SPONSORED NOTICE OF CLAIMED INVESTIGATION FOR A NEW DRUG

As previously mentioned, an IND is sponsored either by a drug company that enlists a group of investigators to conduct the study or by a physician. The physician-sponsored IND is the route taken if an investigator wishes to study a drug that no drug company wishes to sponsor. These so-called orphan drugs may have useful medical applications but for only a limited number of patients, which makes them unfavorable candidates for the costly IND–NDA process. In these instances, a simple abbreviated form of IND submission is acceptable, and the sponsoring physician deals directly with the FDA. This enables the FDA to accumulate data on the safety and efficacy of the drug for that kind of use that can be shared with other physicians.

In nuclear medicine practice there arises, occasionally, the need to use a non-NDA-approve radiopharmaceutical or an approved agent for an unapproved use or different route of administration. In such instances the question of the need to file a physician-sponsored IND also arises. Depending on the circumstances of use, composition of the radiopharmaceutical, or type of radioactive materials license, an IND may or may not be required. This topic, with specific examples, is covered in detail in an article by Swanson and Lieto.[1]

REGULATORY CONTROL OF RADIOPHARMACEUTICALS

The regulation of radiopharmaceuticals has a fairly complicated history, beginning with the Food, Drug, and Cosmetic Act of 1938, which applied to all drugs including radiopharmaceuticals. Because of their radioactive nature, however, radiopharmaceuticals were also controlled by the US Atomic Energy Commission (AEC). Under the Atomic Energy Act of 1954, the AEC was authorized to license the possession, use, and transfer of by-product material, i.e., radioisotopes produced in a nuclear reactor. Radioactive biologicals were controlled under the Public Health Service Act of 1944 by the Bureau of Biologics of the FDA. In 1963, after enactment of the Kefauver-Harris Amendments of 1962, the FDA allowed a temporary exemption for radioactive new drugs and biologics from new drug (IND) requirements, provided they were being shipped in complete conformity with the regulations issued by the AEC in 10 CFR 30-36. The purpose of the temporary exemption was to allow for the continued availability of radiopharmaceuticals while the FDA and AEC explored new ways to avoid unnecessary duplication of regulatory control. The exemption applied only to drugs manufactured from reactor-produced radionuclides. It did not include naturally occurring or accelerator-produced radionuclides. The 1963 exemption was revoked, in part, on November 3, 1971 (37 FR 21026), in which the FDA commissioner added a new section 310.503 (formerly 130.49) to Title 21 CFR, listing specific reactor-produced isotopes that, for certain stated uses, were no longer exempt from new drug regulations. The new drugs listed in section 310.503 were those that the AEC determined had well-established uses, and therefore manufacturers and distributors should submit adequate evidence of safety and effectiveness for use as recommended in their labeling. The agencies also concluded that these drugs should not be distributed under investigational use labeling when actually intended for routine use in medical practice.

A transition period followed this order that allowed manufacturers to continue commercial distribution of radiopharmaceuticals only for those drugs for which an NDA, biologic product license, or IND was submitted to the FDA. A final order was issued on July 25, 1975, that terminated the 1963 exemption. Accordingly, all radiopharmaceuticals after this date came under the full authority of the FDA, similar to all nonradioactive drugs.

On January 19, 1975, the AEC was superseded by the US NRC and the US Energy Research and Development Administration (ERDA). Reactor-produced radiopharmaceuticals are currently regulated by the NRC. The NRC does not regulate naturally occurring and accelerator-produced products. These are regulated by the states.

In many instances the NRC's authority is transferred to the states to control the use of reactor-produced material. These so-called agreement states number 27 and are listed in Table 18-1. In summary, the NRC regulates reactor-produced material only, nonagreement states regulate accelerator products only, and agreement states regulate all materials.

TABLE 18-1. LIST OF NRC AGREEMENT STATES

Alabama	Nebraska
Arizona	Nevada
Arkansas	New Hampshire
California	New Mexico
Colorado	New York
Florida	North Carolina
Georgia	North Dakota
Idaho	Oregon
Kansas	Rhode Island
Kentucky	South Carolina
Louisiana	Tennessee
Maryland	Texas
Mississippi	Utah
	Washington

This list is current as of July 22, 1985.

REGULATORY AUTHORITY OF THE FOOD AND DRUG ADMINISTRATION AND NUCLEAR REGULATORY COMMISSION

After termination of the 1963 exemption for radiopharmaceuticals from IND regulations, the FDA stated that it would regulate the safety and efficacy of radioactive drugs with respect to patients. At the same time, the NRC withdrew from regulating radioactive drug safety and efficacy and stated that it would regulate the radiation safety of the workers and the public.

In 1979 the NRC published the following three-part policy statement that it developed to guide its regulation of the medical uses of radioisotopes (44 FR 8242, effective February 9, 1979):

1. The NRC will continue to regulate the medical uses of radioisotopes as necessary to provide for the radiation safety of workers and the general public.
2. The NRC will regulate the radiation safety of patients where justified by the risk to patients and where voluntary standards or compliance with these standards is inadequate.
3. The NRC will minimize intrusion into medical judgements affecting patients and into other areas traditionally considered to be a part of the practice of medicine.

It states further in 44 FR 8242 that

> ... the NRC intends not to exercise regulatory control in those areas (regarding patients) where, upon careful examination, it determines that there are adequate regulations by other Federal or State agencies or well administered professional standards. The Commission recognizes that the FDA regulates the manufacture, interstate distribution, investigational and research use of drugs, including radiopharmaceuticals, but does not have the authority to restrict the routine use of drugs to the procedures (described in the product labeling) that FDA has approved as safe and effective. The NRC sees itself as the only Federal Agency that is currently authorized to regulate the *routine use* of radioactive drugs from the standpoint of reducing unnecessary radiation exposure to patients.

LICENSING AND REGULATIONS GOVERNING THE USE OF RADIOPHARMACEUTICALS

The regulations that govern the medical use of radionuclides are contained in the Code of Federal Regulations, Title 10, Part 35, Human Uses of By-product Material, and Title 10, Part 20, Standards for Protection Against Radiation. Part 35 contains the criteria for licensing persons to receive, possess, and use by-product material in humans. Part 20 pertains primarily to radiation safety and contains the standards and requirements for protecting the licensee and the public against radiation hazards.

Radioactive Material Licenses

The types of NRC licenses issued for the use of radioactive material are categorized as follows:

1. General license for in vitro use
2. Specific licenses
   A. Limited scope: Physician private practice
   B. Limited scope: Institutional
   C. Broad scope: Institutional

General License

In accordance with 10 CFR 31.11, the general license for in vitro use is issued to physicians, veterinarians, clinical labs, or hospitals for radioactive material, not for administration to humans or animals. It is subject to the following possession limits: I-125, I-131, C-14, and Se-75, not more than 10 μCi/U; H-3, not more than 50 μCi/U; Fe-59, not more than 20 μCi/U; and not more than 200 μCi total of I-125, I-131, Se-75, and Fe-59.

Specific Licenses

The specific license of *limited scope for individual physicians* authorizes a physician or groups of physicians to possess and use radionuclides in the licensee's office practice outside of a medical institution. Licenses issued to physicians for private practice specify the radionuclides and the clinical uses that may be performed by the physician to whom the license is issued. It is not required that a radiation safety committee be formed. The private practice license does not permit other physicians to obtain clinical radionuclide training and experience under it. Section 35.12 of 10 CFR 35 outlines specific requirements for this type of license. The physician(s) must submit an application that documents evidence of training and experience for the proposed use of radioactive material in human subjects.

Specific licenses of *limited scope issued to institutions* are issued in accordance with 10 CFR 30.32 and specify the radionuclides and the clinical uses that may be performed by physicians named on the institution's license. The regulations in 10 CFR 35.22 require an institutional licensee to have a radiation safety committee to evaluate all proposals for clinical research and diagnostic and therapeutic uses of radionuclides within the institution. Membership of the committee must include at least the following: an authorized user for each type of use permitted by the license, a representative of the nursing staff, a representative of the institution's management, and a radiation safety officer.

Physicians designated as authorized users in the license must show evidence of training and experience in the proposed use of radionuclides. The physicians named on the institution's license conduct their programs with the approval of the radiation safety committee. Institutional licenses provide a means whereby nonapproved physicians under the supervision of physicians named on the license may obtain basic clinical radionuclide training and experience that may enable them to qualify as individual users. It is important to note that the physician trainee can qualify only to the extent that the authorized user is qualified.

Specific licenses of *broad scope* for medical use are issued in accordance with 10 CFR 33.12. A broad license authorizes multiple quantities and types of by-product material for unspecified uses, and is issued to institutions that (1) have had previous experience operating under a specific institutional license of limited scope and (2) are engaged in medical research as well as routine diagnosis and therapy using radionuclides. Such programs operate under the supervision of a radiation safety committee.

Individual users are not named on the broad license nor are radionuclides limited to specified uses. Individual users and procedures are approved by the institution's radiation safety committee. Physicians may obtain basic and clinical radionuclide training and experience in the use of radiopharmaceuticals in such programs. Broad licenses are usually not appropriate for most institutions except those associated with a university medical school.

The application for a specific license must generally include a description of the radioactive materials needed and their intended uses as well as the qualifications of the personnel and the facilities available. The publication entitled *Guide for the Preparation of Applications for Medical Programs, Regulatory Guide 10.8*,[2] should be obtained from the NRC before completion and submission of an application for a specific license. This publication contains a license application (Form NRC-313) and instructions on the type and extent of information that must be submitted to NRC based on the nature of by-product materials the applicant has requested to use. Model procedures for a radiation safety program are also included that the applicant can adopt directly or use to develop site-specific procedures.

According to the revised regulations, effective April 1, 1987, once a license is granted, licensees will be able to alter their safety procedures following internal review and approval by the Radiation Safety Committee and not be restricted to only those procedures described in the license application. The proposed changes of course must comply with the regulations. This change was instituted to allow medical licensees to modify their radiation safety procedures, facilities, and equipment, so they can make prompt use of new methods to meet the changing needs of patient care services. Four types of program changes, however, will still require formal license amendments according to 10 CFR 35.13: (1) addition of new authorized users, change of radiation safety officer or teletherapy physicist, (2) new type of use, for example, adding therapy procedures to an imaging only license, (3) ordering of by-product material in excess of the amount, or radionuclide or form different than authorized on the current license, and (4) new location of use.

TYPE OF USE

The application procedure for any specific license has been simplified by the NRC grouping of various human use procedures into six *types of use* categories, formerly called groups. The types of use categories are organized such that a license approval for any one use within a category automatically grants approval for all other uses within that category if specified in the license application.

Listed in 10 CFR Part 35 the six types of use are: (1) under 35.100, *Uptake, Dilution, and Excretion* ("old" Group I): use of radiopharmaceuticals for uptake, dilution and excretion studies, (2) under 35.200, *Imaging and Localization* ("old" Groups II and III): use of radiopharmaceuticals, generators, and reagent kits for imaging and localization studies, (3) under 35.300, *Radiopharmaceuticals for Therapy* ("old" Groups IV and V), (4) under 35.400, *Sources for Brachytherapy* ("old" Group VI): sealed source needles and seeds of Cs-137, Co-60, Au-198, Ir-192, Sr-90, and I-125 used for interstitial, intracavitary, or superficial radiation treatment, (5) under 35.500, *Sealed Sources for Diagnosis* (new group): sealed sources of I-125, Am-241, or Gd-153 for bone mineral analysis and I-125 portable imagers, and (6) under 35.600, *Teletherapy* (new group): sealed sources of Co-60 and Cs-137 in teletherapy units.

The types of radiopharmaceuticals used in the first three *types of use* categories are no longer listed in the regulations but can be obtained from NRC regional offices on request. The reader is referred to Table 1-3 in Chapter 1 for a list of approved radiopharmaceuticals and uses. One should note under category 3, Radiopharmaceuticals for Therapy, that radiation safety instruction must be provided for all personnel caring for a patient receiving radiopharmaceutical therapy according to Part 35.310. A brief discussion can be found in Chapter 8 under safety considerations in radioiodine therapy.

There is a major advantage to these *types of use* categories. When the FDA approves or exempts a new radiopharmaceutical, it is reviewed by the NRC for the radiation safety of workers and the general public and then is usually placed in one of the categories and generally will not require a license amendment before use if a license includes that category. This eliminates much of the need for an institution to amend its license each time a new radiopharmaceutical is approved by the FDA.

Special considerations regarding the use of radiopharmaceuticals in nuclear medicine are as follows: the licensee shall (1) elute generators and prepare reagent kits according to the instructions of the manufacturer, (2) measure the Mo-99 concentration in each generator eluate, (3) prohibit administration to patients of Tc-99m containing more than 0.15 microcurie of Mo-99 per millicurie of Tc-99m, and (4) maintain the Mo-99 test records for 2 years for NRC inspection. The records must include, for each elution of Tc-99m, the measured activity of Tc-99m in millicuries and Mo-99 in microcuries, the ratio of these measures expressed as microcuries of Mo-99 per millicurie of Tc-99m, the time and date of the measurement, and the initials of the individual who made the measurement. *Note*: The test for aluminum ion in the generator eluate is required by the US Pharmacopeia (USP) to be not more than 10 micrograms of Al ion per milliliter of generator eluate.

As cited in 10 CFR 35.205, the administration of a radioactive gas or aerosol must be conducted in a room at negative pressure compared to surrounding rooms so that maximum permissible concentrations in air are not exceeded (Table 18–2). The system used must be vented directly to the outside atmosphere or collected for decay in a shielded container. Precautionary measures must be considered in the event of an accidental spill of radioactive gas into a room. Calculations must be made based on the maximum amount of activity used, room air volume, and exhaust rate and recorded for future reference (see Chapter 10 for examples). Based on these calculations, safety procedures to be followed in the event of a spill must be instituted and posted in the area of use. Collection system operation must be checked each month and ventilation rates in areas of use checked each six months.

A licensee who is licensed to use by-product material for use according to one or more of the *types of use* categories is also authorized by 10 CFR 35.57 to receive, possess, and use calibration and reference standards as follows:

1. Any by-product material listed in 35.100 and 35.200 with
   A. A half-life not longer than 100 days in individual amounts not to exceed 15 mCi
   B. A half-life greater than 100 days in individual amounts not to exceed 200 μCi each
2. Tc-99m in individual amounts not to exceed 50 mCi
3. Any by-product material in sealed sources in amounts not to exceed 15 mCi per source supplied by a licensed manufacturer

If sources in amounts exceeding the aforementioned limits are used, they must be specifically identified within the by-product materials license. Radiation safety and handling instructions supplied by the manufacturer with a sealed source must be maintained and followed for the duration of source use.

According to 10 CFR 35.59 leak tests must be conducted on sealed sources except for the following: by-product material (1) with half-life less than 30 days, (2) consisting only of a gas, (3) containing 100 μCi or less of beta-gamma material or 10 μCi or less of alpha-emitting material, (4) consisting of Ir-192 seeds encased in nylon ribbon or (5) stored sources not being used. If leak tests are required they must be conducted at 6 month intervals unless otherwise specified, by a method capable of detecting 0.005 μCi of material on the sample. Procedures for handling leaky sources can be found in 10 CFR 35.59. Leak test records must be maintained for 5 years. Sealed sources must be inventoried quarterly. Inventory records must be maintained for 5 years and include the source identity, activity, location, model or serial number and signature of the Radiation Safety Officer. Areas where sealed sources are stored must be surveyed quarterly and survey records kept for 2 years.

PREPARATION OF RADIOPHARMACEUTICAL DOSAGES

The terms "dose" and "dosage" are to be distinguished in nuclear medicine. The word "dose" is used to indicate quantities of radiation absorbed dose or dose equivalent that are measured with the base unit of rad or rem. The word "dosage" is used to indicate quantities of radioactivity that are measured with the base unit curie. As cited in 10 CFR 35.53 the requirements for preparing radiopharmaceutical dosages for diagnostic and therapeutic procedures in nuclear medicine are as follows:

1. Measures all dosages containing more than 10 μCi before use

2. Measure all dosages intended to be 10 µCi or less to verify that they do not exceed 10 µCi
3. Retain written records for 2 years which list the
   A. Generic name, trade name, or abbreviation of the radiopharmaceutical, its lot number, radionuclide and expiration date
   B. Patient's name and identification number
   C. Prescribed dosage and activity of the dosage at the time of measurement or a notation that it is less than 10 µCi
   D. Date and time of measurement
   E. Initials of the individual making the record

SYRINGE AND VIAL SHIELDS

Radiopharmaceuticals are contained in vials and dosages are dispensed in syringes. In accordance with 10 CFR 35.60 and 35.61, individuals who prepare a radiopharmaceutical kit shall use a syringe shield and individuals administering a radiopharmaceutical dosage shall use a syringe shield unless contraindicated for the particular patient. The syringe or syringe shield label must show the radiopharmaceutical name or its abbreviation, the clinical procedure to be performed, or the patient's name. Radiopharmaceutical vials shall be kept in radiation shields which are labeled with the radiopharmaceutical name or its abbreviation.

RADIATION MEASURING INSTRUMENTS

Regulations regarding calibration and check of dose calibrators and survey instruments are listed in 10 CFR Parts 35.50 and 35.51, respectively. Detailed procedures for these instruments can be found in Chapter 6 under instrument quality control.

MISADMINISTRATION OF RADIOPHARMACEUTICALS

Regulations regarding reports and records of diagnostic and therapeutic misadministration of radiopharmaceuticals are listed in 10 CFR 35.33. A detailed discussion of misadministration reporting can be found in Chapter 5.

TRAINING AND EXPERIENCE REQUIREMENT FOR MEDICAL USE OF BY-PRODUCT MATERIAL

Human use of by-product material must be carried out by or under the supervision of a physician who is duly authorized by proper training and experience in basic radionuclide handling techniques and in the clinical management of patients to whom radiopharmaceuticals have been administered. Various training requirements are outlined in 10 CFR Part 35 according to the *types of uses* previously discussed.

TRAINING FOR UPTAKE, DILUTION, AND EXCRETION STUDIES

The requirements listed in 10 CFR 35.910 are as follows:

To conduct such studies in humans an authorized user must be a physician who:

1. Is certified in
   A. Nuclear medicine by the American Board of Nuclear Medicine;
   B. Diagnostic radiology by the American Board of Radiology; or
   C. Diagnostic radiology or radiology by the American Osteopathic Board of Radiology; or
2. Has had classroom and laboratory training in basic radioisotope handling techniques applicable to the use of prepared radiopharmaceuticals, and supervised clinical experience as follows

A. 40 hours of classroom and laboratory training that includes: radiation physics and instrumentation; radiation protection; mathematics pertaining to the use and measurement of radioactivity; radiation biology; and radiopharmaceutical chemistry; and
B. 20 hours of supervised clinical experience under the supervision of an authorized user and that includes: examining patients and reviewing their case histories to determine their suitability for radioisotope diagnosis, limitations or contraindications; selecting the suitable radiopharmaceuticals and calculating and measuring the dosage; administering dosages to patients and using syringe radiation shields; collaborating with the authorized user in the interpretation of radioisotope test results; and patient followup; or
3. Has successfully completed a six-month training program in nuclear medicine as part of a training program that has been approved by the Accreditation Council for Graduate Medical Education and that included classroom and laboratory training, work experience, and supervised clinical experience in all the topics identified in item 2 above.

TRAINING FOR IMAGING AND LOCALIZATION STUDIES

The requirements listed in 10 CFR 35.920 are as follows:

To conduct such studies in humans an authorized user of a radiopharmaceutical, generator, or reagent kit must be a physician who:

1. Is certified in
   A. Nuclear medicine by the American Board of Nuclear Medicine;
   B. Diagnostic radiology by the American Board of Radiology; or
   C. Diagnostic radiology or radiology by the American Osteopathic Board of Radiology; or
2. Has had classroom and laboratory training in the basic radioisotope handling techniques applicable to the use of prepared radiopharmaceuticals, generators, and reagent kits, supervised work experience, and supervised clinical experience as follows
   A. 200 hours of classroom and laboratory training that includes: radiation physics and instrumentation; radiation protection; mathematics pertaining to the use and measurement of radioactivity; radiopharmaceutical chemistry; and radiation biology; and
   B. 500 hours of supervised work experience under the supervision of an authorized user that includes: ordering, receiving, and unpacking radioactive materials safely and performing the related radiation surveys; calibrating dose calibrators and diagnostic instruments and performing checks for proper operation of survey meters; calculating and safely preparing patient dosages; using administrative controls to prevent the misadministration of by-product material; using procedures to contain spilled by-product materials safely and using proper decontamination procedures; and eluting Tc-99m from generator systems, measuring and testing the eluate for Mo-99 and alumina contamination, and processing the eluate with reagent kits to prepare Tc-99m labeled radiopharmaceuticals; and
   C. 500 hours of supervised clinical experience under the supervision of an authorized user that includes: examining patients and reviewing their case histories to determine their suitability for radioisotope diagnosis, limitations, or contraindications; selecting the suitable

radiopharmaceuticals and calculating and measuring the dosages; administering dosages to patients and using syringe radiation shields; collaborating with the authorized user in the interpretation of radioisotope test results; and patient followup; or

3. Has successfully completed a six-month training program in nuclear medicine that has been approved by the Accreditation Council for Graduate Medical Education and that included classroom and laboratory training, work experience, and supervised clinical experience in all the topics identified in item 2 above.

TRAINING FOR THERAPEUTIC USE OF RADIOPHARMACEUTICALS

The requirements listed in 10 CFR 35.930 are as follows;

To conduct such studies in humans an authorized user of therapeutic radiopharmaceuticals must be a physician who

1. Is certified by
   A. The American Board of Nuclear Medicine; or
   B. The American Board of Radiology in radiology or therapeutic radiology; or
2. Has had classroom and laboratory training in basic radioisotope handling techniques applicable to the use of therapeutic radiopharmaceuticals, and supervised clinical experience as follows
   A. 80 hours of classroom and laboratory training that includes: radiation physics and instrumentation; radiation protection; mathematics pertaining to the use and measurement of radioactivity; and radiation biology; and
   B. supervised clinical experience under the supervision of an authorized user at a medical institution that includes: use of I-131 for diagnosis of thyroid function and the treatment of hyperthyroidism or cardiac dysfunction in 10 individuals; and use of I-131 for treatment of thyroid carcinoma in 3 individuals.

Documenting Training and Experience

Form NRC-313, *Application for Materials License: Medical*, contains Supplements A and B, which document training and experience (Fig. 18-1). Supplement A lists specific training and experience, and Supplement B is a preceptor statement to document clinical experience.

Certification by a medical specialty board will be accepted as evidence that a physician has had adequate training and experience. Physicians who wish to qualify on the basis of board certification need only complete items 1, 2, and 3 on Supplement A. Other applications should submit Supplements A and B with all items completed. A separate Supplement B should be completed and signed by each preceptor who provided training or supervised experience.

NUCLEAR PHARMACY PRACTICE

Nuclear pharmacy practice standards have been prepared by the Section on Nuclear Pharmacy, Academy of Pharmacy Practice of the American Pharmaceutical Association. The standards supplement the competency-based practice standards for pharmacy in general and serve to delineate those areas of responsibility that are unique to nuclear pharmacy. The standards are intended to provide a sound guideline for nuclear pharmacists in their specialty practice. Additionally, they provide the practical foundation upon which the competency-based nuclear pharmacy certification examination is derived. Although the standards may be useful to other individuals who prepare radioactive material for human use, it is not the intent of these standards to govern the activities of these individuals.

Within the practice standards, nuclear

FORM NRC-313M-SUPPLEMENT A (8-78)	U.S. NUCLEAR REGULATORY COMMISSION
	TRAINING AND EXPERIENCE
	AUTHORIZED USER OR RADIATION SAFETY OFFICER

1. NAME OF AUTHORIZED USER OR RADIATION SAFETY OFFICER	2. STATE OR TERRITORY IN WHICH LICENSED TO PRACTICE MEDICINE

3. CERTIFICATION

SPECIALTY BOARD A	CATEGORY B	MONTH AND YEAR CERTIFIED C

4. TRAINING RECEIVED IN BASIC RADIOISOTOPE HANDLING TECHNIQUES

FIELD OF TRAINING A	LOCATION AND DATE(S) OF TRAINING B	TYPE AND LENGTH OF TRAINING	
		LECTURE/LABORATORY COURSES (Hours) C	SUPERVISED LABORATORY EXPERIENCE (Hours) D
a. RADIATION PHYSICS AND INSTRUMENTATION			
b. RADIATION PROTECTION			
c. MATHEMATICS PERTAINING TO THE USE AND MEASUREMENT OF RADIOACTIVITY			
d. RADIATION BIOLOGY			
e. RADIOPHARMACEUTICAL CHEMISTRY			

5. EXPERIENCE WITH RADIATION. *(Actual use of Radioisotopes or Equivalent Experience)*

ISOTOPE	MAXIMUM AMOUNT	WHERE EXPERIENCE WAS GAINED	DURATION OF EXPERIENCE	TYPE OF USE

Figure 18-1. A. Form NRC 313M, Supplement A: Training and Experience Requirements.

FORM NRC-313M-SUPPLEMENT B	U. S. NUCLEAR REGULATORY COMMISSION
(8-78)	

PRECEPTOR STATEMENT

Supplement B must be completed by the applicant physician's preceptor. If more than one preceptor is necessary to document experience, obtain a separate statement from each.

1. APPLICANT PHYSICIAN'S NAME AND ADDRESS	KEY TO COLUMN C
FULL NAME	**PERSONAL PARTICIPATION SHOULD CONSIST OF:**
	1-Supervised examination of patients to determine the suitability for radioisotope diagnosis and/or treatment and recommendation for prescribed dosage.
STREET ADDRESS	2-Collaboration in dose calibration and actual administration of dose to the patient including calculation of the radiation dose, related measurements and plotting of data.
CITY / STATE / ZIP CODE	3-Adequate period of training to enable physician to manage radioactive patients and follow patients through diagnosis and/or course of treatment.

2. CLINICAL TRAINING AND EXPERIENCE OF ABOVE NAMED PHYSICIAN

ISOTOPE A	CONDITIONS DIAGNOSED OR TREATED B	NUMBER OF CASES INVOLVING PERSONAL PARTICIPATION C	COMMENTS (Additional information or comments may be submitted in duplicate on separate sheets.) D
I-131 or I-125	DIAGNOSIS OF THYROID FUNCTION		
	DETERMINATION OF BLOOD AND BLOOD PLASMA VOLUME		
	LIVER FUNCTION STUDIES		
	FAT ABSORPTION STUDIES		
	KIDNEY FUNCTION STUDIES		
	IN VITRO STUDIES		
OTHER			
I-125	DETECTION OF THROMBOSIS		
I-131	THYROID IMAGING		
P-32	EYE TUMOR LOCALIZATION		
Se-75	PANCREAS IMAGING		
Yb-169	CISTERNOGRAPHY		
Xe-133	BLOOD FLOW STUDIES AND PULMONARY FUNCTION STUDIES		
OTHER			
Tc-99m	BRAIN IMAGING		
	CARDIAC IMAGING		
	THYROID IMAGING		
	SALIVARY GLAND IMAGING		
	BLOOD POOL IMAGING		
	PLACENTA LOCALIZATION		
	LIVER AND SPLEEN IMAGING		
	LUNG IMAGING		
	BONE IMAGING		
OTHER			

Figure 18-1. B. Form NRC 313M, Supplement B: Preceptor Statement. *(continued)*

PRECEPTOR STATEMENT (Continued)

2. CLINICAL TRAINING AND EXPERIENCE OF ABOVE NAMED PHYSICIAN (Continued)

ISOTOPE A	CONDITIONS DIAGNOSED OR TREATED B	NUMBER OF CASES INVOLVING PERSONAL PARTICIPATION C	COMMENTS (Additional information or comments may be submitted in duplicate on separate sheets.) D
P-32 (Soluble)	TREATMENT OF POLYCYTHEMIA VERA, LEUKEMIA, AND BONE METASTASES		
P-32 (Colloidal)	INTRACAVITARY TREATMENT		
I-131	TREATMENT OF THYROID CARCINOMA		
	TREATMENT OF HYPERTHYROIDISM		
Au-198	INTRACAVITARY TREATMENT		
Co-60 or Cs-137	INTERSTITIAL TREATMENT		
	INTRACAVITARY TREATMENT		
I-125 or Ir-192	INTERSTITIAL TREATMENT		
Co-60 or Cs-137	TELETHERAPY TREATMENT		
Sr-90	TREATMENT OF EYE DISEASE		
	RADIOPHARMACEUTICAL PREPARATION		
Mo-99/ Tc-99m	GENERATOR		
Sn-113/ In-113m	GENERATOR		
Tc-99m	REAGENT KITS		
Other			

3. DATES AND TOTAL NUMBER OF HOURS RECEIVED IN CLINICAL RADIOISOTOPE TRAINING

4. THE TRAINING AND EXPERIENCE INDICATED ABOVE WAS OBTAINED UNDER THE SUPERVISION OF:
a. NAME OF SUPERVISOR
b. NAME OF INSTITUTION
c. MAILING ADDRESS
d. CITY

5. MATERIALS LICENSE NUMBER(S)

6. PRECEPTOR'S SIGNATURE

7. PRECEPTOR'S NAME (Please type or print)

8. DATE

Figure 18-1. B. *(continued)*

pharmacy is defined as "a patient oriented service that embodies the scientific knowledge and professional judgement required to improve and promote health through assurance of the safe and efficacious use of radioactive drugs for diagnosis and therapy." Additionally, the standards list the following general areas that comprise the practice of nuclear pharmacy.

1. Procurement of radiopharmaceuticals
2. Compounding of radiopharmaceuticals
3. Performance of routine quality control procedures
4. Dispensing of radiopharmaceuticals
5. Distribution of radiopharmaceuticals
6. Implementation of basic radiation protection procedures and practices
7. Consultation and education to the nuclear medicine community, patients, pharmacists, other health professionals and the general public regarding the following:
   A. Physical and chemical properties of radiopharmaceuticals
   B. Phramacokinetics and biodistribution of radiopharmaceuticals
   C. Drug interactions and other factors that alter patterns of distribution.
8. Research and development of new formulations

DEVELOPMENT OF NUCLEAR PHARMACIES

When radioactive drugs first became generally available, they were usually prepared by commercial drug manufacturers under approved NDAs and shipped to users in a form suitable for direct administration to patients. As the use of radioactive drugs increased within hospitals, particularly those with short-lived radionuclides requiring daily preparations, units within hospitals were often created to handle these drugs. In many hospitals those units became part of the pharmacy department or the nuclear medicine department. Such units employing registered pharmacists and other personnel having specialized training and experience in compounding, preparing, storing, and dispensing radioactive drugs became known as "nuclear pharmacies."

Over the years nuclear medicine and nuclear pharmacy services have grown rapidly. Today nuclear pharmacies are located either in hospital pharmacies and nuclear medicine departments or within the local community. The hospital-based nuclear pharmacy provides radiopharmaceutical services to the hospital alone or in some instances to other nearby hospitals as well. Community-based or centralized nuclear pharmacies are usually located in a large city and provide service to several hospitals within the city and to nearby areas. The majority of nuclear pharmacists practice in centralized nuclear pharmacies.

LICENSING OF NUCLEAR PHARMACIES

Nuclear pharmacies are licensed by individual state boards of pharmacy and by the NRC or agreement state agency. The National Association of Boards of Pharmacy (NABP) has developed model regulations for a nuclear pharmacy that may serve as a guideline to state boards in licensing nuclear pharmacies. In general these model regulations outline the requirements necessary for providing radiopharmaceutical services and the training and experience requirements for nuclear pharmacists to obtain a nuclear pharmacy permit. The latter are similar to the requirements set down by the NRC.

Licensing of a nuclear pharmacy by a state board of pharmacy is not required for a hospital-based nuclear medicine pharmacy that provides radiopharmaceuticals only within that institution. These units operate under a physician-authorized user of radioactive material in humans licensed by the NRC or an agreement state. An authorized user may delegate to properly trained individuals (technologists, chemists, pharmacists) certain responsibilities, namely, the preparation and quality control of radiopharmaceuticals and radiation sources, the measurement of radiopharmaceutical doses before administration, the use of appropriate instrumentation for the collection of data to be used by the physician, and the administration of radiopharmaceuticals and radiation from radionuclide sources to patients if permitted under applicable federal, state, or local laws.

Licensing of a facility as a nuclear pharmacy per se by a state board of pharmacy is required for hospital-based nuclear pharmacies and centralized nuclear pharmacies that dispense radiopharmaceuticals to other institutions. In these circumstances, to operate under applicable local laws regulating the practice of pharmacy and medicine may mean that a nuclear pharmacy must be operated under the supervision of a pharmacist registered in the state to practice pharmacy.

NUCLEAR PHARMACIES AND THE FDA

Initially, when nuclear pharmacies were first established, their activities included (1) purchasing a commercially prepared radioactive drug from a drug manufacturer who held an approved NDA and dispensing the drug in its original unopened container, (2) dispensing a single dose from a multiple-dose container of a commercially prepared radioactive drug, and (3) diluting (including adjustments of buffers, bacteriostatic agents, and stabilizers) and repackaging of commercially prepared radioactive drugs for subsequent use or distribution. Eventually, some nuclear pharmacies began preparing their own radioactive drugs and kits for the preparation of Tc-99m radiopharmaceuticals. As the compounding and distribution of radiopharmaceuticals became more widespread, it became apparent that although most nuclear pharmacy activities involved pharmacy practice others appeared to fall under the realm of manufacturing, which required a nuclear pharmacy to register as a drug establishment under Section 510 of the Food, Drug, and Cosmetic Act. Nuclear pharmacies that are required to register under the act as drug manufacturers are subject to compliance with drug listing provisions, current good manufacturing practices, and factory inspections.

Differences of opinion developed among practitioners and the FDA regarding what nuclear pharmacy activities should be regarded as compounding in the normal course of pharmacy practice and what activities should be regarded as manufacturing. To aid the FDA in establishing criteria to determine what activities of a nuclear pharmacy required registration, a subcommittee of the FDA Radiopharmaceuticals Advisory Committee was appointed in October 1975 to consider the issue. The subcommittee gave its report on April 15, 1976, which contained the following recommendations.

In considering which nuclear pharmacy operations should be regulated by the FDA, the subcommittee concluded the following:

1. If the radioactive drug was prepared and dispensed under a prescription, the laws and regulations governing the practice of pharmacy and medicine at the state level should apply, and the nuclear pharmacy should be considered as engaging in the practice of pharmacy.
2. The presence of a third party, however, in the distribution of a prescription drug, between the location where the product is formulated, compounded, or manufactured and the point where it is administered to patients, changes the practice to one of manufacturing.

Examples of this type of situation include one in which a nuclear pharmacy sells radioactive drugs to a second pharmacy for dispensing by the second pharmacy under a prescription and one in which a nuclear pharmacy sells to other pharmacies bulk quantities of nonradioactive kits that it develops. In each case the first pharmacy could be a manufacturer under the act and be required to register under Section 510 of the act.

The subcommittee also recognized that radioactive drugs are often administered by a nuclear medicine unit in a single institution. Such a nuclear medicine unit may operate a nuclear pharmacy and maintain control over any radioactive drug manufactured or compounded within the pharmacy until it is dispensed. Here, the subcommittee concluded that the high level of control exercised over the drug precluded any need for registration. Additional recommendations of the subcommittee were (1) that substantive changes in FDA regulations, as they pertain to true nuclear pharmacies, were not needed and (2) that individual state boards of pharmacy rather than FDA should regulate nuclear pharmacies in the same manner as they now regulate traditional pharmacies that do not compound or dispense radioactive drugs.

In regard to these latter recommendations it should be noted that Section 510 (g) (1) of the act (21 USC 360 (g) (1)) states that

> . . .pharmacies which maintain establishments in conformance with any applicable local laws regulating the practice of pharmacy and medicine are exempt from the drug registration provisions of the act. For the exemption to apply they must be regularly engaged in dispensing prescription drugs or devices, upon prescriptions of practitioners licensed to administer such drugs or devices to patients under the care of such practitioners in the course of their professional practice, and they must not manufacture, prepare, propagate, compound, or possess drugs or devices for sale other than in the regular course of their business of dispensing or selling drugs or devices at retail.

It is the FDA's opinion that nuclear pharmacies are unique in the nature of their practice activities, which does not qualify *all* of them to be exempt from registration as are traditional pharmacies. The FDA regulation of nuclear pharmacies will therefore be based on a reasonable application of the provisions of Section 510 (g) (1) of the act to nuclear pharmacies and a nuclear pharmacy whose activities are consistent with Section 510 (g) (1) of the act; it will be exempt from registering as a drug establishment but will be required to register if its activities fall outside the provisions of Section 510 (g) (1) of the act. The FDA has defined examples of when a nuclear pharmacy must register as a drug establishment.[3]

NUCLEAR PHARMACISTS AS AUTHORIZED USERS

The use of radioactive material in humans is restricted to authorized physicians; however, persons other than physicians can become authorized users of radioactive material. Nuclear pharmacists who operate nuclear pharmacies and dispense radiopharmaceuticals must also be authorized users of radioactive material. The NRC is primarily interested in assuring that nuclear pharmacists are adequately trained and experienced in handling radioactive material in a safe manner. Radiation safety is the NRC's jurisdiction, and their training and experience requirements are designed to ensure that nuclear pharmacists are qualified to serve as radiation safety officers in their practice.

The NRC has determined, according to 10 CFR 35.900, that effective April 1, 1987, an individual who is certified by the Board of Pharmaceutical Specialties in Nuclear Pharmacy satisfies the training and experience requirements necessary to be Radiation Safety Officer (authorized user). Alternatively, the following outline lists the training and experience that the NRC currently finds acceptable for individuals who are named as authorized users on licenses that involve preparing and dispensing radiopharmaceuticals.[4] This criteria evolved pursuant to 10 CFR 30.33, which requires that applicants be qualified by training and experience to use licensed material for the purpose requested in an application, and also from the NRC's guidelines for physicians in hospital nuclear medicine programs because the type of use and the degree of radiation hazard are quite similar.

1. Training in basic radioisotope handling techniques specifically applicable to the use of unsealed sources (200 hours). The training should consist of lectures and laboratory sessions in the following areas:
   A. Radiation physics and instrumentation: 85 hours
   B. Radiation protection: 45 hours
   C. Mathematics of radioactivity use and measurement: 20 hours
   D. Radiation biology: 20 hours
   E. Radiopharmaceutical chemistry: 30 hours

   The training must emphasize radiation physics, instrumentation, and radiation protection, with no less than 130 hours total devoted to these areas.
2. Supervised experience handling unsealed radioactive material under a qualified instructor (500 hours). This experience should cover the type and quantities of by-product material requested in the application and should include the following
   A. Ordering, receiving, surveying, and unpackaging radioactive materials safely
   B. Calibration of dose calibrators, scintillation detectors, and survey meters
   C. Calculation, preparation, and calibration of patient doses including the proper use of syringe shields
   D. Control procedures to prevent mislabeling
   E. Emergency procedures to handle and contain spilled materials safely including related decontamination procedures, survey, and wipe tests
   F. Elution and assay of Tc-99m generators, testing eluate for Mo-99 and alumina contamination, and processing the eluate with reagent kits to prepare Tc-99m radiopharmaceuticals

These are general guidelines concerning acceptable training and experience for authorized user status, but each program of training and experience should be carefully planned and approved by the NRC.

STANDARDS FOR PROTECTION AGAINST RADIATION

The standards for protection against radiation (10 CFR 20) are established so that the total radiation dose to an individual, i.e., radiation worker, does not exceed the limitations of radiation exposure considered to be safe. The regulations in Part 20 apply to all persons who receive, possess, use, or transfer by-product material.

Permissible Doses, Levels, and Concentrations

A *restricted area* is one to which access is controlled by the licensee for the purpose of protecting individuals from exposure to radiation and radioactive material.

An individual in a restricted area may not receive in any one calendar quarter (13 consecutive weeks) a total occupational dose in excess of the following:

1. Whole body, head and trunk, active blood-forming organs, lens of eyes, or gonads.: 1.25 rem
2. Hands and forearms, feet and ankles: 18.75 rem
3. Skin of whole body: 7.5 rem

The whole-body dose may be greater than that listed but shall not exceed 3 rem in any calendar quarter nor can the accumulated whole-body dose exceed $5(N - 18)$ rem where N equals the individual's age in years at his or her last birthday. The reader is referred to Chapter 2 for additional discussion of this topic.

Before an individual is permitted to work in a restricted area he or she must provide a record of previous employment history involving radiation exposure. The purpose of this record is to allow the licensee to calculate the accumulated radiation dose up to the present time to make certain that excess exposure to radiation will not be acquired during the new employment.

An *unrestricted area* is one to which access is not controlled by the licensee for the purpose of protecting individuals from exposure to radiation and radioactive material. There are limits placed on the maximum concentration of airborne radioactivity permissible in the work environment exposed to the general public, i.e., unrestricted area. The maximum permissible concentration (MPC) of a particular radionuclide is that concentration in μCi/ml to which an individual may be continuously exposed for a finite length of time and not exceed the maximum permissible radiation dose allowed for the whole body or a specified critical organ. MPC values calculated for a restricted area are based on exposure 40 hr/wk for 50 wk/yr, and a whole body MPD of 5 rem/yr. MPC values for an unrestricted area are based on continuous exposure 168 hr/wk for 52 wk/yr and a whole body MPD of 0.5 rem/yr. MPC values for several radionuclides used routinely in nuclear medicine are shown in Table 18–2. From a practical standpoint, the MPC values of greatest concern in nuclear medicine are those for radioxenon gas. Detailed discussions regarding radioxenon concentrations can be found in Chapter 10.

Airborne concentrations of radionuclides can be measured with a specially designed and calibrated air sampling monitor or by obtaining a "grab sample" of air from specified areas of a room with an evacuated vial of known volume that is subsequently counted in a calibrated scintillation counter. In accordance with 10 CFR 20.103, the room air-handling system, exhaust hoods, and various traps to remove airborne radioactivity should be designed to maintain contamination levels below 25 percent of the MPC in a restricted area.

Regarding the use of radiation in an unrestricted area, no licensee may create radiation levels that are in excess of 2 mrem in any 1 hour or that could result in an individual receiving a dose in excess of 100 mrem in any 7 consecutive days if the individual were continuously present (10 CFR 20.105b). This regulation has special significance regarding radiation exposure to individuals from patients being treated with a radiation source.

There are three groups of individuals that are likely to be exposed to a treated pa-

TABLE 18–2. MAXIMUM PERMISSIBLE CONCENTRATIONS IN AIR AND WATER FOR SEVERAL RADIONUCLIDES IMPORTANT TO NUCLEAR MEDICINE

	MPC (μCi/ml)			
	Restricted Area		*Unrestricted Area*	
Radionuclide	*Air*	*Water*	*Air*	*Water*
H-3[a]	5×10^{-6}	1×10^{-1}	2×10^{-7}	3×10^{-3}
I-125[a]	5×10^{-9}	4×10^{-5}	8×10^{-11}	2×10^{-7}
I-131[a]	9×10^{-9}	6×10^{-5}	1×10^{-10}	3×10^{-7}
Ra-226[a]	3×10^{-11}	4×10^{-7}	3×10^{-12}	3×10^{-8}
Tc-99m[a]	4×10^{-5}	2×10^{-1}	1×10^{-6}	6×10^{-3}
Xe-127[b]	1×10^{-6}	—	3×10^{-8}	—
Xe-133[a]	1×10^{-5}	—	3×10^{-7}	—

[a]From 10 CFR 20, Appendix B.
[b]From George DL: Permissible concentration in air of xenon-127: Concise communication. J Nucl Med 19:105, 1978.

tient, namely, nurses, immediate family members, and patients in adjacent rooms. Under specific radiation safety procedures referenced in a license, nurses and visitors may enter the restricted area of an implant therapy patient. For nurses and family members the regulation limits contact time to 50 hours, i.e., 100 mrem/2mR/hr.* Because adjacent patients cannot limit their exposure time, the exposure rate must be reduced below 2 mR/hr for these individuals. Adjacent patients may be expected to be exposed continuously for 7 consecutive days (168 hours). The maximum exposure rate for an adjacent patient may thus be 0.6 mR/hr, i.e, 100 mrem/168 hr. One should be aware, however, that such individuals are not radiation workers and that their total-body exposure must not exceed 500 mrem/yr according to 10 CFR 20.105 (a).

Patients with radiation sources may have exposure levels in excess of 2 mR/hr. Under these circumstances the contact time for nurses and visitors must be limited so that no more than 2 mR exposure is received in any 1 hour. The time of visitation may be extended, however, if the inverse square law is applied. Consider the following example.

Problem:

A survey meter reading at the bedside (1 m away) of a patient treated with I-131 is 15 mR/hr. What length of time can a visitor or a nurse safely remain at the bedside of the patient?

Solution:

$$15 \text{ mR}/60 \text{ min} = 2 \text{ mR}/x \text{ min}$$
$$x = 8 \text{ min (out of every hr at 1 m)}$$

If this were the case, the visitor would be required to leave for 52 minutes but may return for 8 minutes more during the next hour, etc. A visitor who maintains a 2-m distance from the patient, however, would be allowed to remain for 32 minutes according to the inverse square law. If the radioactive source is being metabolized and excreted from the patient, then the radiation exposure will decrease proportionally, and subsequent visitation times could be lengthened after new survey measurements.

The limits on the release of radioactive waste into effluents to unrestricted areas (sewers and atmosphere) are discussed in Chapter 5. One should note that excreta from individuals undergoing medical diagnosis or therapy with radioactive materials is exempt from any regulations in 10 CFR 20 and may be disposed of through the usual sewer systems.

Precautionary Measures

Personnel Monitoring. Personnel-monitoring equipment, e.g., film badges, pocket dosimeters, ring badges, designed for measuring radiation doses shall be worn by individuals who (1) enter a restricted area and will likely receive a dose in any calendar quarter in excess of 25 percent of the total occupational dose (MPD) given previously, (2) are under 18 years of age and who enter a restricted area and are likely to receive a dose in any calendar quarter in excess of 5 percent of the MPD, or (3) enter a high-radiation area.

Radiation Areas, Caution Signs, and Labels. There are basic signs, symbols, and labels used to warn individuals that radiation is present in a container, work area, or room. In general all signs and labels bear the radiation symbol shown in Figure 18–2. It is a three-bladed design in a magenta or purple color on a yellow background. The signs used are as follows:

1. *Caution: Radiation Area* is a sign displayed at a radiation area that is producing radiation levels such that the body could receive from 5.0 mrem to 100 mrem in any 1 hour or 100 mrem in 5 consecutive days.
2. *Caution: High Radiation Area* is a sign displayed in a high-radiation area that

---

*Note: 1 mR/hr = 1 mrem/hr for x- and gamma radiation

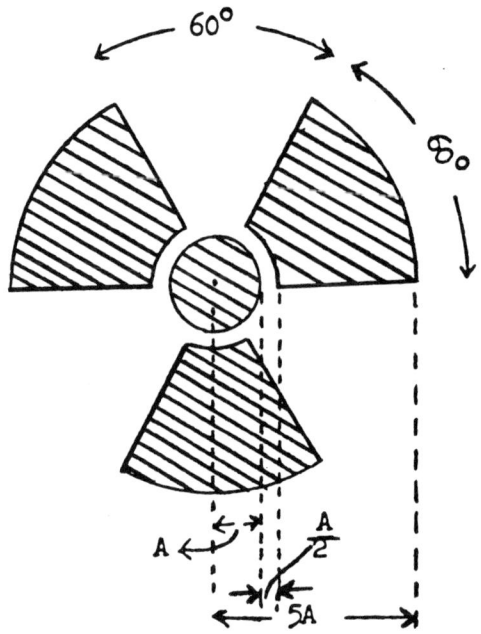

Figure 18-2. Standard radiation symbol. The cross-hatched area is magenta or purple; the background is yellow. (From 10 CFR 20.203.)

is producing radiation levels in excess of 100 mrem in 1 hour. High-radiation areas must be monitored and have controlled access.

3. *Caution: Radioactive Materials* is a sign displayed wherever licensed material is stored that contains radioactive material in amounts exceeding ten times the quantities specified in 10 CFR 20, Appendix C. A summary of Appendix C radionuclides used in nuclear medicine is shown in Table 18-3. Each container of radioactive material shall bear a label displaying the radiation symbol and the words *Caution: Radioactive Material* unless it does not contain licensed material greater than the quantities listed in Appendix C, 10 CFR 20, or greater than the applicable concentrations listed in Appendix B, Table I, Column 2, 10 CFR 20 (Table 18-2, this chapter, Restricted Area–Water).

When an empty uncontaminated container is disposed of into an unrestricted area, i.e., regular trash, the radiation symbol and words should be removed or defaced to indicate that it no longer contains radioactive material.

Wipe Tests

Wipe tests for the detection of removable radioactive contamination are required for several areas in nuclear medicine and nuclear pharmacy practice. These areas and the maximum permissible limits of radioactive contamination are summarized in Table 18-4 and are discussed in the following section.

Receipt of Radioactive Material

The NRC regulations found in 10 CFR 20.205 describe the types and quantities of radioactive material that must be monitored by a wipetest upon receipt. In summary, the following must be monitored in nuclear medicine: items in liquid form (except Mo/Tc generators), items with half-lives greater than or equal to 30 days, and items containing greater than 100 mCi. Specific items requiring monitoring in nuclear medicine are 100 mCi I-131 and Tc-99m (instant only); 10 mCi of I-125,

TABLE 18-3. SUMMARY LIST OF REACTOR-PRODUCED RADIONUCLIDES USED IN NUCLEAR MEDICINE THAT APPEAR IN APPENDIX C, 10 CFR 20

Radionuclides	Microcuries
Cr-51	1000
Co-58	10
I-125	1
I-131	1
Mo-99	100
P-32	10
Se-75	10
Tc-99m	100
Tc-99	10
Tl-201	100
Xe-133	100

TABLE 18-4. WIPE TESTS FOR CONTAMINATION CONTROL OF RADIOACTIVE MATERIAL

Contamination Area: External Surface	Maximum Permissible Limits
Packages received (10 CFR 20.205)	0.01 μCi (22,000 dpm)/100 cm^2
Packages to be shipped (49 CFR 173.443)	0.001 μCi (2,200 dpm)/100 cm^2 (beta-gamma)
	220 dpm/100 cm^2 (alpha)
Work areas[a] (Regulatory Guide 10.8, Appendix I)	200 dpm/100 cm^2
Sealed sources, > 100 μCi; $T_{1/2}$ > 30 days (10 CFR 35.59) every 6 months	0.005 μCi

[a]The limit stated for work areas is only a guide and not a hard and fast regulation. The stated limit is quite stringent, and one may submit a more "practical" limit in the license application to the NRC or Agreement State Agency.

H-3, C-14, and S-35; and 1 mCi Yb-169 and Se-75. These items must be monitored for external contamination within 3 hours of receipt during normal working hours and within 18 hours if received after normal working hours. The procedure one should follow is to wipe the entire external surface of the package with an absorbant paper and count in a scintillation counter. External surface contamination should not exceed 0.01 μCi per 100 cm^2 of surface. The sample count is compared with a standard count of the particular radionuclide to determine whether the limit is exceeded. A standard can be prepared by diluting 10 μCi of the particular radionuclide to 1000 ml in a volumetric flask. Remove 1 ml (0.01 μCi) and count in a scintillation counter at least 10,000 counts. Express this in net counts per minute, and use the value to compare with sample counts from package wipe tests.

In addition to wipetests, radioactive packages should be monitored for external radiation levels using a calibrated Geiger–Müller survey meter. Packages that should be monitored are those labeled with the diamond-shaped Department of Transportation (DOT) Radioactive White-I, Yellow-II, or Yellow-III labels. If no DOT label is present or if the package contains a WHITE-I label with only radioimmunoassay materials for in vitro use, it need not be surveyed. Other packages should be surveyed at 1 m away from the package surface and at the package surface. No package shall exceed 200 mR/hr at the surface nor 10 mR/hr at 1 m. The reading at 1 m is known as the transport index (TI). The TI measurement is not required for White-I-labeled packages. The limits for the various DOT labeled packages are listed in Table 18-5. Figure 18-3 illustrates the DOT labels.

Once packages are monitored and surveyed, they can be opened. The quantities appearing on the packing slip should match those received. It is also useful to radioassay vials to ascertain that they contain the correct amount of activity. One should note that 10 CFR 20.205 (d) requires that procedures be established and maintained for safely opening packages of licensed material after receipt.

If excessive radiation levels, surface contaminations, or shortages are found, one must notify the final delivering carrier, and by telephone and telegraph the regional office of the NRC.

Transport of Radioactive Material

For the most part the regulations in this section apply to pharmaceutical manufacturers and nuclear pharmacies that ship radiopharmaceuticals to hospital clinics. Requirements for packaging and transportation of radioactive material are described in DOT regulations 49 CFR, Parts 100 to

TABLE 18-5. LABELING AND RADIATION EXPOSURE LIMITS FOR RADIOACTIVE PACKAGES

Label Required	Limits of Radiation Exposure from the Package	
	TI[a]	At Package Surface
White-I	Not applicable	Less than or equal to 0.5 mR/hr
Yellow-II	Less than 1.0 mR/hr	Greater than 0.5 mR/hr and less than or equal to 50 mR/hr
Yellow-III	Greater than 1.0 mR/hr	Greater than 50 mR/hr

Note: No package shall exceed 200 mR/hr at the package surface nor 10 mR/hr at 1 m.
[a]Transport Index, which is the radiation level in mR/hr at 1 m from the package surface

199, and in an NRC adapted version in 10 CFR 71 and are summarized in a DOT publication.[5] It is worth noting that agreement states reference only DOT and not 10 CFR 71. Specifically, 10 CFR 71.5 states that "each licensee who transports licensed material outside of the confines of its plant or other place of use, or who delivers licensed material to a carrier for transport, shall comply with the applicable requirements of the regulations appropriate to the mode of transport of DOT in 49 CFR Parts 170-189," particularly in the following areas:

1. Packaging: 49 CFR 173, Subparts A and B, and 173.401 through 173.478
2. Marking and labeling: 49 CFR Part 172, Subpart D, and 172.400 through 172.407 and 172.436 through 172.440
3. Placarding: 49 CFR Part 172.500 through 172.519 and 172.556 and Appendices B and C
4. Monitoring: 49 CFR Part 172, Subpart C
5. Accident reporting: 49 CFR Part 171.15 and 171.16
6. Shipping papers: 49 CFR Part 172, Subpart C

DOT requirements do not apply when radiopharmaceuticals are being transported by a physician for his or her medical practice as outlined in Part 71.9.

For purposes of transportation, radio-

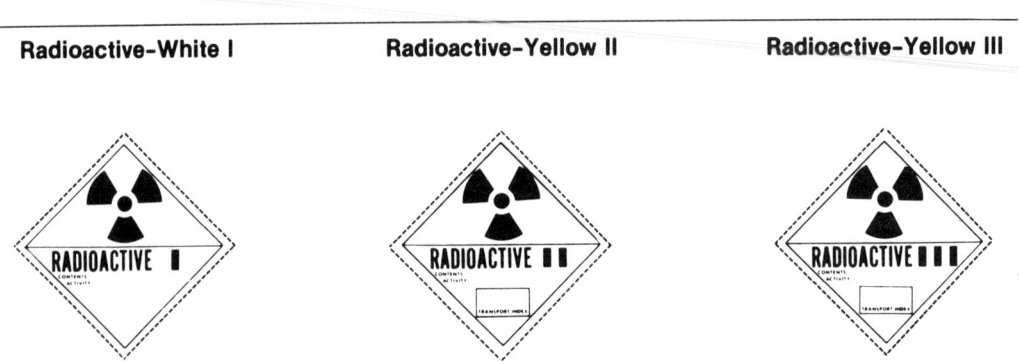

Figure 18-3. DOT labels for radioactive material packages. For all labels, vertical bars on each label are in red. Each label is diamond shaped, 4 inches on each side, and has a black solid-line border one-fourth inch from the edge. The background color of the upper half (within the black line) is white for the *I* label and yellow for the *II* and *III* labels. (From A Review of the Department of Transportation (DOT) Regulations for Transportation of Radioactive Materials, 1983.[5])

active materials are defined as those materials that spontaneously emit ionizing radiation and have a specific activity in excess of 0.002 µCi/g of material. All materials are to some degree radioactive. The demarcation of 0.002 µCi/g allows a distinction between materials not normally considered radioactive and those that are regulated as radioactive in transportation.

Packaging Requirements. Packaging requirements for a radioactive shipment are determined by the form, type, and quantity of radionuclide being shipped.

The two forms of radionuclide are special form and normal form. Special-form radioactive material is material that may present a direct radiation hazard if released from the package but little hazard resulting from contamination because of it being in a nondispersible solid form or sealed in a durable capsule. Special-form materials are much less likely to spread contamination in the event of package failure. The regulations therefore generally allow substantially larger quantities of such materials to be placed in a given package than when the materials are in normal form. Normal-form radioactive materials may be solid, liquid, or gaseous and include any material that has not been qualified as special form. Radiopharmaceuticals are normal-form materials.

There are four types of packages: "type A," "type B," "excepted," and "strong, tight." Package specifications are described in 49 CFR Parts 173.401 through 173.478. Radiopharmaceuticals are generally shipped from the supplier (pharmaceutical manufacturer or nuclear pharmacy) to the hospital in type A packaging.

The quantity of a particular type of radionuclide that can be shipped in a type A package is listed in Table 18–6. Every radio-

TABLE 18-6. TYPE A PACKAGE QUANTITY LIMITS FOR RADIONUCLIDES USED IN NUCLEAR MEDICINE

Radionuclide	Activity in Curies		
	A_1 (Special Form)	A_2 (Normal Form)	Limited Shipment Quantity[a]
Co-57	90	90	0.009
Co-58	20	20	0.002
Cr-51	600	600	0.060
Cs-137	30	10	0.001
Fe-59	10	10	0.001
Ga-67	100	100	0.010
I-123	50	50	0.005
I-125	1000	70	0.007
I-131	40	10	0.001
In-111	30	25	0.0025
Mo-99	100	20	0.002
P-32	30	30	0.003
Se-75	40	40	0.004
Tc-99m	100	100	0.010
Tc-99	1000	25	0.0025
Tl-201	200	200	0.020
Xe-127 (uncompressed)	70	70	0.070
Xe-133 (uncompressed)	1000	1000	0.100
Yb-169	70	70	0.007

[a]Solids and liquids, $A_2 \times 10^{-4}$; gases, $A_2 \times 10^{-3}$. (From 49 CFR 173.421.)
(From 49 CFR 173.435.)

nuclide is now assigned an A_1 and an A_2 value. The A_1 and A_2 system now replaces the transport group system that was used previously for limitations on radioactive materials shipped in normal form. The A_1 and A_2 values are simply the maximum activity (in curies) of that radionuclide that may be transported in a type A package.

Quantities exceeding type A package limits require type B packaging. The A_1 values are for radionuclides in special form and A_2 values for radionuclides in normal form.

Certain quantities of radioactive material are excepted from some of the DOT requirements that apply to type A packages. These exceptions include not having to provide specification packaging, shipping papers, certification, marking, or labeling. There are a number of conditions, however, that must be met as outlined in 49 CFR 173.421. They are as follows:

1. Not to exceed limited shipment quantities (list in Table 18-6)
2. Must be packed in strong, tight packages that will not leak any radioactive material during normal transport conditions
3. The radiation level at any point on the external surface of the package cannot exceed 0.5 mR/hr
4. The external surface of package must be free of significant removable contamination (Table 18-4)
5. The outside of the inner packaging, or if there is no inner packaging, the outside of the packaging itself bears the marking *radioactive*
6. A description of the contents on a document that is in or on the package or forwarded with it. The document must include the name of the consignee or consignor and the statement, "this package conforms to the conditions and limitations specified in 49 CFR 173.421 for excepted radioactive material, limited quantity, n.o.s., UN 2910."

Transport Index. The TI is the highest dose rate at 1 m away from any accessible exterior surface of a package of radioactive material. The TI limits are listed in Table 18-5.

The transport index system is designed to control the radiation level resulting from accumulations of multiple numbers of packages in the transportation environment. The regulations require that the carrier shall maintain certain prescribed separation distances between radioactive material packages and other areas occupied by persons and photographic film (because film may be fogged by radiation). No package offered for transport may have a TI exceeding 10. The TI per package limit is decreased, however, to 3 for packages carried aboard passenger-carrying aircraft. TI's of 10 and 3 are based on standards for limiting personnel exposure and to prevent fogging of fast photographic film. The total of the TI of all packages in any single transport vehicle or storage location generally may not exceed 50. The transport index system provides control by the carrier over the radiation exposures to personnel handling the packages and to casually exposed persons in the vicinity of accumulations of packages.

Warning Labels. Each package of radioactive material, unless excepted, must be labeled on two opposite sides with a distinctive warning label. Each of the three label types bears the unique trefoil symbol (Fig. 18-3) recommended by the International Commission on Radiation Protection (ICRP) in 1956. The labels alert persons that the package contains radioactive materials and that the package may require special handling. A label with an all-white background color indicates that the external radiation level is low and no special handling is required. If the upper half of the label is yellow, this signifies more precaution and higher radiation levels. Radiation level limits for these labels are listed in Table 18-5.

The following items must be entered in the blank spaces on the warning label:

1. Contents: The name of the radionuclide or its appropriate symbol, e.g., Molybdenum-99 or ^{99}Mo

2. Activity: Limits of activity shall be expressed in units of curie, millicurie, microcurie, or their abbreviations Ci, mCi, or µCi, respectively.
3. TI: the value measured with an appropriate survey meter, preferably an ionization chamber, at 1 m from the external surface rounded up to the next highest tenth mR/hr (not required for White-I labels).

Placarding. The shipper of radioactive material packages, by rail or highway, must apply the RADIOACTIVE placard to the transport vehicle if any package on board bears a Radioactive Yellow-III label. The format for the placard is shown in Figure 18-4. The placard must appear on four sides of the vehicle.

Monitoring. Any package of radioactive material offered for transportation must be wipetested for removable contamination on its external surface in accordance with 49 CFR 173.443. The limits are shown in Table 18-4.

Other Package Requirements. There are several additional marking requirements for radioactive material packages. A package in excess of 110 pounds must have its gross weight marked on the outside of the package; the words *Type A* or *Type B* when appropriate must be lettered (1/2 inch high) on the outside of the package; and exported packages must be marked *USA*. The proper shipping name and identification number must also appear on the outside of the package. For radiopharmaceuticals this would appear as "RADIOACTIVE MATERIAL, n.o.s., UN 2982." Additionally, liquid radioactive material must be packaged with enough absorbant material to absorb at least twice the volume of liquid. Finally, the outside of each package must contain a security seal that is not readily breakable and that will give evidence that the package has not been illicitly opened.

Shipping Papers. Shipping papers must be included with transported radioactive material as described in 49 CFR 172.200 through 172.204. The information required on the shipping papers is important to the carrier and consignee. It also is of value to emergency response personnel in the event of an accident. Among the information required are the shipping name and identification number, radionuclides contained in the package, physical and chemical form, activity, category of RADIOACTIVE labels applied to the package, TI for radioactive Yellow-II or -III packages, and other identification markings shown on the package.

Accident Reporting. According to 49 CFR 171.15 and 171.16, the carrier of radioactive material must assure that DOT and the shipper will be notified in the event of fire, breakage, spillage, or suspected radioactive contamination involving the shipment. Carriers must also assure that vehicles, areas, or equipment in which radioactive material may have spilled are not placed in service

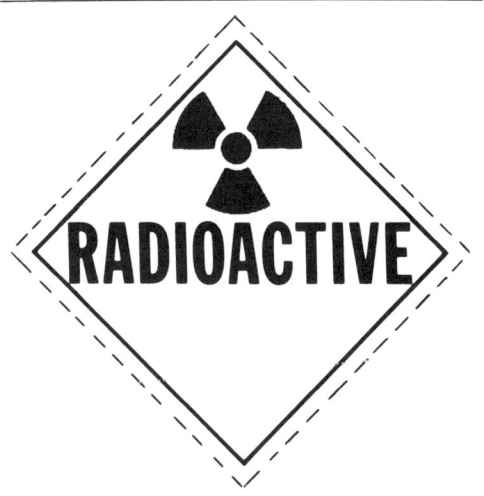

Figure 18-4. Radioactive placard used on transport vehicles (rail or highway) if any radioactive material package on board bears a Radioactive Yellow-III label. The background color for the black trefoil in the upper half of this 12- by 12-inch placard is yellow.

again until they have been surveyed and decontaminated.

Summary of Radioactive Material Shipment. Materials that contain less than the limited quantities shown in Table 18-6 and that have less than 0.5 mR/hr at the surface with no significant external contamination may be shipped in a strong, tight package that will prevent leakage during normal shipment. No outer label is required, but the inner container must be labeled RADIOACTIVE.

Materials that contain more than the limited quantity but no more than the A_2 quantity may be shipped in a type A package. A surface wipetest must be performed to ensure no significant removable contamination and the package surveyed at the surface and at 1 m to determine the TI. The package is labeled with two warning labels, White-I or Yellow-II or -III, one each on opposite sides. The labels are filled in with the name or symbol of the radionuclide, its activity, and the TI. The package must have a security seal and be accompanied by shipping papers.

Empty, reuseable packages such as those used to deliver radiopharmaceutical doses from a nuclear pharmacy to a hospital should be surveyed inside and out before they are returned to the shipper and have any external RADIOACTIVE signs removed if no activity is present.

Monitoring Procedures for Work Areas

To help control the extent of contamination with radioactive material and to help maintain a safe working environment, routine radiation contamination surveys are essential. This will provide some assurance that workers are not being exposed unnecessarily to high doses of radiation because of inadequately shielded sources or poor working habits. Requirements for area surveys and wipe tests are listed in 10 CFR 35.70 as follows:

1. Survey, using a survey instrument capable of detecting 0.1 mR/hr
    A. At the end of each day: All areas where radiopharmaceuticals are prepared or administered
    B. Once each week: All areas where radiopharmaceuticals or radiopharmaceutical waste is stored
2. Notify the Radiation Safety Officer if the established dose rate trigger level is exceeded in the survey
    Note: An acceptable trigger level is 2 mR/hr at 30 cm
3. Wipe test, using a procedure capable of detecting 2000 disintegrations per minute
    A. Once each week: All areas where radiopharmaceuticals are routinely prepared, administered, or stored
4. Notify the Radiation Safety Officer if the established removable contamination trigger level is exceeded
    Note: An acceptable trigger level is 500 dpm/100 cm^2
5. A record of each survey shall be retained for 2 years and must include the survey date, a plan of each area surveyed, the trigger level established for each area, the detected dose rate at several points in each area expressed in millirem per hour of the removable contamination in each area expressed in disintegrations per minute per 100 square centimeters, the instrument used to make the survey or analyze the samples, and the initials of the individual who performed the survey

POSTING REQUIREMENTS

In accordance with 10 CFR 19.11, a licensee shall post current copies of the following documents to employees: the regulations in 10 CFR Part 19, Notices, Instructions, and Reports to Workers; inspections and 10 CFR Part 20, Standards for Protection Against Radiation; the license, license conditions, and appropriate documents and amendments; the operating procedures applicable to licensed activities; and any notice of violation involving radiologic

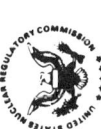

Figure 18-5. NRC-3 Form: Notice to Employees.

working conditions and the response from the licensee.

If posting of these documents is not practicable, the licensee may post a notice that describes the document and states where it may be examined. Additionally, each licensee shall post form NRC-3, *Notice to Employees*, or a similar form required by agreement states. This form (Fig. 18-5) should be posted at locations that permit employees to observe a copy on the way to or from their place of work.

RECORDS

Written records are required for a number of activities involving the use of radioactive material. Some of these records must be kept available for reference and inspection by the NRC for a number of years. Records do accumulate, however, and one may wish to dispose of those that are outdated and have limited usefulness.

Those records that must be kept for definite time periods are as follows:

1. Receipt of radioactive material, from disposal of material: 2 years
2. Radiopharmaceutical dosage assays: 2 years
3. Molybdenum-99 breakthrough assay: 2 years
4. Dose calibrator quality control tests: 2 years
5. Survey instrument calibration: 2 years
6. Sealed source 6 month leak tests: 5 years
7. Sealed source storage area quarterly surveys: 2 years
8. Sealed source quarterly inventory: 5 years

REFERENCES

1. Swanson DP, Lieto RP: The submission of IND applications for radiopharmaceutical research: When and why. J Nucl Med 25:714, 1984
2. Guide for the Preparation of Applications for Medical Programs: Draft Regulatory Guide 10.8, US NRC, Washington, DC, August 1985
3. Nuclear Pharmacy Guideline: Criteria for determining when to register as a drug establishment. Division of Drug Labeling Compliance (HFN-310), Center for Drugs and Biologics, FDA, Washington, DC, May 1984
4. Guide for the Preparation of Applications for Nuclear Pharmacy Licenses, Appendix A: US NRC, August 1985
5. A Review of the Department of Transportation (DOT) Regulations of Transportation of Radioactive Materials: US DOT, Washington, DC, 1983

Index

Page numbers followed by t refer to tables.

Abscess
  formation, 392
  identification, radionuclide imaging
    Ga-67, 402
    In-111 leukocytes, 406
Accelerators, 55
Accuracy of dose calibrators, 137
ACD
  in platelet labeling, 398
  in red cell labeling, 413
Active transport
  brain uptake of drugs, 149, 150
  drug transport from CSF, 162
  kidney excretion of drugs, 317
  myocardial uptake of drugs, 211
  thyroid uptake of drugs, 181
Activity. *See* Radioactivity
Adrenal gland imaging
  adrenal cortex, 459
  adrenal medulla, 460
  radiopharmaceuticals, development, 459, 460
Aerosols, radioactive
  delivery systems, 259
  lung ventilation imaging, 258
Agreement states, list of, 475
ALARA, 6
Albumin, aggregated, I-131, 238
Albumin, aggregated, Tc-99m
  biodistribution, 241
  dosage, 263
  kits, lung imaging, 238, 240
  lung clearance and metabolism, 245
  lung imaging, 263
  mechanism of localization, 242
  particle hardness, 244
  particle size and number, 239, 242
  particle toxicity, 246
  preparation, 239
  radiation dose, 10
Albumin, Cr-51
  gastrointestinal protein loss, 451
Albumin, I-125
  dosage forms, 420
  labeling site, protein molecules, 420
  plasma volume measurement, 415
  preparation, 420
  properties, 420
  quality control, 420
Albumin, I-131
  brain imaging, 149, 151
  cisternography, 159, 161
  liver studies, 275
Albumin microspheres, Tc-99m
  biodistribution, 241
  dosage, 10, 263
  kit, 239, 240
  lung clearance and metabolism, 245
  lung imaging, 263
  mechanism of localization, 242
  particle hardness, 244
  particle size and number, 239, 242
  preparation, 239
  radiation dose, 10
Albumin, Tc-99m
  biologic properties, 217
  cisternography, 159
  myocardial blood pool imaging, 217
  dosage, 10
  radiation dose, 10
Albumin, Tc-99m, electrolytic, 217
Alpha decay, 26
Alpha particles, 34
Aluminum ion
  assay for, in generators, 65

Aluminum ion *(cont.)*
    chelation by EDTA, 81
    effect on Tc-99m sulfur colloid, 281
Annihilation reaction, 23
Antibodies, monoclonal
    development, 465–469
    radiolabeling, 467
    structure, 467
Antigen, 137
ARDS, 268
Artificial cerebrospinal fluid, preparation, 163
Ascorbic acid
    antioxidant in Tc-99m kits, 88
    reaction with free-radicals, 88
    stabilizer in bone kits, 360
Aseptic techniques in nuclear pharmacy, 106
Atoms. *See* Nuclides

Becquerel
    discovery of radioactivity, 28
    unit of radioactivity, defined, 29
BET, 135
Beta decay. *See* Radioactive decay
Beta particles
    mass–energy equivalence, 18
    interactions with matter, 35
Binding energy
    electron shell, 14
    nuclear, 18, 19
Biological half-life, 76
Blood-brain barrier, 147, 148, 150
Blood volume measurement
    Cr-51 red cell labeling, 412
    principle, 412, 413
Bolton–Hunter reagent, 93
Bonding, in radiopharmaceuticals, 80, 81
Bone
    clinical evaluation, 366
    composition, 351
    formation, 352, 353
    physiologic anatomy, 351
    surface area, 353
Bone imaging
    indications, 366
    procedure, 367
    scan interpretation, 371
Bone imaging kits, formulation, 356
Bone imaging radiopharmaceuticals
    altered biodistribution, 365
    development, 353
Bone marrow
    colloid distribution, 296
    imaging, radiopharmaceuticals used, 296
    physiologic anatomy, 295
Bone marrow imaging
    indications, 308
    procedure, 309
    radiopharmaceuticals, 309
    scan interpretation, 310
Bone scans
    absent kidney, 370
    avascular hip necrosis, 373

inflammatory disease, 374
    metastatic prostate carcinoma, 371, 372
    normal, pediatric, 368, 369
    osteomyelitis, 373
    SPECT, 375
Brachytherapy, 478
Brain
    arterial circulation, 148
    blood-brain barrier, 147, 148, 150
    blood perfusion, 147
    clinical evaluation, 164
    imaging study, 148
    radiopharmaceuticals, 149, 167
        development, 149
        mechanisms of localization, 154
Brain death, 174
Brain imaging
    clinical procedures, 164
    delayed images, 165
    flow studies, 165
Brain scans
    brain death, 174
    cerebrovascular accident, 167, 168
    meningioma, 169, 170

Calcium-45, -47, in bone imaging, 354
Carbon isotopes, 20t
Carbon-11
    decay scheme, 23
    nuclear properties, 27
Carbon-11 deoxyglucose, 147, 151, 157
Carbon-14 deoxyglucose, 151, 156, 157
Cardiac shunt study, 222
Carrier, chemical
    defined, 33
    effect on Tc-99m labeling, 68, 69
Cerebrospinal fluid (CSF)
    artificial, composition, 163
    clinical evaluation, 164
    formation, 158
    pressure, 158
    volume, 158
Cerebrovascular accident, 168
Cesium-129, myocardial imaging, 212
Chelate, defined, 81
Chemical purity, 65, 134
Chloramine-T, in radioiodination, 92
Cholecystitis, 308, 309
Chromatography. *See also* Radiochemical purity
    artifacts, 131
    gel and ion exchange, 130–132
    ITLC, 126
    miniaturized, Tc-99m radiopharmaceuticals, 129, 130
    paper, 126
    radiochromatogram analysis, 128
    techniques and pitfalls, 129
Chromic phosphate. *See* Phosphorus-32
Chromium-51
    decay scheme, 24
    nuclear properties, 27
Chromium-51 albumin. *See* Albumin, Cr-51

Chromium-51 chromic chloride
  gastrointestinal protein loss, 451
Chromium-51 red blood cells
  cohort and random labeling, 421
  dosage, 10
  half-life, 423
  in vivo crossmatch, 422
  labeling technique, 412–414
  mean life, 423
  radiation dose, 10, 423
Cisternogram
  NPH, 173
  normal study, 172
  CNS atrophy, 174
Cisternography. See also CSF scans
  agents, development, 159
  drug transport mechanisms, 161, 162
  overpressure, 163
    methods, 163
    artificial CSF, 163
  precautions, 161
    limulus test, 162
    pyrogen reactions, 162
  radiopharmaceuticals, 160
Clearance, renal, 318
Clinical evaluation
  bone, 366
  brain, 164
  cerebrospinal fluid, 164
  genitourinary system, 337
  heart, 222
  hepatobiliary system, 300
  kidney, 337
  lung, 259
  thyroid, 198
CNS atrophy, 174
Cobalt-57, -58
  nuclear properties, 27
  production, 54
Cobalt–57, –58, –60 cyanocobalamin
  chemical structure, 428
  dosage, 425
  preparation and properties, 427
  radiation dose, 8, 428
  Schilling test, 425, 426
Collimators, gamma camera, 45
Compartment, defined, 411
Competitive binding assay, 435
Complexing agents
  chemical structure, 87
  influence on Tc-99m hydrolysis, 89
  function in Tc-99m kits, 86
Compton scatter, 36, 37
Crohn's disease, 452
CSF. *See* Cerebrospinal fluid
CSF rhinorrhea, 176
CSF scans
  CNS atrophy, 174
  CSF rhinorrhea, 176
    normal study, 175
    CSF leak, 176
  normal cisternogram, 172
  normal pressure hydrocephalus (NPH), 173

Curie, 29, 47
Cyanocobalamin. *See also* Cobalt-57, -58, -60
    cyanocobalamin
  metabolism, 423–425
  test for deficiency, 423
    Schilling test, 425
    dual isotope test, 426
Cyclotrons, 55

Dacryocystography, 9, 453, 454
Decay constant
  defined, 29
  related to half-life, 30
Decay schemes, 22
  described, 22
  radionuclide
    carbon-11, 23
    chromium-51, 24
    gallium-67, 383
    indium-111, 389
    iodine-123, 188
    iodine-125, 187
    iodine-131, 186
    mercury-203, 22, 25
    molybdenum-99, 25, 60, 81
    phosphorus-32, 22
    radium-226, 26
    technetium-99m, 152
Decay tables
  construction, 32
  postcalibration decay factors, 33
  precalibration decay factors, 33
  uses in radioactivity calculations, 32
Deoxyglucose, radiolabeled
  C-11, C-14, F-18, in brain studies, 151
  mechanism of localization, 156
  metabolism, 156
Dimercaptosuccinic acid. *See also* Technetium-99m
    succimer
  chemical structure, 87, 321
Disse's space, 274
DMSA. *See* Technetium-99m succimer
Dose calibrator
  accuracy determination, 136, 137
  calibration, 103
  geometry test, 142
  linearity test, 138
    decay method, 139
    shielding method, 140
  precision test, 138
  principle of operation, 39
  quality control, 135
  use in nuclear pharmacy, 103
Dosimetry, 56
DOT regulations, 493
Drug regulations, FDA, 473
DTPA. *See also* Technetium-99m pentetate;
    Indium-111 pentetate
  chemical structure, 87

EDTA
  aluminum chelate, Tc-99m sulfur colloid, 81

EDTA (cont.)
    calcium chelate, structure, 81
    chromium-51, GFR studies, 322
    gallium-67 chelate, 379
    ligand exchange with Tc-HIDA, 289
    stabilizer in Tc-99m sulfur colloid, 277
    use in Tc-99m red blood cell labeling, 218, 219
Effective half-life, 76
EHDP. See Technetium-99m etidronate
Einstein, 17
Ejection fraction, myocardial, 230
Electrolysis
    in radioiodinations, 93
    in technetium reduction, 82
Electron capture decay, 23
Elliott's B solution. See Cerebrospinal fluid, artificial, composition
Emergency procedures, radioactive spill, 119
Emission computed tomography
    camera studies, 4
    imaging technique, 5
Endotoxins, 134
Energy
    atomic, 14–18
        nuclear energy levels, 16
        orbital energy levels, 14
    beta particle energy spectrum, 21
    gamma ray, 35
    nuclear binding energy, 18
    related to mass, 17
Ethylenediamine tetraacetic acid. See EDTA
Extraction ratio, renal, 318
Eye, lacrimal gland imaging, 9, 453

FDA regulations. See also Regulatory control of radiopharmaceuticals, NRC
    drug regulations, historical development, 473
    IND, 474
    radiopharmaceuticals, 475, 476
Ferrokinetic studies, 429
    ferrous citrate Fe-59, 429
    iron metabolism, 429, 430
    iron utilization, 430
    plasma iron clearance, 429
    plasma iron turnover rate, 430
Fibrinogen. See Iodine-125 fibrinogen
Fission, 54
Fluorine-18
    bone imaging, 354
    mechanism of localization in bone, 79
    nuclear properties, 27
Fluorine-18 deoxyglucose, 147, 157
Fluorine-18 sodium fluoride, 354
Foreign labeling, 78
Food and Drug Administration. See also FDA regulations
    authority, compared with NRC, 476
    nuclear pharmacies, regulation, 487
    radiopharmaceuticals regulations, 476

Free radicals, Tc-99m radiopharmaceuticals degradation, 8

Gallate, 382
Gallbladder. See Hepatobiliary system, clinical evaluation
Gallium-67
    chemistry, 379
    decay scheme, 383
    dosage forms, 386
    nuclear properties, 27
    radiopharmaceuticals, development, 380
    tissue distribution, effect of scandium, 383
Gallium-72, bone studies, 354
Gallium citrate, Ga-67
    altered biodistribution, effect of drugs, 387
    binding to transferrin, 382
    biodistribution, 382, 384, 385
    chemical state in vitro, effect of pH and citrate concentration, 382
    chemical structure, 381
    dosage, 8, 401
    excretion, 384
    localization in normal, tumor, and abscess tissue, 384, 385
    production and properties, 381
    radiation dose, 8, 387
Gallium hydroxide, 382
Gallium-67 imaging
    indications, 401
    procedure, 401
    scan interpretation, 401
Gallium-67 scans
    lymphoma, 402
    normal scan, 403
    occult abscess, 404
    SPECT, 405
Gallium-68 radiopharmaceuticals, 386, 387
Gamma camera, 46
Gamma energy spectrum, 42
Gamma rays
    energy calculations, 35
    interactions with matter, 35–37
Gamma ray dose constant, $51t$
Gastric emptying studies
    geometric mean, 450
    procedures, 449, 450
    radiopharmaceuticals, 450
    rationale, 449
Gastroesophageal reflux studies
    indications, 445
    procedure, 445
    reflux index, 449
    study interpretation, 448
Gastrointestinal bleeding studies
    indications, 443
    procedure, 444
    radiopharmaceuticals, 444, 445
    scan interpretation

cecal carcinoma, Tc-RBC, 448
normal scan, Tc-SC, 446
sigmoid bleed, Tc-SC, 447
Gastrointestinal protein loss
Cr-51 albumin and chromic chloride, 451
rationale and procedure, 451
Geiger–Mueller detectors, principle of operation, 39
Geiger–Mueller monitor, use in nuclear pharmacy, 104
Geiger–Mueller survey meter
quality control, 143
use in nuclear pharmacy, 104
Gelatin stabilizer, Tc-sulfur colloid, 277, 280
General license, 476
Generators
disposal, 74
germanium-68/gallium-68, 386
molybdenum-99/technetium-99m
aluminum test, 65
commercial systems, 63
eluate radioassay, 64
elution efficiency, 72
expiration time of eluate, 67
mole fraction, technetium, 67, 68
moly-99 breakthrough, 65, 66
operation, 61
problems, 63
production, 60
quality control, 64–66
regulations for use in nuclear medicine, 478
technetium content in eluate, 67, 68
yield, 62, 72
secular equilibrium, 74
tantalum-193/gold-195m, 231
tin-113/indium-113m, 388
transient equilibrium, 70
types, 60t
yttrium-87/strontium-87m, 354
Generator kinetics. *See* Generator physics
Generator physics
equations, 70–74
secular equilibrium, 73, 74
transient equilibrium, 70–72
Genitourinary system, 315
clinical evaluation, 337
reflux, 341, 344
residual bladder urine, 339
VCUG, 341, 344
Gentisic acid
antioxidant in Tc-99m kits, 89
reaction with free-radicals, 89
stabilizer, bone kits, 360
Geometric mean, gastric emptying studies, 450
Geometry test, dose calibrators, 142
GFR. *See* Glomerular filtration rate
Glomerular filtration rate (GFR), 318, 327
Gluceptate. *See* Technetium-99m gluceptate
Glucoheptonate. *See* Technetium-99m gluceptate
Glucoheptonic acid, chemical structure, 321
Gold-195m, myocardial perfusion studies, 231

Gold-198 colloid
liver studies, 275, 276
lymph node scanning, 458
Grave's disease, 204

Half-life
biological, 75–76
calculation, 30
definition, 30
effective, 75–76
graphical determination, 30
ideal, for diagnostic imaging, 76
physical, 75–76
related to decay constant, 30
Half-value layer
calculation, 51
graphical determination, 52
radionuclides, 51t
related to shielding of Tc-99m and I-131, 98, 99
Heart
altered distribution of radiopharmaceuticals, 220
clinical evaluation, 222
electrolyte kinetics, 211
Heart imaging
cardiac shunt study, 222
infarct avid agents, 214
infarct imaging, 224, 225
perfusion agents, 212
perfusion imaging, 226
ejection fraction, 230
equilibrium technique, 231
first pass technique, 231
myocardial ischemia, 227
radionuclide angiogram, 232
radionuclide ventriculography, 230
physiologic considerations, 211
radionuclides used, 212t
Hemacytometer in particle analysis, 133
Henderson–Hasselbalch equation, 317
HEPA filters, laminar air flow hoods, 102
Hepatobiliary agents
biologic properties, 289
chemical structures, 288, 289
development, 286
excretion requirements, 289
mechanism of localization, 290
radiation dose, 291, 292
Hepatobiliary system, *clinical evaluation*, 300
Hepatobiliary system imaging
indications, 300
procedure, 300
radiopharmaceuticals, 286, 300
scan interpretation, 303
acute cholecystitis, 308, 309
normal study, 307
obstruction, 310, 311
Hepatocytes, 273, 275
Herpes encephalitis, brain scan, 170
High radiation area, signs, 491

HIPDM, I-123
  brain imaging, 151
  mechanism of localization, 157
Hippuran. See Iodine-131 o-iodohippurate
HMDP. See Technetium-99m oxidronate
Hoods
  exhaust, 101
  fume, 101
  laminar air flow, 101, 102
HSA. See Albumin entries
Hybridomas, 467
Hydrocephalus, 173
Hydrolyzed technetium, 89
Hydroxyapatite, 351, 352, 364
Hydroxymethylene diphosphonate. See Technetium-99m oxidronate
Hyperthyroidism, I-131 treatment, 203
Hypoxanthene-aminopterin-thymidine (HAT), 468

Imaging agents, diagnostic
  ideal properties, 75
  use in nuclear medicine, 2
Immunoglobulin. See Antibodies, monoclonal
IMP. See Iodine-123 iodoamphetamine
IND. See Investigational new drug
Indium chemistry, 379, 388
Indium-111
  agents, cisternography, 159, 160
  decay scheme, 309
  physical properties, 27, 389
  radiopharmaceuticals, development, 388
Indium-111 acetylacetone, 399
Indium-111 chloride
  abscess localization, 406
  preparation and properties, 390
Indium-111 leukocytes
  biodistribution, 396
  dosage, 405
  labeling efficiency, 395
  labeling mechanism, 397
  radiation dose, 396
  radiolabeling method, 394, 395
  viability, 395
Indium-111 leukocyte imaging
  compared to Ga-67 citrate, 397
  indications, 404
  procedure, 404
  scan interpretation, 406
    abscess localization, 406
    tissue distribution, 406
Indium-111 lymphocytes, radiation dose, risk factor, 397
Indium-111 oxine
  chemical structure, 393
  leukocyte labeling, 392, 395
  preparation and properties, 393
Indium-111 pentetate (DTPA)
  biodistribution, 329
  biological properties, 390
  chemical structure, 391

CSF studies, 167, 172–174
gastric emptying studies, 450
GFR measurements, 322
preparation, 390
quality control, 390
renal excretion mechanism, 329
stability, 329
Indium-111 platelets
  clinical use, 399
  labeling method, 398, 400
  radiation dose, 399
Indium-111 tropolone, 399
Indium-113m
  generator, 388
  nuclear properties, 27
  radiolabeled agents, 388
Infarct imaging, 224
Inflammation
  causes, 391
  detection, In-111 leukocytes, 404
Interactions of radiation with matter
  alpha particles, 34
  gamma rays, 35–37
  negatrons, 35
  positrons, 34
Internal conversion, 25
Intrinsic factor, 424, 426
Inulin, C-14, GFR studies, 322
Investigational new drug (IND)
  physician sponsored, 474
  procedures for, 474
In vitro tests, 435
In vivo crossmatch, red blood cells, 422
In vivo function agents
  ideal properties, 75
  use in nuclear medicine, 4
Iodide
  oxidation
    effect of pH, 90
    retardation by thiosulfate, 90
  Lugol's solution, 193
  saturated solution of potassium iodide (SSKI), 193
  solution chemistry, 90
  thyroid blocking dose, 193
Iodide, radioactive
  concentration in salivary, gastric, mammary, and sweat glands, 196
  daily turnover in body, 183
  development, for thyroid studies, 184
  dosage forms, 190
  distribution in body, 197
  handling methods, 190t
  metabolism, 192
  placental uptake, 196
  production and properties, 185
  radiation dose, 8, 197
  renal clearance, 192
  solution chemistry, 189
  solutions, stabilization, 190
  thyroid metabolism, 182
  urinary excretion, 193

Iodination reactions
  mechanism of, in protein labeling, 420
  methods, 91
Iodine monochloride
  production, 92
  radioiodinating agent, 92
Iodine-123
  decay scheme, 188
  impurities, comparison of production methods, 187
  production and physical properties, 27, 90, 186, 187, 188
  purity, 124, 187
  radiation dose, 8, 197
  thyroid imaging, 198, 201
Iodine-123 iodoamphetamine
  brain imaging, 151
  mechanism of localization, 157
Iodine-123 orthoiodohippuric acid, 325
Iodine-125
  decay scheme, 187
  measurement, effect of container configuration, 143
  production and physical properties, 27, 90, 185, 186
  radiation dose, 8, 197
  thyroid imaging, 198
Iodine-125 albumin. See Albumin, I-125
Iodine-125 fibrinogen
  detection of deep venous thrombosis, 454
  dosage, 454
  preparation, 455
  radiation dose, 8, 458
  radioiodination method, 93
Iodine-125 HSA. See Albumin, I-125
Iodine-131
  decay scheme, 186
  iodide capsule statistical analysis, 191
  measurement, effect of container configuration, 143
  production and properties, 27, 90, 185, 186
  radiation dose, 8, 197
  thyroid imaging, 198, 201
Iodine-131 albumin. See Albumin, I-131
Iodine-131 albumin, aggregated, 238
Iodine-131 albumin colloid, 276
Iodine-131 iodocholesterol
  chemical structure, 460
  dosage, 460
  production and properties, 459
  quality control, 459
  radiation dose, 460
  rationale for use, 79
Iodine-131 orthoiodohippuric acid
  altered biodistribution, 336
  biodistribution, 323
  chemical structure, 320, 322
  chromatography of, 323
  decomposition, 125, 323
  development of, 319
  ERPF measurements with, 324
  preparation and properties, 322
  protein binding, 323
  purity, 124, 323
  radiation dose, 9, 326
  radiochemical impurities, 323
  radioiodination method, 94
  renal excretion mechanism, 323
  renal excretion rate, 325
  renal extraction efficiency, 323
  renal function evaluation, 325
Iodine-131 iodopyracet
  chemical structure, 320
  kidney evaluation with, 319
Ionization chamber, 38
Iothalamic acid, I-131
  chemical structure, 320
  GFR measurement with, 322
Iothalamate sodium, I-125, -131
  biodistribution mechanism, 327
  GFR measurement with, 327
  preparation and properties, 327
Iron ascorbic acid complex. See Technetium-99m
Iron-59
  iron metabolism, 429
  production and properties, 27, 429
  radiation dose from, 431
Iron-59 ferrous citrate
  chemical structure, 429
  dosage, 429
  preparation and properties, 429
  radiation dose, 9, 431
Iron metabolism, 429
Iron utilization, 430
Isobars, 13
Isomers, 14
Isomeric transition, 24
Isotones, 14
Isotopes, 13
Isotope dilution analysis, 412
Isotopic labeling
  defined, 77
  radionuclides used in, 78t

Jaundice, effect on excretion of Tc-99m IDA compounds, 291
Joints, bone scanning, degenerative joint disease, 367
Joliot, Frederic and Irene Curie, 1

Kidney
  clearance, 318
  clinical evaluation, 337
  excretion
    mechanisms, 316
    Tc-hepatobiliary agents, 291, 311
  extraction ratio, 318
  physiologic anatomy, 315
  renal blood flow, 319
  thallium-201 uptake, 213
Kidney imaging
  indications, 337

Kidney imaging *(cont.)*
  procedures, 337
  radiopharmaceuticals
    agents, chemical structure, 320, 321
    agents of choice, 341
    development, 319
  study interpretation, 343
    differential kidney function, 339, 343
    diuretic renogram, 342, 343
    ERPF, 339
    kidney transplant renogram, 340, 341
    perfusion studies, 337, 338
    renal scans, 338, 339, 345, 346
    renograms, 338, 340, 341
Kits, Tc-99m. *See also* Technetium
  commercial products, comparison
    bone agents, 358t
    heart agents, 215t
    kidney agents, 330t
    liver–spleen agents, 278t–279t
    lung agents, 240t–241t
  impurities, 87–89, 129–131
  labeling chemistry, 86–89
  production methods, 82, 83
  quality control, 129–131
Krypton-81m
  dosage, 9
  lung imaging, 248, 263
  production and properties, 27, 250
  radiation dose, 9
Kupffer's cells, 272

Lactoferrin, Ga-67 binding, 385, 386
Lactoperoxidase, 92
LAL. *See* Limulus test
Laminar flow hoods, 102
Lasix, use in diuretic renogram, 342
Leak tests, sealed sources, regulatory requirements, 479
Leukocytes
  abscess formation, 392
  in inflammation, 391, 392
  life time, 391
  number, 396
  radiolabeling methods, 392
  types, 391
Leukocytes, In-111. *See* Indium-111
Licensing of radioactive material, 476
  application, 483–485
  type of use, radioactive material, 478
  types of licenses, 476–478
Ligands. *See* Complexing agents
Limulus test, 135, 162
Linear accelerator, 55, 56
Linear energy transfer, 34
Linearity test
  dose calibrators, 138
    decay method, 139
    shielding method, 140
Lipophilic compounds, brain imaging, 157
Liver
  endothelial cells, 272
  hepatocytes, 273
  Kupffer's cells, 272
  physiologic anatomy, 271–275
  sinusoidal cells, 272
Liver imaging
  indications, 297
  procedure, 297
  radiopharmaceuticals, 297
  scan interpretation, 298
Liver scans, hepatobiliary
  acute cholecystitis, 308
  acute gangrenous cholecystitis, 309
  normal, 307
  obstruction, 310, 311
Liver scans, perfusion–static
  cyst, 303, 304
  hepatocellular disease, 305, 306
  normal, 298, 299
  SPECT, 300
  tumor, 301, 302
Logit-log plot, TSH-RIA, 441
Lugol's solution
  adrenal cortex imaging, 460
  adrenal medulla imaging, 462
  fibrinogen I-125 uptake study, 455
  thyroid blockade, 193
Lung
  airways, 236
  clinical evaluation, 259
  vasculature, 236
Lung imaging
  adverse reactions, 246, 263
  indications, 259
  interpretation, 261
  perfusion agents, development, 238
  perfusion–ventilation methods, 248
  procedures, 260
  radiopharmaceuticals, 263
  ventilation agents, 247, 249
Lung imaging kits, 240–241
Lung scan, liver uptake, 244
Lung scan, perfusion–ventilation
  normal, 261, 262
  obstructive pulmonary disease, 266, 267
  pulmonary embolism, 264, 265
  pulmonary hypertension, 261
  right-to-left cardiac shunt, 268
Lung ventilation. *See* Lung imaging
Lymph node scanning, 458
Lysosomes, influence on Ga-67 localization, 385

Mass number, 13
Maximum permissible concentration
  defined, 490
  radioactive waste calculations, 116
  radionuclides in nuclear medicine, 490t
Maximum permissible dose, 48
Mean life, 31
Meckel's diverticulum
  imaging of, 452
  incidence, 451

INDEX 509

methods of detection, 451
Tc-99m pertechnetate in, 451
Medical Internal Radiation Dose Committee, 57
Medronate. *See* Technetium-99m medronate
Meningioma, 169
Mercury-197, nuclear properties, 27
Mercury-203
  decay scheme, 22, 25
  nuclear properties, 27
Mercury-197, -203 chlormerodrin
  brain imaging with, 149, 151
  chemical structure, 321
  kidney studies with, 320
Metaiodobenzylguanidine, I-131
  adrenal medulla imaging, 461
  chemical structure, 461
  development, 461
  dosage, 462
  properties, 461
  radiation dose, 462
Metastable state, defined, 24
Methimazole
  effect on thyroid gland, 199, 200
  in thyroid therapy, 205
Methotrexate, influence on Ga-67 distribution, 387
Methylene diphosphonate. *See also* Technetium-99m medronate
  chemical structure, 87
MDP. *See* Technetium-99m medronate
MIBG. *See* Metaiodobenzylguanidine
Microcurie, 29
Microspheres, albumin. *See also* Technetium
  cardiac shunt evaluation, 268
  kit, Tc-99m labeling, 240
  preparation, 239
Millicurie, 29
MIRD. *See* Medical Internal Radiation Dose Committee
Misadministration, radiopharmaceutical, 120
Molecular weight, of drug molecules
  effect on distribution in CSF, 161
  effect on hepatobiliary excretion, 289
  effect on kidney excretion, 317
Molybdenum-99
  breakthrough test, 65
  impurity, Tc-99m generator, 66–67
  molybdate, liver studies, 275
  nuclear properties, 27
Monitoring, radioactive material
  permissible dose levels and concentrations, 489, 490
  personnel, 491
  transportation requirements, 494, 497
  work areas, 498
MPD. *See* Maximum permissible dose
Multigated acquisition (MUGA), cardiac blood pool study, 222
Myocardial imaging
  ischemia, 227, 229
  perfusion studies, 226
  radionuclide angiogram, 232
  radionuclide ventriculography, 230

Negatrons, 35
Negatron decay, 20
Nephron anatomy, 316
Neutrino
  described, 21
  role in beta decay, 21
New drug application, 474
Nitrogen-13, nuclear properties, 78
Nitrogen purging
  effect on stability of stannous pyrophosphate solution, 84
  removal of oxygen from water, 84
Nomogram, pediatric dosages, 115
Nonisotopic labeling, 78
NP-59, I-131
  adrenal cortex imaging, 460
  chemical structure, 460
  dosage, 460
  preparation, properties, quality control, 459, 460
  radiation dose, 460
Notice to employees, NRC-3 form, 499
Nuclear energy, 17
Nuclear forces, 18
Nuclear magnetic resonance, 1
Nuclear medicine
  defined, 1
  procedures, 2
    imaging, 2
    in vitro studies, 5
    in vivo function studies, 4
    therapy, 5
Nuclear pharmacies
  development, 486
  FDA regulations, 487
  licensing, 486
Nuclear pharmacists, authorized user status, 485
  training requirements for, 489
Nuclear pharmacy
  definition, 486
  floor plan, 97
  hoods, 102
  hot sinks, 101
  shielding and storage equipment, 98
  standards of practice, 482
  supplies, 104
  techniques used in handling radioactive material, 106
Nuclear pharmacy functions
  compounding of radiopharmaceuticals, 110
  Tc-99m kit preparation, 112
  dispensing radiopharmaceuticals, 113
    pediatric dosages, 114
  purchase and receipt of radiopharmaceuticals, 109
  quality control, 115
  radionuclide waste disposal, 116
  record keeping, 117
Nuclear reactor, 55
Nuclear regulatory commission
  authority, compared with FDA, 476
  regulation of radiopharmaceuticals, 476
Nuclides
  chart of, 15

Nuclides (cont.)
  definition, 13
  mass and energy relationship, 17
  properties, 14

Opsonins, 284
Organ radiation dose, radiopharmaceuticals, $8t$–$11t$
Organification, iodine in thyroid gland, 182–183
Osteomyelitis
  bone imaging, differentiation from cellulitis, 366
  bone scan of, 373
Overpressure cisternography, 163
Oxidation
  stannous ion, 88
  stannous pyrophosphate, 84
  Tc-99m pyrophosphate, 359
  Tc-99m radiopharmaceuticals, 87
Oxidronate. See also Technetium-99m oxidronate
  chemical structure, 87
Oxine, 379
  Ga-68 complex, 386
  In-111 complex, 393, 397
Oxygen, dissolved, reduction of, by nitrogen gas, 84

Packages, radioactive
  receipt procedures, 110–111
  requirements for, DOT, 493–498
Pair production, 37
Para-aminohippuric acid
  chemical structure, 320
  renal clearance, 317, 319
Parathyroid imaging
  clinical evaluation, 464
  procedures, 463, 464
  radiopharmaceuticals, 463
  rationale, 463
Particle accelerator, 55
Particles
  analysis
    lung radiopharmaceuticals, 242
    liver radiopharmaceuticals, 276, 280, 283
  number
    lung scanning, pulmonary hypertension, 246
    pediatric lung scans, 246
Particle toxicity, lung scanning, 246
Partition of drugs into brain, 157
Passive transport, 316
Pediatric dosage
  lung scanning, particle number, 246
  nomogram, 115
Pentetate. See Technetium-99m pentetate
Pentetic acid, chemical structure, 321
Perchlorate
  brain imaging, dosage, 153
  effect on pertechnetate distribution, 153
  thyroid gland
    effect on iodide trapping, 184
Perchlorate washout test, 199, 200
Personnel monitoring, 51, 491

pH
  brain fluid, 157
  cerebrospinal fluid, artificial, 163
  Henderson–Hasselbalch equation, 317
  importance in protein iodination, 91
  influence on radioiodide stability, 90
  influence on Tc-99m hydrolysis, 89
  range of, in radiopharmaceuticals, 134
Phagocytosis, of radiocolloids, 271–273
Phosphorus-32
  decay scheme, 22
  handling, radiation dose to fingers, 463
  nuclear properties, 27
  radiation exposure from plastic syringes, 108
  therapeutic use, 462
Phosphorus-32 chromic phosphate
  compared with sodium phosphate P-32, 463
  liver studies, 275
  production and properties, 463
  therapeutic use, 463
Phosphorus-32 sodium phosphate
  compared with chromic phosphate P-32, 463
  production and properties, 462
  radiation dose, 463
  therapeutic use, polycythemia, 462
Photoelectric effect, 35
Photon
  defined, 35
  energy, 35
  ideal energy, diagnostic radionuclides, 76
  interactions with matter, 35–38
Physical half-life
  radionuclides, diagnostic imaging, 76
  related to effective half-life, 76–77
Pinocytosis in brain, 148, 150
PIPIDA. See Technetium-99m iprofenin
Placarding in radiopharmaceutical transport, 497
Plasma iron
  clearance, 429
  turnover rate, 430
Plasma volume measurement
  methods, 415, 417
  worksheet for, 419
Platelets. See also Indium-111 platelets
  formation and function, 398
  labeling, 398
Plummer's disease, 205
Pluronic F-68, 239
Polycythemia vera, P-32 therapy, 462
Pool, defined, 411
Positrons, 34
Positron decay
  annihilation reaction, 23
  mechanism, 22
Positron emitting nuclides, 78
Posting requirements, NRC-3 form, notice to employees, 498
Potassium-43, myocardial imaging, 212
Potassium iodide, protection of thyroid gland
  adrenal cortex imaging, 460
  fibrinogen I-125 uptake study, 435
  thyroid blockade, 193

INDEX 511

Precision test, dose calibrator, 138
Propylthiouracil (PTU)
    considerations in thyroid treatment with I-131, 205
    effect on thyroid uptake, 184
Protein iodination
    general methods, 91
    mechanism of, 420
Protein losing enteropathy, 451
PTU. See Propylthiouracil
Pulmonary hypertension, precautions in lung scanning, 346
Pulse height analyzer, 42
Purity of radiopharmaceuticals, 124
Pyrogens
    defined, 134
    detection, LAL test, 135
    test report, rabbit test, 136
Pyrophosphate, stannous
    kits
        labeling red blood cells, 215
        labeling Tc-99m, 215
        stability, 85
    toxicity, 220
Pyrophosphoric acid, chemical structure, 87

Quality control
    chemical purity, 134
    chromatography
        column, 130, 132
        techniques and pitfalls, 129, 131
        thin-layer and paper, 126–130
    pH, 134
    pyrogens, 134
    radioactivity measurements, 133
    radiochemical purity, 124
    radionuclidic purity, 124
    sterility, 134
    visual inspection, particle size, color, 133
Quality factors, radiation, 48

RAD, 47
Radiation
    defined, 19
    detection, 38
    dosimetry, 56, 57
    interactions with matter, 34–35
    measurement, 46
    units, 47–48
Radiation area, 491
Radiation emergency procedures, 119
Radiation detection instrumentation
    ion collection methods, 38
    scintillation methods, 40
Radiation dose
    calculations methods, 56–57
    radiopharmaceuticals, routine use, $8t–11t$
Radiation exposure
    effect of shielding, 107

techniques to limit, 108
unshielded syringes and vials, 107
Radiation monitoring
    devices for, 53
    methods, 51, 52
Radiation protection
    calculations, 50
    half-value layer in, 51
    maximum permissible dose (MPD), 48
    protection guides, 48
    techniques for
        time, distance, and shielding, 49, 50
Radiation protection guides, 48
Radiation, range in tissue, 49
Radiation safety regulations, 473, 489
Radiation safety techniques, 106
Radiation shielding
    dispensing area shield, 101
    storage equipment, 98–100
    syringe and vial shields, 101, 107
Radiation surveys
    radioactive packages
        receipt, 492
        shipment, 493
    records, 500
    wipe tests, 493
    work areas, 498
Radiation symbol, 492
Radioactive concentration
    calculations, 33
    carrier added, 34
    carrier free, 33
    no carrier added, 34
    specific activity, 33
    specific concentration, 33
Radioactive decay
    alpha decay, 26
    causes, 19, 20
    electron capture decay, 23
    negatron decay, 20
    neutron-proton ratio, 20
    positron decay, 22
Radioactive gases and aerosols, regulations for use in nuclear medicine, 479
Radioactive material
    techniques for handling in nuclear pharmacy, 106
    transfer to authorized recipient, 118
Radioactive material, human use, training requirements, for, 480–485
Radioactive waste, disposal, 116
Radioactivity
    calculations, 29
    decay constant, 29
    decay law, 28
    decay tables, 32
    defined, 28
    half-life, 30
    measurement, 36
    units for, 29
Radioaerosol ventilation imaging, 258
Radioassay tests, in vitro
    competitive protein binding assay, 435

Radioassay tests, in vitro *(cont.)*
  principle, 435
  radioimmunoassay, 436
  thyroxine assay, 438
  TSH assay, 438
Radiochemical purity
  causes, 125
  definition, 124
  methods
    column chromatography, 130
    thin-layer and paper, 126, 127
    pitfalls, 129
  purity limits of selected radiopharmaceuticals, 127t
Radiocolloids, development, 275
Radioimmunoassay (RIA)
  antibody production, 436
  antigen-antibody separation methods, 437
  development, 436
  haptens, 437
  principle, 435
  substrates, 437
  thyroxine RIA, 438
  TSH RIA, 438
Radioiodinations
  mechanisms, 90
  methods, 90–93
  protein, 90
  yields, 92–93
Radiolysis
  effect on generator yield, 63
  free-radical degradation of Tc-99m agents, 88
Radionuclide(s)
  defined, 14
  ideal properties, diagnostic, 76t
  production methods, 53–55
    particle accelerator, 54, 55
    nuclear reactor, 54, 55
  used in nuclear medicine, 27t
Radionuclide generators, 59
Radionuclide measurement, effect of container configuration, 143
Radionuclidic purity
  causes, 124
  defined, 124
  measurement techniques, 124
Radiopharmaceutical
  chemical bonding in, 80, 81
  chemical and physical forms, 7
  compounding, 110
    control records, 113
    Tc-99m kit preparation, 112
  definition, 2
  development, 77–80
  dispensing
    dosage calculation, 114
    labels, 113
    pediatric dosage, 114
    prescription orders, 114
  distribution patterns, diagnostic imaging, 2
  ideal properties, 75–77
  misadministration
    diagnostic and therapeutic, 120
    records, 120
  procurement and receipt
    inventory records, 111
    ordering requirements, 110
    surveys and wipe tests, 110
  quality control
    biologic considerations, 134
    definition and scope, 123
    pharmaceutical considerations, 133
    radiation considerations, 124
    radiochemical purity, 124
    radionuclidic purity, 124
  routes of administration, 7
  routine use, 8t–11t
  transfer of, records, 118
  unique properties, 7
  use in nuclear medicine, 6
  waste disposal
    methods and limits, 116, 117
    records, 118
Radium-226, decay scheme, 26
RBE (relative biologic effectiveness), 47
Records, receipt, use and survey of radioactive material, 500
Red blood cell, labeling. *See* Technetium-99m red blood cells
Red cell volume
  methods, 412
  worksheet for, 416
Red cell survival, 420–422
Reference standards
  authorization to receive, use, and possess, 479
  dose calibrator, 137
Regulatory control of radiopharmaceuticals, NRC
  dosage preparation requirements, 479
  historical review, 475
  radioactive aerosols and gases requirements, 479
  syringe shields requirements, 480
  Tc-99m generator quality control requirements, 478
REM (roentgen equivalent man), 47
Renal blood flow, 319
Renal scans
  differential kidney function, 343
  diuretic renogram, 342
  hydronephrosis, 339
  normal renal scan, Tc-DMSA, 345
  perfusion study, renal artery stenosis, 338
  reflux, 344
  renal disease, liver uptake of Tc-DMSA, 333
  renal mass, 346
  renal transplant, hepatobiliary excretion of Tc-GH, 335
  transplant renogram, 340
Renogram
  evaluation, 324
  I-131 hippuran, 325
Resolving time, scintillation counter, 129
Restricted area, 489
Reticuloendothelial system blockade, 285, 286

INDEX 513

Rf, 128
Roentgen, 47
Rose bengal
  biliary excretion, 290
  I-131 labeled, 286
Rubidium-81, myocardial imaging, 212

S value, radiation dose estimates, 56
Salivary gland imaging, 452
Scandium, effect on Ga-67 distribution, 383
Schilling test
  intrinsic factor in, 426
  methods, 425, 426
  pitfalls and precautions, 426, 427
Scintillation counter quality control, 143
Scintillation detectors
  gamma camera, 46
  photomultiplier tube, 41
  principle of operation, 40
  probe, 44
  pulse height analysis, 42
  spectrometer, 42
  well counter, 43
Scintillation uptake probe, 44
Scintillation well counter, 43
  use in nuclear pharmacy, 104
Scrotal imaging, 346, 347
Sealed sources, wipe testing, 110, 492
Secular equilibrium
  defined, 73
  Rb-81/Kr-81m generator, 73
Selenium-75
  nuclear properties, 27
  selenomethionine, pancreas agent, 79
Shielding
  considerations of HVL for Tc-99m and I-131, 99
  formula for calculations, 50
  lead bricks, 98
  lead L-block dispensing station, 99, 101
  lead vial shields, 98
  radiopharmaceutical syringe shields, 98
Skeletal imaging. *See* Bone
Skin blood flow measurement, 465
Sodium atom, structural diagram, 14
Sodium-potassium-ATPase pump, 211
Sodium chromate, Cr-51
  dosage forms, 415
  quality control, 415
  production and properties, 415
Space, defined, 411
Specific activity, 33
Specific concentration, 33
Specific gamma ray dose constant, 50
Specific licenses, 477
SPECT imaging, 4, 5
Spectrometer, 42
Spills, radioactive material, 119
Spleen imaging agents, 293
Spleen, physiologic anatomy, 292
Spleen scan, accessory spleen, 312

Spleen (**specific**) imaging, 304
  indications, 304
  procedure, 305
  radiopharmaceuticals, 306
  scan interpretation, 307
    accessory spleen, 312
Standards for protection against radiation
  caution signs and labeling, 491
  monitoring requirements, work areas, 498
  permissible dose levels and concentrations, 489, 490
  personnel monitoring, 491
  posting requirements, notice to employees, 499
  radioactive packages
    monitoring, 493
    wipe tests, limits, 492, 493
Stannous pyrophosphate kit, 83
Stannous ion. *See* Tin
Sterility tests, 134
Strontium-85, -87m, 354
Survey meter
  calibration, 144, 145
  monitoring radioactive shipments, 110, 493
  use in nuclear pharmacy, 104
Syringe shields, 99, 101, 106, 107, 480

Tantalum syringe shield, 99
Technetium
  chemistry, 82
  complexes, radiolytic decomposition, 88
  dimeric structure in complexes, 89
  discovery, 81
  hydrolysis, 89
  hydrolyzed-reduced impurity, 89
  kits
    labeling with Tc-99m, 86
    production, 82
    reduction by stannous ion, 87
  ligand complexation, 89
  oxidation, 87
  pertechnetate impurity, Tc-99m radiopharmaceuticals, 87
  properties, 82
  reduction, 82
  syringe shields for, 98
  valence (oxidation) states, 82, 86
Technetium albumin. *See also* Albumin, Tc-99m
  effect of carrier Tc-99 on labeling, 68
Technetium carrier, effect on Tc-99m labeling, 68
Technetium-99m
  decay scheme, 152
  expiration time in generator eluate, 67
  generator, 59
  mole fraction in generator, 67
  nuclear properties, 27
  radioassay, effect of container configuration, 143
Technetium-99m albumin aggregated. *See* Albumin, aggregated, Tc-99m
Technetium-99m albumin colloid, 276
Technetium-99m antimony sulfide colloid
  dosage, 459

Technetium-99 antimony sulfide colloid (cont.)
 lymph node scanning, 458
 preparation and properties, 459
 radiation dose, 459
Technetium-99m BIDA. See Technetium-99m
 butilfenin
Technetium-99m butilfenin
 distribution and excretion, 290, 291
 radiation dose, 292
Technetium-99m DIDA. See Technetium-99m
 etilfenin
Technetium-99m DISIDA. See Technetium-99m
 disofenin
Technetium-99m disofenin
 distribution and excretion, 290, 291
 radiation dose, 292
Technetium-99m DTPA. See Technetium-99m
 pentetate
Technetium-99m etidronate
 adsorption on hydroxyapatite, 364
 altered biodistribution, 365
 blood clearance, 362, 363
 bone localization mechanism, 362, 364
 bone uptake, 355, 363
 chemical structure, 357
 development, 355
 dosage, 10, 367
 in vitro stability, effect of ascorbic acid, 360
 kits, 358
 myocardial uptake, 214
 preparation and properties, 356
 radiation dose, 10, 364
Technetium-99m etilfenin
 distribution and excretion, 290, 291
 radiation dose, 292
Technetium-99m gluceptate
 biodistribution, 334
 brain imaging, compared with Tc-99m DTPA, 150, 151
 chemical structure, 335
 dosage, 10
 hepatobiliary excretion, in renal transplant, 335
 kidney localization, 334
 kit, 330
 mechanism of renal excretion, 334
 myocardial uptake, 214
 preparation and properties, 328, 334
 radiation dose, 10, 336
 renal imaging, compared Tc-DTPA and Tc-DMSA, 328
 use in kidney studies, 335
Technetium-99m HIDA. See Technetium-99m
 lidofenin
Technetium-99m HAM. See Albumin
 microspheres, Tc-99m
Technetium-99m HM-PAO, brain imaging, 151
Technetium-99m iprofenin
 distribution and excretion, 290, 291
 radiation dose, 292
Technetium-99m iron ascorbate, 321
Technetium-99m lidofenin
 chemical structure, 289
 distribution and excretion, 290, 291
 properties, 289
 radiation dose, 292
Technetium-99m MAA. See Albumin, aggregated, Tc-99m
Technetium-99m medronate
 adsorption on hydroxyapatite, 364
 altered biodistribution, 365
 biodistribution and excretion, 361
 blood clearance, 362, 363
 bone localization mechanisms, 362, 364
 chemical structure, 357, 361
 development, 355
 dosage, 10, 367
 kits, 358
 myocardial uptake, 214
 preparation and properties, 356
 radiation dose, 10, 364
Technetium-99m microspheres. See Albumin
 microspheres, Tc-99m
Technetium-99m oxidronate
 adsorption on hydroxyapatite, 364
 altered biodistribution, 365
 biodistribution and excretion, 361
 blood clearance, 363
 bone localization mechanism, 363
 bone uptake, 361, 363
 chemical structure, 87
 development, 356
 dosage, 10, 367
 kit, 358
 preparation and properties, 357
 radiation dose, 10, 364
Technetium-99m pentetate
 altered biodistribution, 336
 biodistribution, 327
 brain imaging, compared with Tc-99m GH, 150, 151
 dosage, 10
 gastric emptying studies, 450
 GFR measurement, 322
 kits, 330
 mechanism of renal excretion, 327
 production and properties, 327, 328
 radiation dose, 10, 329
 renal imaging, compared with Tc-DMSA and Tc-GH, 328
 use in kidney evaluation, 328
Technetium-99m pentetate aerosol
 administration system, 259
 dosage, 10, 258
 particle size, 258
 rate of lung clearance, 259
 use in lung scanning, 259
Technetium-99m pertechnetate
 biologic distribution, 152
 brain imaging, compared with Tc-GH and DTPA, 150, 151
 dacryocystography, 453
 first use in scanning, 150
 impurity in bone imaging radiopharmaceuticals, 125, 126

impurity in Tc-99m kits, 87
Meckel's diverticulum, 451
parathyroid imaging, 463
physical properties, 152
radiation dose, 153, 154
salivary gland imaging, 452
Technetium-99m PIPIDA. *See* Technetium-99m iprofenin
Technetium-99m polyphosphate
  chemical structure, 357
  development, 355
Technetium-99m purity, 124
Technetium-99m pyridoxylidene glutamate (PYG), 287
Technetium-99m pyrophosphate
  altered biodistribution, 218, 365
  biologic properties, 215, 361
  blood clearance, 362
  bone uptake, 355, 363
  chemical structure, 357
  compared with Tc-99m diphosphonates, 355
  development, 355
  dosage, 10, 367
  infarct avid imaging, 214
  kits, 215, 358
  labeling efficiency, effect of Sn:Tc molar ratio, 359
  myocardial uptake and mechanism of localization, 214, 216
  preparation and properties, 215, 356
  radiation dose, 10, 217
Technetium-99m red blood cells
  altered biodistribution of, 220
  biologic properties, 220
  development, 294
  effect of carrier Tc-99, 294
  gastrointestinal bleeding studies, 444, 448
  heat damaged
    mechanism of localization, 295
    plasma half-life, 294
    preparation, 294
    spleen imaging, 294
  kit preparation, 294
  labeling mechanism, 219
  labeling methods
    in vitro, 218
    in vivo, 218
    modified in vivo, 219
    whole blood, 219
  radiation dose, 220, 221
Technetium-99m resin, cation exchange
  gastric emptying studies, 450
  preparation, 450
Technetium-99m succimer (DMSA)
  biodistribution, 331
  chemical structure, 332
  dosage, 11
  kidney localization, 331
  kit, 330
  liver uptake, secondary to renal failure, 333
  mechanism of renal excretion, 328, 331

radiation dose, 11, 333
renal imaging, compared with Tc-DTPA and Tc-GH, 328
stability, 329
use in kidney studies, 332
Technetium-99m sulfur colloid
  adverse reactions, 286
  biodistribution, factors affecting, 283
  blood clearance rate, 283, 284
  development, liver studies, 276
  dosage, 11, 297
  flocculation, 281
  gastric emptying studies, 450
  gastroesophageal reflux studies, 445
  kits, 278, 279
  mechanism of localization, 284
  metabolic fate, 284
  microscopic appearance, 280
  particle size, 283
  preparation, 277, 278
  radiation dose, 11, 286
  stability, factors affecting, 279
Teletherapy, 478
Testicular scan, 346
Thallium-201
  biologic distribution, 213
  blood disappearance curves, 226
  myocardial localization mechanism, 213
  parathyroid imaging, 463
  production and properties, 27, 212
  purity, 124
  radiation dose, 11, 213
  SPECT imaging, 228
  thyroid imaging, 201
  time course in myocardium, 229
Thrombus detection, deep venous, fibrinogen uptake study, 454
Thyroid carcinoma, I-131 treatment, 206
Thyroid, *clinical evaluation*, 198
Thyroid gland
  evaluation, 181
  hormone production, 182
  iodine metabolism, 182
  physiology, 181
Thyroid hormone production, 181, 182
Thyroid imaging
  indications, 201
  procedure, 201
  radiopharmaceuticals, 201
  scan interpretation
    cold nodule, 202
    Grave's disease, 204
    hot nodule, 203
    multinodular goiter, 203, 205
    normal study, 202
    total body scan, 206
Thyroid stimulating hormone RIA
  principle, 438
  procedure, 440
  standard curve, 441
Thyroid therapy
  indications, 207

Thyroid therapy (cont.)
  procedures
    Grave's disease, 204
    Plummer's disease, 205
  safety considerations, 207
  treatment evaluation, 207
Thyroid uptake study
  clinical indications, 198
  effect of drugs, 195
  effect of stable iodide, 193
  effect of thiocyanate and PTU, 184
  interpretation, 199
  perchlorate washout test, 199, 200
  procedure, 194, 199
  radiopharmaceuticals, 184, 193, 194, 199
Thyroxine RIA
  principle of test, 438
  standard curve for, 439
  step-wise procedure, 438
Tin
  assay for, in radiopharmaceuticals, 85
  metabolism and excretion, 85, 86
  stannous ion
    hydrolysis, 89
    oxidation, 88
    use in Tc-99m kits, 86-89
  tissue distribution, 86
  toxicity, 85, 86
Tin-113, 74, 388
TLD, 52
Total body imaging, 379, 401
Tracer, defined, 411
Training requirements, authorized user
  medical use of by-product material, 480-482
  nuclear pharmacist, 489
Transferrin
  indium-111 complex, 159
  influence on leukocyte labeling, 395
  molecular weight, 159
Transient equilibrium
  defined, 70
  Mo-99/Tc-99m generator, 71
Transport index, 494, 496
Transport of radioactive material
  accident reporting, 497
  labeling requirements, 494, 496
  monitoring requirements, 494, 497
  packaging requirements, 495
  shipping papers, 497
  transport index, 496
Traps, charcoal, xenon administration systems, 256
Tropolone, platelet labeling, 399
TSH, 183
  stimulation of thyroid gland, 204

Unrestricted area, 490
USP, radiochemical purity of radiopharmaceuticals, 127t

Venous thrombosis detection
  I-125 fibrinogen uptake study, 454
  leg marking positions, 456, 457
Ventilation imaging. *See* Lung imaging
Ventriculography, heart studies, 230
Vitamin B-12 deficiency, tests for, 423. *See also* Cyanocobalamin
Voiding cystourethrogram, 341, 344
Volume of distribution, 319

Wipe tests, receipt of radioactive material, 110, 492

Xenon, radioactive
  biodistribution, 250, 251
  charcoal trapping, 256
  lung ventilation imaging, 248
  maximum permissible concentration, 257
  packaging and storage, 251
  patient administration systems, 254, 255
  radiation dose, 11, 251
  retention by unit dose vials, 254
  safety calculation, restricted and unrestricted areas, 254
Xenon-127
  dosage, 11
  lung imaging, 248, 263
  maximum permissible concentration, 257
  production and properties, 27, 249, 250
  radiation dose, 11, 251
Xenon-133
  dosage, 11
  lung imaging, 248, 263
  maximum permissible concentration, 257
  production and properties, 27, 249, 250
  radiation dose, 11, 251
Xenon-133 in saline, skin blood flow measurement, 465
Xenon-135, properties, 249, 250

Ytterbium-169 pentetate, cisternography, 159, 161
Yttrium-87/strontium-87m generator, 354

Zirconium oxide, tin-113/indium-113m generator, 388